Molecular and Integrative Toxicology

Series Editors

Jamie C. DeWitt
East Carolina University
Greenville, NC, USA

Sarah Blossom
Arkansas Children's Hospital Research Institute
Little Rock, AR, USA

More information about this series at http://www.springer.com/series/8792

Bernhard Michalke

Editor

Selenium

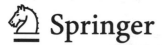 Springer

Editor
Bernhard Michalke
Research Unit: Analytical BioGeoChemistry
Helmholtz Zentrum München – German Research Center
for Environmental Health GmbH
Neuherberg, Germany

ISSN 2168-4219   ISSN 2168-4235   (electronic)
Molecular and Integrative Toxicology
ISBN 978-3-030-07026-7   ISBN 978-3-319-95390-8   (eBook)
https://doi.org/10.1007/978-3-319-95390-8

This Springer imprint is published by the registered company Springer Nature Switzerland AG
The registered company address is: Gewerbestrasse 11, 6330 Cham, Switzerland

Editorial

Selenium

The element Selenium has experienced a unique consideration among elements relevant to life. Selenium was discovered by the Swedish medical doctor and chemical scientist Jöns Jakob Berzelius in 1817, and he named the new element after the Latin expression for moon (Selene).

For long time, selenium was considered to be a toxic substance, since in the 1930s, veterinarians in the Great Plains identified high levels of selenium in plants fed to cattle for alkalinity and blind ataxia of these animals. Conversely, in the 1950s, a research group reported that selenium prevented necrotic liver degeneration, and another group found selenium deficiency as cause for weakness of calves. Following such early reports, during several decades, researchers from institutions all over the world begun studies on the benefits of selenium supplementation on the performance and health, first of dairy cattle, but then increasingly studying human health and even more, specific selenium-related molecular mechanisms and pathways using animal and cell culture experiments. In parallel, epidemiological study designs on various population groups, either Se-deficient or Se-exposed, were reported.

Selenium has been attributed to a couple of health benefits such as prevention of some cancer forms, heart disease, and other cardiovascular or muscle disorders, inhibiting viral expression, delaying AIDS symptoms in HIV positive humans, slowing the aging process, or being involved in male reproduction and immune function.

This book—being published within the Springer Toxicology Series—is intended to provide current information on research in the rapidly developing selenium field, on the one side being centered around the health benefits attributed to selenium but, on the other side, also reporting about research related to toxicological aspects.

It starts with a comprehensive overview on selenium research and proceeds with chapters reporting how Se may be taken up, by enlightening its bio-accessibility and dietary aspects, the latter in turn being related to selenium in soil and plants. A next section of the book covers selenium related to genes, proteins, pathways, and its metabolism followed from health effects. These include the involvement in redox systems and the protective role of Se against oxidative stress, having close correlation to inflammation, thyroid, or disease protection. Neurological aspects are also a matter of particular interest. Selenium is of paramount importance during infantile neurodevelopment, and it is discussed being crucial after stroke or in autism. Respective chapters in this book spot light on these issues. As an interesting counterpoint, a chapter focuses on detrimental effects on peripheral nerves and from an epidemiological viewpoint about neurotoxicity of some inorganic selenium forms. A further paragraph with various chapters is centered around selenium and cancer. The roles of specific seleno-compounds like selenoprotein P or seleno-cysteine in cancer are discussed aside from aspects of cell proliferation, cytotoxicity, and finally the action of selenium in radiotherapy. A couple of chapters are dedicated to selenium and various diseases, including cardiovascular diseases, diabetes, muscle disease, de-balanced immune response, or risks of Se-deficiency. Important aspects of selenium biology are also addressed regarding new health challenges, e.g., caused by Se-nanoparticles or interactions of selenium with other trace elements, vitamins, or pharmaceuticals. It is fundamental for the above chapters to have knowledge about cellular bioavailability and cytotoxicity, ruled out on cell culture experiments, and in general, information about reliable selenium analytics. The latter must include solid analytical approaches, validated selenium speciation techniques, and biomonitoring studies. Each of these aspects is concerned within individual chapters of this book.

Although this book cannot cover all aspects in the wide selenium field, I think it nevertheless covers a comprehensive and relevant range of topics being of interest to the reader. It will be a success of this book when, specifically, young researchers are motivated to focus their new ideas and research into selenium biochemistry and related health effects. However, it will be also within the intention of this book to provide updated information from selenium research to all interested readers, either being already settled in this fast-growing field or whether still being at the beginning of their professional career and looking for an interesting research topic for their scientific journey.

Neuherberg, Germany   Bernhard Michalke

Contents

Contributors

Jan Aaseth Innlandet Hospital Trust, Kongsvinger, Norway

Inland Norway University of Applied Sciences, Terningen Arena, Elverum, Norway

Yasumi Anan Laboratory of Health Chemistry, Showa Pharmaceutical Sciences, Tokyo, Japan

Josiane Arnaud Institute of Biology and Pathology, University Hospital of Grenoble and Alpes, Grenoble, France

Mireille Baltzinger Université de Strasbourg, CNRS, Architecture et Réactivité de l'ARN, IBMC-15, Strasbourg, France

Geir Bjørklund Council for Nutritional and Environmental Medicine, Mo i Rana, Norway

Mikael Björnstedt Division of Pathology F42, Department of Laboratory Medicine, Karolinska Institutet, Karolinska University Hospital Huddinge, Stockholm, Sweden

Regina Brigelius-Flohé German Institute of Human Nutrition Potsdam-Rehbrücke, Nuthetal, Germany

Jens Buentzel Klinik für Hals-Nasen-Ohren-Heilkunde, Südharz Klinikum, Nordhausen, Germany

Francisco Carrilho Department of Endocrinology, Diabetes and Metabolism, Centro Hospitalar e Universitário de Coimbra, Coimbra, Portugal

Laurent Chavatte Centre International de Recherche en Infectiologie, CIRI, Lyon, France

Inserm U1111, Lyon, France

CNRS, Ecole Normale Supérieure de Lyon, Université de Lyon 1, UMR5308, Lyon, France

Marcus Conrad Helmholtz Zentrum München, Institute of Developmental Genetics, Neuherberg, Germany

Marc Dauplais Laboratoire de Biochimie, Ecole Polytechnique, CNRS, Université Paris-Saclay, Palaiseau Cedex, France

Laboratoire de Biochimie, Ecole Polytechnique, CNRS UMR7654, Palaiseau Cedex, France

Franziska Ebert Department of Food Chemistry, Institute of Nutritional Science, University of Potsdam, Potsdam, Germany

Tommaso Filippini CREAGEN, Environmental, Genetic and Nutritional Epidemiology Research Center; Section of Public Health, Department of Biomedical, Metabolic and Neural Sciences, University of Modena and Reggio Emilia, Modena, Italy

Noelia Fradejas-Villar Institut für Biochemie und Molekularbiologie, Rheinische Friedrich-Wilhelms-Universität Bonn, Bonn, Germany

Roland Gärtner Klinikum der Universität München—Medizinische Klinik und Polyklinik IV, Endokrinologie, Munich, Germany

Thomas Göen Friedrich-Alexander-Universität Erlangen-Nürnberg, Institut und Poliklinik für Arbeits-, Sozial-und Umweltmedizin, Erlangen, Germany

Annette Greiner Friedrich-Alexander-Universität Erlangen-Nürnberg, Institut und Poliklinik für Arbeits-, Sozial-und Umweltmedizin, Erlangen, Germany

Viktor A. Gritsenko Institute of Cellular and Intracellular Symbiosis, Russian Academy of Sciences, Orenburg, Russia

Kaixun Huang Hubei Key Laboratory of Bioinorganic Chemistry and Materia Medica, School of Chemistry and Chemical Engineering, Huazhong University of Science and Technology, Wuhan, China

Irina Ingold Helmholtz Zentrum München, Institute of Developmental Genetics, Neuherberg, Germany

Anna P. Kipp Department of Molecular Nutritional Physiology, Institute of Nutritional Sciences, Friedrich Schiller University Jena, Jena, Germany

Lyudmila L. Klimenko Institute of chemical Physics of N. N. Semenov of the Russian Academy of Sciences, Moscow, Russia

Solveigh C. Koeberle Department of Molecular Nutritional Physiology, Institute of Nutritional Sciences, Friedrich Schiller University Jena, Jena, Germany

Myriam Lazard Laboratoire de Biochimie, Ecole Polytechnique, CNRS, Université Paris-Saclay, Palaiseau Cedex, France

Laboratoire de Biochimie, Ecole Polytechnique, CNRS UMR7654, Palaiseau Cedex, France

Xin Gen Lei Department of Animal Science, Cornell University, Ithaca, NY, USA

Alain Lescure Université de Strasbourg, CNRS, Architecture et Réactivité de l'ARN, UPR 9002, IBMC-15, Strasbourg, France

Xinli Li Department of Nutrition and Food Hygiene, School of Public Health, Medical College of Soochow University, Suzhou, Jiangsu, China

Jessica Mandrioli Department of Neurosciences, Azienda Ospedaliero-Universitaria di Modena, Sant Agostino Estense Hospital, Modena, Italy

Aksana N. Mazilina Institute of Chemical Physics of N. N. Semenov of the Russian Academy of Sciences, Moscow, Russia

Clinical Hospital No 123 Federal Medical-Biological Agency of Russia, Moscow, Russia

Miguel Melo Department of Endocrinology, Diabetes and Metabolism, Centro Hospitalar e Universitário de Coimbra, Coimbra, Portugal

Faculty of Medicine, University of Coimbra, Coimbra, Portugal

Instituto de Investigação e Inovação em Saúde (I3S), Porto, Portugal

Institute of Pathology and Immunology of the University of Porto, Porto, Portugal

Soeren Meyer Department of Food Chemistry, Institute of Nutritional Science, University of Potsdam, Potsdam, Germany

Bernhard Michalke Research Unit: Analytical BioGeoChemistry, Helmholtz Zentrum München – German Research Center for Environmental Health GmbH, Neuherberg, Germany

Oliver Micke Klinik für Strahlentherapie und Radioonkologie, Franziskus Hospital Bielefeld, Bielefeld, Germany

Sougat Misra Division of Pathology F42, Department of Laboratory Medicine, Karolinska Institutet, Karolinska University Hospital Huddinge, Stockholm, Sweden

Ralph Mücke Strahlentherapie RheinMainNahe, Bad Kreuznach, Germany

Sandra M. Müller Department of Food Chemistry, Institute of Nutritional Science, University of Potsdam, Potsdam, Germany

Yasumitsu Ogra Laboratory of Toxicology and Environmental Health, Graduate School of Pharmaceutical Sciences, Chiba University, Chiba, Japan

Théophile Ohlmann Centre International de Recherche en Infectiologie, CIRI, Lyon, France

Inserm U1111, Lyon, France

CNRS, Ecole Normale Supérieure de Lyon, Université de Lyon 1, UMR5308, Lyon, France

Pierre Plateau Laboratoire de Biochimie, Ecole Polytechnique, CNRS, Université Paris-Saclay, Palaiseau Cedex, France

Kostja Renko Institut für Experimentelle Endokrinologie, Charité—Universitäts medizin Berlin, Berlin, Germany

Lutz Schomburg Charité—Universitätsmedizin Berlin, Institut für Experimentelle Endokrinologie, Berlin, Germany

Ulrich Schweizer Institut für Biochemie und Molekularbiologie, Rheinische Friedrich-Wilhelms-Universität Bonn, Bonn, Germany

Tanja Schwerdtle Department of Food Chemistry, Institute of Nutritional Science, University of Potsdam, Potsdam, Germany

TraceAge—DFG Research Unit on Interactions of Essential Trace Elements in Healthy and Diseased Elderly, Potsdam-Berlin-Jena, Germany

Arun Kumar Selvam Division of Pathology F42, Department of Laboratory Medicine, Karolinska Institutet, Karolinska University Hospital Huddinge, Stockholm, Sweden

Margarita G. Skalnaya Peoples' Friendship University of Russia (RUDN University), Moscow, Russia

Anatoly V. Skalny Yaroslavl State University, Yaroslavl, Russia

Peoples' Friendship University of Russia (RUDN University), Moscow, Russia

All-Russian Research Institute of Medicinal and Aromatic Plants (VILAR), Moscow, Russia

Yiqing Song Department of Epidemiology, Richard M. Fairbanks School of Public Health, Indiana University, Indianapolis, IN, USA

Liqin Su Department of Soil Quality and Health Monitoring, National Institute of Environmental Health, Chinese Center for Disease Control and Prevention, Beijing, China

Noriyuki Suzuki Laboratory of Toxicology and Environmental Health, Graduate School of Pharmaceutical Sciences, Chiba University, Chiba, Japan

Alexey A. Tinkov Yaroslavl State University, Yaroslavl, Russia

Peoples' Friendship University of Russia (RUDN University), Moscow, Russia

Institute of Cellular and Intracellular Symbiosis, Russian Academy of Sciences, Orenburg, Russia

Aristidis M. Tsatsakis Department of Forensic Sciences and Toxicology, University of Crete, Heraklion, Greece

Peter van Dael DSM Nutritional Products, Kaiseraugst, Switzerland

Mara Ventura Department of Endocrinology, Diabetes and Metabolism, Centro Hospitalar e Universitário de Coimbra, Coimbra, Portugal

Marco Vinceti CREAGEN, Environmental, Genetic and Nutritional Epidemiology Research Center; Section of Public Health, Department of Biomedical, Metabolic and Neural Sciences, University of Modena and Reggio Emilia, Modena, Italy

Department of Epidemiology, Boston University School of Public Health, Boston, MA, USA

Caroline Vindry Centre International de Recherche en Infectiologie, CIRI, Lyon, France

Inserm U1111, Lyon, France

CNRS, Ecole Normale Supérieure de Lyon, Université de Lyon 1, UMR5308, Lyon, France

Ivana Vinković Vrček Institute for Medical Research and Occupational Health, Zagreb, Croatia

Jennifer Weuve Department of Epidemiology, Boston University School of Public Health, Boston, MA, USA

Philip J. White Ecological Science Group, The James Hutton Institute, Dundee, UK

Weili Zhang State Key Laboratory of Cardiovascular Disease, FuWai Hospital, National Center for Cardiovascular Diseases, Peking Union Medical College and Chinese Academy of Medical Sciences, Beijing, China

Xi Zhang Clinical Research Unit, Xin Hua Hospital Affiliated to Shanghai Jiao Tong University School of Medicine, Shanghai, China

Ji-Chang Zhou School of Public Health (Shenzhen), Sun Yat-sen University, Shenzhen, China

Molecular Biology Laboratory, Shenzhen Center for Chronic Disease Control, Shenzhen, China

Jun Zhou Hubei Key Laboratory of Bioinorganic Chemistry and Materia Medica, School of Chemistry and Chemical Engineering, Huazhong University of Science and Technology, Wuhan, China

Ester Zito Dulbecco Telethon Institute at IRCCS-Istituto di Ricerche Farmacologiche Mario Negri, Milan, Italy

Part I
Overview

Keshan and Kashin-Beck disease were the first diseases recognized to be associated with selenium deficiency in humans.

The Keshan disease is an endemic cardiomyopathy observed in 1935 in the Keshan county in the Heilongjiang province in China (Yang et al. 1988), reviewed in Loscalzo (2014). Samples of heart tissue of patients who had died from Keshan disease showed similarities with samples from sheep with white muscle disease appearing when animals were raised on selenium-deficient meadows. The livestock could be protected from the disease by adding selenium to the diet (Muth et al. 1958). Selenium deficiency was made responsible for the Keshan disease too, and selenium supplementation as sodium selenite proved to be lifesaving (Ge and Yang 1993). Infection of mice with a Coxsackie virus isolated from a Keshan disease victim led to a severe heart pathology, especially when the animals were selenium deficient or had their GPX1 deleted (Ge and Yang 1993). Moreover, under these conditions the avirulent form of the virus mutated to a virulent form (Beck et al. 1995). This acquisition of virulence could be attributed to point mutations in the viral genome, presumably resulting from the mutagenic potential of hydroperoxides, which were not adequately metabolized in the selenium-deficient animals or by the lack of GPX1. Collectively, these observations support the conclusion that selenium, via GPX-dependent hydroperoxide removal, dampens any overreaction of the innate immune response and also prevents the collateral damage typically associated with the oxidative burst against bacterial or viral infections.

The Kashin-Beck disease is an endemic degenerative osteoarthropathy present in selenium-deficient areas, not only in China. The etiology is largely unknown, but the mycotoxin T-2 (trichothecene mycotoxin) might be an important risk factor apart from selenium deficiency (Stone 2009). As mechanism, an inhibition of aggrecan synthesis in chondrocytes, and promotion of aggrecanases and production of pro-inflammatory cytokines by T-2, which can be blocked by selenium, is being discussed (Chen et al. 2006).

With the early detection of links between selenium intakes and disease it became likely that selenium is not only essential for grazing livestock but also for humans. Also for long known to be toxic, selenium became an issue of fierce debates about its risks and benefits. The scope of this chapter is to present the consensus achieved on selenium requirements of humans, to briefly compile the functions of selenoproteins putatively involved in expected benefits, and to discuss the underlying mechanisms.

Nutritional Requirements and Recommendations

Dietary reference intakes (DRI) and tolerable upper intake levels (UL) vary between geographic areas. Up to 2015 the recommendation of the German, Austrian, and Swiss nutritional societies (DACH) was 30–70 µg/day and then was enhanced to 60 (female) and 70 (male) µg/day (Kipp et al. 2015). Other European countries recommend 40–75 µg/day, the UK for example 75 for males and 60 for females. This roughly corresponds to the recommendation of respective institutions in Australia and New Zealand of 2006 (www.nrv.gov.au/nutrients/selenium). The European Food Safety Authority (EFSA) recommends 55 µg/day (UL 300), as does the Food and Nutrition Board (FNB) of the Institute of Medicine (IOM) of the USA (UL 400). The World Health Organization (WHO) suggests 26 for females and 34 for males.

Patients receiving parenteral nutrition (PN) are at risk to become selenium deficient. Even cardiomyopathic symptoms similar to those seen in Keshan disease have been observed (Fleming et al. 1982; Johnson et al. 1981). Symptoms could be reversed by selenium (Reeves et al. 1989). The requirements of patients are difficult to estimate since it may depend on the illness, surgery, length of hospital stay, PN at home, and more. The American Society for Parenteral and Enteral Nutrition (ASPEN) suggests 60–100 µg/day according to a review by Shenkin (2009). The related European Society (ESPEN) recommends 32–71 µg/day for adults (Staun et al. 2009).

The Chemical Nature of Selenium Compounds

Main nutritional sources of selenium are crop plants. The Se content varies depending on the Se content in the soil they are growing on. Cereals contain selenite, selenomethionine (SeMet), and selenocysteine (Sec), wheat contains also Se-methyl-Sec. Nuts contain mainly SeMet, Brazil nuts up to 2.5 µg/g. Se-rich vegetables are broccoli, cabbage, onions, and garlic. They contain Se-methyl-Sec, SeMet, and selenate, which can be enriched by growing these vegetables on Se-enriched soil (Fairweather-Tait et al. 2010; Rayman 2008). Sec and SeMet are present in meat and fish (0.1–4 µg/g), and selenite also in tuna and crustaceans. Selenium-enriched dietary supplements (garlic, yeast) apart from SeMet, Sec, and γ-glutamyl-Se-methyl-Sec also contain inorganic compounds such as selenite and selenite (Ip et al. 2000). Milk and dairy products contain Sec and selenate, if cows are supplemented with selenium-enriched yeast and also SeMet. Eggs mainly contain Sec and SeMet. The content depends on the feeding of the hens and can reach up to 0.5 mg/kg (Fairweather-Tait et al. 2010; Rayman 2008). (For more details see Chaps. 2, 3, 20, and 25)

Selenium as Part of Selenoproteins

Physiologically, selenium and selenium compounds are not effective as such, but selenium has to be incorporated into proteins as selenocysteine (for details see Chap. 4). The human genome contains 25 genes for selenoproteins. These proteins are involved in redox homeostasis, redox regulation of signaling cascades and transcription factors, and thyroid hormone metabolism, but the function is not yet known for about 50% of them. Known functions are listed and described in

Brigelius-Flohé and Flohé (2017) and Labunskyy et al. (2014). The nomenclature of selenoproteins has recently been harmonized (Gladyshev et al. 2016). Selenoproteins with known enzyme function are named according to these functions, as before: TXNRD1–3 (thioredoxin reductase 1–3), GPX1–4 and 6 (glutathione peroxidases), DIO1–3 (iodothyronine deiodinase 1–3), MSRB1 (methionine sulfoxide reductase B1), and SEPHS2 (selenophosphate synthetase 2). Selenoproteins without known functions were previously named "selenoprotein," followed by a letter. They now are characterized by the root symbol SELENO followed by the same letter, e.g., SELENOP for selenoprotein P.

Biomarkers of the Selenium Status

To get an idea about the selenium status of individuals, plasma selenium levels have often been used. However, the different forms of selenium found in plasma are functionally not equally identical. Inorganic and organic compounds of selenium absorbed from food are metabolized in the liver into selenide (H_2Se), the selenium form required for incorporation into selenoproteins as Sec. Also SeMet can be metabolized into selenide. However, if applied in excess, it is unspecifically incorporated into plasma proteins instead of methionine. As such it is functionally not active, but contributes to the plasma selenium status. In order to get information on the biologically relevant selenium content, selenoproteins are determined that fulfill two requirements: (1) responsiveness to already minor selenium deficiency and (2) easy availability. Two selenoproteins fulfill these criteria: GPX3 and SELENOP, the main selenoproteins in plasma. Both together constitute a concentration of 80–90 µg selenium/L (Burk et al. 2001). SELENOP can be measured by immunoassay (Combs Jr. et al. 2011; Hollenbach et al. 2008; Hybsier et al. 2017), and GPX3 via its activity (Flohé and Günzler 1984). For long plasma GPX3 has been considered the biomarker of choice. More recently, however, SELENOP has been promoted, since the selenium level required for reaching the plateau of SELENOP is 110–125 ng/mL, which can be reached by a selenium intake of about 100 µg/day, whereas that for maximal GPX3 activity was only 70–90 ng/mL (Fairweather-Tait et al. 2011; Hurst et al. 2010). However, the selenium status varies in different parts of the world and depends on the dietary selenium intake. In a Chinese study with an average intake of 10 µg/day, 37 µg/day as SeMet was sufficient to optimize GPX3, whereas of selenite 66 µg was needed. SELENOP did not reach a maximum with these doses (Xia et al. 2005). In the following study, in subjects with a baseline intake of 14 µg selenium/day, a supplementation of 49 and 35 µg/day of SeMet was found to optimize SELENOP and GPX3 levels, respectively. From these findings, about 75 µg/day as SeMet was postulated for US residents (Xia et al. 2010). Thus, SELENOP appears to be the most suitable biomarker for the selenium status. (For more details see Chap. 23)

Selenium and Cancer

An epidemiological link between a suboptimal selenium status and an increased cancer incidence and mortality was reported already in the late 1960s (Shamberger and Frost 1969). The so-called Linxian trial was among the first large randomized, double-blind, primary prevention studies investigating a putative prevention of cancer by vitamins and trace elements. A mixture of selenium, vitamin E, and β-carotene, called factor D, significantly reduced cancer mortality, most significantly mortality from gastric cancer (Blot et al. 1993). Although selenium was not given as a single component, according to subsequent studies, it appeared to have the most pronounced effects. 10 years after completion of the Linxian trial, reduction in mortality remained 5% for total and 11% for gastric cancer. Considering age, the effect of factor D was much stronger in individuals younger than 55 but almost absent in subjects older than 55 years. Obviously the stage of cancer played a role.

In the nutritional prevention of cancer (NPC) trial, 1312 patients with a history of basal cell or squamous cell carcinomas of the skin were supplemented with 200 μg yeast-based organic selenium per day for 4.5 years (Clark et al. 1996). The supplementation did not significantly affect the primary end point (incidence of skin cancer), but significantly reduced total cancer mortality and development of lung, colorectal, and prostate cancers. This result was weakened by a reevaluation, which revealed that only those participants entering the study with a low selenium status (<106 ng/mL) experienced a reduction in the incidence of total and prostate cancer, whereas in those with a higher status (>122 ng/mL) the incidence was non-significantly increased (Duffield-Lillico et al. 2002). A second reevaluation revealed an increased risk of skin cancer in patients with a high Se status (>123.2 ng/mL) (Duffield-Lillico et al. 2003). Thus, a selenium status of around 122 ng/mL was considered to be optimal. In a substudy, patients were supplemented with either 200 or 400 μg/day selenium as selenium-enriched yeast. The 200 μg treatment significantly decreased total cancer incidence by 25%, whereas 400 μg had no effect (Reid et al. 2008). Thus, a high and long-term dosage does not necessarily have a beneficial effect.

These early overall promising results were compromised by the second large clinical trial, the Selenium and Vitamin E Cancer Prevention Trial (SELECT). It was based on the positive outcome of the NPC study and was undertaken to further corroborate the prevention of prostate cancer by selenium. 35,533 men were supplemented with 200 μg selenium per day in the form of L-selenomethionine alone or in combination with vitamin E (400 IU/d of all rac-α-tocopheryl acetate). After 5.5 years of supplementation, a benefit of selenium on the incidence of prostate cancer or other cancers was not observed (Lippman et al. 2009). Instead, vitamin E increased prostate cancer risk and selenium diabetes type 2, although both not significantly. In contrast to the NPC study participants entered the SELECT study with a relatively optimal selenium status of 136 ng/mL (range 122–152), which might explain the failure of selenium supplementation.

In the population-based Swedish Mammography cohort study, a high dietary intake of selenium was associated with better survival of women diagnosed with invasive breast cancer (Harris et al. 2012). Estimation of the daily intake was started before breast cancer diagnosis. With 20–27 µg/day, it was generally low. However, in the group of women in the highest quartile of selenium intake ($\geq$27.7 µg/day) the breast cancer death with 81 cases was lower compared to the lowest quartile ($\leq$20.5 µg/day) with 123 deaths after 12 years' observation. This indicates that selenium is effective in persons with a low selenium intake.

In the European Prospective Investigation into Cancer and Nutrition (EPIC) study it was investigated whether the selenium status was associated with hepatobiliary cancers. Cases were diagnosed 6 years after blood collection. The selenium serum level in the third tertile ($\geq$94.5 ng/mL) correlated with the highest SELENOP concentration (6.4 mg/L) and was significantly associated with a lower hepatocellular carcinoma development. The postulated optimal selenium level of $\geq$122 ng/mL was not reached, indicating that a marginally low selenium status still exists in the Western European population. Nevertheless, the study shows that serum levels of selenium and SELENOP are suitable markers for the selenium status and its association with liver cancer at least (Hughes et al. 2016). Another examination of EPIC samples revealed that higher selenium and SELENOP levels were associated with a lower risk to develop colon cancer which, however, was significant only in women (Hughes et al. 2015).

Selenoproteins and Cancer

GPX2 is upregulated in several human tumors, including colorectal cancer, Barrett's esophagus, squamous cell carcinoma, and lung adenocarcinomas in smokers (Brigelius-Flohé and Kipp 2009; Brigelius-Flohé and Maiorino 2013). Regarding the regulation of GPX2 expression by cancer-linked transcription factors (Brigelius-Flohé and Kipp 2009) and the fact that HT29 cancer cells lacking GPX2 injected into nude mice developed significantly smaller tumors than those from WT cells, a pro-carcinogenic role of GPX2 has been suggested (Banning et al. 2008). This conclusion has been supported by its regulation by Nrf2 which is generally protective, but also tumor cells profit from protective enzymes (Brigelius-Flohé et al. 2012).

Two recent studies in mice underline a dual role of GPX2 in cancer. In inflammation-triggered colon carcinogenesis in GPX2 KO and WT mice, GPX2 acted anti-inflammatory and, thus, reduced tumor numbers in WT. However, tumor size was larger in WT mice indicating that GPX2 supported tumor growth as observed in the xenograft model (Banning et al. 2008). When colorectal cancer (CRC) was initiated spontaneously (AOM model), KO mice developed fewer adenoma than WT mice. This was explained by an apoptotic removal of AOM-initiated cells in GPX2 KO mice (Müller et al. 2013).

In sum, GPX2 might act preventive at early stages of cancer if driven by inflammation. If cancer cells are already initiated and should be removed by apoptosis, the presence of GPX2 rather supports cancer cell growth (Brigelius-Flohé and Kipp 2016). Related functions of other GPXs have recently been reviewed (Kipp 2017).

Based on these findings GPX2 was tested as suitable prognostic biomarker. In patients with urothelial carcinoma a low GPX2 level was associated with an advanced tumor status and an unfavorable clinical outcome (Chang et al. 2015). In contrast, high GPX2 was associated with a poor prognosis in patients with castration-resistant prostate cancer (Naiki et al. 2014), with hepatocellular carcinoma (Liu et al. 2017a) and with gastric carcinoma (Liu et al. 2017b).

From these and additional animal studies (Brigelius-Flohé and Kipp 2016) it can be concluded that a benefit of selenium supplementation and especially of GPX2 expression in cancer may depend on (1) the basal selenium status, (2) the chemical form and dosage of the applied selenium, (3) the type and stage of cancer, and (4) the involvement of inflammation.

Selenium in Inflammation and Immune Response

Selenium and Inflammatory Diseases

Patients with chronic inflammation have a lower selenium status than healthy controls. This holds true for patients with cystic fibrosis (Michalke 2004), rheumatoid arthritis (Canter et al. 2007), and inflammatory bowel disease (IBD) (Kuroki et al. 2003; Ojuawo and Keith 2002). In a more recent study serum selenium was measured in 106 IBD patients. Levels from patients were significantly lower than in controls but all below 122 ng/mL. Severity of the disease increased with decreasing serum selenium. An adequate selenium status was suggested to be important to also minimize the risk of CVD, which was increased with increasing inflammatory biomarkers (Castro Aguilar-Tablada et al. 2016).

Asthma is a multifactorial inflammatory syndrome and, thus, has been tried to be treated with selenium. As reported in a systematic Cochrane review (Allam and Lucane 2004), only one double-blind randomized controlled trial (RCT) presented convincing clinical improvement by selenium supplementation (100 μg selenite/day), which, however, could not be verified by individual parameters such as lung function or airway hyper-responsiveness. The increase of serum selenium and platelet GPX activity after supplementation was accompanied by a reduction in irreversible platelet aggregation (Hasselmark et al. 1993). In contrast, a larger randomized double-blind placebo-controlled trial (PCT) supplementing 100 μg selenium-enriched yeast/day for 24 weeks did not find clinical benefits in adult patients with asthma taking inhaled steroids (Shaheen et al. 2007).

Critical illness includes septic shock, systemic inflammatory response syndrome (SIRS), and sepsis. Critically ill patients have an up to 40% decreased plasma selenium status, a decrease in GPX activity, and also loss of SELENOP. The latter for still unknown reasons massively binds to the endothelium (Forceville et al. 2009). Critical illness is the only situation where high doses of selenium are administered for treatment. Up to 1000 μg sodium selenite/day is used for short-term supplementation (Angstwurm and Gaertner 2006; Heyland 2007). A bolus of 2000 μg sodium selenite has been applied over the first 2 h (Manzanares et al. 2011) or an infusion of 4000 µg over the first 24 h in a placebo-controlled randomized double-blind phase II study (Forceville et al. 2007), all without adverse effects. A recent meta-analysis of RCTs has reviewed studies with focus on the effect of selenium supplementation on mortality (Alhazzani et al. 2013). These doses were below or above 500 µg/day, mainly as sodium selenite leading to a statistically significant reduction of mortality. Hardy et al. (2012) summarized evidence for a suggestion for selenium supplementation in critically ill. They recommended 500–1600 µg/day involving an initial loading bolus followed by a continuous daily infusion up to 14 days. Also these doses were considered to be safe. Likely, the bolus in the early phase makes use of the pro-oxidative action of selenite (Spallholz 1994), which may reversibly downregulate pro-inflammatory cytokines by blocking the binding of NF-kB to DNA, by inducing apoptosis in circulating pro-inflammatory cells, and by a probably direct virucidal and bactericidal effect. Later on, selenium becomes incorporated into selenoproteins which generally should act protective (Hardy et al. 2012). The efficacy of parenteral selenium supplementation on clinical outcomes of critically ills was meta-analyzed in nine trials (Huang et al. 2013). All-cause mortality was reduced in patients with sepsis or SIRS by selenium. Subgroup analyses revealed that longer duration, loading bolus, or a high dose of selenium might be associated with a lower mortality risk (Huang et al. 2013). However, the highly expected study conducted by the SepNet Critical Care Trials Group undertaken to confirm the benefit of the infusion of high doses of selenium did not result in an improved outcome in patients with severe sepsis. The administration of high-dose sodium selenite was not supported (Bloos et al. 2016).

Selenium and HIV

Research on a possible effect of selenium in HIV infection is based on the striking findings of the inhibition of symptoms of Keshan disease by preventing the virulence of the involved Coxsackie virus by selenium (see above). Human studies on selenium and HIV/AIDS have been compiled and outcomes summarized recently (Rayman 2012; Stone et al. 2010). Cross-sectional studies revealed that the selenium status decreases in the advanced stages of AIDS in HIV-infected patients, whereas patients in early stages did not differ from controls. Cohort and case-control studies on serum selenium and HIV progression consistently found an association of low-serum selenium with risk of mortality. Randomized control trials described that selenium supplementation in some cases improved the selenium status, increased CD4+ T cell count (a measure for resistance to infection), and reduced morbidity also from comorbidities such as diarrhea (Stone et al. 2010). However, the low number of studies and inconclusive outcomes require additional studies to explore the value of selenium in AIDS therapy. For more details about selenium and inflammation see comprehensive reviews (Hoffmann and Berry 2008; Huang et al. 2012).

Potential Roles of Selenoproteins in Suppressing Inflammation

Lipoxygenases (LOX) and cyclooxygenases (COX) catalyze a realm of inflamma-tory mediators such as prostaglandin (PG), prostacyclin (PC), thromboxane, and leukotrienes (Samuelsson 1983). For being active, the catalytic iron in these enzymes has to be oxidized by a "starting" hydroperoxide, likely a lipophilic hydro-peroxide, which of course can be inhibited by GPXs (Brigelius-Flohé and Flohé 2017; Brigelius-Flohé and Maiorino 2013). Thus, GPXs silence LOX and COX. In selenium deficiency, their expression is reduced and inflammation supported. On the other hand, LOXs can be irreversibly inactivated by their own products (Cashman et al. 1988). Interruption of their activation by enhanced GPX activity can prolong their lifetime, and thus their ability to respond to inflammatory stimuli.

Most of the diseases described here are considered to be somehow caused by or associated with oxidative stress. Therefore, the use of selenium is based on its anti-oxidative capacity. However, there is increasing evidence that H_2O_2 and other hydroperoxides act as signaling molecules (Brigelius-Flohé and Flohé 2011; Murphy et al. 2011). Their concentration is regulated by GPXs, which thus cannot only be considered as antioxidant devices but as regulators. As shown for GPX1 and 4, GPXs can also dampen inflammatory pathways by inhibiting TLR4- or TNFα-mediated activation of NF-kB. The underlying mechanism is an inactivation of pro-tein phosphatases by hydroperoxides (Brigelius-Flohé and Maiorino 2013).

A possible benefit of an increasing selenium status may be the upregulation of TRXRD1. This selenoenzyme targets the HIV-1 protein Tat and, thus, inhibits HIV-1 replication (Kalantari et al. 2008).

More recently, a function of methionine sulfoxide reductase (MSRB1) in immune response has been described (Lee et al. 2013). Macrophages respond to pathogens with a reorganization of the cytoskeleton. MSRB1 together with Mical regulates actin assembly via reversible stereoselective methionine oxidation and reduction, enabling inflammatory processes, such as release of pro-inflammatory cytokines.

Apart from GPX1, GPX4, and MSRB1, other selenoproteins responding to sele-nium in inflammatory cells may be implicated in inflammation. In human peripheral blood mononuclear cells, SELENOW mRNA levels were increased after a 12-week application of a selenium-enriched onion diet (50 µg/day), remained unchanged by supplementation with 50 and 100 µg/day selenium as selenium-enriched yeast, and decreased by 200 µg/day. SELENOR did not respond to any of these diets. mRNA for SELENOS significantly increased after an influenza virus challenge and was, thus, concluded to have a role in immune function (Goldson et al. 2011). SELENOK and SELENOF mRNA as well as plasma selenium status were increased in periph-eral leukocytes in participants of the SELGEN selenium supplementation trial after an intake of 100 µg/day selenium as sodium selenite for 6 weeks (Pagmantidis et al. 2008). The role of selenium in inflammation obviously depends on enzymes. As component of MSRB1 it may support a regular immune response. As part of GPXs it rather dampens it.

Selenium and Cardiovascular Diseases

As known from the Keshan disease, the cardiovascular system can be affected by selenium deficiency. A relationship between serum selenium concentration and cardiovascular disease (CVD) was also found in populations living in countries with low-selenium soil, e.g., Eastern Finland and parts of Germany or Sweden. Respective clinical studies found subnormal serum selenium in patients with acute myocardial infarction (Oster and Prellwitz 1990). In selenium deficiency, lipid peroxides may accumulate in the blood and induce vascular and tissue damage. Since many of the selenoproteins are considered to reduce oxidative stress, prevent oxidative modification of lipids, inhibit platelet aggregation, and reduce inflammation, it was investigated whether selenium might be able to reduce the risk of CVDs.

In a meta-analysis of 25 observational (11 case-control and 14 cohort) studies, a 50% increase in plasma or toenail selenium was found to be associated with a 24% decrease in the risk of coronary artery disease (Flores-Mateo et al. 2006).

Further data come from the NHANES (National Health and Nutrition Examination Survey). Evaluation of NHANES III (survey 1988–1994) revealed a positive association of the serum selenium level with that of total cholesterol, LDL cholesterol, HDL cholesterol, triglycerides, apo B, and apo A1. It was explicitly mentioned that US adults are a selenium-replete population (Bleys et al. 2008).

The analysis of NHANES survey 2003–2004 showed that peripheral arterial disease prevalence decreased with increasing serum selenium levels up to 150–160 ng/mL; above this level the risk increased with further increasing selenium levels. The association was, however, not statistically significant. Nevertheless, it pointed to a U-shaped relationship of the selenium effect (Bleys et al. 2009). Also prevalence of hypertension and risk of hypertonia increased when selenium increased from baseline levels of 137.1–160 ng/mL (Laclaustra et al. 2009). The same was observed regarding selenium and serum lipid levels often made responsible for development of atherosclerosis. The association between selenium and total and LDL-cholesterol (LDL-C) was strong and linear, whereas HDL-cholesterol (HDL-C) reached a plateau at a relatively low selenium level. Triglycerides were regulated in a U-shaped manner (Laclaustra et al. 2010). Thus, there is growing evidence that high selenium can increase serum lipid levels.

In the 2011–2012 NHANES survey, the association of serum selenium and lipids was combined with hypertension as related outcome. Total cholesterol, LDL-C, and triglycerides significantly increased with increasing selenium, LDL-C, however, not linearly. HDL-C did not respond to selenium at all (Christensen et al. 2015). Differences in the associations between selenium and HDL-C and LDL-C between younger and older participants were observed. Thus, age should be taken into account when associations between selenium and lipids are evaluated.

While the correlation studies quoted above suggested a beneficial role of Se in CVD disease, if not given excessively, the outcome of controlled prospective studies was less convincing. The supplementation of 200 µg selenium/day in the NPC trial did not show any overall effect of selenium on CVD incidences and mortality

(Stranges et al. 2006). In the UK PRECISE Pilot randomized trial investigating people with a low selenium status, a 6-month supplementation with 100 or 200 µg selenium/day as selenized yeast decreased serum total and non-HDL cholesterol, whereas 300 µg/day had no effect and even enhanced HDL cholesterol (Rayman et al. 2011).

A meta-analysis of 16 randomized controlled trials published from 1989 to 2015, including SELECT, revealed that we are not yet able to decide whether selenium influences CVD or CHD (coronary heart disease) (Ju et al. 2017). There was no significant effect of Se on mortality, and HDL-, LDL-, or total cholesterol. Results were extremely variable, which was explained by the variable study design. Basal selenium status, if measured, was different, as was the form and dosage of selenium and the duration of supplementation. Only 2 of the 16 studies seemed to show that Se can decrease mortality. However, in these studies selenium was administered together with coenzyme Q10. The meta-analysis clearly shows that selenium alone obviously is not sufficient to reduce CHD mortality.

In short, results of studies based on a hypothesized beneficial effect of selenium on CVD have remained equivocal. At best, selenium supplementation appeared to be beneficial for those with a low baseline level. Supplementation of individuals with an optimal level might rather experience no or negative effects.

Selenium and Thyroid Function

Thyroid gland has the highest selenium content of all tissues and regarding selenium supply is one of the most privileged endocrine organs (Schomburg and Köhrle 2008). Thus, thyroid function is dependent not only on iodine but also on selenium. The active thyroid hormone 3, 3′,5-tri-iodothyronine (T3), is primarily formed from the prohormone thyroxine (tetra-iodothyronine, T4) by the selenoenzymes deiodinase 1 and 2 (DIO1, DIO2). The peripheral DIO3 is responsible for degradation. T4 is cleaved by proteolysis from the protein thyroglobulin (Tg), released into the circulation, and taken up by target cells. Thyronine is iodinated at Tg by thyroid peroxidase (TPO) that utilizes iodide and H_2O_2, the latter being generated by the dual-function NADPH oxidases DUOX1 and DUOX2. To regulate the balance of H_2O_2 concentration, the thyroid gland is equipped with protective selenoproteins comprising GPX1, -3, and -4, TXNRDs, and SELENOP, F, M, and S. The role of selenium in biosynthesis and degradation of thyroid hormones has been amply reviewed (Darras et al. 2015; Mondal et al. 2016; Schomburg 2011; Zavacki et al. 2012).

Autoimmune thyroiditis (AIT) from which 90% is Hashimoto's thyroidism (HT) (presence of antibodies) is a hypothyroidism characterized by infiltration of inflammatory lymphocytes into the thyroid, which destruct thyroid cells and impair thyroid hormone production. Serum levels of thyroid-stimulating hormone (TSH) levels increase, whereas those of free T4 decrease and TPO and Tg antibodies appear. Graves' disease (GD) is a hyperthyroidism caused by thyroid-stimulating antibodies (TS-Abs) produced by B lymphocytes. TS-Abs stimulate the TSH receptor and thereby enhance thyroid hormone synthesis, which is associated with overproduction of H_2O_2 (Duntas 2006).

Effects of variation in dietary intake of selenium on thyroid functions are rarely observed. A combined deficiency of selenium and iodine, as present in some regions of Africa, leads to myxoedematous cretinism (Dumont et al. 1994) and has been discussed to be one of the risk factors for the development of Kashin-Beck disease (Schomburg and Köhrle 2008). However, due to the high hierarchical ranking of DIOs, selenium deficiency does not readily affect their synthesis. Nevertheless, an improvement of AIT by selenium supplementation has been observed (Duntas 2006; Gärtner et al. 2002; Turker et al. 2006). Surprisingly, it later turned out that selenium improved not only impaired thyroid function but also GD (Rayman 2012).

More recent clinical trials in different forms of hypothyroidism were less encouraging. For instance, supplementation of 200 µg selenium/day as selenite had beneficial effects only for AIT patients with high disease activity (Karanikas et al. 2008). Also, a 6-month intake of 166 µg/day of SeMet did only marginally affect the course of euthyroid HT. Thus, short-term supplementation was considered to be ineffective (Esposito et al. 2017). Moreover, hypothyroidic HT patients under long-term levothyroxine treatment had a normal thyroid function and normal selenium status and, almost expectedly, did not convincingly benefit from selenium supplementation (Nourbakhsh et al. 2016). Recent meta-analyses, although confirming some benefit of selenium supplementation in normalizing antibody titers and thyroid function, conclude that the current level of evidence for an efficiency of selenium treatment of HT patients does not allow any reliable decision (Fan et al. 2014; van Zuuren et al. 2013). Almost identically they claim that more high-quality, well-designed, long-term, randomized, controlled, multicenter trials are still needed. One may also underscore that dosages, the nature of selenium compounds applied, and the basal selenium status deserve more attention.

The efficacy of selenium in Graves' disease has gained support by recent studies. A population-based study on patients with newly diagnosed GD, autoimmune overt hypothyroidism (AIH), and euthyroid subjects with high TPO-Ab revealed a significantly lower serum selenium level in newly diagnosed GD and AIH patients than in healthy controls (Bülow Pedersen et al. 2013). In patients with recurrent GD, selenium (100 µg 2×/day for 6 months) decreased free T4 and T3, TSH, and TR-Ab (TSH receptor Ab). Furthermore, selenium was considered to enhance the effects of antithyroid drugs. Nevertheless, more trials were recommended to validate these findings (Wang et al. 2016a).

Selenoproteins and Thyroid Function

As possible mechanism of the efficacy of selenium in thyroid diseases, we can rule out a modulation of DIO activity, unless the patients are severely selenium deficient, as possibly in the African cases. The position of the deiodinases in the hierarchy of selenoproteins is simply too high to make their response to dietary selenium very likely. Moreover, the efficacy of selenium in both hypo- and hyperthyreotic conditions strongly argues against an involvement of the deiodinases in the therapeutic effects of selenium. Instead, a search in PubMed and Cochrane Library about the risk of HT offers a more likely explanation: Selenium optimizes GPX activity and simultaneously reduces TPO-antibody titers and ameliorates hypothyroidism. Optimization of GPX activity was therefore regarded as pivotal. GPX activity is easily manipulated by the selenium status, in particular when the overall activity is dominated by GPX1 and -3, which rank low in the hierarchy of selenoproteins and, thus, readily respond to selenium supply. Selenium proved to be helpful in areas of iodine deficiency or excess and ameliorates diseases associated with hypo- and hyperthyreoidism, as long as these pathologies have an inflammatory component. An intake of 50–100 μg Se/day was concluded to be appropriate to achieve optimum GPX activity (Hu and Rayman 2017). A similar conclusion was drawn in the cross-sectional observational study with 6152 participants in China (Wu et al. 2015). According to the results of this study, a low selenium status is associated with increased prevalence of thyroid diseases.

In short, observed clinical improvements of thyroid diseases appear to be due to optimization of GPXs because of their anti-inflammatory potential. This view has meanwhile been shared by most of the researchers in the field. For more details see Chap. 6.

Selenium in Male Fertility

GPX4 is the only GPX able to reduce not only H_2O_2 but also complex lipid hydroperoxides in membranes. It is highly expressed in testis, specifically in round spermatids (Maiorino et al. 1998), whereas its activity is almost undetectable in mature spermatozoa. The protein, however, is still present: During the late phase of spermiogenesis GPX4 is transformed into an enzymatically inactive structure protein (Ursini et al. 1999). The transformation is triggered by a sudden production of hydroperoxides leading to a loss of glutathione. Selenium in GPX4 becomes oxidized and reacts with other cysteine-rich proteins or with itself and forms the mitochondrial capsule in the midpiece of spermatozoa. If this does not take place, e.g., in selenium deficiency, sperm becomes instable which actually leads to a loss of fertilization capacity (Foresta et al. 2002; Imai et al. 2001).

Decrease in spermatozoal GPX4 is not necessarily caused by Se deficiency. This was observed in a Japanese study, where infertile men with impaired sperm motility had a decreased GPX4 level in spermatozoa but not in leukocytes (Imai et al. 2001). Regulation of GPX4 levels by gonadotropins may rather play the major role (Maiorino et al. 1998). Nevertheless, 100 μg/day was needed to increase sperm motility in subfertile men and enabled 11% of them to gain paternity (Rayman 2000).

In contrast, intake of 300 µg/day not specified selenium-rich diet for 48 weeks did not increase sperm selenium despite a high increase in blood plasma, indicating that dietary selenium does not affect sperm selenium (Hawkes and Turek 2001). An organ ranking high in the hierarchy like testis (Flohé 2009; Behne et al. 1988; Flohé 2007) will be saturated by selenium even at suboptimum supply and cannot benefit from any over-supplementation. Unexpectedly, the intake of 300 µg/day, which is high but still below the upper safe level of 400 µg, decreased sperm motility in these healthy men. This was explained with the administration of 300 µg of pure sodium selenite on day 110 as part of a metabolic tracer study. Selenite could have affected sperm motility via production of oxidative stress (Hawkes and Turek 2001). Since most of the selenium supplements are formulated from high-selenium yeast, the study was repeated, this time with selenium-enriched yeast. Again, selenium supplementation had no effect on sperm selenium, and in contrast to the first study also no effect on sperm motility. It was, thus, concluded that high-selenium yeast at levels near the upper safe limits does not impair sperm quality in healthy men (Hawkes et al. 2009). In addition, these studies point to the possibility that adverse effects might depend on the chemical form of selenium. Thus, there is need to know how different forms of selenium act in vivo.

SELENOP is indispensable for sperm development and function. A knockout in mice dramatically reduced selenium content in testis and impaired male fertility, which could not be restored by selenium supplementation (Burk et al. 2006; Conrad et al. 2005). SELENOP is synthesized in the liver and transported to other organs including testes. There it is taken up by Sertoli cells via the ApoE receptor-2 (Olson et al. 2007) and supplies growing spermatids with selenium. Its concentration in seminal plasma correlated positively with sperm density and the fraction of vital sperm showing that it might have more function than only supporting GPX4 biosynthesis. It has also been discussed as a novel biomarker of sperm quality (Michaelis et al. 2014).

A third selenoprotein is abundantly expressed in elongating spermatids, thioredoxin-glutathione reductase (TGR), a member of the thioredoxin family with a glutaredoxin domain (Su et al. 2005). It has first been found in mice, but later also in humans (Gerashchenko et al. 2010). TGR is located at the site of mitochondrial capsule formation. It can act as disulfide isomerase and correct "incorrectly" formed disulfides. TGR may interact with GPX4 in the formation of disulfide bonds in the structural proteins forming the mitochondrial sheath (Su et al. 2005). A detailed underlying mechanism was not yet studied. Also the function of other selenoproteins found in testes, SELENOF, K, S, V, and W is still waiting to be worked out (Boitani and Puglisi 2008; Ferguson et al. 2006). For more details on selenium and male fertility see Conrad et al. (2015).

Selenium and Diabetes

Insulin resistance (IR), a hallmark for type 2 diabetes mellitus (T2DM), is considered to be associated with oxidative stress. According to its postulated antioxidative function, selenium was found to improve glucose metabolism in animal models (for review see Zhou et al. 2013). Based on such findings, a secondary analysis of the NPC trial was conducted. A statistically significant increase of T2DM was observed in patients in the highest tertile of the selenium plasma level (>121.6 ng/mL) (Stranges et al. 2007). Similar findings were also observed in the SELECT, although the increased incidence of diabetes was not significant (Lippman et al. 2009). The link between selenium and diabetes was investigated in several studies in the following years. These have been summarized and discussed by Rayman and Stranges (2013).

A beneficial effect of dietary selenium intake up to 1.6 µg/kg/day on insulin resistance was observed in the Newfoundland population. Above this cutoff, the effect disappeared (Wang et al. 2017). A meta-analysis of five observational studies with 13,460 participants found a higher prevalence of T2DM in the highest category of serum selenium (>132.5 ng/mL) compared to the lowest (<97.5 ng/mL) and a nonlinear dose-response relationship. Associations were positive with low- and high-serum selenium levels and T2DM pointing to a U-shape function of selenium (Wang et al. 2016b). A positive correlation between dietary selenium intake and prevalence of T2DM was also described in a cross-sectional study with 5423 individuals (Wei et al. 2015). In a case-control study the positive association between serum selenium and T2DM disappeared after adjusting for insulin resistance and obesity, but not in the quartile with the highest selenium (>104.5 ng/mL) (Lu et al. 2016). Adenoma development was studied in patients with colonoscopic removal of colorectal adenomas and a supplementation with 200 µg selenized yeast/day. Selenium did not prevent colorectal adenomas, but had some benefit in patients with baseline advanced adenomas. Increase in T2DM was described to be similar to other trials. Thus, selenium was not recommended for preventing colorectal adenomas in selenium-adequate individuals (Thompson et al. 2016).

A recent study addressed the question whether human obesity might be associated with changes in H_2O_2 metabolism in visceral and subcutaneous fat depots and whether these changes are linked to development of insulin resistance. To this end, 43 non-diabetic men undergoing abdominal surgeries were recruited. In participants with abdominal obesity, SOD was upregulated and H_2O_2 accumulated in the visceral fat depot despite an increased catalase activity (Akl et al. 2017). All three parameters correlated positively with IR. The findings are in line with animal studies (see Chap. 17) and confirm the earlier findings of the need for an intact H_2O_2 pathway for intact insulin signaling (see below).

Selenoproteins and Diabetes

When the XinGen Lei group tried to create a super-healthy mouse by overexpression of GPX1, expected to counteract all kinds of oxidative stress, completely unexpected observations were made. Mice became obese, were hyperglycemic, hyper-insulinemic, and insulin-resistant, and had elevated leptin levels. In addition, they developed T2DM (McClung et al. 2004). In line with these findings, in mice with a knockout of GPX1 insulin sensitivity was improved (Loh et al. 2009). Also SELENOP induced insulin resistance (Misu et al. 2010) indicating that more than one selenoprotein might contribute to glucose metabolism.

The underlying mechanism may well be an "over-scavenging" of H_2O_2 which is needed for insulin signaling as known for more than 30 years now (Czech et al. 1974; May and de Haen 1979) and only recently detected to be NOX4 derived (Wu and Williams 2012). Insulin-mediated H_2O_2 production inhibits protein phosphatases like PTEN or PTP1B by oxidation of thiol groups. The phosphatases counteract and regulate protein kinases, e.g., PI3K or Akt needed in the insulin pathway. If phosphatases are not inhibited by H_2O_2, kinases cannot stay phosphorylated and thus not active. The cascade is blocked and insulin resistance created. For more details see Steinbrenner (2013). In sum, the insulin pathway turns out to be redox controlled and the selenium-dependent peroxidases are likely in charge of fine-tuning the signaling cascade.

SELENOS (previously called Tanis) has gained great interest in the last years. It is a membrane protein with receptor functions at the cell surface. SELENOS interacts with a high number of proteins, and contributes to many pathways, mainly connected to protein transport. Most interestingly, SELENOS is regulated by glucose, dysregulated in diabetes, and obviously promotes development of insulin resistance. Apart from diabetes, SELENOS has connections to CVD, metabolic disorders, AIT, inflammation, and cancer (reviewed in Liu and Rozovsky 2015). Research is ongoing and may be SELENOS will contribute to find answers to the question how selenium act in human health and disease.

Conclusion

Although the gain of knowledge over the last years is quite large, the evidence for a therapeutic value of selenium for human health is yet not convincing. The variety in the outcomes of human studies makes it difficult to provide recommendations. Most of the studies described here end with the conclusion that more, larger, and more rigorous studies are required. They also should be better comparable regarding chemical form and dosage of selenium, and duration of a supplementation. Nevertheless, some important observations have been made. Mainly subjects with a low selenium status profit from a supplementation. The optimal plasma selenium status in most studies was around 120 ng/L. A lower one increased the risk of developing, e.g., cancer and cardiovascular diseases, a higher one cancer, CVD, and diabetes, which means that selenium can have negative effects at a low and a high status, the so-called U-shape. If it turns out that the level of 120 ng/L is optimal, indeed, this will make the situation much easier. Only subjects with a status lower than the optimum should get supplements being aware that this comes on top of that what they get from the diet anyway. Those with the optimum or higher should not take supplements. An exception is patients with critically illness. A positive result of the last years, however, is the consensus about the increase of the RDI for selenium.

A remaining problem is the limited knowledge about the functions of about half of the selenoproteins. This should be solved as far as possible. Without knowing the biological functions of all of them, we will not understand what selenium can do for our health.

References

Akl MG, Fawzy E, Deif M, Farouk A, Elshorbagy AK. Perturbed adipose tissue hydrogen peroxide metabolism in centrally obese men: association with insulin resistance. PLoS One. 2017;12:e0177268.

Alhazzani W, Jacobi J, Sindi A, Hartog C, Reinhart K, Kokkoris S, Gerlach H, Andrews P, Drabek T, Manzanares W, Cook DJ, Jaeschke RZ. The effect of selenium therapy on mortality in patients with sepsis syndrome: a systematic review and meta-analysis of randomized controlled trials. Crit Care Med. 2013;41:1555–64.

Allam MF, Lucane RA. Selenium supplementation for asthma. Cochrane Database Syst Rev. 2004:CD003538.

Angstwurm MW, Gaertner R. Practicalities of selenium supplementation in critically ill patients. Curr Opin Clin Nutr Metab Care. 2006;9:233–8.

Banning A, Kipp A, Schmitmeier S, Loewinger M, Florian S, Krehl S, Thalmann S, Thierbach R, Steinberg P, Brigelius-Flohé R. Glutathione peroxidase 2 inhibits cyclooxygenase-2-mediated migration and invasion of HT-29 adenocarcinoma cells but supports their growth as tumors in nude mice. Cancer Res. 2008;68:9746–53.

Beck MA, Shi Q, Morris VC, Levander OA. Rapid genomic evolution of a non-virulent coxsackievirus B3 in selenium-deficient mice results in selection of identical virulent isolates. Nat Med. 1995;1:433–6.

Behne D, Hilmert H, Scheid S, Gessner H, Elger W. Evidence for specific selenium target tissues and new biologically important selenoproteins. Biochim Biophys Acta. 1988;966:12–21.

Bleys J, Navas-Acien A, Stranges S, Menke A, Miller ER 3rd, Guallar E. Serum selenium and serum lipids in US adults. Am J Clin Nutr. 2008;88:416–23.

Bleys J, Navas-Acien A, Laclaustra M, Pastor-Barriuso R, Menke A, Ordovas J, Stranges S, Guallar E. Serum selenium and peripheral arterial disease: results from the national health and nutrition examination survey, 2003–2004. Am J Epidemiol. 2009;169:996–1003.

Bloos F, Trips E, Nierhaus A, Briegel J, Heyland DK, Jaschinski U, Moerer O, Weyland A, Marx G, Grundling M, Kluge S, Kaufmann I, Ott K, Quintel M, Jelschen F, Meybohm P, Rademacher S, Meier-Hellmann A, Utzolino S, Kaisers UX, Putensen C, Elke G, Ragaller M, Gerlach H, Ludewig K, Kiehntopf M, Bogatsch H, Engel C, Brunkhorst FM, Loeffler M, Reinhart K, for SepNet Critical Care Trials, G. Effect of sodium selenite administration and procalcitonin-guided therapy on mortality in patients with severe sepsis or septic shock: a randomized clinical trial. JAMA Intern Med. 2016;176:1266–76.

Blot WJ, Li JY, Taylor PR, Guo W, Dawsey S, Wang GQ, Yang CS, Zheng SF, Gail M, Li GY, et al. Nutrition intervention trials in Linxian, China: supplementation with specific vitamin/mineral combinations, cancer incidence, and disease-specific mortality in the general population. J Natl Cancer Inst. 1993;85:1483–92.

Boitani C, Puglisi R. Selenium, a key element in spermatogenesis and male fertility. Adv Exp Med Biol. 2008;636:65–73.

Brigelius-Flohé R, Flohé L. Basic principles and emerging concepts in the redox control of transcription factors. Antioxid Redox Signal. 2011;15(8):2335–81.

Brigelius-Flohe R, Flohe L. Selenium and redox signaling. Arch Biochem Biophys. 2017;617:48–59.

Brigelius-Flohe R, Kipp A. Glutathione peroxidases in different stages of carcinogenesis. Biochim Biophys Acta. 2009;1790:1555–68.

Brigelius-Flohé R, Kipp AP. Glutathione peroxidase 2, a selenoprotein exhibiting a dual personality in preventing and promoting cancer. In: Hatfield DL, Schweizer U, Tsuji PA, Gladyshev VN, editors. Selenium. Its molcular biology and role in human health. New York: Springer; 2016. p. 451–62.

Brigelius-Flohe R, Maiorino M. Glutathione peroxidases. Biochim Biophys Acta. 2013;1830:3289–303.

Brigelius-Flohe R, Muller M, Lippmann D, Kipp AP. The yin and yang of nrf2-regulated selenoproteins in carcinogenesis. Int J Cell Biol. 2012;2012:486147.

Bülow Pedersen I, Knudsen N, Carle A, Schomburg L, Kohrle J, Jorgensen T, Rasmussen LB, Ovesen L, Laurberg P. Serum selenium is low in newly diagnosed Graves' disease: a population-based study. Clin Endocrinol. 2013;79:584–90.

Burk RF, Hill KE, Motley AK. Plasma selenium in specific and non-specific forms. Biofactors. 2001;14:107–14.

Burk RF, Olson GE, Hill KE. Deletion of selenoprotein P gene in the mouse. In: Hatfield DL, Berry MJ, Gladyshev VN, editors. Selenium. Its molecular biology and role in human health. New York: Springer; 2006. p. 111–22.

Canter PH, Wider B, Ernst E. The antioxidant vitamins A, C, E and selenium in the treatment of arthritis: a systematic review of randomized clinical trials. Rheumatology (Oxford). 2007;46:1223–33.

Cashman JR, Lambert C, Sigal E. Inhibition of human leukocyte 5-lipoxygenase by 15-HPETE and related eicosanoids. Biochem Biophys Res Commun. 1988;155:38–44.

Castro Aguilar-Tablada T, Navarro-Alarcon M, Quesada Granados J, Samaniego Sanchez C, Rufian-Henares JA, Nogueras-Lopez F. Ulcerative colitis and Crohn's disease are associated with decreased serum selenium concentrations and increased cardiovascular risk. Nutrients. 2016;8:E780.

Chang IW, Lin VC, Hung CH, Wang HP, Lin YY, Wu WJ, Huang CN, Li CC, Li WM, Wu JY, Li CF. GPX2 underexpression indicates poor prognosis in patients with urothelial carcinomas of the upper urinary tract and urinary bladder. World J Urol. 2015;33:1777–89.

Chen J, Chu Y, Cao J, Yang Z, Guo X, Wang Z. T-2 toxin induces apoptosis, and selenium partly blocks, T-2 toxin induced apoptosis in chondrocytes through modulation of the Bax/Bcl-2 ratio. Food Chem Toxicol. 2006;44:567–73.

Christensen K, Werner M, Malecki K. Serum selenium and lipid levels: associations observed in the National Health and Nutrition Examination Survey (NHANES) 2011–2012. Environ Res. 2015;140:76–84.

Clark LC, Combs GF Jr, Turnbull BW, Slate EH, Chalker DK, Chow J, Davis LS, Glover RA, Graham GF, Gross EG, Krongrad A, Lesher JL Jr, Park HK, Sanders BB Jr, Smith CL, Taylor JR. Effects of selenium supplementation for cancer prevention in patients with carcinoma of the skin. A randomized controlled trial. Nutritional Prevention of Cancer Study Group. JAMA. 1996;276:1957–63.

Combs GF Jr, Watts JC, Jackson MI, Johnson LK, Zeng H, Scheett AJ, Uthus EO, Schomburg L, Hoeg A, Hoefig CS, Davis CD, Milner JA. Determinants of selenium status in healthy adults. Nutr J. 2011;10:75.

Conrad M, Moreno SG, Sinowatz F, Ursini F, Kolle S, Roveri A, Brielmeier M, Wurst W, Maiorino M, Bornkamm GW. The nuclear form of phospholipid hydroperoxide glutathione peroxidase is a protein thiol peroxidase contributing to sperm chromatin stability. Mol Cell Biol. 2005;25:7637–44.

Conrad M, Ingold I, Buday K, Kobayashi S, Angeli JP. ROS, thiols and thiol-regulating systems in male gametogenesis. Biochim Biophys Acta. 2015;1850:1566–74.

Czech MP, Lawrence JC Jr, Lynn WS. Evidence for the involvement of sulfhydryl oxidation in the regulation of fat cell hexose transport by insulin. Proc Natl Acad Sci U S A. 1974;71:4173–7.

Darras VM, Houbrechts AM, Van Herck SL. Intracellular thyroid hormone metabolism as a local regulator of nuclear thyroid hormone receptor-mediated impact on vertebrate development. Biochim Biophys Acta. 2015;1849:130–41.

Duffield-Lillico AJ, Reid ME, Turnbull BW, Combs GF Jr, Slate EH, Fischbach LA, Marshall JR, Clark LC. Baseline characteristics and the effect of selenium supplementation on cancer incidence in a randomized clinical trial: a summary report of the Nutritional Prevention of Cancer Trial. Cancer Epidemiol Biomark Prev. 2002;11:630–9.

Duffield-Lillico AJ, Dalkin BL, Reid ME, Turnbull BW, Slate EH, Jacobs ET, Marshall JR, Clark LC, Nutritional Prevention of Cancer Study, G. Selenium supplementation, baseline plasma selenium status and incidence of prostate cancer: an analysis of the complete treatment period of the Nutritional Prevention of Cancer Trial. BJU Int. 2003;91:608–12.

Dumont JE, Corvilain B, Contempre B. The biochemistry of endemic cretinism: roles of iodine and selenium deficiency and goitrogens. Mol Cell Endocrinol. 1994;100:163–6.

Duntas LH. The role of selenium in thyroid autoimmunity and cancer. Thyroid. 2006;16:455–60.

Esposito D, Rotondi M, Accardo G, Vallone G, Conzo G, Docimo G, Selvaggi F, Cappelli C, Chiovato L, Giugliano D, Pasquali D. Influence of short-term selenium supplementation on the natural course of Hashimoto's thyroiditis: clinical results of a blinded placebo-controlled randomized prospective trial. J Endocrinol Investig. 2017;40:83–9.

Fairweather-Tait SJ, Collings R, Hurst R. Selenium bioavailability: current knowledge and future research requirements. Am J Clin Nutr. 2010;91:1484S–91S.

Fairweather-Tait SJ, Bao Y, Broadley MR, Collings R, Ford D, Hesketh JE, Hurst R. Selenium in human health and disease. Antioxid Redox Signal. 2011;14:1337–83.

Fan Y, Xu S, Zhang H, Cao W, Wang K, Chen G, Di H, Cao M, Liu C. Selenium supplementation for autoimmune thyroiditis: a systematic review and meta-analysis. Int J Endocrinol. 2014;2014:904573.

Ferguson AD, Labunskyy VM, Fomenko DE, Arac D, Chelliah Y, Amezcua CA, Rizo J, Gladyshev VN, Deisenhofer J. NMR structures of the selenoproteins Sep15 and SelM reveal redox activity of a new thioredoxin-like family. J Biol Chem. 2006;281:3536–43.

Fleming CR, Lie JT, McCall JT, O'Brien JF, Baillie EE, Thistle JL. Selenium deficiency and fatal cardiomyopathy in a patient on home parenteral nutrition. Gastroenterology. 1982;83:689–93.

Flohe L. Selenium in mammalian spermiogenesis. Biol Chem. 2007;388:987–95.

Flohe L. The labour pains of biochemical selenology: the history of selenoprotein biosynthesis. Biochim Biophys Acta. 2009;1790:1389–403.

Flohé L, Günzler WA. Assays of glutathione peroxidase. Methods Enzymol. 1984;105:114–21.

Flores-Mateo G, Navas-Acien A, Pastor-Barriuso R, Guallar E. Selenium and coronary heart disease: a meta-analysis. Am J Clin Nutr. 2006;84:762–73.

Forceville X, Laviolle B, Annane D, Vitoux D, Bleichner G, Korach JM, Cantais E, Georges H, Soubirou JL, Combes A, Bellissant E. Effects of high doses of selenium, as sodium selenite, in septic shock: a placebo-controlled, randomized, double-blind, phase II study. Crit Care. 2007;11:R73.

Forceville X, Mostert V, Pierantoni A, Vitoux D, Le Toumelin P, Plouvier E, Dehoux M, Thuillier F, Combes A. Selenoprotein P, rather than glutathione peroxidase, as a potential marker of septic shock and related syndromes. Eur Surg Res. 2009;43:338–47.

Foresta C, Flohe L, Garolla A, Roveri A, Ursini F, Maiorino M. Male fertility is linked to the selenoprotein phospholipid hydroperoxide glutathione peroxidase. Biol Reprod. 2002;67:967–71.

Gärtner R, Gasnier BC, Dietrich JW, Krebs B, Angstwurm MW. Selenium supplementation in patients with autoimmune thyroiditis decreases thyroid peroxidase antibodies concentrations. J Clin Endocrinol Metab. 2002;87:1687–91.

Ge K, Yang G. The epidemiology of selenium deficiency in the etiological study of endemic diseases in China. Am J Clin Nutr. 1993;57:259S–63S.

Gerashchenko MV, Su D, Gladyshev VN. CUG start codon generates thioredoxin/glutathione reductase isoforms in mouse testes. J Biol Chem. 2010;285:4595–602.

Gladyshev VN, Arner ES, Berry MJ, Brigelius-Flohe R, Bruford EA, Burk RF, Carlson BA, Castellano S, Chavatte L, Conrad M, Copeland PR, Diamond AM, Driscoll DM, Ferreiro A, Flohe L, Green FR, Guigo R, Handy DE, Hatfield DL, Hesketh J, Hoffmann PR, Holmgren A, Hondal RJ, Howard MT, Huang K, Kim HY, Kim IY, Kohrle J, Krol A, Kryukov GV, Lee BJ, Lee BC, Lei XG, Liu Q, Lescure A, Lobanov AV, Loscalzo J, Maiorino M, Mariotti M, Sandeep Prabhu K, Rayman MP, Rozovsky S, Salinas G, Schmidt EE, Schomburg L, Schweizer U, Simonovic M, Sunde RA, Tsuji PA, Tweedie S, Ursini F, Whanger PD, Zhang Y. Selenoprotein gene nomenclature. J Biol Chem. 2016;291:24036–40.

Goldson AJ, Fairweather-Tait SJ, Armah CN, Bao Y, Broadley MR, Dainty JR, Furniss C, Hart DJ, Teucher B, Hurst R. Effects of selenium supplementation on selenoprotein gene expression and response to influenza vaccine challenge: a randomised controlled trial. PLoS One. 2011;6:e14771.

Hardy G, Hardy I, Manzanares W. Selenium supplementation in the critically ill. Nutr Clin Pract. 2012;27:21–33.

Harris HR, Bergkvist L, Wolk A. Selenium intake and breast cancer mortality in a cohort of Swedish women. Breast Cancer Res Treat. 2012;134:1269–77.

Hasselmark L, Malmgren R, Zetterstrom O, Unge G. Selenium supplementation in intrinsic asthma. Allergy. 1993;48:30–6.

Hawkes WC, Turek PJ. Effects of dietary selenium on sperm motility in healthy men. J Androl. 2001;22:764–72.

Hawkes WC, Alkan Z, Wong K. Selenium supplementation does not affect testicular selenium status or semen quality in North American men. J Androl. 2009;30:525–33.

Heyland DK. Selenium supplementation in critically ill patients: can too much of a good thing be a bad thing? Crit Care. 2007;11:153.

Hoffmann PR, Berry MJ. The influence of selenium on immune responses. Mol Nutr Food Res. 2008;52:1273–80.

Hollenbach B, Morgenthaler NG, Struck J, Alonso C, Bergmann A, Kohrle J, Schomburg L. New assay for the measurement of selenoprotein P as a sepsis biomarker from serum. J Trace Elem Med Biol. 2008;22:24–32.

Hu S, Rayman MP. Multiple nutritional factors and the risk of Hashimoto's thyroiditis. Thyroid. 2017;27:597–610.

Huang Z, Rose AH, Hoffmann PR. The role of selenium in inflammation and immunity: from molecular mechanisms to therapeutic opportunities. Antioxid Redox Signal. 2012;16:705–43.

Huang TS, Shyu YC, Chen HY, Lin LM, Lo CY, Yuan SS, Chen PJ. Effect of parenteral selenium supplementation in critically ill patients: a systematic review and meta-analysis. PLoS One. 2013;8:e54431.

Hughes DJ, Fedirko V, Jenab M, Schomburg L, Meplan C, Freisling H, Bueno-de-Mesquita HB, Hybsier S, Becker NP, Czuban M, Tjonneland A, Outzen M, Boutron-Ruault MC, Racine A, Bastide N, Kuhn T, Kaaks R, Trichopoulos D, Trichopoulou A, Lagiou P, Panico S, Peeters PH, Weiderpass E, Skeie G, Dagrun E, Chirlaque MD, Sanchez MJ, Ardanaz E, Ljuslinder I, Wennberg M, Bradbury KE, Vineis P, Naccarati A, Palli D, Boeing H, Overvad K, Dorronsoro M, Jakszyn P, Cross AJ, Quiros JR, Stepien M, Kong SY, Duarte-Salles T, Riboli E, Hesketh JE. Selenium status is associated with colorectal cancer risk in the European prospective investigation of cancer and nutrition cohort. Int J Cancer. 2015;136:1149–61.

Hughes DJ, Duarte-Salles T, Hybsier S, Trichopoulou A, Stepien M, Aleksandrova K, Overvad K, Tjonneland A, Olsen A, Affret A, Fagherazzi G, Boutron-Ruault MC, Katzke V, Kaaks R,

Boeing H, Bamia C, Lagiou P, Peppa E, Palli D, Krogh V, Panico S, Tumino R, Sacerdote C, Bueno-de-Mesquita HB, Peeters PH, Engeset D, Weiderpass E, Lasheras C, Agudo A, Sanchez MJ, Navarro C, Ardanaz E, Dorronsoro M, Hemmingsson O, Wareham NJ, Khaw KT, Bradbury KE, Cross AJ, Gunter M, Riboli E, Romieu I, Schomburg L, Jenab M. Prediagnostic selenium status and hepatobiliary cancer risk in the European Prospective Investigation into Cancer and Nutrition cohort. Am J Clin Nutr. 2016;104:406–14.

Hurst R, Armah CN, Dainty JR, Hart DJ, Teucher B, Goldson AJ, Broadley MR, Motley AK, Fairweather-Tait SJ. Establishing optimal selenium status: results of a randomized, double-blind, placebo-controlled trial. Am J Clin Nutr. 2010;91:923–31.

Hybsier S, Schulz T, Wu Z, Demuth I, Minich WB, Renko K, Rijntjes E, Kohrle J, Strasburger CJ, Steinhagen-Thiessen E, Schomburg L. Sex-specific and inter-individual differences in bio-markers of selenium status identified by a calibrated ELISA for selenoprotein P. Redox Biol. 2017;11:403–14.

Imai H, Suzuki K, Ishizaka K, Ichinose S, Oshima H, Okayasu I, Emoto K, Umeda M, Nakagawa Y. Failure of the expression of phospholipid hydroperoxide glutathione peroxidase in the sper-matozoa of human infertile males. Biol Reprod. 2001;64:674–83.

Ip C, Birringer M, Block E, Kotrebai M, Tyson JF, Uden PC, Lisk DJ. Chemical speciation influ-ences comparative activity of selenium-enriched garlic and yeast in mammary cancer preven-tion. J Agric Food Chem. 2000;48:2062–70.

Johnson RA, Baker SS, Fallon JT, Maynard EP 3rd, Ruskin JN, Wen Z, Ge K, Cohen HJ. An occidental case of cardiomyopathy and selenium deficiency. N Engl J Med. 1981;304:1210–2.

Ju W, Li X, Li Z, Wu GR, Fu XF, Yang XM, Zhang XQ, Gao XB. The effect of selenium supple-mentation on coronary heart disease: a systematic review and meta-analysis of randomized controlled trials. J Trace Elem Med Biol. 2017;44:8–16.

Kalantari P, Narayan V, Natarajan SK, Muralidhar K, Gandhi UH, Vunta H, Henderson AJ, Prabhu KS. Thioredoxin reductase-1 negatively regulates HIV-1 transactivating protein Tat-dependent transcription in human macrophages. J Biol Chem. 2008;283:33183–90.

Karanikas G, Schuetz M, Kontur S, Duan H, Kommata S, Schoen R, Antoni A, Kletter K, Dudczak R, Willheim M. No immunological benefit of selenium in consecutive patients with autoim-mune thyroiditis. Thyroid. 2008;18:7–12.

Kipp AP. Selenium-dependent glutathione peroxidases during tumor development. Adv Cancer Res. 2017;136:109–38.

Kipp AP, Strohm D, Brigelius-Flohe R, Schomburg L, Bechthold A, Leschik-Bonnet E, Heseker H. Revised reference values for selenium intake. J Trace Elem Med Biol. 2015;32:195–9.

Kuroki F, Matsumoto T, Iida M. Selenium is depleted in Crohn's disease on enteral nutrition. Dig Dis. 2003;21:266–70.

Labunskyy VM, Hatfield DL, Gladyshev VN. Selenoproteins: molecular pathways and physiologi-cal roles. Physiol Rev. 2014;94:739–77.

Laclaustra M, Navas-Acien A, Stranges S, Ordovas JM, Guallar E. Serum selenium concentrations and hypertension in the US Population. Circ Cardiovasc Qual Outcomes. 2009;2:369–76.

Laclaustra M, Stranges S, Navas-Acien A, Ordovas JM, Guallar E. Serum selenium and serum lip-ids in US adults: National Health and Nutrition Examination Survey (NHANES) 2003–2004. Atherosclerosis. 2010;210:643–8.

Lee BC, Peterfi Z, Hoffmann FW, Moore RE, Kaya A, Avanesov A, Tarrago L, Zhou Y, Weerapana E, Fomenko DE, Hoffmann PR, Gladyshev VN. MsrB1 and MICALs regulate actin assem-bly and macrophage function via reversible stereoselective methionine oxidation. Mol Cell. 2013;51:397–404.

Lippman SM, Klein EA, Goodman PJ, Lucia MS, Thompson IM, Ford LG, Parnes HL, Minasian LM, Gaziano JM, Hartline JA, Parsons JK, Bearden JD 3rd, Crawford ED, Goodman GE, Claudio J, Winquist E, Cook ED, Karp DD, Walther P, Lieber MM, Kristal AR, Darke AK, Arnold KB, Ganz PA, Santella RM, Albanes D, Taylor PR, Probstfield JL, Jagpal TJ, Crowley JJ, Meyskens FL Jr, Baker LH, Coltman CA Jr. Effect of selenium and vitamin E on risk of prostate cancer and other cancers: the selenium and Vitamin E Cancer Prevention Trial (SELECT). JAMA. 2009;301:39–51.

Liu J, Rozovsky S. Membrane-bound selenoproteins. Antioxid Redox Signal. 2015;23:795–813.

Liu T, Kan XF, Ma C, Chen LL, Cheng TT, Zou ZW, Li Y, Cao FJ, Zhang WJ, Yao J, Li PD. GPX2 overexpression indicates poor prognosis in patients with hepatocellular carcinoma. Tumour Biol. 2017a;39:1010428317700410.

Liu D, Sun L, Tong J, Chen X, Li H, Zhang Q. Prognostic significance of glutathione peroxidase 2 in gastric carcinoma. Tumour Biol. 2017b;39:1010428317701443.

Loh K, Deng H, Fukushima A, Cai X, Boivin B, Galic S, Bruce C, Shields BJ, Skiba B, Ooms LM, Stepto N, Wu B, Mitchell CA, Tonks NK, Watt MJ, Febbraio MA, Crack PJ, Andrikopoulos S, Tiganis T. Reactive oxygen species enhance insulin sensitivity. Cell Metab. 2009;10:260–72.

Loscalzo J. Keshan disease, selenium deficiency, and the selenoproteome. N Engl J Med. 2014;370:1756–60.

Lu CW, Chang HH, Yang KC, Kuo CS, Lee LT, Huang KC. High serum selenium levels are associated with increased risk for diabetes mellitus independent of central obesity and insulin resistance. BMJ Open Diabetes Res Care. 2016;4:e000253.

Maiorino M, Wissing JB, Brigelius-Flohé R, Calabrese F, Roveri A, Steinert P, Ursini F, Flohé L. Testosterone mediates expression of the selenoprotein PHGPx by induction of spermatogenesis and not by direct transcriptional gene activation. FASEB J. 1998;12:1359–70.

Manzanares W, Biestro A, Torre MH, Galusso F, Facchin G, Hardy G. High-dose selenium reduces ventilator-associated pneumonia and illness severity in critically ill patients with systemic inflammation. Intensive Care Med. 2011;37:1120–7.

May JM, de Haen C. The insulin-like effect of hydrogen peroxide on pathways of lipid synthesis in rat adipocytes. J Biol Chem. 1979;254:9017–21.

McClung JP, Roneker CA, Mu W, Lisk DJ, Langlais P, Liu F, Lei XG. Development of insulin resistance and obesity in mice overexpressing cellular glutathione peroxidase. Proc Natl Acad Sci U S A. 2004;101:8852–527.

Michaelis M, Gralla O, Behrends T, Scharpf M, Endermann T, Rijntjes E, Pietschmann N, Hollenbach B, Schomburg L. Selenoprotein P in seminal fluid is a novel biomarker of sperm quality. Biochem Biophys Res Commun. 2014;443:905–10.

Michalke B. Selenium speciation in human serum of cystic fibrosis patients compared to serum from healthy persons. J Chromatogr A. 2004;1058:203–8.

Misu H, Takamura T, Takayama H, Hayashi H, Matsuzawa-Nagata N, Kurita S, Ishikura K, Ando H, Takeshita Y, Ota T, Sakurai M, Yamashita T, Mizukoshi E, Honda M, Miyamoto K, Kubota T, Kubota N, Kadowaki T, Kim HJ, Lee IK, Minokoshi Y, Saito Y, Takahashi K, Yamada Y, Takakura N, Kaneko S. A liver-derived secretory protein, selenoprotein P, causes insulin resistance. Cell Metab. 2010;12:483–95.

Mondal S, Raja K, Schweizer U, Mugesh G. Chemistry and biology in the biosynthesis and action of thyroid hormones. Angew Chem Int Ed Engl. 2016;55:7606–30.

Muller MF, Florian S, Pommer K, Osterhoff M, Esworthy RS, Chu FF, Brigelius-Flohe R, Kipp AP. Deletion of glutathione peroxidase-2 inhibits azoxymethane-induced colon cancer development. PLoS One. 2013;8:e72055.

Murphy MP, Holmgren A, Larsson NG, Halliwell B, Chang CJ, Kalyanaraman B, Rhee SG, Thornalley PJ, Partridge L, Gems D, Nystrom T, Belousov V, Schumacker PT, Winterbourn CC. Unraveling the biological roles of reactive oxygen species. Cell Metab. 2011;13:361–6.

Muth OH, Oldfield JE, Remmert LF, Schubert JR. Effects of selenium and vitamin E on white muscle disease. Science. 1958;128:1090.

Naiki T, Naiki-Ito A, Asamoto M, Kawai N, Tozawa K, Etani T, Sato S, Suzuki S, Shirai T, Kohri K, Takahashi S. GPX2 overexpression is involved in cell proliferation and prognosis of castration-resistant prostate cancer. Carcinogenesis. 2014;35:1962–7.

Nourbakhsh M, Ahmadpour F, Chahardoli B, Malekpour-Dehkordi Z, Nourbakhsh M, Hosseini-Fard SR, Doustimotlagh A, Golestani A, Razzaghy-Azar M. Selenium and its relationship with selenoprotein P and glutathione peroxidase in children and adolescents with Hashimoto's thyroiditis and hypothyroidism. J Trace Elem Med Biol. 2016;34:10–4.

Ojuawo A, Keith L. The serum concentrations of zinc, copper and selenium in children with inflammatory bowel disease. Cent Afr J Med. 2002;48:116–9.

Olson GE, Winfrey VP, Nagdas SK, Hill KE, Burk RF. Apolipoprotein E receptor-2 (ApoER2) mediates selenium uptake from selenoprotein P by the mouse testis. J Biol Chem. 2007;282:12290–7.

Oster O, Prellwitz W. Selenium and cardiovascular disease. Biol Trace Elem Res. 1990;24:91–103.

Pagmantidis V, Meplan C, van Schothorst EM, Keijer J, Hesketh JE. Supplementation of healthy volunteers with nutritionally relevant amounts of selenium increases the expression of lymphocyte protein biosynthesis genes. Am J Clin Nutr. 2008;87:181–9.

Rayman MP. The importance of selenium to human health. Lancet. 2000;356:233–41.

Rayman MP. Food-chain selenium and human health: emphasis on intake. Br J Nutr. 2008;100:254–68.

Rayman MP. Selenium and human health. Lancet. 2012;379:1256–68.

Rayman MP, Stranges S. Epidemiology of selenium and type 2 diabetes: can we make sense of it? Free Radic Biol Med. 2013;65:1557–64.

Rayman MP, Stranges S, Griffin BA, Pastor-Barriuso R, Guallar E. Effect of supplementation with high-selenium yeast on plasma lipids: a randomized trial. Ann Intern Med. 2011;154:656–65.

Reeves WC, Marcuard SP, Willis SE, Movahed A. Reversible cardiomyopathy due to selenium deficiency. J Parenter Enteral Nutr. 1989;13:663–5.

Reid ME, Duffield-Lillico AJ, Slate E, Natarajan N, Turnbull B, Jacobs E, Combs GF Jr, Alberts DS, Clark LC, Marshall JR. The nutritional prevention of cancer: 400 mcg per day selenium treatment. Nutr Cancer. 2008;60:155–63.

Samuelsson B. From studies of biochemical mechanism to novel biological mediators: prostaglandin endoperoxides, thromboxanes, and leukotrienes. Nobel Lecture, 8 December 1982. Biosci Rep. 1983;3:791–813.

Schomburg L. Selenium, selenoproteins and the thyroid gland: interactions in health and disease. Nat Rev Endocrinol. 2011;8:160–71.

Schomburg L, Köhrle J. On the importance of selenium and iodine metabolism for thyroid hormone biosynthesis and human health. Mol Nutr Food Res. 2008;52:1235–46.

Schwarz K, Foltz CM. Selenium as an integral part of factor 3 against dietary necrotic liver degeneration. J Am Chem Soc. 1957;79:3292–3.

Shaheen SO, Newson RB, Rayman MP, Wong AP, Tumilty MK, Phillips JM, Potts JF, Kelly FJ, White PT, Burney PG. Randomised, double blind, placebo-controlled trial of selenium supplementation in adult asthma. Thorax. 2007;62:483–90.

Shamberger RJ, Frost DV. Possible protective effect of selenium against human cancer. Can Med Assoc J. 1969;100:682.

Shenkin A. Selenium in intravenous nutrition. Gastroenterology. 2009;137:S61–9.

Spallholz JE. On the nature of selenium toxicity and carcinostatic activity. Free Radic Biol Med. 1994;17:45–64.

Staun M, Pironi L, Bozzetti F, Baxter J, Forbes A, Joly F, Jeppesen P, Moreno J, Hebuterne X, Pertkiewicz M, Muhlebach S, Shenkin A, Van Gossum A. ESPEN Guidelines on Parenteral Nutrition: home parenteral nutrition (HPN) in adult patients. Clin Nutr. 2009;28:467–79.

Steinbrenner H. Interference of selenium and selenoproteins with the insulin-regulated carbohydrate and lipid metabolism. Free Radic Biol Med. 2013;65:1538–47.

Stone R. Diseases. A medical mystery in middle China. Science. 2009;324:1378–81.

Stone CA, Kawai K, Kupka R, Fawzi WW. Role of selenium in HIV infection. Nutr Rev. 2010;68:671–81.

Stranges S, Marshall JR, Trevisan M, Natarajan R, Donahue RP, Combs GF, Farinaro E, Clark LC, Reid ME. Effects of selenium supplementation on cardiovascular disease incidence and mortality: secondary analyses in a randomized clinical trial. Am J Epidemiol. 2006;163:694–9.

Stranges S, Marshall JR, Natarajan R, Donahue RP, Trevisan M, Combs GF, Cappuccio FP, Ceriello A, Reid ME. Effects of long-term selenium supplementation on the incidence of type 2 diabetes: a randomized trial. Ann Intern Med. 2007;147:217–23.

Su D, Novoselov SV, Sun QA, Moustafa ME, Zhou Y, Oko R, Hatfield DL, Gladyshev VN. Mammalian selenoprotein thioredoxin-glutathione reductase. Roles in disulfide bond formation and sperm maturation. J Biol Chem. 2005;280:26491–8.

Thompson PA, Ashbeck EL, Roe DJ, Fales L, Buckmeier J, Wang F, Bhattacharyya A, Hsu CH, Chow HH, Ahnen DJ, Boland CR, Heigh RI, Fay DE, Hamilton SR, Jacobs ET, Martinez ME, Alberts DS, Lance P. Selenium supplementation for prevention of colorectal adenomas and risk of associated type 2 diabetes. J Natl Cancer Inst. 2016;108:djw152.

Turker O, Kumanlioglu K, Karapolat I, Dogan I. Selenium treatment in autoimmune thyroiditis: 9-month follow-up with variable doses. J Endocrinol. 2006;190:151–6.

Ursini F, Heim S, Kiess M, Maiorino M, Roveri A, Wissing J, Flohe L. Dual function of the selenoprotein PHGPx during sperm maturation. Science. 1999;285:1393–6.

Wang L, Wang B, Chen SR, Hou X, Wang XF, Zhao SH, Song JQ, Wang YG. Effect of selenium supplementation on recurrent hyperthyroidism caused by graves' disease: a prospective pilot study. Horm Metab Res. 2016a;48:559–64.

Wang XL, Yang TB, Wei J, Lei GH, Zeng C. Association between serum selenium level and type 2 diabetes mellitus: a non-linear dose-response meta-analysis of observational studies. Nutr J. 2016b;15:48.

Wang Y, Lin M, Gao X, Pedram P, Du J, Vikram C, Gulliver W, Zhang H, Sun G. High dietary selenium intake is associated with less insulin resistance in the Newfoundland population. PLoS One. 2017;12:e0174149.

Wei J, Zeng C, Gong QY, Yang HB, Li XX, Lei GH, Yang TB. The association between dietary selenium intake and diabetes: a cross-sectional study among middle-aged and older adults. Nutr J. 2015;14:18.

Wu X, Williams KJ. NOX4 pathway as a source of selective insulin resistance and responsiveness. Arterioscler Thromb Vasc Biol. 2012;32:1236–45.

Wu Q, Rayman MP, Lv H, Schomburg L, Cui B, Gao C, Chen P, Zhuang G, Zhang Z, Peng X, Li H, Zhao Y, He X, Zeng G, Qin F, Hou P, Shi B. Low population selenium status is associated with increased prevalence of thyroid disease. J Clin Endocrinol Metab. 2015;100:4037–47.

Xia Y, Hill KE, Byrne DW, Xu J, Burk RF. Effectiveness of selenium supplements in a low-selenium area of China. Am J Clin Nutr. 2005;81:829–34.

Xia Y, Hill KE, Li P, Xu J, Zhou D, Motley AK, Wang L, Byrne DW, Burk RF. Optimization of selenoprotein P and other plasma selenium biomarkers for the assessment of the selenium nutritional requirement: a placebo-controlled, double-blind study of selenomethionine supplementation in selenium-deficient Chinese subjects. Am J Clin Nutr. 2010;92:525–31.

Yang GQ, Ge KY, Chen JS, Chen XS. Selenium-related endemic diseases and the daily selenium requirement of humans. World Rev Nutr Diet. 1988;55:98–152.

Zavacki AM, Marsili A, Larsen PR. Control of thyroid hormone activation and inactivation by the iodothyronine deiodinase family of selenoenzymes. In: Hatfield DL, Berry MJ, Gladyshev VN, editors. Selenium. Its molecular biology and role in human health. New York: Springer; 2012. p. 369–82.

Zhou J, Huang K, Lei XG. Selenium and diabetes--evidence from animal studies. Free Radic Biol Med. 2013;65:1548–56.

van Zuuren EJ, Albusta AY, Fedorowicz Z, Carter B, Pijl H. Selenium supplementation for Hashimoto's thyroiditis. In: Cochrane Database Syst Rev; 2013. p. CD010223.

Part II
Bioaccessibility and Dietary Aspects of Selenium

Chapter 2
Selenium in Soils and Crops

Philip J. White

Abstract Edible crops are the foundation of food chains for humans and livestock. However, although selenium (Se) is an essential nutrient for animals, it is not required by plants. Selenium is acquired and metabolised by plants because of its chemical similarity to sulphur. This chapter first describes how geology, climate and soil chemistry affect the concentration and forms of Se in soils and, consequently, their uptake by crops. It then describes the metabolism of Se in plants and the prevalent chemical forms of Se in edible crops, particularly those contributing substantially to human nutrition, such as cereals, potatoes, alliums and brassicaceous vegetables. Finally it describes strategies to biofortify edible crops with Se using agronomic approaches, such as the application of Se fertilisers, and how these might be complemented by selecting or breeding genotypes with a greater ability to acquire Se and distribute it to edible tissues.

Keywords Agronomy · Allium · Biofortification · Brassica · Breeding · Cereal · Fertiliser · Glucosinolate · Speciation

Introduction

Selenium (Se) is a chalcogen (Group 16) element with chemical properties similar to sulphur (S). It is an essential mineral nutrient for humans and livestock, but excessive dietary Se intakes can be toxic (White and Broadley 2009; Fairweather-Tait et al. 2011; Fordyce 2013; Roman et al. 2014; Schomburg and Arnér 2017). Recommended minimal daily Se intakes for humans are 40–75 µg d^{-1}, depending upon age and gender, and regular intakes greater than 400–1000 µg d^{-1} are potentially harmful (Fairweather-Tait et al. 2011; Fordyce 2013; Roman et al. 2014; White 2016b; Schomburg and Arnér 2017). The corresponding recommendations for Se concentrations in livestock feed are greater than 50–100 µg kg^{-1} and less than 1–5 mg kg^{-1} (Dhillon and Dhillon 2003; Fordyce 2013; Sunde et al. 2017).

P. J. White (✉)
Ecological Science Group, The James Hutton Institute, Dundee, UK
e-mail: philip.white@hutton.ac.uk

© Springer International Publishing AG, part of Springer Nature 2018
B. Michalke (ed.), *Selenium*, Molecular and Integrative Toxicology,
https://doi.org/10.1007/978-3-319-95390-8_2

Selenium is required for a variety of biochemical and physiological functions in humans, who have 25 genes encoding selenoproteins containing the Se-amino acid selenocysteine (SeCys). With the exception of Selenoprotein P (SELENOP), which has a role in Se transport, all these selenoproteins are enzymes with redox activities (Labunskyy et al. 2014; Roman et al. 2014; Wrobel et al. 2016; Schomburg and Arnér 2017). They include three thyroid protein deiodinases (Dio1, Dio2, Dio3), which activate and inactivate thyroid hormones; five glutathione peroxidises (GPX1, GPX2, GPX3, GPX4, GPX6), which protect tissues from oxidative damage caused by hydrogen peroxide and prevent lipid peroxidation, SelH, which regulates glutathione synthesis; three thioredoxin reductases (Txrnd1, Txrnd3, TGR), which reduce organoselenium compounds to provide selenide for the synthesis of selenoproteins; selenophosphate synthetase (SPS2), which is also involved in the synthesis of selenophosphate, Sep15, which has a role in protein folding in the endoplasmic reticulum (ER), SELENOM, which rearranges disulphide bonds in ER-localised proteins, SELENOK and SELENOS, which are implicated in degradation of misfolded proteins, SELENON, which has a role in regulating intracellular Ca^{2+} fluxes; a methionine sulphoxide reductase (MsrB1), which repairs oxidised methionines and is implicated in actin reorganisation; an ethanolaminephosphotransferase (SELENOI); and several proteins with unknown function (SELENOO, SELENOT, SELENOV, SELENOW).

Insufficient dietary Se intakes can result in thyroid malfunction, cretinism, cardiomyopathy, immune dysfunction, bone defects, inflammation, male infertility and, possibly, increased risk of some cancers in humans (Fairweather-Tait et al. 2011; Rayman 2012; Fordyce 2013; Labunskyy et al. 2014; Roman et al. 2014; Schomburg and Arnér 2017). It is estimated that the diets of up to one billion people might lack sufficient Se, often because the Se content of their food, whether based on plant or animal products, is restricted by low Se phytoavailability in the soils where their food is produced (Combs 2001; White and Broadley 2009; Fairweather-Tait et al. 2011; Fordyce 2013; Joy et al. 2015). Increasing dietary Se intakes of these individuals can improve their Se status and their health (Fairweather-Tait et al. 2011; Hurst et al. 2013; Alfthan et al. 2015). By contrast, excessive consumption of Se by humans and livestock can occur when forage, feed or food crops are produced on seleniferous soils with high Se phytoavailability (Dhillon and Dhillon 2003; Fordyce 2013; Schomburg and Arnér 2017). Livestock diseases associated with excessive Se intakes include "blind staggers", which include symptoms of impaired vision, low appetite and circular meandering, and "alkali disease", which includes symptoms of emaciation, hoof and bone defects, loss of vitality and hair loss (Dhillon and Dhillon 2003; Fordyce 2013; Schomburg and Arnér 2017). Similarly, Se toxicity in humans is associated with nausea, fatigue, dermatitis, loss of nails and hair, and garlicky breath (Dhillon and Dhillon 2003; Fordyce 2013; Huang et al. 2013).

Edible crops supply most of the Se in human diets either directly or indirectly (Fig. 2.1; Fairweather-Tait et al. 2011; Fordyce 2013; ODS 2016; White 2016b). The main forms of Se in human diets are SeCys and selenomethionine (SeMet), proteins containing these Se-amino acids, and their metabolites, such as Se-methyl-selenocysteine (SeMSeCys) and γ-glutamyl-Se-methyl-selenocysteine (γ-GluSeMSeCys), although the amounts of selenate and selenite can also be signifi-

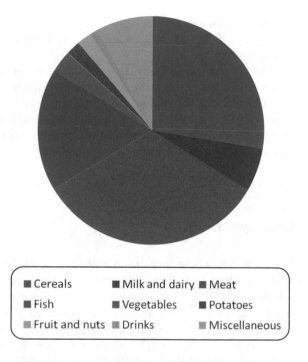

Fig. 2.1 Sources of selenium in the diets of UK adults as a proportion of their mean daily intake of 48 μg selenium. Data are from Bates et al. (2014), as presented by White (2016b)

■ Cereals   ■ Milk and dairy ■ Meat
■ Fish   ■ Vegetables   ■ Potatoes
■ Fruit and nuts ■ Drinks   ■ Miscellaneous

cant (Fairweather-Tait et al. 2011; Schomburg and Arnér 2017). However, Se is not an essential element for plants, although it can benefit their growth and survival under some circumstances (Pilon-Smits et al. 2009; El Mehdawi and Pilon-Smits 2012; Feng et al. 2013; White 2016a, 2017). Selenium is taken up, metabolised and distributed within plants because of its chemical similarity to S (White 2016a, 2017; Schiavon and Pilon-Smits 2017). Excessive Se accumulation is toxic to most plants because the nonspecific replacement of cysteine and methionine by SeCys and SeMet in proteins impairs their activities and leads to biochemical and physiological malfunction (Brown and Shrift 1982; White et al. 2004; Van Hoewyk 2013; Dimkovikj et al. 2015). In addition, Se can cause oxidative stress, which results in damage to proteins and lipids, leading to aberrant metabolism, respiration, photosynthesis and cellular homeostasis (Van Hoewyk 2013, 2016; Dimkovikj et al. 2015). Although plant species differ in their ability to tolerate Se in their tissues, most edible crops are classified as "non-accumulator" species. They cannot tolerate tissue Se concentrations greater than 10–100 μg g^{-1} dry matter (DM) and cannot grow on seleniferous soils (Rosenfeld and Beath 1964; White et al. 2004, 2007a; Fordyce 2013; White 2016a, 2017). Although a few edible crops, including alliums and brassicaceous species, termed "Se-accumulator" species, can tolerate tissue Se concentrations approaching 1 mg g^{-1} DM and are able to grow on seleniferous soils (White et al. 2004, 2007a; Dhillon and Bañuelos 2017), none can tolerate tissue Se concentrations greater than this and, therefore, none can be termed a "Se-hyperaccumulator" (Reeves and Baker 2000; White 2016a). A Se-hyperaccumulator is defined as a plant with a leaf Se concentration >1 mg g^{-1} DM when sampled from its natural environment (Reeves and Baker 2000; White

2016a). Indeed, although the trait of Se-hyperaccumulation has evolved independently in plant lineages several times, it has been reported in fewer than 60 plant species (White 2016a).

This chapter first describes how geology, climate and soil chemistry affect the concentration and forms of Se in soils and, consequently, their uptake by crops. It then describes the metabolism of Se in plants and the prevalent chemical forms of Se in edible crops. Finally, it describes strategies to biofortify edible crops with Se using agronomic approaches, such as the application of Se fertilisers, and how these might be complemented by selecting or breeding genotypes with a greater ability to acquire Se and distribute it to edible tissues.

Selenium in Soil

The Se concentrations in plants are determined by Se phytoavailability in the soil solution, which is governed by geology, climate and soil chemistry (White et al. 2007b; Winkel et al. 2015; Sun et al. 2016; Jones et al. 2017; Statwick and Sher 2017). Differences in soil Se phytoavailability account for most of the variations in Se concentrations in a particular edible crop both among and within countries (Ihnat 1989; Broadley et al. 2006; Williams et al. 2009; Fairweather-Tait et al. 2011; Lee et al. 2011; Fordyce 2013; Garrett et al. 2013; Hurst et al. 2013; Joy et al. 2015; Ates et al. 2016; dos Reis et al. 2017; Kumssa et al. 2017).

Most soils have Se concentrations between 0.01 and 2.0 mg kg^{-1} (Dhillon and Dhillon 2003; Fordyce 2013; Pilbeam et al. 2015), and the S/Se quotient of agricultural soils approximates 500–3000 g S g^{-1} Se (Bisbjerg 1972). However, soils associated with particular geological formations or climatic conditions can have Se concentrations up to 1200 mg kg^{-1} (Oldfield 2002; Dhillon and Dhillon 2003; Fordyce 2013; Pilbeam et al. 2015). These seleniferous soils are toxic to many plants, and support a unique flora (Rosenfield and Beath 1964, Dhillon and Dhillon 2003; White 2016a). Seleniferous soils are widespread across, for example, the Great Plains of the USA and Canada, the Punjab of India, the central belt of China, South America, Australia and Russia (Oldfield 2002; Dhillon and Dhillon 2003; Fordyce 2013; Pilbeam et al. 2015; dos Reis et al. 2017). Considerable heterogeneity in total Se concentrations in soils is observed at both continental and regional scales (Oldfield 2002; GEMAS 2014; Sun et al. 2016; Jones et al. 2017). In non-seleniferous soils there is often a linear relationship between phytoavailable and total Se in soils, which results in a linear increase in Se concentrations in plant tissues when Se fertilisers are applied to crops grown on these soils (Broadley et al. 2010; Chilimba et al. 2012; Bañuelos et al. 2016; Statwick and Sher 2017), but there is often little relationship between phytoavailable and total Se in seleniferous soils (Statwick and Sher 2017).

In principle, soil Se can originate from both local processes, such as the weathering of parent rocks, and distant processes through atmospheric deposition of Se from anthropogenic activities, such as the combustion of fossil fuels, and natural sources, such as volcanic eruptions and Se volatilisation by living organisms (Fordyce 2013; Sun et al. 2016; Bañuelos et al. 2017). Geology appears to be the most important factor affecting soil Se concentration at the regional scale (Dhillon and Dhillon 2014; Sun et al. 2016; Jones and Winkel 2017). Since the radii of Se^{2-} (0.191 nm) and S^{2-} (0.174 nm) are similar, Se can replace S in sulphide minerals in unweathered rocks and mineral ores (White et al. 2004; Fordyce 2013). Selenium concentrations in igneous rocks generally range from 0.05 to 0.09 mg kg^{-1} and those in metamorphic rocks from 0.02 to 10 mg kg^{-1} (Bisbjerg 1972; Fordyce 2013; Sun et al. 2016). Selenium is also present in all sedimentary rocks formed during the Carboniferous to Quaternary Periods as a result of weathering and erosion of rocks, atmospheric deposition and marine bioaccumulation of Se, but is most abundant in shales formed during the Late Cretaceous to early Tertiary Periods. Sedimentary rocks can have Se concentrations from 0.03 to 6500 mg kg^{-1} (White et al. 2004; Fordyce 2013; Pilbeam et al. 2015; Sun et al. 2016). Soils lacking Se are mostly derived from igneous rocks (Hartikainen 2005), whereas the large Se concentrations of many seleniferous soils, such as those in China and the USA, derive from sedimentary rock originating in the Cretaceous Period (Fordyce 2013; Pilbeam et al. 2015; Bañuelos et al. 2017; Statwick and Sher 2017).

Other soils are thought to derive much of their Se from the atmosphere (Winkel et al. 2015; Sun et al. 2016; Jones et al. 2017). Atmospheric deposition of Se is estimated to be between 1.4 and 5.0 g Se ha^{-1} y^{-1}, which is mainly deposited by rainwater (Winkel et al. 2015). About half the atmospheric Se arises from natural processes, such as volcanic eruptions, erosion of mineral dust and Se volatilisation by organisms, and climatic factors, such as aridity and precipitation, can have large effects on soil Se concentrations across a continent (Fordyce 2013; Winkel et al. 2015; Sun et al. 2016). For example, Se volatilisation by microorganisms and atmospheric Se deposition in precipitation during the East Asian summer monsoon and in dry deposition during the East Asian winter monsoon appear to determine the distribution of Se in surface soils across China, rather than simply local geology (Sun et al. 2016).

Anthropogenic inputs also contribute significantly to the Se content of soils. These can arise from the combustion of fossil fuels, the use of fertilisers, lime and manures in agriculture, and the disposal of coal-generated fly ash, mine tailings and sewage sludge to land (Dhillon and Dhillon 2003; Broadley et al. 2006; White et al. 2007b; Fordyce 2013; Winkel et al. 2015). The significant effect of industrialisation on Se deposition has been documented in the Se content of historical plant and soil samples (Haygarth et al. 1993; Bowley et al. 2017). Selenium can also accumulate in agricultural soils through the application of Se fertilisers to crops (White et al. 2007b) or irrigation with Se-rich water (Dhillon and Dhillon 2003). Ammonium sulphate fertilisers can contain up to 36 mg Se kg^{-1} (Bisbjerg 1972). Phosphate rocks can contain up to 178 mg Se kg^{-1} and single-superphosphate fertilisers up to 25 mg Se kg^{-1}, whereas triple-superphosphate fertilisers contain less than 4 mg Se kg^{-1} (Bisbjerg 1972; Charter et al. 1995).

Selenium is naturally present in one of the four oxidation states: +6 (selenate), +4 (selenite), 0 (elemental Se) and −2 (selenide). Plant roots can take up selenate, selenite and organoselenium compounds, such as SeCys and SeMet, from the soil solution, but are unable to take up selenides or colloidal elemental Se (White et al. 2007b; White 2016a). The amount and chemical forms of Se in the soil solution will depend upon a variety of soil factors including pH, redox potential, organic matter and clay content, and the presence of competing anions such as sulphsate and phosphate (Fig. 2.2; Mikkelsen et al. 1989; Dhillon and Dhillon 2003; White et al. 2007b; Fordyce 2013; Pilbeam et al. 2015; Winkel et al. 2015; Ros et al. 2016; Supriatin et al. 2016; Jones and Winkel 2017; Jones et al. 2017; Li et al. 2017). These, in turn, are influenced by soil moisture and by the physical, chemical and biological properties of the soil, which are determined both by the weather and by environmental conditions that govern paedogenesis (Jones and Winkel 2017). Selenate (SeO_4^{2-}) is the main water-soluble form of Se in oxic soils (pH + pE > 15), whilst selenite (SeO_3^{2-}, $HSeO^{3-}$, H_2SeO_3) predominates in anaerobic soils with a neutral to acidic pH (pH + pE = 7.5–15). Selenate is relatively mobile in the soil solution, but selenite is strongly absorbed by iron and aluminium oxides/hydroxides and, to a lesser extent, by clays and organic matter (Fordyce 2013; Pilbeam et al. 2015). The retention of selenate and selenite by soils increases with soil acidification and Se uptake by plants is correspondingly reduced with decreasing pH of the soil solution (Hurst et al. 2013; Bowley et al. 2017; Li et al. 2017). Selenides (Se^{2-}) are present only in severely anaerobic, and often acidic, soils (pH + pE < 7.5). Organoselenium compounds, such as SeMet, selenocystine ($SeCys_2$), methaneseleninic acid (MeSOOH) and trimethylselenonium (Me_3Se^+), are present in small concentrations in the soil solution as a result of degradation of organic

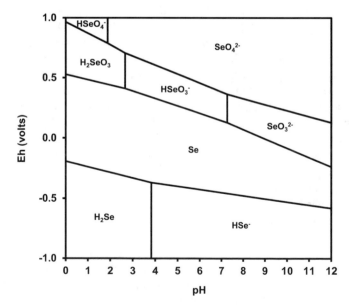

Fig. 2.2 The effects of redox potential (Eh) and pH on selenium speciation in an aqueous system containing 1 μM Se. Each line in the diagram represents an equilibrium between the oxidised form written above the line and the reduced form written below it, or the protonated form written on the left and the unprotonated form written on the right. Figure adapted from Mikkelsen et al. (1989) by White et al. (2007b)

material and biological activities (Li et al. 2017). Since plant roots can affect rhizosphere chemistry through the release of protons, organic compounds and enzymes that degrade organic material, they can influence the forms of Se present in the soil solution and their ability to acquire Se (White et al. 2013; Jin et al. 2017; Jones and Winkel 2017). Differences in root exudates have been observed both among and within plant species (White et al. 2013). Root exudates also affect the biology of the rhizosphere, which can again influence the forms of Se present in the soil solution and Se phytoavailability at the field scale indirectly (Winkel et al. 2015; Jones and Winkel 2017; Li et al. 2017).

Selenium Uptake and Metabolism in Crops

The uptake of selenate across the plasma membrane of root cells is catalysed by high-affinity, H^+/sulphate symporters, homologous to AtSULTR1;1 and AtSULTR1;2 of the model brassicaceous plant Arabidopsis (*Arabidopsis thaliana* [L.] Heynh.; Sors et al. 2005; White et al. 2007b; Shinmachi et al. 2010; Gigolashvili and Kopriva 2014; White 2016a). However, although selenate and sulphate share the same transporters, increasing rhizosphere selenate concentrations often increases S uptake because Se accumulation in plant tissues results in transcriptional changes resembling those induced by S starvation (White et al. 2004; El Kassis et al. 2007; Hsu et al. 2011; Boldrin et al. 2016; Drahoňovský et al. 2016; Schiavon et al. 2016; White 2016a, 2017). In Arabidopsis, AtSULTR1;2 catalyses most of the selenate uptake by roots of S-replete plants (Shibagaki et al. 2002; El Kassis et al. 2007; Barberon et al. 2008), but if a plant lacks sufficient S for optimal growth, or if its tissue Se concentration increases, the contribution of AtSULTR1;1 to the uptake of selenite increases (El Kassis et al. 2007; Rouached et al. 2008; Shinmachi et al. 2010). By contrast, increasing sulphate in the rhizosphere tends to reduce selenate uptake as a consequence of both competition for transport and reduced expression of *AtSULTR1;1*. The uptake of selenite as $HSeO_3^-$ is probably catalysed by members of the phosphate transporter Pht1 family (Zhang et al. 2014; Song et al. 2017) and the uptake of selenite as H_2SeO_3 is most likely catalysed by aquaporins, such as the rice OsNIP2;1 transporter (Zhao et al. 2010). It is likely that plant roots take up SeCys and SeMet through transporters for Cys and Met (Kikkert and Berkelaar 2013; White 2016a). Plant species differ in their capacity to take up Se under identical environmental conditions, the Se/S selectivity of the complement of Se transporters present in the plasma membrane of root cells, and the response of the complement of Se transporters in the plasma membrane of root cells to plant S nutritional status and Se supply (White et al. 2004, 2007a, b; Drahoňovský et al. 2016; White 2016a).

Following its uptake into root cells, selenate moves through the symplast to the stele and is loaded into the xylem for transport to the shoot, whereas selenite is converted to organoselenium compounds (White et al. 2004; Li et al. 2008; Wang et al. 2015). Members of the ALMT family of transporters (organic acid transporters) are believed to load selenate into the xylem, although the activities of AtSULTR2;1, AtSULTR2;2 and AtSULTR3;5 might affect the rate of xylem loading by controlling the uptake of selenate into pericycle and xylem parenchyma cells (Kataoka et al. 2004a; Takahashi et al. 2011; Gigolashvili and Kopriva 2014). The expression of *AtSULTR2;1* and *AtSULTR2;2*, and their homologues in many crop species, is induced by S starvation and by increasing Se supply (Takahashi et al. 2000; Van Hoewyk et al. 2008; Hsu et al. 2011; Gigolashvili and Kopriva 2014; Schiavon et al. 2016), whereas their homologues in Se-hyperaccumulator species are expressed constitutively (Cabannes et al. 2011; Schiavon et al. 2015).

Most Se is present in the xylem as selenate, but small amounts of SeMet and selenomethionine Se oxide (SeOMet) have also been reported (Li et al. 2008; White 2016a). Following its delivery to the shoot via the xylem, selenate enters leaf cells through SULTR transporters in their plasma membranes (Fig. 2.3; Takahashi et al. 2011; Gigolashvili and Kopriva 2014). In most plants, selenate is sequestered in the vacuoles of cells within the vasculature and leaf mesophyll (Ximénez-Embún et al. 2004; Mazej et al. 2008; Wang et al. 2015). The transporters catalysing selenate influx to vacuoles are unknown, but homologues of AtSULTR4;1 and AtSULTR4;2

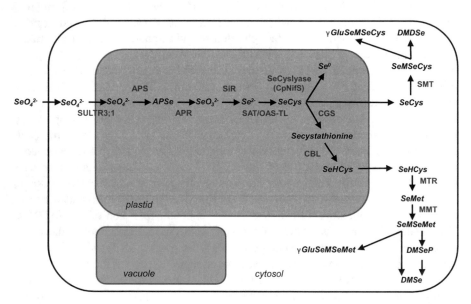

Fig. 2.3 Generalised scheme of selenium metabolism in the leaves of higher plants. Abbreviations: *SeO₄²⁻* selenate, SULTR3; 1 transporter on plastid membrane, *APS* adenosine triphosphate sulphurylase, *APSe* adenosine 5'-phosphoselenate, *APR* adenosine 5'-phosphosulphate reductase, *SeO₃²⁻* selenite, *SiR* sulphite reductase, Se²⁻ *selenide*, *SAT/OAS-TL* cysteine synthase, which contains both serine acetyl transferase (SAT) and O-acetylserine (thiol) lyase (OAS-TL) subunits, *SeCys* selenocysteine, *CGS* cystathionine γ-synthase, *CBL* cystathionine β-lyase, *SeHCys* selenohomocysteine, *MTR* methionine synthase, *SeMet* selenomethionine, *cpNifS* chloroplast SeCys lyase, *Se⁰* elemental Se, *SMT* selenocysteine methyltransferase, *SeMSeCys* Se-methylselenocysteine, *γ-GluSeMSeCys* γ-glutamyl-SeMSeCys, *DMDSe* dimethyl diselenide, *SeMSeMet* Se-methylselenomethionine, *MMT* S-adenosyl-methionine:methionine methyl transferase, *γ-GluSeMSeMet* γ-glutamyl-SeMSeMet, *DMSeP* dimethyl selenonium propionate, *DMSe* dimethyl selenide. Figure from White (2017)

are thought to catalyse the efflux of selenate from the vacuole (Kataoka et al. 2004b; Gigolashvili and Kopriva 2014). The expression of genes encoding these transporters is upregulated by both S starvation and Se accumulation in most plants (White 2016a; Bowley et al. 2017), but their expression is constitutively high in Se-hyperaccumulator species (Freeman et al. 2010; White 2016a, 2017). Selenium is readily redistributed in the phloem as selenate, SeMet and SeMSeCys (Carey et al. 2012). In Arabidopsis, AtSULTR1;3 appears to catalyse selenate uptake into the phloem (Yoshimoto et al. 2003), whilst amino acid transporters might load seleno-amino acids into the phloem (Tegeder 2014). Again, the expression of genes encoding homologues of AtSULTR1;3 is upregulated by the accumulation of Se in plants (Boldrin et al. 2016).

Most of what is known about Se metabolism in plants is based on knowledge of the analogous S metabolism (Fig. 2.3; White et al. 2007b; Pilon-Smits and LeDuc 2009; White and Broadley 2009; Winkel et al. 2015; White 2016a, 2017; Schiavon and Pilon-Smits 2017). Following its uptake by leaf cells, selenate probably enters plastids through homologues of the Arabidopsis AtSULTR3;1 transporter, where it is activated by adenosine triphosphate sulphurylase (APS) to form adenosine 5′-phosphoselenate (APSe), which is reduced to selenite by adenosine 5′-phospho-sulphate reductase (APR) using reduced glutathione as the electron donor. The conversion of selenate to selenite appears to be the rate-limiting step in the assimilation of Se into organic compounds (Pilon-Smits et al. 1999b). It is also possible for Se to be converted to selenoglutathione and selenolipids from APSe, following the analogous S metabolic pathways (Duncan et al. 2017). Selenite might be reduced to selenide either enzymatically by sulphite reductase (SiR), although it is unclear whether this enzyme actually has selenite reductase activity (González-Morales et al. 2017; Van Hoewyk and Çakir 2017), or non-enzymatically by interaction with reduced glutathione. Selenide is then converted to SeCys by the enzyme complex cysteine synthase, which contains both serine acetyl transferase (SAT) and O-acetylserine (thiol) lyase (OAS-TL) subunits. The conversion of SeCys to SeMet proceeds via selenocystathionine and selenohomocysteine (SeHCys) and is catalysed by cystathionine γ-synthase (CGS), cystathionine β-lyase (CBL) and methionine synthase (MTR). In some plant species, including brassicaceous vegetables, selenohomolanthionine (SeHLan) and its derivatives can be formed from SeHCys (Fig. 2.4; Ogra et al. 2007; Ouerdane et al. 2013; Duncan et al. 2017). SeCys can also be converted to selenocystine (SeCys$_2$), which is a major organoselenium compound present in many eudicot species (Drahoňovský et al. 2016), including the Se-hyperaccumulator *Cardamine hupingshanensis* (Yuan et al. 2013).

The enzymes catalysing Se metabolism are encoded by small multigene families. For example, the Arabidopsis genome contains four genes encoding APS (one, APS2, is found in both plastids and cytosol, Bohrer et al. 2015), three genes encoding APR, one gene encoding SiR, five genes encoding SAT, nine genes encoding OAS-TL, two genes encoding CGS, one gene encoding CBL and three genes encoding MTR (Hesse et al. 2004; Bermúdez et al. 2013; Schiavon et al. 2015). In most plant species the expression of genes encoding enzymes involved in the primary S/Se assimilation pathway are upregulated when plants become

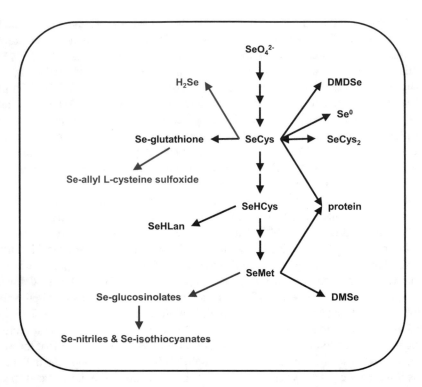

Fig. 2.4 Generalised scheme for the incorporation of selenocysteine (SeCys) and selenomethionine (SeMet) into proteins and the production of elemental selenium (Se^0); the volatiles dimethyl diselenide (DMDSe), dimethyl selenide (DMSe) and hydrogen selenide (H_2Se); the secondary metabolites selenocystine ($SeCys_2$) and selenohomolanthionine (SeHLan); and the characteristic organoselenium compounds of alliums (Se-allyl L-cysteine sulfoxide) and brassicas (Se-glucosinolates, Se-nitriles and Se-isothiocyanates)

S deficient or when Se supply is increased, but in Se-hyperaccumulator species genes encoding APS, APR, SAT/OAS-TL and MTP show constitutively high expression (Van Hoewyk et al. 2005, 2008; Freeman et al. 2010; White 2016a).

In the cytoplasm, SeCys and SeMet can be converted to SeMSeCys and Se-methylselenomethionine (SeMSeMet) through the activities of SeCys methyl-transferase (SMT) and S-adenosyl-methionine: methionine methyl transferase (MMT), respectively (Fig. 2.3; Sors et al. 2005; White et al. 2007b; Pilon-Smits and LeDuc 2009; Van Hoewyk 2013; Winkel et al. 2015; White 2016a; Guignardi and Schiavon 2017). However, many plants, including Arabidopsis, do not possess genes encoding functional SMT (Lyi et al. 2005; Van Hoewyk 2013; Zhao et al. 2015) and have few genes encoding MMT, Arabidopsis having only one (Tagmount et al. 2002). Nevertheless, large concentrations of SeMSeCys are found in Poales (Drahoňovský et al. 2016) and in alliums and brassicas fertilised with selenate or selenite (Birringer et al. 2002; Lyi et al. 2005; Fairweather-Tait et al. 2011; Ouerdane et al. 2013; White 2016a). Both SeMSeCys and SeMSeMet can be conjugated with glutamate to form γ-GluSeMSeCys or γ-glutamyl-SeMSeMet (γ-GluSeMSeMet), or converted to dimethyl selenide (DMSe) or dimethyl diselenide (DMDSe) and volatilised (Sors et al. 2005; White et al. 2007b; Pilon-Smits and LeDuc 2009; Van Hoewyk 2013; Winkel et al. 2015; Guignardi and Schiavon 2017). The production of DMSe in non-accumulator and accumulator species appears to be limited by the conversion of SeCys to SeMet (Van Huysen et al. 2003; Pilon-Smits and LeDuc 2009). DMDSe is formed by converting MSeCys to methylselenocysteine selenoxide (MSeCysSeO), MeSeCysSeO to methaneselenol (CH_3SeH) catalysed by cysteine sulphoxide lyase, and thence to DMDSe (Winkel et al. 2015; Guignardi and Schiavon 2017). SeMSeMet can be converted to DMSe via the conventional S volatilisation pathway or via dimethyl selenonium propionate (DMSeP), which is a major organoselenium compound in Poales and various other plant species (Guignardi and Schiavon 2017), to DMSe (Grant et al. 2004; Winkel et al. 2015; White 2016a; Guignardi and Schiavon 2017). Plant species differ greatly in their ability to volatilise Se (Terry et al. 1992; Pilon-Smits et al. 1999a; de Souza et al. 2000). The predominant volatile organoselenium compound produced by non-accumulator species is generally DMSe, whereas that produced by Se-hyperaccumulator species is DMDSe (Pilon-Smits and LeDuc 2009; White 2017).

Selenate is often the most abundant form of Se in non-accumulator plants (Fairweather-Tait et al. 2011; Drahoňovský et al. 2016; White 2016a, 2017). The most abundant organoselenium compounds differ between plant species, growth conditions and tissue samples (Fairweather-Tait et al. 2011; Ouerdane et al. 2013; Bañuelos et al. 2015; White 2016a, 2017). When grown in non-seleniferous soils, without the addition of Se fertilisers, SeMet is often the most abundant organoselenium compound in edible seeds and cereal grains, in leafy vegetables and potato tubers, and in carrot roots, although substantial concentrations of SeMSeCys and γ-GluSeMSeCys have been found in alliums (Fairweather-Tait et al. 2011; White 2016a; Ruszczynska et al. 2017). By contrast, large concentrations of SeMSeCys have been reported in shoots of vegetables fertilised with selenite (Sugihara et al. 2004; Mazej et al. 2008; Schiavon et al. 2016; Mahn 2017; Wiesner-Reinhold et al. 2017; Ruszczynska et al. 2017), in tubers of selenised potato (Gionfriddo et al. 2012) and in seeds of selenised legumes (Smrkolj et al. 2007; Shao et al. 2014), whereas large concentrations of both SeMSeCys and γ-GluSeMSeCys have been reported in selenised allium crops (Birringer et al. 2002; Sugihara et al. 2004; White et al. 2007b; Fairweather-Tait et al. 2011; Pilbeam et al. 2015; White 2016a, 2017; Ruszczynska et al. 2017).

In addition to the replacement of S by Se in the primary metabolites described above, SeCys can be converted to elemental Se and alanine by selenocysteine lyase in the cytosol or plastids (Van Hoewyk et al. 2005; White 2016a, 2017; Guignardi and Schiavon 2017), and Se can be incorporated into secondary metabolites, such as selenoglutathione, which is probably synthesised from SeCys, glutamate and glycine through the activities of γ-glutamylcysteinesynthetase and glutathione synthetase (Crawford et al. 2000; Pivato et al. 2014), and selenoglucosinolates, which are synthesised from SeMet (Matich et al. 2012, 2015; Ouerdane et al. 2013). The complement, and biosynthesis, of secondary Se metabolites appears to be analogous to their S counterparts (Fig. 2.4).

Alliums (e.g. chive, garlic, elephant garlic, leek, scallion, onion) and brassica-ceous vegetables (e.g. broccoli, Brussels sprouts, cabbage, cauliflower, Chinese cabbage, cress, horseradish, Indian mustard, kale, radish, turnip, watercress, white mustard) are characterised by elaborate S/Se secondary metabolism and accumulate large-shoot Se and S concentrations (White et al. 2004, 2007a,b; White 2016a; González-Morales et al. 2017; Wiesner-Reinhold et al. 2017). Although alliums do not volatilise Se very effectively, they have a considerable capacity to methylate SeCys, resulting in large-tissue Se, SeMSeCys and γ-GluSeMSeCys concentra-tions, especially when selenised (Birringer et al. 2002; Fairweather-Tait et al. 2011; White 2016a, 2017; 2017; González-Morales et al. 2017; Puccinelli et al. 2017; Ruszczynska et al. 2017). The volatile sulphur compounds that are characteristic of alliums are derived from glutathione, from which sulphoxides (methiin, alliin, propiin, isoalliin, ethiin, butiin) and, subsequently, thiosulphinates are produced (González-Morales et al. 2017). Although the application of selenate can increase the concentrations of these compounds in alliums, excessive tissue Se concentrations have the opposite effect (González-Morales et al. 2017). In addition to being the precursor of SeMSeCys and γ-GluSeMSeCys (Fig. 2.3), SeCys can be converted to elemental Se in alliums, be incorporated into proteins or be the precursor of selenoglutathione, Se-allyl-L-cysteine sulphoxide and hydrogen selenide (Fig. 2.4). It can also be converted to SeMet, which can be incorporated into proteins or metabolised to DMSe (Figs. 2.3 and 2.4).

Brassicas constitute about 10% of the world's vegetable production (Wiesner-Reinhold et al. 2017). Glucosinolates create the sharp taste of brassicaceous vegetables and when plants are injured they are converted to compounds such as indoles and isothiocyanates through the action of myrosinase (Agerbirk and Olsen 2012). Three classes of glucosinolates have been reported in brassicas: indolic glucosinolates, which are derived from tryptophan; aromatic glucosinolates, which are derived from phenylalanine and tyrosine; and aliphatic glucosinolates, which are derived from alanine, leucine, isoleucine, valine or methionine (Agerbirk and Olsen 2012). Selenium does not appear to be incorporated into the isocyanate group of glucosinolates, although their precursors appear to be present in brassicas, and all selenoglucosinolates appear to be derived from SeMet (Fig. 2.4; Matich et al. 2012, 2015; Ouerdane et al. 2013). Aliphatic selenoglucosinolates (methylselenoglucosinolates) and their metabolites (methylselenonitriles and methylselenoisothiocyanates) have been reported in several brassicaceous vegetables fertilised with selenate (Matich et al. 2012, 2015; Ouerdane et al. 2013; Wiesner-Reinhold et al. 2017).

The application of Se to brassicas results in complex changes in gene expression and in the secondary metabolism of Se and S (Schiavon et al. 2016). Although selenate applications can increase S uptake and, thereby, increase concentrations of total glucosinolates and sulphoraphane (a degradation product of the aliphatic glucosinolate glucoraphanin), excessive tissue Se accumulation generally results in their reduction and a reduction in myrosinase activity (Robbins et al. 2005; Hsu et al. 2011; Ramos et al. 2011b; Barickman et al. 2013; Sepúlveda et al. 2013; Matich et al. 2015; Huang et al. 2016; Tian et al. 2016; Mahn 2017). The effects of

Se biofortification on tissue S, amino acid, glutathione and glucosinolate concentrations also differ depending upon whether the Se fertiliser is supplied to leaves or roots (Schiavon et al. 2016). Foliar application of selenate to radish led to greater leaf S, glutathione, SeMSeCys and glucosinolate (glucophoranin, glucobrassicin) concentrations, whereas when selenate was supplied in the nutrient solution to plants growing hydroponically, increasing selenate concentration resulted in an increase in leaf S and SeMSeCys concentrations but a reduction in leaf cysteine, glutathione and glucosinolate (glucoraphasatin, glucobrassicin) concentrations (Schiavon et al. 2016). Such observations illustrate the complex interactions between Se and S in their uptake, transport between tissues, and metabolism.

Biofortification of Edible Crops

It is estimated that the diets of up to one billion people across the world lack sufficient Se for optimal health (Combs 2001). Strategies to increase dietary Se intakes of Se-deficient populations include Se supplementation with pills and tonics, food fortification through the addition Se to flours, cooking ingredients or processed foods, and biofortification, the combination of effective agronomy with improved genotypes to produce crops with greater Se concentrations in their edible portions (Broadley et al. 2006; White and Broadley 2009; Fairweather-Tait et al. 2011; White 2016a,b, 2017). Since low dietary Se intakes of both humans and livestock are generally associated with crop production on soils with little phytoavailable Se, the application of Se fertilisers is fundamental to Se biofortification of edible crops (Broadley et al. 2006; White and Broadley 2009; Alfthan et al. 2015; Joy et al. 2015; White 2016a). The use of Se fertilisers to increase Se concentrations in edible crops has been particularly successful in increasing dietary Se intakes and human Se status in Finland (Alfthan et al. 2015). It has also been used to increase Se concentrations in diverse plant products, including processed foods, bread and tea (Broadley et al. 2006; Hart et al. 2011; Lazo-Vélez et al. 2015; Wu et al. 2015), through the application of Se fertilisers, and animal products, such as meat and eggs (Fisinin et al. 2009), through Se-enriched forage or feed in several countries. The complementary development of crop genotypes that acquire more of the Se applied and accumulate more of the Se acquired in their edible portions improves the efficiency by which Se fertilisers are used in the Se biofortification of edible crops (White and Broadley 2009; White 2016a, 2017).

Many studies over the last two decades have examined the potential of different chemical forms of Se and contrasting application methods of Se fertilisers for Se biofortification of edible crops (Broadley et al. 2006; Wu et al. 2015; Ros et al. 2016; Bañuelos et al. 2017). In essence, Se fertilisers can be added either to the soil or to the substrate of crops grown in fields and glasshouses, supplied in the nutrient solution of hydroponically grown crops, or sprayed onto foliage or fruit (Broadley et al. 2006; White and Broadley 2009; Pilbeam et al. 2015; Wu et al. 2015; Ros et al.

2016; Bañuelos et al. 2017). A further strategy is to apply a Se fertiliser coating to pelletised seed, which has successfully increased Se concentrations in herbage from grasslands and in produce for humans (Pilbeam et al. 2015; Ros et al. 2016; Puccinelli et al. 2017).

When crops are grown in the field, the application of Se fertilisers to the soil is generally recommended, especially when crops are likely to experience water and heat stress (Lyons et al. 2005; Bañuelos et al. 2017). Although foliar applications of Se fertilisers have successfully increased Se concentrations in many crops, excessive Se concentrations causing phytotoxicity are more likely when Se fertilisers are applied directly to foliage than when applied to the soil (Bañuelos et al. 2017). Inorganic potassium, sodium or barium salts of selenate or selenite are often applied directly to the soil in granular or blended forms or as high-volume liquid drenches (Gupta and Gupta 2002; Broadley et al. 2006, 2010; Pilbeam et al. 2015; Wu et al. 2015; Bañuelos et al. 2017). Soluble selenate fertilisers are generally more effective in increasing Se concentrations in crops because the Se is available immediately to crops, but the application of selenite or less soluble forms of selenate, such as $BaSeO_4$, can provide longer lasting effects (Gupta and Gupta 2002; Broadley et al. 2006; White and Broadley 2009; Pilbeam et al. 2015; Ros et al. 2016). The addition of Se-rich plant material to soils has also been used successfully, and provides phytoavailable Se for several years after application (Bañuelos et al. 2015, 2016, 2017). The efficiency of acquisition of Se by crops from Se fertilisers applied to soil depends upon the crop, the form of Se applied, the application method, the amount of Se applied and the timing of the Se fertiliser application, with crops acquiring from less than 1% to over 50% of the Se fertiliser applied (Broadley et al. 2006; Pilbeam et al. 2015; Ros et al. 2016; Li et al. 2017). The efficiency of Se acquisition will be affected by weather conditions and soil chemistry, losses due to leaching and volatilisation, retention in the soil, and activities of soil biota (Ros et al. 2016; Li et al. 2017). It can also be affected by the timing, form and amounts of N, P, K and S fertilisers both directly, by competition with Se for uptake, and indirectly, through changes in soil chemistry or plant growth and metabolism (Ros et al. 2016; Bañuelos et al. 2017).

Foliar applications of solutions containing selenate or selenite have successfully increased the Se concentration of many crops, including cereals, legumes, leafy vegetables (including brassicas and alliums), potatoes, carrots and soft fruit (Gupta and Gupta 2002; Broadley et al. 2006; Wu et al. 2015; Ros et al. 2016; Bañuelos et al. 2017; Puccinelli et al. 2017). In general the application of Se fertilisers to foliage is more efficient than applications to the soil, both in terms of the amount of fertiliser required to achieve a particular target for Se biofortification and in the recovery of fertiliser Se in produce (Ros et al. 2016; González-Morales et al. 2017). However, care must be taken when applying Se fertilisers to foliage to avoid phytotoxicity and to prevent losses to the environment by ensuring sufficient leaf surface area and avoiding windy or rainy days (Bañuelos et al. 2017).

The most efficient strategy to biofortify glasshouse vegetables and soft fruit with Se is to provide selenate to crops grown hydroponically (Ros et al. 2016; Puccinelli et al. 2017; Wiesner-Reinhold et al. 2017). This system allows control of the timing, amounts and chemical forms of Se delivered to crops and, thereby, the chemical forms and concentrations of Se plant tissues and can be easily adapted for different crop species to achieve target Se concentrations in their edible portions (Puccinelli et al. 2017).

Recently, there has been a substantial effort to identify crop genotypes that accumulate more Se in their edible portions that could be used directly in Se biofortification programmes and in studies to determine the genetic basis of increased Se accumulation to enable marker-assisted breeding of genotypes with greater Se biofortification potential (White and Broadley 2009; Pilbeam et al. 2015; White 2016a, 2017). Genetic variation has been reported in grain Se concentration of major cereals, including bread wheat (*Triticum aestivum* L.), durum wheat (*Triticum turgidum* L.), rice (*Oryza sativa* L.), millet (*Setaria italica* [L.] P. Beauv.; Liu et al. 2016), barley (*Hordeum vulgare* L.) and oats (*Avena sativa* L.); in seed Se concentration of common legumes, such as chickpea (*Cicer arietinum* L.), lentil (*Lens culinaris* Medik.), mung bean (*Vigna radiata* [L.] R.Wilczek) and soybean (*Glycine max* [L.] Merr.); in tuber Se concentration of potato (*Solanum tuberosum* L.); in fruit Se concentration of tomato (*Solanum lycopersicum* L.) and pepper (*Capsicum annuum* L.); in leafy vegetables, such as onions (*Allium cepa* L.), broccoli (*Brassica oleracea L.* Italica Group), cauliflower (*B. oleracea* L. Botrytis Group), kale (*B. oleracea* L. Acephala Group), Chinese cabbage (*B. rapa* L.), Indian mustard (*Brassica juncea* [L.] Czern.), lettuce (*Lactuca sativa* L.) and chicory (*Cichorium intybus* L.); and in tea (*Camelia sinensis* [L.] Kuntze, Zhao et al. 2016). Research on the genetics of Se accumulation in edible portions has highlighted the importance of genes encoding transporters catalysing Se uptake and movement within the plant and genes involved in both primary and secondary Se metabolism, but there is still much work to be done before this knowledge can be applied practically (Ramos et al. 2011a; Chao et al. 2014; Ramamurthy et al. 2014; White 2016a, 2017).

Acknowledgement This work was supported by the Rural and Environment Science and Analytical Services Division (RESAS) of the Scottish Government.

References

Agerbirk N, Olsen CE. Glucosinolate structures in evolution. Phytochemistry. 2012;77:16–45.

Alfthan G, Eurola M, Ekholm P, et al. Effects of nationwide addition of selenium to fertilizers on foods, and animal and human health in Finland: from deficiency to optimal selenium status of the population. J Trace Elem Med Biol. 2015;31:142–7.

Ates D, Sever T, Aldemir S, et al. Identification QTLs controlling genes for Se uptake in lentil seeds. PLoS One. 2016;11(3):e0149210. https://doi.org/10.1371/journal.pone.0149210.

Bañuelos GS, Arroyo I, Pickering IJ, Yang SI, Freeman JL. Selenium biofortification of broccoli and carrots grown in soil amended with Se-enriched hyperaccumulator *Stanleya pinnata*. Food Chem. 2015;166:603–8.

Bañuelos GS, Arroyo IS, Dangi SR, Zambrano MC. Continued selenium biofortification of carrots and broccoli grown in soils once amended with Se-enriched *S. pinnata*. Front Plant Sci. 2016;7:1251. https://doi.org/10.3389/fpls.2016.01251.

Bañuelos GS, Lin Z-Q, Broadley M. Selenium biofortification. In: EAH P-S, LHE W, Lin Z-Q, editors. Selenium in plants: molecular, physiological, ecological and evolutionary aspects. Cham, Switzerland: Springer; 2017. p. 231–55.

Barberon M, Berthomieu P, Clairotte M, et al. Unequal functional redundancy between the two *Arabidopsis thaliana* high-affinity sulphate transporters *SULTR1;1* and *SULTR1;2*. New Phytol. 2008;180:608–19.

Barickman TC, Kopsell DA, Sams CE. Selenium influences glucosinolate and isothiocyanates and increases sulphur uptake in *Arabidopsis thaliana* and rapid-cycling *Brassica oleracea*. J Agric Food Chem. 2013;61:202–9.

Bates B, Lennox A, Prentice A, et al. National diet and nutrition survey: results from years 1-4 (combined) of the rolling programme (2008/2009–2011/2012). London: Public Health England; 2014.

Bermúdez MA, Páez-Ochoa MA, Gotor C, et al. *Arabidopsis* S-sulfocysteine synthase activity is essential for chloroplast function and long-day light-dependent redox control. Plant Cell. 2013;22:403–16.

Birringer M, Pilawa S, Flohé L. Trends in selenium biochemistry. Nat Prod Rep. 2002;19:693–718.

Bisbjerg B. Riso report no. 200: Studies on selenium in plants and soils. Copenhagen, Danish Atomic Energy Comission Research Establishment Riso, Denmark; 1972.

Bohrer A-S, Kopriva S, Takahashi H. Plastid-cytosol partitioning and integration of metabolic pathways for APS/PAPS biosynthesis in *Arabidopsis thaliana*. Front Plant Sci. 2015;5:751. https://doi.org/10.3389/fpls.2014.00751.

Boldrin PF, de Figueiredo MA, Yang Y, et al. Selenium promotes sulfur accumulation and plant growth in wheat (*Triticum aestivum*). Physiol Plant. 2016;158:80–91.

Bowley HE, Mathers AW, Young SD, et al. Historical trends in iodine and selenium in soil and herbage at the Park Grass Experiment, Rothamsted Research, UK. Soil Use Manag. 2017;33:252–62.

Broadley MR, White PJ, Bryson RJ, et al. Biofortification of UK food crops with selenium. Proc Nutr Soc. 2006;65:169–81.

Broadley MR, Alcock J, Alford J, et al. Selenium biofortification of high-yielding winter wheat (*Triticum aestivum* L.) by liquid or granular Se fertilisation. Plant and Soil. 2010;332:5–18.

Brown TA, Shrift A. Selenium: toxicity and tolerance in higher plants. Biol Rev. 1982;57:59–84.

Cabannes E, Buchner P, Broadley MR, et al. A comparison of sulfate and selenium accumulation in relation to the expression of sulfate transporter genes in *Astragalus* species. Plant Physiol. 2011;157:2227–39.

Carey A-M, Scheckel KG, Lombi E, et al. Grain accumulation of selenium species in rice (*Oryza sativa* L.). Environ Sci Technol. 2012;46:5557–64.

Chao D-Y, Baraniecka P, Danku J, et al. Variation in sulfur and selenium accumulation is controlled by naturally occurring isoforms of the key sulfur assimilation enzyme ADENOSINE 5′-PHOSPHOSULFATE REDUCTASE2 across the Arabidopsis species range. Plant Physiol. 2014;166:1593–608.

Charter RA, Tabatabai MA, Schafer JW. Arsenic, molybdenum, selenium and tungsten contents of fertilizers and phosphate rocks. Commun Soil Sci Plant Anal. 1995;26:3051–62.

Chilimba ADC, Young SD, Black CR, et al. Agronomic biofortification of maize with selenium (Se) in Malawi. Field Crop Res. 2012;125:118–28.

Combs GF. Selenium in global food systems. Br J Nutr. 2001;85:517–47.

Crawford NM, Kahn ML, Leustek T, et al. Nitrogen and sulfur. In: Buchanan BB, Gruissem W, Jones RL, editors. Biochemistry and molecular biology of plants. Rockville, MD: American Society of Plant Physiologists; 2000. p. 786–849.

de Souza MP, Pilon-Smits EAH, Terry N. The physiology and biochemistry of selenium volatilization by plants. In: Raskin I, Ensley BD, editors. Phytoremediation of toxic metals: using plants to clean-up the environment. New York: Wiley; 2000. p. 171–90.

dos Reis AR, El-Ramady H, Santos EF, et al. Overview of selenium deficiency and toxicity worldwide: affected areas, selenium-related health issues, and case studies. In: EAH P-S, LHE W, Lin Z-Q, editors. Selenium in plants: Molecular, physiological, ecological and evolutionary aspects. Cham, Switzerland: Springer; 2017. p. 209–30.

Dhillon KS, Bañuelos GS. Overview and prospects of selenium phytoremediation approaches. In: EAH P-S, LHE W, Lin Z-Q, editors. Selenium in plants: molecular, physiological, ecological and evolutionary aspects. Cham, Switzerland: Springer; 2017. p. 277–321.

Dhillon KS, Dhillon SK. Distribution and management of seleniferous soils. Adv Agron. 2003;79:119–84.

Dhillon KS, Dhillon SK. Development and mapping of seleniferous soils in northwestern India. Chemosphere. 2014;99:56–63.

Dimkovikj A, Fisher B, Hutchison K, et al. Stuck between a ROS and a hard place: Analysis of the ubiquitin proteasome pathway in selenocysteine treated *Brassica napus* reveals different toxicities during selenium assimilation. J Plant Physiol. 2015;181:50–4.

Drahoňovský J, Száková J, Mestek O, et al. Selenium uptake, transformation and inter-element interactions by selected wildlife plant species after foliar selenate application. Environ Exp Bot. 2016;125:12–9.

Duncan EG, Maher WA, Jagtap R, et al. Selenium speciation in wheat grain varies in the presence of nitrogen and sulphur fertilisers. Environ Geochem Health. 2017;39:955–66.

El Kassis E, Cathala N, Rouached H, et al. Characterization of a selenate-resistant Arabidopsis mutant. Root growth as a potential target for selenite toxicity. Plant Physiol. 2007;143:1231–41.

El Mehdawi AF, Pilon-Smits EAH. Ecological aspects of plant selenium hyperaccumulation. Plant Biol. 2012;14:1–10.

Fairweather-Tait SJ, Bao Y, Broadley MR, et al. Selenium in human health and disease. Antioxid Redox Signal. 2011;14:1337–83.

Feng R, Wei C, Tud S. The roles of selenium in protecting plants against abiotic stresses. Environ Exp Bot. 2013;87:58–68.

Fisinin VI, Papazyan TT, Surai PF. Producing selenium-enriched eggs and meat to improve the selenium status of the general population. Crit Rev Biotechnol. 2009;29:18–28.

Fordyce FM. Selenium deficiency and toxicity in the environment. In: Selinus O, Alloway B, Centeno JA, et al., editors. Essentials of medical geology, revised edn. Dordrecht: Springer; 2013. p. 375–416.

Freeman JL, Tamaoki M, Stushnoff C, et al. Molecular mechanisms of selenium tolerance and hyperaccumulation in *Stanleya pinnata*. Plant Physiol. 2010;153:1630–52.

Garrett RG, Gawalko E, Wang N, et al. Macrorelationships between regional-scale field pea (*Pisum sativum*) selenium chemistry and environmental factors in western Canada. Can J Plant Sci. 2013;93:1059–71.

GEMAS [GEochemical Mapping of Agricultural and grazing land Soil]. The GEMAS periodic table of elements at high resolution. 2014. http://gemas.geolba.ac.at/Download/GEMAS_Periodic_Table_of_Elements_High_resolution.pdf (Accessed 26 November 2017).

Gigolashvili T, Kopriva S. Transporters in plant sulphur metabolism. Front Plant Sci. 2014;5:422. https://doi.org/10.3389/fpls.2014.00442.

Gionfriddo E, Naccarato A, Sindona G, et al. A reliable solid phase microextraction-gas chromatography–triple quadrupole mass spectrometry method for the assay of selenomethionine and selenomethylselenocysteine in aqueous extracts: difference between selenized and not-enriched selenium potatoes. Anal Chim Acta. 2012;747:58–66.

González-Morales S, Pérez-Labrada F, García-Enciso EL, et al. Selenium and sulfur to produce *Allium* functional crops. Molecules. 2017;22:558. https://doi.org/10.3390/molecules22040558.

Grant TD, Montes-Bayón M, LeDuc D, et al. Identification and characterization of Se-methyl selenomethionine in *Brassica juncea* roots. J Chromatogr A. 2004;1026:159–66.

Guignardi Z, Schiavon M. Biochemistry of plant selenium uptake and metabolism. In: EAH P-S, LHE W, Lin Z-Q, editors. Selenium in plants: molecular, physiological, ecological and evolutionary aspects. Cham, Switzerland: Springer; 2017. p. 21–34.

Gupta UC, Gupta SC. Quality of animal and human life as affected by selenium management of soils and crops. Commun Soil Sci Plant Anal. 2002;33:15–8.

Hart DJ, Fairweather-Tait SJ, Broadley MR, et al. Selenium concentration and speciation in bio-fortified flour and bread: retention of selenium during grain biofortification, processing and production of Se-enriched food. Food Chem. 2011;126:1771–8.

Hartikainen H. Biogeochemistry of selenium and its impact on food chain quality and human health. J Trace Elem Med Biol. 2005;18:309–18.

Haygarth PM, Cooke AI, Jones KC, et al. Long-term change in the biogeochemical cycling of atmospheric selenium: deposition to plants and soil. J Geophys Res. 1993;98:16769–76.

Hesse H, Kreft O, Maimann S, et al. Current understanding of the regulation of methionine biosynthesis in plants. J Exp Bot. 2004;55:1799–808.

Hsu F-C, Wirtz M, Heppel SC, et al. Generation of Se-fortified broccoli as functional food: impact of Se fertilization on S metabolism. Plant Cell Environ. 2011;34:192–207.

Huang K, Lin JC, Wu QY, et al. Changes in sulforaphane and selenocysteine methyltransferase transcript levels in broccoli treated with sodium selenite. Plant Mol Biol Report. 2016;34:807–14.

Huang Y, Wang Q, Gao J, et al. Daily dietary selenium intake in a high selenium area of Enshi, China. Nutrients. 2013;5:700–10.

Hurst R, Siyame EWP, Young SD, et al. Soil-type influences human selenium status and underlies widespread selenium deficiency risks in Malawi. Sci Rep. 2013;3:1425. https://doi.org/10.1038/srep01425.

Ihnat M. Plants and agricultural materials. In: Ihnat M, editor. Occurrence and distribution of selenium. Boca Raton, FL: CRC Press; 1989. p. 33–105.

Jin K, White PJ, Whalley WR, et al. Shaping an optimal soil by root-soil interaction. Trends Plant Sci. 2017;22:823–9.

Joy EJM, Broadley MR, Young SD, et al. Soil type influences crop mineral composition in Malawi. Sci Total Environ. 2015;505:587–95.

Jones GD, Winkel LHE. Multi-scale factors and processes controlling selenium distributions in soils. In: EAH P-S, LHE W, Lin Z-Q, editors. Selenium in plants: molecular, physiological, ecological and evolutionary aspects. Cham, Switzerland: Springer; 2017. p. 3–20.

Jones GD, Droz B, Greve P, et al. Selenium deficiency risk predicted to increase under future climate change. Proc Natl Acad Sci U S A. 2017;114:2848–53.

Kataoka T, Hayashi N, Yamaya T, et al. Root-to-shoot transport of sulfate in Arabidopsis. Evidence for the role of SULTR3;5 as a component of low-affinity sulfate transport system in the root vasculature. Plant Physiol. 2004a;136:4198–204.

Kataoka T, Watanabe-Takahashi A, Hayashi N, et al. Vacuolar sulphate transporters are essential determinants controlling internal distribution of sulfate in Arabidopsis. Plant Cell. 2004b;16:2693–704.

Kikkert J, Berkelaar E. Plant uptake and translocation of inorganic and organic forms of selenium. Arch Environ Contam Toxicol. 2013;65:458–65.

Kumssa DB, Joy EJM, Young SD, et al. Variation in the mineral element concentration of *Moringa oleifera* Lam. and *M. stenopetala* (Bak. f.) Cuf.: Role in human nutrition. PLoS One. 2017;12(4):e0175503. https://doi.org/10.1371/journal.pone.0175503.

Labunskyy VM, Hatfield DL, Gladyshev VN. Selenoproteins: molecular pathways and physiological roles. Physiol Rev. 2014;94:739–77.

Lazo-Vélez MA, Chávez-Santoscoy A, Serna-Saldivar SO. Selenium-enriched breads and their benefits in human nutrition and health as affected by agronomic, milling, and baking factors. Cereal Chem J. 2015;92:134–44.

Lee S, Woodward HJ, Doolittle JJ. Selenium uptake response among selected wheat (*Triticum aestivum*) varieties and relationship with soil selenium fractions. Soil Sci Plant Nutr. 2011;57:823–32.

Li H-F, McGrath SP, Zhao F-J. Selenium uptake, translocation and speciation in wheat supplied with selenate or selenite. New Phytol. 2008;178:92–102.

Li Z, Liang DL, Peng Q, et al. Interaction between selenium and soil organic matter and its impact on soil selenium bioavailability: a review. Geoderma. 2017;295:69–79.

Liu MX, Zhang ZW, Ren GX, et al. Evaluation of selenium and carotenoid concentrations of 200 foxtail millet accessions from China and their correlations with agronomic performance. J Integr Agric. 2016;15:1449–57.

Lyi SM, Heller LI, Rutzke M, et al. Molecular and biochemical characterization of the selenocysteine Se-methyltransferase gene and Se-methylselenocysteine synthesis in broccoli. Plant Physiol. 2005;138:409–20.

Lyons GH, Judson GJ, Ortiz-Monasterio I, Genc Y, Stangoulis JC, Graham RD. Selenium in Australia: selenium status and biofortification of wheat for better health. J Trace Elem Med Biol. 2005;19:75–82.

Mahn A. Modelling of the effect of selenium fertilization on the content of bioactive compounds in broccoli heads. Food Chem. 2017;233:492–9.

Matich AJ, McKenzie MJ, Lill RE, et al. Selenoglucosinolates and their metabolites produced in *Brassica* spp. fertilised with sodium selenate. Phytochemistry. 2012;75:140–52.

Matich AJ, McKenzie MJ, Lill RE, et al. Distribution of selenoglucosinolates and their metabolites in Brassica treated with sodium selenate. J Agric Food Chem. 2015;63:1896–905.

Mazej D, Osvald J, Stibilj V. Selenium species in leaves of chicory, dandelion, lamb's lettuce and parsley. Food Chem. 2008;107:75–83.

Mikkelsen RL, Page AL, Bingham FT. Factors affecting selenium accumulation by agricultural crops. In: Jacobs LW, Chang AC, Dowdy RH, et al., editors. Selenium in agriculture and the environment. Soil science society of america, special publication, vol. 23; 1989. p. 65–94.

ODS [Office of Dietary Supplements]. Selenium: dietary supplement fact sheet. Health Information. US Department of Health and Human Services, National Institutes of Health, Office of Dietary Supplements, Washington, DC; 2016.

Ogra Y, Kitaguchi T, Ishiwata K, et al. Identification of selenohomolanthionine in selenium-enriched Japanese pungent radish. J Anal At Spectrom. 2007;22:1390–6.

Oldfield JE. Selenium world atlas. Selenium-tellurium development association. 2002. http://www.369.com.cn/En/Se%20Atlas%202002.pdf (Accessed 26 November 2017).

Ouerdane L, Aureli F, Flis P, et al. Comprehensive speciation of low-molecular weight selenium metabolites in mustard seeds using HPLC-electrospray linear trap/orbitrap tandem mass spectrometry. Metallomics. 2013;5:1294–304.

Pilbeam DJ, Greathead HMR, Drihem K. Selenium. In: Barker AV, Pilbeam DJ, editors. A handbook of plant nutrition. 2nd ed. Boca Raton, FL: CRC Press; 2015. p. 165–98.

Pilon-Smits EAH, LeDuc DL. Phytoremediation of selenium using transgenic plants. Curr Opin Biotechnol. 2009;20:207–12.

Pilon-Smits EAH, de Souza MP, Hong G, et al. Selenium volatalization and accumulation by twenty aquatic plant species. J Environ Qual. 1999a;28:1011–8.

Pilon-Smits EAH, Hwang SB, Lytle CM, et al. Overexpression of ATPsulphurylase in *Brassica juncea* leads to increased selenite uptake. Reduction and tolerance. Plant Physiol. 1999b;119:123–32.

Pilon-Smits EAH, Quinn CF, Tapken W, et al. Physiological functions of beneficial elements. Curr Opin Plant Biol. 2009;12:267–74.

Pivato M, Fabrega-Prats M, Masi A. Low-molecular-weight thiols in plants: functional and analytical implications. Arch Biochem Biophys. 2014;560:83–99.

Puccinelli M, Malorgio F, Pezzarossa B. Selenium enrichment of horticultural crops. Molecules. 2017;22:933. https://doi.org/10.3390/molecules22060933.

Ramamurthy RK, Jedlicka J, Graef GL, et al. Identification of new QTLs for seed mineral, cysteine, and methionine concentrations in soybean [*Glycine max* (L.) Merr.]. Mol Breed. 2014;34:431–45.

Ramos SJ, Rutzke MA, Hayes RJ, et al. Selenium accumulation in lettuce germplasm. Planta. 2011a;233:649–60.

Ramos SJ, Yuan Y, Faquin V, et al. Evaluation of genotypic variation of broccoli (Brassica oleracea var. italic) in response to selenium treatment. J Food Agric Chem. 2011b;59:3657–65.

Rayman MP. Selenium and human health. Lancet. 2012;379:1256–68.

Reeves RD, Baker AJM. Metal-accumulating plants. In: Raskin I, Ensley BD, editors. Phytoremediation of toxic metals: using plants to clean up the environment. New York: Wiley; 2000. p. 193–229.

Robbins RJ, Keck AS, Banuelos G, et al. Cultivation conditions and selenium fertilization alter the phenolic profile, glucosinolate, and sulforaphane content of broccoli. J Med Food. 2005;8:204–14.

Roman M, Jitaru P, Barbante C. Selenium biochemistry and its role for human health. Metallomics. 2014;6:25–54.

Ros G, van Rotterdam A, Bussink D, et al. Selenium fertilization strategies for bio-fortification of food: an agro-ecosystem approach. Plant and Soil. 2016;1:99–112.

Rosenfeld I, Beath OA. Selenium: Geobotany, biochemistry, toxicity, and nutrition. New York: Academic Press; 1964.

Rouached H, Wirtz M, Alary R, et al. Differential regulation of the expression of two high-affinity sulfate transporters, SULTR1.1 and SULTR1.2, in Arabidopsis. Plant Physiol. 2008;147:897–911.

Ruszczynska A, Konopka A, Kurek E, et al. Investigation of biotransformation of selenium in plants using spectrometric methods. Spectrochim Acta B. 2017;130:7–16.

Schiavon M, Pilon-Smits EAH. The fascinating facets of plant selenium accumulation–biochemistry, physiology, evolution and ecology. New Phytol. 2017;213:1582–96.

Schiavon M, Pilon M, Malagoli M, et al. Exploring the importance of sulphate transporters and ATPsulphurylases for selenium hyperaccumulation – comparison of *Stanleya pinnata* and *Brassica juncea* (Brassicaceae). Front Plant Sci. 2015;6:2. https://doi.org/10.3389/fpls.2015.00002.

Schiavon M, Berto C, Malagoli M, et al. Selenium biofortification in radish enhances nutritional quality via accumulation of methyl-selenocysteine and promotion of transcripts and metabolites related to glucosinolates, phenolics, and amino acids. Front Plant Sci. 2016;7:1371. https://doi.org/10.3389/fpls.2016.01371.

Schomburg L, Arnér ESJ. Selenium metabolism in herbivores and higher trophic levels including mammals. In: EAH P-S, LHE W, Lin Z-Q, editors. Selenium in plants: molecular, physiological, ecological and evolutionary aspects. Cham, Switzerland: Springer; 2017. p. 123–39.

Sepúlveda I, Barrientos H, Mahn A, et al. Changes in SeMSC, glucosinolates and sulforaphane levels, and in proteome profile in broccoli (*Brassica oleracea* var. *italica*) fertilized with sodium selenate. Molecules. 2013;18:5221–34.

Shao SX, Mi XB, Ouerdane L, et al. Quantification of Se-methylselenocysteine and its γ-glutamyl derivative from naturally Se-enriched green bean (*Phaseolus vulgaris vulgaris*) after HPLC-ESI-TOF-MS and orbitrap MSn-based identification. Food Anal Methods. 2014;7:1147–57.

Shibagaki N, Rose A, McDermott JP, et al. Selenate-resistant mutants of *Arabidopsis thaliana* identify *Sultr1;2*, a sulfate transporter required for efficient transport of sulfate into roots. Plant J. 2002;29:475–86.

Shinmachi F, Buchner P, Stroud JL, et al. Influence of sulfur deficiency on the expression of specific sulfate transporters and the distribution of sulfur, selenium, and molybdenum in wheat. Plant Physiol. 2010;153:327–36.

Smrkolj P, Osvald M, Osvald J, et al. Selenium uptake and species distribution in selenium-enriched bean (*Phasolus vulgaris* L.) seeds obtained by two different cultivations. Eur Food Res Technol. 2007;225:233–7.

Song Z, Shao H, Huang H, et al. Overexpression of the phosphate transporter gene OsPT8 improves the Pi and selenium contents in *Nicotiana tabacum*. Environ Exp Bot. 2017;137:158–65.

Sors TG, Ellis DR, Salt DE. Selenium uptake, translocation, assimilation and metabolic fate in plants. Photosynth Res. 2005;86:373–89.

Statwick J, Sher AA. Selenium in soils of western Colorado. J Arid Environ. 2017;137:1–6.

Sugihara S, Kondo M, Chihara Y, et al. Preparation of selenium-enriched sprouts and identification of their selenium species by high-performance liquid chromatography-inductively coupled plasma mass spectrometry. Biosci Biotechnol Biochem. 2004;68:193–9.

Sun G-X, Meharg AA, Li G, et al. Distribution of soil selenium in China is potentially controlled by deposition and volatilization? Sci Rep. 2016;6:20953. https://doi.org/10.1038/srep20953.

Sunde RA, Li J-L, Taylor RM. Insights for setting of nutrient requirements, gleaned by comparison of selenium status biomarkers in turkeys and chickens versus rats, mice, and lambs. Adv Nutr. 2017;7:1129–38.

Supriatin S, Weng L, Comans RNJ. Selenium-rich dissolved organic matter determines selenium uptake in wheat grown on low-selenium arable land soils. Plant and Soil. 2016;408:73–94.

Tagmount A, Berken A, Terry N. An essential role of S-adenosyl-Lmethionine: L-methionine S-methyltransferase in selenium volatilization by plants. Methylation of selenomethionine to selenium-methyl-L-seleniummethionine, the precursor of volatile selenium. Plant Physiol. 2002;130:847–56.

Takahashi H, Watanabe-Takahashi A, Smith FW, et al. The roles of three functional sulphate transporters involved in uptake and translocation of sulphate in *Arabidopsis thaliana*. Plant J. 2000;23:171–82.

Takahashi H, Kopriva S, Giordano M, et al. Sulfur assimilation in photosynthetic organisms: molecular functions and regulations of transporters and assimilatory enzymes. Annu Rev Plant Biol. 2011;62:157–84.

Tegeder M. Transporters involved in source to sink partitioning of amino acids and ureides: opportunities for crop improvement. J Exp Bot. 2014;65:1865–78.

Terry N, Carlson C, Raab TK, et al. Rates of selenium volatilization among crop species. J Environ Qual. 1992;21:341–4.

Tian M, Xu X, Liu Y, et al. Effect of Se treatment on glucosinolate metabolism and health-promoting compounds in the broccoli sprouts of three cultivars. Food Chem. 2016;190:374–80.

Van Hoewyk D. A tale of two toxicities: malformed selenoproteins and oxidative stress both contribute to selenium stress in plants. Ann Bot. 2013;112:965–72.

Van Hoewyk D. Defects in endoplasmic reticulum-associated degradation (ERAD) increase selenate sensitivity in Arabidopsis. Plant Signal Behav. 2016;13:e1171451. https://doi.org/10.10 80/15592324.2016.1171451.

Van Hoewyk D, Çakir O. Manipulating selenium metabolism in plants: a simple twist of metabolic fate can alter selenium tolerance and accumulation. In: EAH P-S, LHE W, Lin Z-Q, editors. Selenium in plants: molecular, physiological, ecological and evolutionary aspects. Cham, Switzerland: Springer; 2017. p. 165–76.

Van Hoewyk D, Garifullina GF, Ackley AR, et al. Overexpression of AtCpNifS enhances selenium tolerance and accumulation in Arabidopsis. Plant Physiol. 2005;139:1518–28.

Van Hoewyk D, Takahashi H, Hess A, et al. Transcriptome and biochemical analyses give insights into selenium-stress responses and selenium tolerance mechanisms in Arabidopsis. Physiol Plant. 2008;132:236–53.

Van Huysen T, Abdel-Ghany S, Hale KL, et al. Overexpression of cystathionine-γ-synthase enhances selenium volatilisation in *Brassica juncea*. Planta. 2003;218:71–8.

Wang P, Menzies NW, Lombi E, et al. Synchrotron-based X-ray absorption near-edge spectroscopy imaging for laterally resolved speciation of selenium in fresh roots and leaves of wheat and rice. J Exp Bot. 2015;66:4795–806.

White PJ. Selenium accumulation by plants. Ann Bot. 2016a;117:217–35.

White PJ. Biofortification of edible crops. In: eLS. Chichester: Wiley; 2016b. https://doi.org/10.1002/9780470015902.a0023743.

White PJ. The genetics of selenium accumulation in plants. In: EAH P-S, LHE W, Lin Z-Q, editors. Selenium in plants: Molecular, physiological, ecological and evolutionary aspects. Cham, Switzerland: Springer; 2017. p. 143–63.

White PJ, Broadley MR. Biofortification of crops with seven mineral elements often lacking in human diets – iron, zinc, copper, calcium, magnesium, selenium and iodine. New Phytol. 2009;182:49–84.

White PJ, Bowen HC, Parmaguru P, et al. Interactions between selenium and sulphur nutrition in *Arabidopsis thaliana*. J Exp Bot. 2004;55:1927–37.

White PJ, Bowen HC, Marshall B, et al. Extraordinarily high leaf selenium to sulphur ratios define 'Se-accumulator' plants. Ann Bot. 2007a;100:111–8.

White PJ, Broadley MR, Bowen HC, et al. Selenium and its relationship with sufur. In: Hawkesford MJ, de Kok LJ, editors. Sulfur in plants - an ecological perspective. Dordrecht: Springer; 2007b. p. 225–52.

White PJ, George TS, Gregory PJ, et al. Matching roots to their environment. Ann Bot. 2013;112:207–22.

Wiesner-Reinhold M, Schreiner M, Baldermann S, et al. Mechanisms of selenium enrichment and measurement in brassicaceous vegetables, and their application to human health. Front Plant Sci. 2017;8:1365. https://doi.org/10.3389/fpls.2017.01365.

Williams PN, Lombi E, Sun GX, et al. Selenium characterization in the global rice supply chain. Environ Sci Technol. 2009;43:6024–30.

Winkel LH, Vriens B, Jones GD, et al. Selenium cycling across soil-plant-atmosphere interfaces: a critical review. Nutrients. 2015;7:4199–239.

Wrobel JK, Power R, Toborek M. Biological activity of selenium: revisited. IUMB Life. 2016;68:97–105.

Wu Z, Bañuelos GS, Lin Z-Q, et al. Biofortification and phytoremediation of selenium in China. Front Plant Sci. 2015;6:136. https://doi.org/10.3389/fpls.2015.00136.

Ximénez-Embún P, Alonso I, Madrid-Albarráan Y, et al. Establishment of selenium uptake and species distribution in lupine, Indian mustard, and sunflower plants. J Agric Food Chem. 2004;52:832–8.

Yoshimoto N, Inoue E, Saito K, et al. Phloem localizing sulfate transporter, Sultr1;3, mediates re-distribution of sulphur from source to sink organs in Arabidopsis. Plant Physiol. 2003;131:1511–7.

Yuan LX, Zhu YY, Lin ZQ, et al. A novel selenocystine-accumulating plant in selenium-mine drainage area in Enshi, China. PLoS One. 2013;8:e65615. https://doi.org/10.1371/journal.pone.0065615.

Zhang L, Hu B, Li W, et al. OsPT2, a phosphate transporter, is involved in the active uptake of selenite in rice. New Phytol. 2014;201:1183–91.

Zhao D-Y, Sun F-L, Zhang B, et al. Systematic comparisons of orthologous selenocysteine methyltransferase and homocysteine methyltransferase genes from seven monocots species. Nat Sci Biol. 2015;7:210–6.

Zhao H, Huang J, Li Y, et al. Natural variation of selenium concentration in diverse tea plant (*Camellia sinensis*) accessions at seedling stage. Sci Hortic. 2016;198:163–9.

Zhao XQ, Mitani N, Yamaji N, et al. Involvement of silicon influx transporter OsNIP2;1 in selenite uptake in rice. Plant Physiol. 2010;153:1871–7.

Chapter 3
Dietary Aspects for Selenium and/or Selenium Compounds

Lutz Schomburg

Abstract The essential trace element selenium is present in our diet in different forms and concentrations. An insufficiently low intake will cause a status of selenium deficiency that is associated with an increased risk for developing certain diseases including cancer, infectious, autoimmune and other diseases. On the other hand, an acute or chronic over-supplementation with high amounts of selenium will likewise challenge our health, and signs of selenosis may develop that include nail and hair loss besides other symptoms. The human organism has developed a number of biochemical pathways safeguarding a prioritised supply of the most important tissues and organs with the essential trace element in order to avoid the development of health-relevant states of selenium deficiency or selenosis. This chapter highlights some of the underlying mechanisms, scientific achievements and open questions regarding the role of selenium in the human diet and its metabolism.

Keywords Cancer · Thyroid · Nutrition · Vegetarian · Selenosis · Deficiency

"Being alive and kicking means you have to eat. In fact, all life must feed. For most creatures, this exigency of survival is simple, if not always easy. Sometimes, food is merely elusive. Sometimes, it runs away. Sometimes, it fights back" (slightly modified from the book: Vegetarian and Plant-Based Diets in Health and Disease Prevention, (C) 2017, Elsevier Inc., ISBN: 978-0-12-803,968-7, Foreword by David L. Katz, Derby, CT, US).

Selenium (Se) is part of our food and an essential trace element for mammals. This notion may appear trivial at first sight, but highlights two important features of Se as a micronutrient; Se is essential, i.e. for us there is no growth, life and fertility without a sufficiently high Se supply, and Se is a trace element, i.e. it is needed in small amounts only. If these small quantities are not provided by our regular food,

L. Schomburg (✉)
Charité—Universitätsmedizin Berlin, Institut für Experimentelle Endokrinologie,
Berlin, Germany
e-mail: lutz.schomburg@charite.de

© Springer International Publishing AG, part of Springer Nature 2018
B. Michalke (ed.), *Selenium*, Molecular and Integrative Toxicology,
https://doi.org/10.1007/978-3-319-95390-8_3

we are insufficiently supplied, i.e. Se deficient. If the intake surpasses reasonable limits, we are at the risk of developing signs and symptoms of toxicity from surplus Se, i.e. we develop Se overload, called selenosis. The obvious challenge for us is finding the right balance of Se intake, i.e. a sufficiently high amount without being at risk for selenosis. The quantity needed varies according to other parameters like health status, age and stress, and our body is able to a certain extent to adapt its Se metabolism dynamically to the actual Se availability and our current needs. Besides the thresholds of extreme Se intakes that define deficiency or selenosis, there is a range of safe intakes that seem to support our health and exert mainly beneficial metabolic effects. However, the exact boundaries of this range cannot easily be determined. The characteristics of such an optimal intake would be defined by clinical studies in which a population is either actively supplemented or not with Se (intervention trials), or in observational studies, in which disease incidences are related to the Se status percentiles at study entry. In view of the support of antioxidative defence systems and thyroid hormone activity control by selenoproteins, this optimal range of Se intake and Se status may not be a constant figure but rather depend on the increased and changing requirements of an ageing and disease-prone organism. From these considerations, we may conclude that there will likely be no globally applicable level of best Se intake, but rather an optimal range of intakes that depends on personal health status and age-dependent parameters and challenges.

Defining the Boundaries of Safe and Health-Supporting Se Intake

The optimally needed level of Se intake for maintaining health and avoiding Se-dependent disease risks can be determined with some certainty in a straightforward way, i.e. by analysing disease incidences in relation to Se intake or Se status in suitable cohort studies. Two areas of clinical research shall serve here as paradigmatic examples that have yielded respective insights, i.e. oncology and thyroidology.

As first example, the two large cancer prevention studies in the USA aiming to reduce cancer risk by supplemental Se nicely showed that some protection was exerted in the first study (the so-called NPC trial Clark et al. 1996), but not in the second study (the so-called SELECT study, similar design as NPC Klein et al. 2011). The major difference in both studies was the baseline Se status of the participants, which differed considerably (on average 113 μg/L in the NPC trial vs. 135 μg/L in SELECT) (Hatfield and Gladyshev 2009). Moreover, only the subjects in the lowest two tertiles of plasma Se in the successful NPC trial showed reduced cancer risk upon Se supplementation (Duffield-Lillico et al. 2003). These findings collectively indicate that subjects with plasma Se concentrations exceeding 123 μg/L (threshold between middle and high tertiles in NPC) may not profit from supplemental Se intake with respect to their prostate cancer risk. However, in how far this threshold also applies to other cancer types, and in how far it is the same threshold in other populations and especially in women in general, remains to be determined. In addition, it is unclear whether there was also some modifying effect of the slightly different selenocompounds used (Se-rich yeast vs. pure selenomethionine).

As second example, it is long known that a Se deficit constitutes a risk factor for thyroid diseases (Corvilain et al. 1993; Kohrle et al. 2005; Schomburg 2011). Several studies have shown an increased goitre or nodule risk in women with low Se intake or status (Derumeaux et al. 2003; Rasmussen et al. 2011). A recent comparison of a high number of subjects residing in neighbouring areas of different habitual Se intakes in China showed strongly increased thyroid disease rates in the population with lower plasma Se concentrations (median and interquartile range; 57.4 [39.4, 82.1] µg/L) as compared to the subjects in the better supplied area (103.6 [79.7, 135.9] µg/L) (Wu et al. 2015). Again, these data point to an advisable range of Se intakes for achieving health-promoting plasma concentrations of >100 µg/L as the requirement for a beneficial Se status. The average Se status of subjects residing in many areas of Africa, Asia or Europe is below this threshold, implying that an increased Se intake may reduce their cancer and thyroid disease risk. However, it is difficult to assess whether one is reaching this plasma Se concentration based on theoretical assumptions alone or based on data of the Se content of the meals consumed. Analytical measurements of biomaterial, preferentially blood samples, are needed for a better understanding of the personal Se supply and status. In addition, supplementation studies need to report final serum or plasma Se concentrations, which will enable a better assessment of the effects of certain supplements and dosages. A well-controlled supplementation trial comparing 200 and 400 µg of Se-rich yeast per day, similar protocol as the NPC trial, reported an increase of plasma Se concentrations from 115 µg/L to 200 and 250 µg/L, respectively, stabilising after approx. 1 year (Reid et al. 2008). This experience indicates that a constant supplementation increases serum or plasma Se concentrations relatively predictable, and that a supplementation of an already well-supplied cohort of subjects with 200 or 400 µg Se/day may cause a Se status that is beyond the threshold needed and that has been associated with adverse health effects in other studies (Fig. 3.1).

The Threat of Exaggerated Se Intake, i.e. Selenosis

The level at which Se intake may become toxic can be deduced with some certainty from published case reports of selenosis or from an in-depth analysis of clinical trials that are conducted in areas with already high habitual Se intakes, or from the high Se areas in China, where intakes of >1 mg Se/day are reported (Yang et al. 1989). Currently, the widely accepted tolerable upper limit is in the range of 400 µg/day, the no observed adverse effect level is at 800 µg/day and the lowest observed adverse effect level starts at around 900 µg/day, respectively (Monsen 2000). However, the evidence for these thresholds is limited and incomplete, as neither the nature of the specific selenocompounds nor the characteristic of the subject consuming the micronutrient are taken into account. The figures may be different for

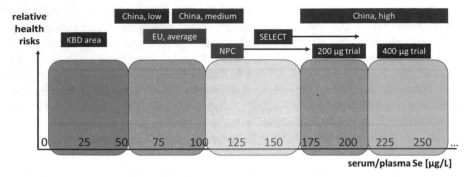

Fig. 3.1 Schematic drawing indicating the average serum or plasma Se concentration ranges in different clinical studies mentioned in the text. Subjects residing in the Se-poor Keshan disease belt in China show serum Se concentrations of around 20 µg/L only (Yao et al. 2011). A recent analysis on thyroid disease compared two areas in China (Wu et al. 2015) with serum Se concentrations spanning the range typically observed in European subjects (Hughes et al. 2015). In comparison, probands in the NPC supplementation study (Clark et al. 1996) had a higher Se status, but still considerably lower than in the follow-up SELECT study (Hatfield and Gladyshev 2009). Daily supplementation with 200 or 400 µg Se-rich yeast increased the plasma Se concentrations in the US participants (Reid et al. 2008) into ranges formerly only known from the very-Se-rich areas in China (Yang et al. 1989). The colour code indicating relative health risk is an estimation by the author and not (yet) strictly based on clinical evidence

inorganic versus organic selenocompounds, or for young and healthy versus elderly subjects. It is conceivable from studies in model systems that the chemical nature of Se makes a huge difference (Hoefig et al. 2011; Marschall et al. 2016). A high intake of selenomethionine is inserted directly and efficiently by regular translation into many newly synthesised proteins, while high amounts of selenite may not accumulate in the body but rather become excreted fast once a saturating biosynthesis of selenoproteins is reached. But often, neither the concentration nor the molecular nature of the selenocompounds of a given food item is known. The problem of a varying Se content of certain food items poses serious problems and has already been reported as a reason for selenosis in rare cases of high consumption of, e.g., paranuts (Senthilkumaran et al. 2012). More problematic are nutritional supplements in case the production occurs in error causing too high Se contents in the products; a recent report on a misformulated supplement affected around 100 healthy subjects, developing hair and nail loss and a number of long-lasting side effects after consuming daily supplements containing up to >30 mg (!) Se/daily dose (Morris and Crane 2013). This report indicates that even daily intakes of around 500 times the recommended daily intake of 60–70 µg/day (Kipp et al. 2015) do not directly cause fatalities but rather reversible health problems. On the other hand, recent reports on supplemental Se intake that are suspected to potentially increase type 2 diabetes mellitus or cancer risk raise concerns with respect to slightly exceeding the regular habitual Se intake (Jablonska and Vinceti 2015). Whether these concerns are justified is the subject of current preclinical and clinical analyses. A recent large-scale and high-quality analysis indicated an opposite relation between

Se intake and carbohydrate metabolism and body weight, i.e. the CODING study, highlighting that a Se deficit may constitute a hunger signal, and a sufficiently high Se intake may protect from metabolic disease and support a healthier body composition profile (Wang et al. 2016). Probably again, the concerns of selenosis are justified for populations on already high habitual basic Se intake, but with no relevance for health risks for the majority of subjects residing in Africa, Asia or Europe (please also compare Fig. 3.1).

The Quest for Finding an Optimal Se Intake and Se Status

The studies mentioned above indicate that an insufficient Se intake confers certain health risks, and that the threshold at which Se intake may become toxic and causing side effects is ill defined and controversially discussed. The optimal intake is somewhere in between the extreme values that have been reported, but its exact range is difficult to determine and may depend on a number of characteristics like the exact nature of the dietary Se sources, the age and health of the subject, sex-specific oddities in Se metabolism and other parameters. The strong differences in average Se intakes in different populations ranging from less than 50 μg/day in most European countries to more than 200 μg/day in Venezuela or even to >1 mg/day in the Se-rich areas in China argue for very efficient metabolic pathways protecting from selenosis and efficiently utilising the available Se for supporting human health. Two hierarchical principles of Se metabolism are largely responsible for the dynamic adaptations controlling the Se status, relating to the prioritised supply of essentially needed selenoproteins over dispensable ones, and to the hierarchically preferred supply of important endocrine organs and brain over other tissues in times of poor supply (Schomburg and Schweizer 2009). In addition, the decline of selenoprotein biosynthesis rates in face of ample Se supply leading to a plateauing effect on circulating selenoproteins with increasing Se intake protects efficiently from the development of selenosis over a wide intake range (Xia et al. 2010). The selenoprotein translation machinery is thus somehow subject to feedback regulation, protecting itself from exaggerated selenoprotein biosynthesis. From these studies and theoretical considerations it can be concluded that the attempts to raising awareness of Se as an important trace element are to be supported. An increased intake if residing in a Se-poor area would rather cause positive health benefits and reduced disease risks with little or no negative side effects, as the organism is able to prevent itself from selenosis, but not to avoid Se deficiency if the trace element is not provided in sufficient amounts. Nevertheless, an analysis of the current Se status in a given subject remains the most meaningful measure in order to counsel on the diet and adapt the intake to reach the desired supply. From both the cancer prevention and thyroid disease data (above) along with a growing number of additional clinical studies on the interaction of Se with disease risks, it appears advisable to aim for a plasma Se concentration of >100 μg/L. This level is rarely reached in Europeans, as seen in a recent multinational epidemiological analysis reporting an average serum Se concentration in the healthy probands from ten European countries of around 85 µg/L (Hughes et al. 2015). The only positive exception in Europe is Finland, where a systematic enrichment of the mineral fertilisers is in place since more than 30 years. This brave endeavour has successfully increased the average daily Se intake of the Finnish population from 25 µg/day to around 80 µg/day, corresponding to an increase in plasma Se concentrations from 0.9 to 1.4 µM (from 71 to 111 µg/L) (Alfthan et al. 2015).

Health Benefits and Limits of Optimising the Se Intake

However, as often in nutrition research, the reader should not consult this chapter with exaggerated expectations. It appears as a disease of our times that one does expect certain daily food components to provide good health and protection from disease, i.e. being responsible for maintaining fitness and youth despite a sedentary, largely indoor lifestyle and adverse general nutrition pattern in combination with the inevitable process of ageing. Such an approach would be expecting too much from a single micronutrient (Ioannidis 2013). The trace element Se may contribute to our health but it is not a medicinal product. The misunderstanding of the role of our nutrition and the far-reaching expectations are no novel phenomenon, but have already been put forward by Hippocrates, father of medicine, 431 B.C: *Let food be thy medicine and medicine be thy food*. With all due respect, I tend not to agree, for our nutrition cannot fulfil this requirement. Yet, avoiding a Se deficit by a balanced nutrition that is taking a sufficiently high Se content into account is an important factor for staying fit, alive and healthy, and probably for avoiding premature ageing and age-related declining body functions. However a definite health claim for supplemental Se intake, i.e. an intake surpassing our basal requirement in order to help curing diseases in an adjuvant mode, is also possible and first results have been reported (Angstwurm et al. 2007; Brodin et al. 2015). However, this line of research on the application of Se supplements is relatively novel, and not yet supported by a sufficient number of solid clinical studies.

The Path of Selenium into Our Food

Plants accumulate Se mainly from soil. However, especially in fortification studies, also the absorption through the leaves is possible, e.g. by foliar application of selenate solutions (Sindelarova et al. 2015). Soil Se is of geochemical origin or introduced into soil through raining or by fertilisation (Winkel et al. 2015). There are several soil-plant-specific parameters that affect Se uptake and metabolism: acidity of the soil in conjunction with aeration and general soil watering, basic soil Se concentrations and the dominant chemical forms of Se present as well as plant-specific parameters including species-dependent uptake mechanisms with respect to the different Se forms (White 2016). Intra-plant transport and accumulation processes and plant Se sensitivity are giving rise to indifferent, tolerant and even super-accumulating species. The latter are known as excellent options for covering the Se requirement of Se-deficient subjects, e.g. of vegetarians living in areas of a generally low Se status. Nevertheless, especially these super-accumulators are directly dependent on soil quality and soil Se concentrations; the South-American paranuts, well known for their potential richness in Se reaching concentrations of up to 1000 ppm, depend heavily on the particular area where the trees are grown. The Se concentration of a given Brazil or paranut cannot be predicted and may range from almost minute background concentrations to amounts that need to be considered dangerous and toxic if several nuts per day are consumed (Chang et al. 1995). A better labelling of the Se content of paranuts and other potentially super-accumulating foodstuff is clearly needed.

Another well-characterised application of Se super-accumulating plants in conjunction with soil microorganisms is soil remediation of Se-contaminated areas (Wu 2004). Dry soils tend to become more and more trace element and mineral laden. Water resources are sometimes sparse and agricultural use for a lucrative and fruitful production of products from such land is very restricted. Super-accumulating plant species, such as brassica ssp., offer here a biological and efficient option for specifically reducing high Se concentrations from the soil, and open the perspective of using these Se-rich plants as specifically valuable nutrients for export into Se-poor areas for the consumption by subjects with otherwise insufficient intake (Wiesner-Reinhold et al. 2017). At the same time, a detoxification of the soil for agricultural purposes and the cultivation of less tolerant plants are enabled.

There are also efficient ways of improving the Se content of foodstuff produced in areas with typically low soil Se availability. One of the must illustrative examples is given by the Finish experience over the last 30 years (Aro et al. 1995). In 1985, Finland started to systematically enriching its agricultural fertilisers with selenate. Due to a lack of experience with such a population-wide intervention strategy, the dosage needed for achieving the desired daily Se intake had to be dynamically adapted to the developing Se status in the Finish population. Starting with around 5 mg/kg fertiliser, and not reaching the desired average Se intake of 70 µg/day in an average subject, the authorities and the expert committee decided to increase the supplemental Se content of the fertilisers. However, a few years later, daily Se intake surpassed the targeted threshold of average daily Se intake slightly. Consequently, it needed to be reduced again, and a final adaption of the Se content in fertilisers took place. Now, Finland has reached the desired average Se intake of around 70–80 µg/day, and the general improvement of health in the Finish population over the last decades supports the measures taken, even though the particular contribution of Se cannot be worked out as the full population was exposed to supplemental Se and no control group is available (Alfthan et al. 2015; Aro et al. 1995). One could ask why Se enrichment of the population was not attempted by directly supplementing a specific food item with the essential trace element, as, e.g., done in relation to iodine by fortifying table salt with the health-relevant micronutrient (Farebrother et al. 2015). There are two obvious advantages of using the plant in between the inorganic mineral fertiliser and the human recipient; a grossly miscalculated dosage would harm the plant first and prevent the human population of becoming exposed and potentially poisoned, and secondly the relatively cheap inorganic selenate becomes converted by the plant into potentially better and more efficiently metabolised organic selenocompounds.

Major Forms and Amount of Selenium in the Different Food Items

The Se content of food depends on the specific soil characteristics where it is grown and the particular plant characteristics (White 2016; Winkel et al. 2015). The major form of Se in the different plant parts depends on the biosynthetic pathways dominating the respective cells and tissues. Uptake of selenate appears to be mediated by using the root sulphate transport system utilising members of the family of the plant sulphate/selenate cotransporters (Sultr1;1 and Sultr1;2) (Schiavon and Pilon-Smits 2017). Consequently, in the roots, there is—depending on the kinetics of biotransformation—some of the originally accumulated soil Se sources detectable. The plant biosynthesis machinery for methionine does not discriminate between sulphur and Se, which leads to selenomethionine (SeMet) as one major anabolic plant metabolite. However, SeMet is not only used for protein biosynthesis but also further metabolised, giving rise to different relative amounts of methylated and further modified SeMet derivatives. High Se accumulation in plants apparently provides some protection from herbivores (Quinn et al. 2010). By different enzymatic conversions, SeMet can be methylated or otherwise modified, and transformed into Se-methyl selenocysteine and selenocysteine (SeCys) and several derivatives thereof. Again, further reaction products may be generated from SeMet and SeCys, finally leading to a complex pattern of Se-containing amino acids and their derivatives (Ogra and Anan 2012). Unfortunately, our current knowledge on the physiological effects of the different plant-derived selenocompounds is sparse.

Besides plants, also yeast can use inorganic Se forms to convert them into organic selenocompounds (Kieliszek et al. 2015). Often, therefore, Se-enriched yeast is commercially promoted as a very natural source (termed "bio-Se"). However, again the exact pattern of different selenocompounds in yeast is variable, depending on the particular yeast strain used and the culture conditions including the Se source provided, growth temperature, growth speed, pH value and dissolved oxygen level in the culture medium (Suhajda et al. 2000). It is for these reasons that, e.g., the large prostate cancer prevention trial SELECT preferred using the exactly defined SeMet as Se source instead of Se-enriched yeast, even though the prior successful NPC study used a Se-enriched yeast preparation (Lippman et al. 2005).

The variability of different selenocompounds in animal-derived food items is less complex than in plants, and the contents are more uniform. Two amino acids prevail, i.e. SeMet and SeCys (Bierla et al. 2008). Depending on the Se status of the animals and their particular diet, the relative proportion is largely determined by the degree of plant-derived versus animal-derived food items. The former are rich sources of SeMet and Se-methyl selenocysteine and further modified derivatives of these two amino acids, whereas animal-derived Se mainly consists of SeCys and to a smaller extent SeMet, but very few other selenocompounds. Consequently, the sensitivity of animals to selenosis on the one hand and the essentiality of Se as a trace element on the other hand safeguard a balanced Se concentration in animal-derived products, well suited for a safe supply of humans with the essential trace element. Vegetarians face a diet with higher variation of the Se content, where the Se intake can hardly be predicted, and are often at risk of developing very low Se status (Hoeflich et al. 2010). Therefore, vegetarians, and especially vegans, constitute a relevant risk group for low Se supply and Se deficiency.

Fate of Selenium in the Human Body

In humans, biosynthesis of the essentially needed selenoproteins is the prioritised fate of Se acquired from the diet (Schomburg and Schweizer 2009). Studies in model organisms and cell culture have shown that almost all dietary selenocompounds can be finally used for the generation of the tRNA carrying SeCys and thus for selenoprotein biosynthesis (Takahashi et al. 2017). The intestinal absorption rates of the different selenocompounds differ slightly, and depend on health state, sex, age, Se status and other individual parameters. However, after successful absorption, the major metabolic pathway in humans is exerted by hepatocytes and their biosynthesis of hepatic selenoproteins and selenoprotein P (SELENOP), respectively, which is used as a systemic carrier for a targeted distribution of Se throughout the body, especially to the privileged sites (Burk and Hill 2009). In blood, there are two actively secreted selenoproteins that dominate circulating Se concentrations, i.e. the kidney-derived extracellular glutathione peroxidase (GPX3), which itself depends on liver-derived SELENOP for biosynthesis (Renko et al. 2008), and SELENOP itself as the Se-specific transport protein (Burk and Hill 2009). Besides these SeCys-containing actively secreted selenoproteins, a fraction of SeMet-containing proteins can be found (Combs Jr et al. 2011). Importantly, the amount of SeMet-containing proteins depends directly on the uptake of SeMet via the nutrition and the Se status of the individual. In conditions of relative Se deficiency, as is found in large areas of Europe, Africa and Asia, the relative fraction of SeMet-containing selenoproteins in comparison to the SeCys-containing selenoproteins GPX3 and SELENOP is relatively small. In contrast, in subjects with a relatively high regular Se supply, such as in large areas of, e.g., the USA, Canada or Japan, the SeCys-containing selenoproteins are expressed to a maximal level, and dietary derived SeMet is not needed for further generation of tRNA-Sec, causing relatively high insertion of SeMet instead of Met during regular protein biosynthesis (Schrauzer 2003). Hereby, a relatively high fraction of SeMet-containing proteins both intracellular and in the circulation is generated. It is estimated that in a well-supplied individual approx. 1 in 8000 methionines is replaced by a SeMet residue (Burk et al. 2001). Besides serving as a readily available Se reservoir, the SeMet-containing proteins seem not to fulfil a specific function, which is not surprising in view of the random insertion process. Surplus Se can be excreted via different routes. Under normal conditions, two different selenosugars are secreted via the urine, namely methyl 2-acetamido-2-deoxy-1-seleno-ß-d-galactosamine and the glucosamine variant (SeGalNAc and SeGluNAc), whereas under high Se intake also dimethyl selenide via breath and trimethyl selenonium via the urine represent secretion products (Kobayashi et al. 2002). Especially the volatile dimethyl selenide constitutes the repulsive smelling selenocompound that is characteristic for Se poisoning and that is used as a typical diagnostic marker of selenosis (Fig. 3.2).

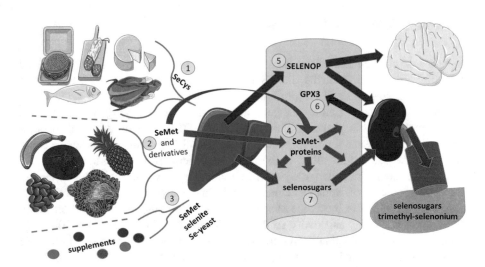

Fig. 3.2 Simplified scheme of the metabolism of dietary and supplemental selenocompounds by the human body. Se is taken up from the daily nutrition or from supplements. Animal-derived foodstuff mainly contains SeCys and a number of less abundant selenocompounds like SeMet, derivatives of these amino acids and other endogenous metabolites (1). Plant-derived Se mainly consists of SeMet, Se-methylselenocysteine and derivatives of these two amino acids (2). Supplemental Se is provided in the form of inorganic selenite or selenate, as SeMet or Se-enriched yeast (3). SeMet can be loaded on Met-tRNA and inserted in an unregulated way into any growing peptide chain, thereby replacing regular methionine residues and establishing a reserve pool of readily available Se (4), whereas other selenocompounds are subject to more intensive metabolism. Liver is responsible for the majority of circulating SELENOP biosynthesis that contains up to 10 SeCys residues per molecule and enables tissue-specific Se supply and preferential Se transport to brain (5). The other circulating selenoprotein is GPX3, mainly originating from the kidney (6). The major route of regulated excretion of surplus Se occurs as a component of selenosugars that can be transferred into urine for disposal (7). Figure generated with the support of graphics provided by Servier Medical Art, a service to medicine provided by Les Laboratoires Servier

Specific Dietary or Supplemental Se Requirements in Health and Disease

Selenoproteins take advantage of the chemical properties of Se as part of their enzymatically active centre and are mainly implicated in different redox reactions (Steinbrenner et al. 2016). As catalysts, selenoproteins cycle through different chemical states, requiring co-factors for returning to the reduced form. As such, the GPX depends on the glutathione (GSH) and di-glutathione (GS-SG) redox system as co-factor, and similarly the thioredoxin reductases depend on the monomeric reduced and dimeric oxidised thioredoxin proteins (TXN-SH/TXN-S-S-TXN). The oxidised and reducing substrate for the deiodinases (DIO) has not yet finally been identified, but likely also belongs to the group of small protein thiols, probably in an DIO-isoform-specific manner (Schweizer et al. 2017). Collectively, Se used for selenoprotein-dependent catalysis of redox reactions is not consumed during the reactions and therefore Se is not a substrate or an "antioxidant" that needs to be supplemented in stoichiometric amounts to the diet once higher redox activities by selenoproteins are required in specific health or disease circumstances. Nevertheless, Se is needed for the regular biosynthesis of selenoproteins and for replenishing lost Se during metabolism, and an insufficient intake may cause selenoprotein deficiency and thereby insufficient protection by these components of our antioxidative defence system (McCann and Ames 2011).

As the Se requirement needs to be covered by the diet, it is conceivable that the quality of the food consumed determines our Se intake. The agricultural production in North America is mainly located in areas of high soil Se concentrations, causing plant and animal food items to containing ample Se amounts, and a replete Se status of most US Americans results (Hargreaves et al. 2014). Similarly, populations residing in coastal areas or islands often have a relatively high fish intake, again leading to a sufficient Se supply (Hansen et al. 2004). In contrast, large areas of the world have low Se in soil, especially in higher altitudes such as Tibet or Nepal (Schulze et al. 2014). Here, the low Se content of the local food items is causing endemic Se deficiency, such as Kashin-Beck or Keshan disease (Yao et al. 2011). First insights into an endemic health risk by a combined low Se and iodine intake, causing myxedematous cretinism, have been reported from Central Africa (Contempre et al. 1991). Here, some systematic supplementation efforts have been installed preventing the disease in especially sensible risk groups such as children and the elderly. Also in Europe, the average regular Se intake is below the amount that is considered optimal (Stoffaneller and Morse 2015; Hughes et al. 2015). Besides Finland, there is no other country at present where systematic measures are taken in order to counteract this obvious insufficient supply.

Plants form the basic nutrition also for the breeding of farm animals, i.e. cattle, pigs, sheep, chicken and other less intensively used species. In areas with sufficient soil Se, both humans and animals receive the essentially needed micronutrient in sufficient amounts. In contrast, in areas of low soil Se concentrations, the animals may also develop Se-deficiency syndromes such as white muscle disease or blind stagger (Lenz and Lens 2009). Moreover, when consumed by humans, these farm animals do not constitute an ample source of Se. The risk of health-relevant Se deficit is long known by farmers implicated in intensive and industrial-like animal production, and thus the feed is enriched and supplemented with essential micronutrients such as certain minerals and vitamins (Stewart et al. 2012). Consequently, there are two groups of humans at risk of insufficient Se intake, i.e. populations living in areas of low soil Se in general, especially when Se supplements are not used in breeding of farm animals, and vegetarians living in areas of low soil Se, also in developed countries such as in Europe (Judd et al. 1997; Hoeflich et al. 2010). It appears of high importance to take respective measures for improving their Se intake, for educating on the potential health risks of a regularly low Se intake and for offering natural and vegetarian products suitable to correcting the deficits.

A second important reason for insufficient Se intake is a decreased absorption of dietary Se due to disease. Especially chronic diseases are associated with a high tonus of pro-inflammatory cytokines that are known to reduce hepatic Se metabolism and bioconversion, e.g. in sepsis (Renko et al. 2009). Similarly, total parenteral nutrition may cause specific deficiencies in certain micronutrients if the nutrition is not correctly formulated and composed (Abrams et al. 1992; Oguri et al. 2012). Also newborns, especially preterm children, depend on formula nutrients and thus on a kind of synthetic diet that needs to be composed according to the actual needs of the child, which in nature is usually guaranteed through feedback mechanisms within the mother by actively adapting the milk quality according to the developmental stage and age of the newborn. Severe Se deficiency may develop if infection and preterm birth coincide (Wiehe et al. 2016), necessitating specific care and supply. Moreover, during pregnancy in general, Se seems to become redistributed from mother to the growing foetus (Ambroziak et al. 2017). Consequently, if the mother is not well supplied with the essentially needed micronutrient, she may develop a state of Se deficiency, which is a risk factor for the health of the mother, for the birth process and for health and development of the newborn baby (Polanska et al. 2016).

Finally, the elderly who are often also multi-morbid and subject to polypharmacy may develop a low Se intake in combination with age- and medication-dependent disruption of the regular selenoprotein biosynthesis. There are respective reports on disrupting effects of the class of lipid-lowering statin drugs (Moosmann and Behl 2004), antibiotics of the aminoglycoside family (Handy et al. 2006) or even the widespread anti-diabetes drug metformin (Speckmann et al. 2009). In how far combinations of such medication may act in synergism and impair regular Se metabolism and selenoprotein biosynthesis in a health-relevant manner is largely unexplored and constitutes one of the research focuses in current studies. Especially an ageing organism may display an increased requirement for antioxidative protection due to the many noxae that are accumulating during life, including the increased generation of pro-oxidative processes causing protein aggregation and declining repair activities. In how far an age-adapted increase of Se supply in the elderly would constitute a health-relevant measure remains to be evaluated.

Conclusions

Collectively, our current knowledge highlights that dietary Se supply differs strongly between different populations and between individuals, depending on the quality and Se contents of the food items consumed. Moreover, the health status of an individual modifies Se metabolism, as well as a number of less well-characterised parameters like sex, age, medication, genotype and others which all have an impact on the organification rate of dietary or supplemental Se sources. As the Se content of a given food item cannot be predicted precisely as it depends on the soil or food quality that was available during growth or breeding, there is no easy and reliable way of Se status assessment except for laboratory-based analyses. Overt signs of Se deficiency or selenosis only develop when Se intake strongly deviates from normal, which is rarely the case. It is therefore difficult to determine and maintain an optimal Se intake. Two reasonable approaches remain if one wants to be sure not to develop a health-relevant Se deficiency or selenosis, i.e. either providing a serum or plasma sample for analytical Se measurement or choosing one's diet wisely and consuming a variety of different food items, thereby avoiding a one-sided and potentially severely poor or highly enriched nutritional pattern of selenocompounds. In certain areas of central Asia and Africa, the habitual low Se supply is a serious health issue and needs to be addressed more seriously. In more developed societies, even though a number of well-conducted clinical studies indicate some health risks related to low Se intake, there is little evidence for a general Se deficit. Yet, certain circumstances seem to require a higher than normal intake, e.g. in chronic diseases, during one-sided or parenteral nutrition, in pregnancy and probably during growth in childhood and for a healthy ageing in the elderly. However, a solid database for far-reaching conclusions is not yet at hand, and additional cross-sectional and prospective clinical studies are needed to provide the insights necessary for a better counselling on this easily controlled and eminent important health and nutrition issue. With the growing choice of Se-enriched food items, we can assume that it will become easier and more convenient to avoiding a health-relevant Se deficit, at least in the industrialised countries. The problem of severe Se deficits in populations residing in poorly developed areas of the world remains as a pressing challenge that needs to be solved for the sake of humanity.

References

Abrams CK, Siram SM, Galsim C, Johnson-Hamilton H, Munford FL, Mezghebe H. Selenium deficiency in long-term total parenteral nutrition. Nutr Clin Pract. 1992;7(4):175–8.

Alfthan G, Eurola M, Ekholm P, Venalainen ER, Root T, Korkalainen K, et al. Effects of nationwide addition of selenium to fertilizers on foods, and animal and human health in Finland: from deficiency to optimal selenium status of the population. J Trace Elem Med Biol. 2015;31:142–7.

Ambroziak U, Hybsier S, Shahnazaryan U, Krasnodebska-Kiljanska M, Rijntjes E, Bartoszewicz Z, et al. Severe selenium deficits in pregnant women irrespective of autoimmune thyroid disease in an area with marginal selenium intake. J Trace Elem Med Biol. 2017;44:186–91.

Angstwurm MW, Engelmann L, Zimmermann T, Lehmann C, Spes CH, Abel P, et al. Selenium in Intensive Care (SIC): results of a prospective randomized, placebo-controlled, multiple-center study in patients with severe systemic inflammatory response syndrome, sepsis, and septic shock. Crit Care Med. 2007;35(1):118–26.

Aro A, Alfthan G, Varo P. Effects of supplementation of fertilizers on human selenium status in Finland. Analyst. 1995;120(3):841–3.

Bierla K, Dernovics M, Vacchina V, Szpunar J, Bertin G, Lobinski R. Determination of selenocysteine and selenomethionine in edible animal tissues by 2D size-exclusion reversed-phase HPLC-ICP MS following carbamidomethylation and proteolytic extraction. Anal Bioanal Chem. 2008;390(7):1789–98.

Brodin O, Eksborg S, Wallenberg M, Asker-Hagelberg C, Larsen EH, Mohlkert D, et al. Pharmacokinetics and toxicity of sodium selenite in the treatment of patients with carcinoma in a Phase I Clinical Trial: The SECAR Study. Nutrients. 2015;7(6):4978–94.

Burk RF, Hill KE. Selenoprotein P-expression, functions, and roles in mammals. Biochim Biophys Acta. 2009;1790(11):1441–7.

Burk RF, Hill KE, Motley AK. Plasma selenium in specific and non-specific forms. Biofactors. 2001;14(1-4):107–14.

Chang JC, Gutenmann WH, Reid CM, Lisk DJ. Selenium content of Brazil nuts from two geographic locations in Brazil. Chemosphere. 1995;30(4):801–2.

Clark LC, Combs GF Jr, Turnbull BW, Slate EH, Chalker DK, Chow J, et al. Effects of selenium supplementation for cancer prevention in patients with carcinoma of the skin. A randomized controlled trial. Nutritional Prevention of Cancer Study Group. JAMA. 1996;276(24):1957–63.

Combs GF Jr, Watts JC, Jackson MI, Johnson LK, Zeng H, Scheett AJ, et al. Determinants of selenium status in healthy adults. Nutr J. 2011;10:75.

Contempre B, Vanderpas J, Dumont JE. Cretinism, thyroid hormones and selenium. Mol Cell Endocrinol. 1991;81(1–3):C193–5.

Corvilain B, Contempre B, Longombe AO, Goyens P, Gervydecoster C, Lamy F, et al. Selenium and the thyroid—how the relationship was established. Am J Clin Nutr. 1993;57(2):244–8.

Derumeaux H, Valeix P, Castetbon K, Bensimon M, Boutron-Ruault MC, Arnaud J, et al. Association of selenium with thyroid volume and echostructure in 35- to 60-year-old French adults. Eur J Endocrinol. 2003;148(3):309–15.

Duffield-Lillico AJ, Dalkin BL, Reid ME, Turnbull BW, Slate EH, Jacobs ET, et al. Selenium supplementation, baseline plasma selenium status and incidence of prostate cancer: an analysis of the complete treatment period of the Nutritional Prevention of Cancer Trial. BJU Int. 2003;91(7):608–12.

Farebrother J, Naude CE, Nicol L, Andersson M, Zimmermann MB. Iodised salt and iodine supplements for prenatal and postnatal growth: a rapid scoping of existing systematic reviews. Nutr J. 2015;14:89.

Handy DE, Hang G, Scolaro J, Metes N, Razaq N, Yang Y, et al. Aminoglycosides decrease glutathione peroxidase-1 activity by interfering with selenocysteine incorporation. J Biol Chem. 2006;281(6):3382–8.

Hansen JC, Deutch B, Pedersen HS. Selenium status in Greenland Inuit. Sci Total Environ. 2004;331(1–3):207–14.

Hargreaves MK, Liu J, Buchowski MS, Patel KA, Larson CO, Schlundt DG, et al. Plasma selenium biomarkers in low income black and white americans from the southeastern United States. PLoS One. 2014;9(1):e84972.

Hatfield DL, Gladyshev VN. The outcome of Selenium and Vitamin E Cancer Prevention Trial (SELECT) reveals the need for better understanding of selenium biology. Mol Interv. 2009;9(1):18–21.

Hoefig CS, Renko K, Kohrle J, Birringer M, Schomburg L. Comparison of different selenocompounds with respect to nutritional value vs. toxicity using liver cells in culture. J Nutr Biochem. 2011;22(10):945–55.

Hoeflich J, Hollenbach B, Behrends T, Hoeg A, Stosnach H, Schomburg L. The choice of biomarkers determines the selenium status in young German vegans and vegetarians. Br J Nutr. 2010;104(11):1601–4.

Hughes DJ, Fedirko V, Jenab M, Schomburg L, Meplan C, Freisling H, et al. Selenium status is associated with colorectal cancer risk in the European prospective investigation of cancer and nutrition cohort. Int J Cancer. 2015;136(5):1149–61.

Ioannidis JP. Implausible results in human nutrition research. BMJ. 2013;347:f6698.

Jablonska E, Vinceti M. Selenium and human health: witnessing a copernican revolution? J Environ Sci Health C. 2015;33(3):328–68.

Judd PA, Long A, Butcher M, Caygill CP, Diplock AT. Vegetarians and vegans may be most at risk from low selenium intakes. Brit Med J. 1997;314(7097):1834.

Kieliszek M, Blazejak S, Gientka I, Bzducha-Wrobel A. Accumulation and metabolism of selenium by yeast cells. Appl Microbiol Biotechnol. 2015;99(13):5373–82.

Kipp AP, Strohm D, Brigelius-Flohe R, Schomburg L, Bechthold A, Leschik-Bonnet E, et al. Revised reference values for selenium intake. J Trace Elem Med Biol. 2015;32:195–9.

Klein EA, Thompson IM, Tangen CM, Crowley JJ, Lucia MS, Goodman PJ, et al. Vitamin E and the risk of prostate cancer: the Selenium and Vitamin E Cancer Prevention Trial (SELECT). J Am Med Assoc. 2011;306(14):1549–56.

Kobayashi Y, Ogra Y, Ishiwata K, Takayama H, Aimi N, Suzuki KT. Selenosugars are key and urinary metabolites for selenium excretion within the required to low-toxic range. Proc Natl Acad Sci U S A. 2002;99(25):15932–6.

Kohrle J, Jakob F, Contempre B, Dumont JE. Selenium, the thyroid, and the endocrine system. Endocr Rev. 2005;26(7):944–84.

Lenz M, Lens PNL. The essential toxin: The changing perception of selenium in environmental sciences. Sci Total Environ. 2009;407(12):3620–33.

Lippman SM, Goodman PJ, Klein EA, Parnes HL, Thompson IM Jr, Kristal AR, et al. Designing the selenium and Vitamin E Cancer Prevention Trial (SELECT). J Natl Cancer Inst. 2005;97(2):94–102.

Marschall TA, Bornhorst J, Kuehnelt D, Schwerdtle T. Differing cytotoxicity and bioavailability of selenite, methylselenocysteine, selenomethionine, selenosugar 1 and trimethylselenonium ion and their underlying metabolic transformations in human cells. Mol Nutr Food Res. 2016;60(12):2622–32.

McCann JC, Ames BN. Adaptive dysfunction of selenoproteins from the perspective of the triage theory: why modest selenium deficiency may increase risk of diseases of aging. FASEB J. 2011;25(6):1793–814.

Monsen ER. Dietary reference intakes for the antioxidant nutrients: vitamin C, vitamin E, selenium, and carotenoids. J Am Diet Assoc. 2000;100(6):637–40.

Moosmann B, Behl C. Selenoprotein synthesis and side-effects of statins. Lancet. 2004;363(9412):892–4.

Morris JS, Crane SB. Selenium toxicity from a misformulated dietary supplement, adverse health effects, and the temporal response in the nail biologic monitor. Nutrients. 2013;5(4):1024–57.

Ogra Y, Anan Y. Selenometabolomics explored by speciation. Biol Pharm Bull. 2012;35(11):1863–9.

Oguri T, Hattori M, Yamawaki T, Tanida S, Sasaki M, Joh T, et al. Neurological deficits in a patient with selenium deficiency due to long-term total parenteral nutrition. J Neurol. 2012;259(8):1734–5.

Polanska K, Krol A, Sobala W, Gromadzinska J, Brodzka R, Calamandrei G, et al. Selenium status during pregnancy and child psychomotor development-Polish Mother and Child Cohort study. Pediatr Res. 2016;79(6):863–9.

Quinn CF, Freeman JL, Reynolds RJ, Cappa JJ, Fakra SC, Marcus MA, et al. Selenium hyperaccumulation offers protection from cell disruptor herbivores. BMC Ecol. 2010;10:19.

Rasmussen L, Schomburg L, Köhrle J, Pedersen IB, Hollenbach B, Hog A, et al. Selenium status, thyroid volume and multiple nodule formation in an area with mild iodine deficiency. Eur J Endocrinol. 2011;164(4):585–90.

Reid ME, Duffield-Lillico AJ, Slate E, Natarajan N, Turnbull B, Jacobs E, et al. The nutritional prevention of cancer: 400 mcg per day selenium treatment. Nutr Cancer. 2008;60(2):155–63.

Renko K, Werner M, Renner-Müller I, Cooper TG, Yeung CH, Hollenbach B, et al. Hepatic selenoprotein P (SePP) expression restores selenium transport and prevents infertility and motor-incoordination in Sepp-knockout mice. Biochem J. 2008;409(3):741–9.

Renko K, Hofmann PJ, Stoedter M, Hollenbach B, Behrends T, Kohrle J, et al. Down-regulation of the hepatic selenoprotein biosynthesis machinery impairs selenium metabolism during the acute phase response in mice. FASEB J. 2009;23(6):1758–65.

Schiavon M, Pilon-Smits EA. The fascinating facets of plant selenium accumulation—biochemistry, physiology, evolution and ecology. New Phytol. 2017;213(4):1582–96.

Schomburg L. Selenium, selenoproteins and the thyroid gland: interactions in health and disease. Nat Rev Endocrinol. 2011;8(3):160–71.

Schomburg L, Schweizer U. Hierarchical regulation of selenoprotein expression and sex-specific effects of selenium. Biochim Biophys Acta. 2009;1790(11):1453–62.

Schrauzer GN. The nutritional significance, metabolism and toxicology of selenomethionine. Adv Food Nutr Res. 2003;47:73–112.

Schulze KJ, Christian P, Wu LS, Arguello M, Cui H, Nanayakkara-Bind A, et al. Micronutrient deficiencies are common in 6- to 8-year-old children of rural Nepal, with prevalence estimates modestly affected by inflammation. J Nutr. 2014;144(6):979–87.

Schweizer U, Towell H, Vit A, Rodriguez-Ruiz A, Steegborn C. Structural aspects of thyroid hormone binding to proteins and competitive interactions with natural and synthetic compounds. Mol Cell Endocrinol. 2017;458:57–67.

Senthilkumaran S, Balamurugan N, Vohra R, Thirumalaikolundusubramanian P. Paradise nut paradox: alopecia due to selenosis from a nutritional therapy. Int J Trichology. 2012;4(4):283–4.

Sindelarova K, Szakova J, Tremlova J, Mestek O, Praus L, Kana A, et al. The response of broccoli (Brassica oleracea convar. italica) varieties on foliar application of selenium: uptake, translocation, and speciation. Food Addit Contam Part A Chem Anal Control Expo Risk Assess. 2015;32(12):2027–38.

Speckmann B, Sies H, Steinbrenner H. Attenuation of hepatic expression and secretion of selenoprotein P by metformin. Biochem Biophys Res Commun. 2009;387(1):158–63.

Steinbrenner H, Speckmann B, Klotz LO. Selenoproteins: antioxidant selenoenzymes and beyond. Arch Biochem Biophys. 2016;595:113–9.

Stewart WC, Bobe G, Pirelli GJ, Mosher WD, Hall JA. Organic and inorganic selenium: III. Ewe and progeny performance. J Anim Sci. 2012;90(12):4536–43.

Stoffaneller R, Morse NL. A review of dietary selenium intake and selenium status in Europe and the Middle East. Nutrients. 2015;7(3):1494–537.

Suhajda A, Hegoczki J, Janzso B, Pais I, Vereczkey G. Preparation of selenium yeasts I. Preparation of selenium-enriched Saccharomyces cerevisiae. J Trace Elem Med Biol. 2000;14(1):43–7.

Takahashi K, Suzuki N, Ogra Y. Bioavailability comparison of nine bioselenocompounds in vitro and in vivo. Int J Mol Sci. 2017;18(3):506. https://doi.org/10.3390/ijms18030506.

Wang Y, Gao X, Pedram P, Shahidi M, Du J, Yi Y, et al. Significant beneficial association of high dietary selenium intake with reduced body fat in the CODING Study. Nutrients. 2016;8(1):E24. https://doi.org/10.3390/nu8010024.

White PJ. Selenium accumulation by plants. Ann Bot. 2016;117(2):217–35.

Wiehe L, Cremer M, Wisniewska M, Becker NP, Rijntjes E, Martitz J, et al. Selenium status in neonates with connatal infection. Br J Nutr. 2016;116(3):504–13.

Wiesner-Reinhold M, Schreiner M, Baldermann S, Schwarz D, Hanschen FS, Kipp AP, et al. Mechanisms of selenium enrichment and measurement in brassicaceous vegetables, and their application to human health. Front Plant Sci. 2017;8:1365.

Winkel LH, Vriens B, Jones GD, Schneider LS, Pilon-Smits E, Banuelos GS. Selenium cycling across soil-plant-atmosphere interfaces: a critical review. Nutrients. 2015;7(6):4199–239.

Wu L. Review of 15 years of research on ecotoxicology and remediation of land contaminated by agricultural drainage sediment rich in selenium. Ecotoxicol Environ Saf. 2004;57(3):257–69.

Wu Q, Rayman MP, Lv H, Schomburg L, Cui B, Gao C, et al. Low population selenium status is associated with increased prevalence of thyroid disease. J Clin Endocrinol Metab. 2015;100(11):4037–47.

Xia Y, Hill KE, Li P, Xu J, Zhou D, Motley AK, et al. Optimization of selenoprotein P and other plasma selenium biomarkers for the assessment of the selenium nutritional requirement: a placebo-controlled, double-blind study of selenomethionine supplementation in selenium-deficient Chinese subjects. Am J Clin Nutr. 2010;92(3):525–31.

Yang G, Yin S, Zhou R, Gu L, Yan B, Liu Y. Studies of safe maximal daily dietary Se-intake in a seleniferous area in China. Part II: Relation between Se-intake and the manifestation of clinical signs and certain biochemical alterations in blood and urine. J Trace Elem Electrolytes Health Dis. 1989;3(3):123–30.

Yao YF, Pei FX, Kang PD. Selenium, iodine, and the relation with Kashin-Beck disease. Nutrition. 2011;27(11-12):1095–100.

Part III
Genes, Proteins, Pathways, and Metabolism Related to Selenium

Chapter 4
Contribution of the Yeast *Saccharomyces cerevisiae* Model to Understand the Mechanisms of Selenium Toxicity

Myriam Lazard, Marc Dauplais, and Pierre Plateau

Abstract Selenium (Se) is an essential trace element for mammals. It is involved in redox functions as the amino acid selenocysteine, translationally inserted in the active site of a few proteins. However, at high doses it is toxic and the mechanisms underlying this toxicity are poorly understood. Because of the high level of conservation of its genes and pathways with those of higher organisms and the powerful genetic techniques that it offers, *Saccharomyces cerevisiae* is an attractive model organism to study the molecular basis of Se toxicity. High-throughput technologies developed in this yeast include genome-wide screening of bar-coded systematic deletion sets, as well as whole-transcriptome, -proteome, and -metabolome analysis.

This chapter focuses on the contribution of *S. cerevisiae* to the understanding of the mechanisms of selenocompound toxicity, combining results from classical biochemistry with genome-wide analyses and more detailed gene-by-gene approaches. Experimental data demonstrate that toxicity is compound specific. Inorganic Se induces DNA damage whereas selenoamino acids cause proteotoxicity.

Keywords Selenium · Selenomethionine · Selenocysteine · Selenite · Selenide · Yeast · Genome-wide

Introduction

Selenium (Se) has attracted considerable interest in the last decades for its reported beneficial effects on the prevention of several cancers and other diseases (see chapters Part V – VII) but also from a toxicological perspective because of the narrow margin between intakes that result in efficacy and toxicity. As a trace element, it is required to synthetize a few selenoproteins, in which Se is specifically incorporated as the amino acid selenocysteine (SeCys) (Böck et al. 1991). The translational

M. Lazard (✉) · M. Dauplais · P. Plateau
Laboratoire de Biochimie, Ecole Polytechnique, CNRS, Université Paris-Saclay,
91128 Palaiseau Cedex, France
e-mail: myriam.lazard@polytechnique.edu

© Springer International Publishing AG, part of Springer Nature 2018
B. Michalke (ed.), *Selenium*, Molecular and Integrative Toxicology,
https://doi.org/10.1007/978-3-319-95390-8_4

incorporation of SeCys into a selenoprotein requires an elaborate machinery that uses selenophosphate as Se donor (Turanov et al. 2011). Selenophosphate is synthesized by selenophosphate synthetase from ATP and selenide (H_2Se/HSe^-). In spite of the importance for humans of low levels of Se intake, there is accumulating evidence that adverse health effects are associated with excess dietary Se supplementation (Jablonska and Vinceti 2015). Thus, the safe range of dietary Se intake is still uncertain. Despite its medical importance, our understanding of the molecular mechanisms underlying Se toxic mode of action remains limited.

Both inorganic and organic forms of Se can serve as nutritional source to be used for selenoprotein synthesis. Selenate (SeO_4^{2-}) and selenite (SeO_3^{2-}) are metabolically reduced to selenide, the precursor used for SeCys insertion. Organic selenomethionine (SeMet) can be metabolized, first to SeCys by the transsulfuration pathway then to selenide by selenocysteine β-lyase that degrades SeCys to selenide. Numerous studies were performed to evaluate the cytotoxic effects of different forms of Se in cell culture assays and in animal models. The results obtained in these studies varied considerably depending on chemical form, concentration, exposure time, and type of cells used in the assay (Valdiglesias et al. 2010).

Metabolization of selenocompounds in vivo gives rise to multiple different metabolites (Arnaudguilhem et al. 2012; Preud'homme et al. 2012). Therefore, the biological activity of different Se species depends upon their transformation into different active products (Weekley and Harris 2013). Studies aimed at defining the metabolic pathways used by Se metabolic intermediaries is an important step to better understand both the beneficial and toxic mechanisms of Se in human biology. To this end, the budding yeast *Saccharomyces cerevisiae* is a suitable model. Firstly, this organism, like all fungi and plants, lacks the pathway for the genetically encoded incorporation of SeCys into proteins, which precludes interferences between Se metabolism and function of Se incorporated in the active site of selenoenzymes. Secondly, its ease of manipulation and amenability to genetic modifications make it easy to study strains deleted for individual genes in a particular pathway. Lastly, since *S. cerevisiae* was the first eukaryote to have its complete genome sequenced, it has become a pioneer organism for high-throughput systematic approaches at the genome, transcriptome, and proteome levels (Botstein and Fink 2011). Functional information is available for up to 90% of the nearly 6000 *S. cerevisiae* genes. Moreover, functional pathways that control key aspects of eukaryotic cell biology, including the cell cycle, protein quality control, vesicular transport, and many key signalling pathways, are well conserved between yeast and human (Dolinski and Botstein 2007). Kachroo et al. (2015) showed that a substantial portion (nearly 50% of the tested genes) of conserved genes perform much the same roles in both organisms—to an extent that the protein-coding DNA of a human gene can actually substitute for that of the yeast. It is, thus, expected that knowledge gathered in the yeast model will be relevant to elucidate the toxicity of Se in higher eukaryotes.

Mechanisms of Inorganic Se Toxicity

Inorganic Se is commonly found in four oxidation states: +6 (e.g., selenate), +4 (selenite), 0 (Se⁰, elemental Se), and −2 (selenide) (Cupp-Sutton and Ashby 2016). Inorganic Se compounds do not have specific transporters for uptake in *S. cerevisiae*. Selenate is taken up by sulfate transporters (Cherest et al. 1997) and reduced to selenite by the sulfate reduction pathway (Fig. 4.1). Selenite was shown to be transported by a high-affinity system and a low-affinity system operating at different selenite concentrations (Gharieb and Gadd 2004). These systems were later characterized as the high- and low-affinity phosphate transporters (Lazard et al. 2010). When yeast cells are cultured in a non-glucose medium, selenite is taken up

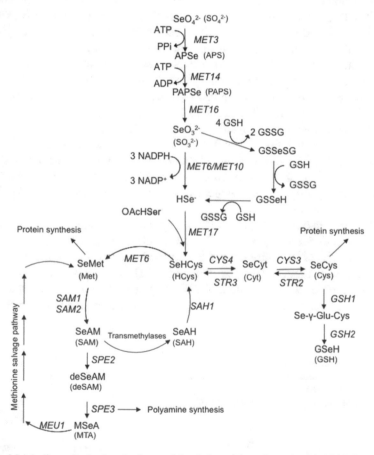

Fig. 4.1 Metabolism of selenium in *S. cerevisiae* (adapted from Lazard et al. 2015; Thomas and Surdin-Kerjan 1997). Names of genes involved in enzymatic reactions are indicated as well as the sulfur-containing analogues (indicated below in brackets). Abbreviations not used in the main text are as follows: *APSe* adenylyl-selenate, *PAPSe* phosphoadenylyl-selenate, *deSeAM* decarboxylated SeAM, *MSeA* methylselenoadenosine, *SeCyt* selenocystathionine, *OAcHSer* O-acetylhomoserine

efficiently by the monocarboxylate transporter Jen1p (McDermott et al. 2010). Elemental selenium, which is insoluble, is not expected to be transported across membranes. Volatile H_2Se is believed to cross membranes by diffusion.

Selenite Toxicity

Selenite was the first Se compound to be extensively studied with respect to its toxicity. In 1941, Painter proposed that selenite reacts with intracellular thiols (RSH) (Painter 1941). Later investigations demonstrated that selenite is reduced by glutathione (GSH) to hydrogen selenide according to the scheme presented in Fig. 4.2a (Ganther 1968; Ganther 1971; Tarze et al. 2007). It first reacts spontaneously with GSH to produce selenodiglutathione (GSSeSG). In the presence of excess glutathione, selenodiglutathione is further reduced into glutathione selenenylsulfide (GSSeH). The latter either spontaneously dismutates into Se^0 and glutathione or is further reduced by glutathione to yield H_2Se/HSe^-. Alternatively, H_2Se can result from the reduction of selenite by other thiols (cysteine, thioredoxin, ...) or can be enzymatically produced by glutathione reductase or thioredoxin reductase (Hsieh and Ganther 1975; Björnstedt et al. 1997). H_2Se/HSe^- is readily oxidized by oxygen with concomitant generation of ROS (Fig. 4.2b) (Chaudiere et al. 1992; Kitahara et al. 1993; Seko and Imura 1997). This reaction produces $Se^{(0)}$, which can be reduced by thiols with regeneration of H_2Se/HSe^- that will initiate a new cycle of oxidation/reduction. These redox cycles consume intracellular antioxidants such as thioredoxin and GSH and, consequently, the reducing cofactor NADPH (Kumar et al. 1992).

Early works in bacterial and cell culture systems indicated that selenite had the potential to produce damage to DNA (Nakamuro et al. 1976). Whiting and coworkers (1980) found that GSH addition to the culture medium enhanced selenite-dependent DNA damage and proposed that this damage might be the result of radical formation in the oxidation of selenide or GSSeH. Garberg et al. found that selenite-induced DNA fragmentation was oxygen dependent and suggested that redox cycles were

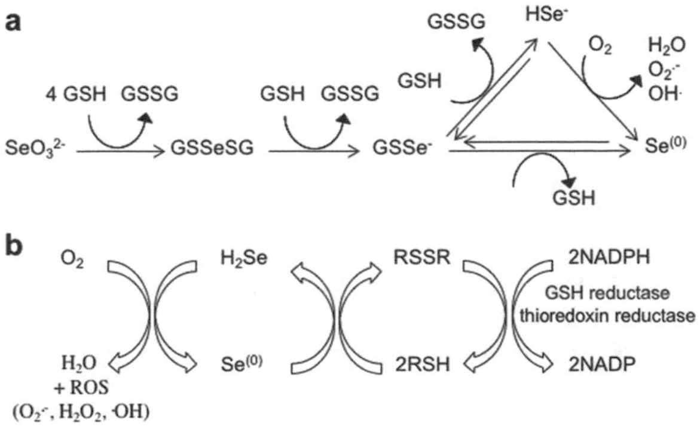

Fig. 4.2 Redox reactions of inorganic selenium compounds. (**a**) Selenite reduction by GSH. (**b**) Selenide redox cycling

involved in these DNA alterations (Garberg and Hogberg 1987; Garberg et al. 1988). Later investigations in a variety of organisms, including budding yeast, confirmed that selenite toxicity involves ROS-dependent DNA strand breaks and/or base oxidations that can lead to cell death (for review, see Letavayová et al. 2006a; Brozmanová et al. 2010; Misra et al. 2015; Herrero and Wellinger 2015).

Cells have evolved a number of mechanisms to detect and repair the various types of damage that occur in DNA (Chalissery et al. 2017). Base lesions produced by oxidative damage are generally recognized and repaired by base excision repair (BER) and nucleotide excision repair (NER) pathways (Boiteux and Guillet 2004). The lesions that block the replicating DNA polymerases, stopping the progression of the replication fork, are overcome by post-replication repair (PRR). This mechanism prevents replication fork collapse by recruiting specialized translesion DNA polymerases that are able to replicate past DNA lesions (Prakash et al. 2005). When DNA polymerase encounters a single-strand break (SSB), collapse of the replication fork generates double-strand breaks (DSB), which are repaired by nonhomologous end joining (NHEJ) and homologous recombination (HR) pathways (Krogh and Symington 2004). HR uses homologous DNA sequences (usually in the sister chromatid) as templates for repairing broken ends. Thus, HR is normally considered to be restricted to S and G2 phases of the cell cycle. DSBs induce the activation of DNA damage checkpoints that stop the progression of the cell cycle and provide additional time for the damage repair process (Foiani et al. 2000). Most of these repair pathways are conserved from prokaryotes to higher eukaryotes.

Studies of yeast deletion mutants have been helpful to determine the genes and pathways involved in the response to selenite. Letavayová et al. showed that selenite induces DSBs and chromosome fragmentation (Letavayová et al. 2008a). Such lesions are expected to be repaired primarily by homologous recombination in yeast. Accordingly, a *rad52* (a key gene in the HR pathway) mutant was found to be hypersensitive to sodium selenite and unable to repair selenite-induced DSBs, whereas inactivation of *YKU70*, a gene involved in NHEJ, showed no effect (Letavayová et al. 2006b, 2008b). Another deletion that confers hypersensitivity to selenite was found in *RAD9*, a DNA-damage checkpoint gene, required for transient cell cycle arrest and activation of DNA repair mechanisms in response to DSBs (Pinson et al. 2000). A recent genome-wide study of yeast gene deletion mutants confirmed the importance of HR in the resistance to selenite exposure (Mániková et al. 2012). Among the 39 mutants identified as highly sensitive, 9 corresponded to deletions in genes involved in HR (*MMS4, MUS81, RAD50, RAD51, RAD52, RAD54, RAD55, RAD57, XRS2*).

The sensitivity to selenite of specific DNA repair-defective mutants revealed that DNA repair pathways different from HR also contribute to the protection of yeast against selenite exposure. A first study on the role of the BER pathway in the protection against selenite damage found that single mutations in this pathway (*ogg1, ntg1, ntg2,* and *apn1*) did not affect growth in the presence of selenite, whereas a triple *ntg1-ntg2-apn1* mutant was slightly more sensitive than the parental strain (Pinson et al. 2000). Another study (Maniková et al. 2010) confirmed that single mutants in the BER repair pathway were not affected by selenite but that several multiple mutants (*apn1-apn2*, *apn1-tpp1*, *apn1-apn2-tpp1*, *ntg1-ntg2-apn1*) were sensitive to selenite, suggesting that selenite induces DNA base oxidative lesions that are recognized by the BER repair pathway.

Hypersensitivity to selenite was also associated with deletion of several genes involved in the PRR pathway. Pinson et al. showed that a *rev3* mutant was significantly more sensitive to selenite than the wild type (Pinson et al. 2000). *REV3* encodes the catalytic subunit of DNA polymerase ζ (pol ζ), which plays a key role in the replication past DNA lesions during PRR (Rattray and Strathern 2003) and is also involved in the repair of DNA double-strand breaks (Kolas and Durocher 2006). In another genetic context, Seitomer et al. did not observe an effect of the *rev3* deletion but found that hypersensitivity to selenite was associated with deletion of other genes involved in the PRR pathway such as *mms2*, *rad5*, *rad6*, *rad18*, and *rev7*, the gene encoding the regulatory subunit of pol ζ (Seitomer et al. 2008). Analysis of *rad5-rad52* and *rad6-rad52* double mutants revealed a synergistic effect between HR and PRR pathways, suggesting that both pathways are active in the removal of DNA damage induced by selenite (Máníková et al. 2012).

Although DNA repair proteins are necessary for survival to selenite stress, a transcriptome analysis indicated that, apart from a few genes such as *RAD52*, *RDH54*, *RFA1-3*, *RAD6*, and *POL30*, virtually no transcriptional activation was observed for genes involved in DNA repair following selenite treatment (Máníková et al. 2012). This finding is not altogether unexpected, as it has already been shown that transcription of most of the genes involved in protection against DNA damage was not stimulated in response to toxic doses of several DNA-damaging agents (Birrell et al. 2002).

Apart from DNA damage, a large body of evidence also attests that selenite exposure causes an oxidative stress. A yeast genome-wide transcriptome analysis revealed that selenite treatment upregulated genes involved in the oxidative stress response under the control of the Yap1p transcription factor (Salin et al. 2008). Yap1p was itself found to be upregulated at the mRNA level following selenite treatment. Several gene targets of Yap1p, such as *GLR1* and *TRR1*, encoding glutathione reductase and cytosolic thioredoxin reductase, respectively, were found to be strongly upregulated (4- and 14-fold, respectively) by selenite treatment in a Yap1p-dependent manner (Pinson et al. 2000). Upregulation of oxidative stress-responsive genes was also observed in a transcriptome analysis in a different genetic background (Perez-Sampietro et al. 2016). In a genome-wide screen, deletion mutants corresponding to two proteins involved in GSH metabolism, glutathione reductase (*glr1*) and γ-glutamylcysteine synthetase (*gsh1*), were found to be among the most sensitive mutants to selenite (Máníková et al. 2012). In contrast, overexpression of Glr1p, which converts oxidized glutathione (GSSG) back to GSH, was shown to increase cell resistance to selenite (Pinson et al. 2000). In agreement, analysis of single-deletion mutants for selenite sensitivity showed that several genes belonging to the glutathione redox pathway, such as *GSH1*, *GLR1*, *GRX1, GRX2, GRX3, GRX5*, and *YAP1*, are important for tolerance to selenite exposure (Pinson et al. 2000; Seitomer et al. 2008; Lewinska and Bartosz 2008; Izquierdo et al. 2010). The increased sensitivity of mutants in genes involved in

GSH homeostasis is likely linked to the oxidation of GSH by the reductive metabolism of selenite resulting in a severe decrease of the reduced/oxidized ratio of all low-molecular-weight thiols (glutathione, cysteine, homocysteine, γ-glutamyl-cysteine, and cysteinyl-glycine) (Rao et al. 2010).

Deletion of *YCF1*, encoding a vacuolar transporter which detoxifies heavy metals by sequestration in the vacuole as GSH conjugates, confers increased resistance to selenite exposure (Pinson et al. 2000). Conversely, overexpression of Ycf1p exacerbates selenite toxicity (Lazard et al. 2011). Ycf1p was shown to transport the unstable selenodiglutathione (GSSeSG) metabolite of selenite, which is expected to further react with GSH in the vacuole and produce HSe^- and GSSG (see Fig. 4.2). This provides a rationale for the unexpected resistance of the $\Delta ycf1$ mutant. Diffusion of volatile HSe^- to the cytosol, while GSSG is retained in the vacuole, would cause a detrimental cytosolic GSH depletion (Lazard et al. 2011). It was, indeed, shown that the selenite-induced decrease of the GSH/GSSG ratio (Rao et al. 2010) is exacerbated by Ycf1p overexpression (Lazard et al. 2011).

Selenide Toxicity

It is likely that the reduction of selenite into HSe^-, in vivo, followed by redox cycling of selenide in the presence of oxygen and thiols, accounts for selenite-induced DNA damage. Thus, in vitro studies on the mechanism of DNA cleavage by selenite derivatives showed that selenite alone was unable to produce DNA strand breaks (Peyroche et al. 2012). Single-strand breaks were only detected upon addition of GSH or when DNA was incubated in the presence of HSe^-. The reaction was inhibited by mannitol, a hydroxyl radical quencher, but not by superoxide dismutase or catalase, suggesting that selenide reaction with oxygen generated hydroxyl-like radicals. An ˙OH signature could, indeed, be detected by electron spin resonance upon exposure of a solution of hydrogen selenide to O_2. Hydroxyl radicals can cleave a DNA strand by abstracting a hydrogen atom from a deoxyribose sugar in the DNA backbone (Balasubramanian et al. 1998).

In accordance with the idea that H_2Se/HSe^- is the effector of selenite toxicity, a screen of a collection of yeast deletion mutant strains for hypersensitivity to sodium selenide revealed a strong enrichment for HR, DNA-damage checkpoint genes, and GSH redox pathway genes (Peyroche et al. 2012). Thus, the set of genes required for selenide tolerance strongly overlap with that observed to confer protection against selenite (Fig. 4.3), lending support to the assumption that toxicity is exerted by the reduction of inorganic Se to HSe^-.

When SSBs occur during DNA replication (S phase), they can be converted to more lethal DSBs by replication fork collapse, whereas damage occurring after replication is completed leaves cell more time for correction by specialized DNA polymerases and ligases. This may explain the higher sensitivity to selenide of exponentially growing yeast cells compared to nondividing stationary-phase cells

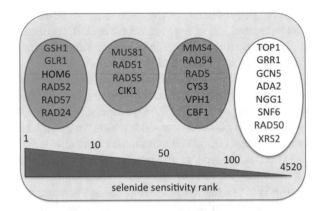

Fig. 4.3 Overlap between mutants sensitive to selenite or selenide. Among the 39 deletion mutants that were defined as selenite hypersensitive in Mániková et al. (2012), 24 were also analyzed in a genome-wide screen for selenide sensitivity. In the latter study, mutants were ranked from 1 (most sensitive) to 4520 (most resistant) (Peyroche et al. 2012). 6 selenite-sensitive mutants rank below 10 (circled in red), 4 rank between 10 and 50 (circled in orange), 6 rank between 50 and 100 (circled in yellow), and 8 (in a blank box) rank higher than 100. Genes involved in GSH metabolism are colored in blue, and those involved in DNA damage response are in red

(Fig. 4.4), as already observed by Letavayová et al. following exposure to selenite (Letavayová et al. 2008a). Consistent with the idea that DSBs are the major cause of selenide-induced lethality, G2/M cell cycle checkpoint is activated by selenide exposure (Peyroche et al. 2012). This results in a cell cycle arrest that prevents cells from undergoing mitosis before damage is repaired. Failure of the repair mechanism results in chromosome fragmentation as observed by a pulsed-field gel electrophoresis analysis.

Altogether, these studies suggest that inorganic Se toxic mechanisms involve reduction to H_2Se, redox cycling of the latter with oxygen and thiols, resulting in redox imbalance and generation of ROS that kill cells mainly through DNA damage.

Mechanisms of Toxicity of Selenoamino Acids

The mechanism of SeMet toxicity is understood less than that of selenite (Kitajima and Chiba 2013; Lazard et al. 2017). Here again, the use of yeast mutants has brought insights into the mechanisms of cytotoxicity. Seitomer et al. (2008) compared the effects of SeMet and selenite on the growth of wild-type yeast cells and mutants affected in the DNA repair and oxidative stress-response pathways. This study indicated the lesser importance of DNA damage in SeMet versus selenite toxicity. In particular, several mutants involved in DNA repair that were shown to be hypersensitive to selenite (*rad9*, *rad18* for instance) displayed wild-type growth rates in the presence of SeMet. Several oxidative stress-responsive genes behaved oppositely under SeMet and selenite exposure. *sod1* and *zwf1* mutants displayed

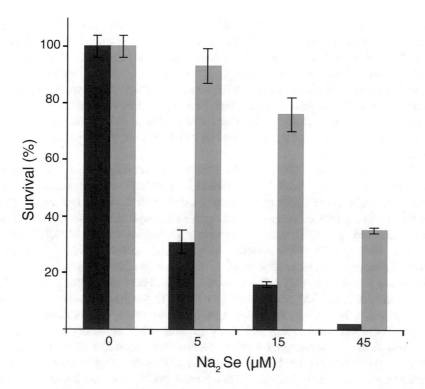

Fig. 4.4 Selenide is less toxic in stationary phase than in exponential phase. Exponentially growing (black bars) or stationary-phase (grey bars) BY4742 cells grown in rich medium (YPGlucose) were exposed for 5 min to the indicated concentrations of sodium selenide (Na$_2$Se). Then, cells were appropriately diluted and plated on YPGlucose-agar. Cell viability was determined after 2-day growth at 30 °C. The results are expressed as percentages of survival compared with control samples incubated in the absence of Na$_2$Se. The error bars represent the range of two independent experiments

sensitivity to SeMet but not to selenite and *yap1*, *glr1*, and *sod2* mutants were sensitive only to selenite. These results indicated that the mechanistic bases of SeMet and selenite toxicities are substantially different.

Because of the chemical similarity between Se and sulfur, most enzymes involved in sulfur metabolism do not discriminate between the two chalcogen elements. Thus, SeMet can be activated and transferred onto tRNA by methionyl-tRNA synthetase or used as substrate for *S*-adenosyl-methionine synthetase with similar efficiency to methionine (Colombani et al. 1975). To obtain high levels of SeMet-containing eukaryotic proteins suitable for X-ray crystallography, several studies have reported the production of yeast SeMet-resistant mutants. These strains have the ability to substitute up to 90% of the protein methioninyl residues by SeMet without strongly affecting cellular growth, indicating that misincorporation of SeMet does not impair protein homeostasis. In particular, Bockhorn et al. (2008) screened a collection of single-gene deletion mutants of *S. cerevisiae* for resistance to SeMet and demonstrated that a mutant lacking cystathionine γ-lyase activity (Δ*cys3*) showed the highest resistance to SeMet. Another mutation that allows a high level of SeMet/methionine substitution was found in the *MUP1* gene, which encodes the high-affinity methionine permease resulting in a reduced methionine (and SeMet) uptake (Kitajima et al. 2010). In another study, Malkowski et al. (2007) constructed a *S. cerevisiae sam1-sam2* mutant, unable to convert SeMet into *S*-adenosylmethionine (SAM). The toxicity of SeMet was dramatically reduced in this mutant, indicating that the cytotoxic compound is a metabolic product of SeMet rather than SeMet itself.

To gain insights into the metabolic product(s) underlying SeMet toxicity, we compared the sensitivity to SeMet of several *S. cerevisiae* mutants compromised in individual pathways of sulfur metabolism (Lazard et al. 2015). To test the effects of Se metabolites produced downstream from *Se*-adenosylmethionine (SeAM) in the polyamine and the methionine salvage pathways, strains deleted for *SPE2*, *SPE3*, *MEU1*, and *MDE1* were used. Δ*meu1* and Δ*mde1* cells accumulate methylthioadenosine and methylthioribulose-1-P, respectively, whereas Δ*spe2* and Δ*spe3* are impaired in polyamine synthesis immediately downstream from SAM and decarboxylated SAM, respectively (see Fig. 4.1). All the mutants behaved as the parental strain, indicating that impairing the polyamine or the methionine salvage pathways did not increase SeMet toxicity. Inhibition of transmethylation reactions resulting from an accumulation of *Se*-adenosylhomocysteine (SeAH) could be another way to induce growth inhibition. Western blotting using antibodies directed against methylated histone H3 shows that SeMet toxicity does not involve a general methylation deficiency (Fig. 4.5). In contrast, impairing the hydrolysis of SeAH, thereby reducing the amount of Se entering the transsulfuration pathway, increased SeMet resistance (Lazard et al. 2015), implying that the toxicity of SeMet involves selenohomocysteine (SeHCys) or its metabolization by the transsulfuration pathway. Because a Δ*cys3* mutant, unable to synthetize SeCys from SeMet, was shown to be resistant to SeMet (Bockhorn et al. 2008), SeCys and/or a downstream metabolite

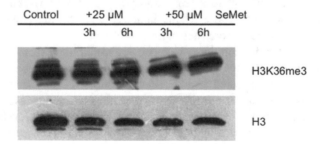

Fig. 4.5 Western blot analysis of histone H3 methylation. Protein extracts were prepared from BY4742 cells grown at 30 °C for 3 h in synthetic minimal medium (SD + 100 μM methionine; Lazard et al. 2015) (control) or for 3 or 6 h in the same medium supplemented with 25 μM or 50 μM SeMet. 10 μg of proteins was loaded on a 12% polyacrylamide gel and analyzed by western blotting using antibodies directed against histone H3 (H3) or histone H3 tri-methylated at position 36 (H3K36me3). Antibodies were purchased from Abcam

might be involved in SeMet toxicity. In contrast to SeMet, there is no published report on SeCys toxicity in *S. cerevisiae*. This is probably due to the rapid reaction of this amino acid with oxygen (half-life is less than 10 min at pH 7). In addition, the very poor transport of oxidized selenocystine across yeast membranes prohibits its use as a precursor of SeCys. Nevertheless, TCEP (tris(2-carboxyethyl)phosphine), a strong reducing agent that does not cross cell membranes, can keep SeCys in the reduced form in the growth medium. As shown in Fig. 4.6a, addition of 1 mM TCEP was able to maintain SeCys reduced for a couple of hours. We used these conditions to show that exposure to SeCys for 2 h, indeed, decreased the viability of yeast cells (Fig. 4.6b).

Recently, we screened a *S. cerevisiae* deletion collection for sensitivity or resistance to SeMet (Plateau et al. 2017). Gene Ontology (GO) analysis revealed that GO terms related to protein metabolic processes were significantly enriched in both the sensitive and resistant datasets (Fig. 4.7). Genes related to ubiquitin-mediated protein degradation, either via the proteasome complex or via the multivesicular body sorting pathway, were overrepresented among deletion mutants sensitive to SeMet. Mutants impaired in the translational process, including ribosomal subunits, proteins necessary for ribosome biogenesis, and several tRNA-modifying enzymes, represented around 50% of the SeMet-resistant dataset. Most of the null allele strains displaying a SeMet-resistant phenotype grew more slowly than the parental strain in the absence of stress, suggesting that a decreased growth rate provides an advantage under SeMet stress.

The importance of mechanisms related to the biosynthesis of proteins and to the removal of damaged proteins suggested that processes involved in protein homeostasis were major targets of SeMet toxicity. In support of this hypothesis, the expression of the chaperone protein Hsp104p, involved in the disaggregation and refolding of aggregated proteins, was shown to be induced upon SeMet exposure (Plateau et al. 2017). Fluorescence microscopy using an Hsp104-GFP construct revealed a dose-dependent accumulation of protein aggregates in cells exposed to increasing concentrations of SeMet. Protein aggregation, as well as SeMet-induced growth inhibition, was suppressed in the presence of cycloheximide, a potent translation initiation inhibitor or in a Δ*cys3* mutant strain in which SeCys cannot be formed from SeMet. Therefore, metabolization of SeMet to SeCys is necessary to generate toxic protein aggregation and SeCys misincorporation in nascent proteins is likely responsible for protein aggregation. In support of this hypothesis, proteomic analyses showed that the selenoamino acids SeMet and SeCys produced from inorganic Se (Bierla et al. 2013) or from SeMet exposure (Plateau et al. 2017) can be incorporated into proteins in the place of methionine and cysteine. In contrast to the seemingly harmless incorporation of SeMet, random replacement of cysteine by the more reactive SeCys is likely to induce misfolding and aggregation by formation of intermolecular or intramolecular selenylsulfide or diselenide bridges.

Low-molecular-weight selenols (RSeH) are also a potential source of toxicity. Indeed, they may react with essential protein thiols or oxidize to form diselenides or mixed selenylsulfides. Thus, mass spectrometry-based metabolomic studies in SeMet-treated cells showed that most of the selenols detected were in the oxidized

A

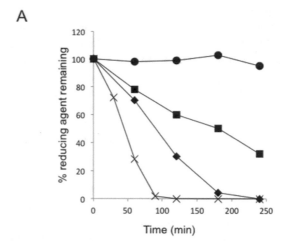

B

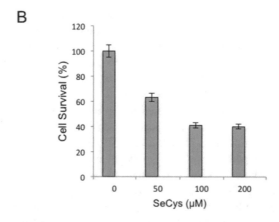

Fig. 4.6 SeCys oxidation and toxicity. (**a**) Time course of the oxidation of a TCEP/SeCys mixture. 0 (●), 50 μM (■), 100 μM (◆), or 200 μM (×) D,L-SeCys was incubated in the presence of 1 mM TCEP, in synthetic minimal medium (SD medium) at 30 °C. With time, SeCys is oxidized by oxygen into selenocystine, which is reduced back to SeCys by TCEP. As a consequence of these reactions, the reducing power of the sample progressively decreases. The concentration of remaining reducing equivalent was determined over time by measuring the absorbance at 412 nm after addition of 5,5′-dithiobis(2-nitrobenzoic acid) (DTNB) to an aliquot of the sample. (**b**) BY4742 cells, exponentially growing in SD medium, were exposed for 2 h to the indicated concentrations of D,L-SeCys, in the presence of 1 mM TCEP. Then, cells were appropriately diluted and plated on YPGlucose-agar. Cell viability was determined after 2-day growth at 30 °C. The results are expressed as percentages compared with survival of control samples incubated in the absence of SeCys. The error bars represent the range of two independent experiments

forms (Rao et al. 2010) and that low-molecular-weight reduced thiols were significantly decreased, with concomitant increase in diselenide and selenylsulfide compounds (Kitajima et al. 2012). Selenol oxidation by oxygen was shown to produce superoxide radicals in vitro and deletion of *SOD1*, the gene coding for superoxide

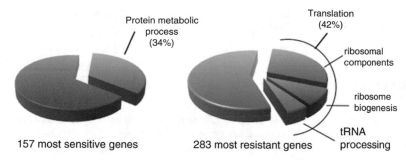

Fig. 4.7 Distribution of SeMet-sensitive and SeMet-resistant mutants according to biological processes affected. Adapted from Plateau et al. (2017). The 157 SeMet-sensitive and 283 SeMet-resistant genes, identified by genome-wide mutant fitness profiling, were analyzed for Gene Ontology (GO) term enrichment

dismutase, was shown to increase SeMet toxicity (Lazard et al. 2015). Therefore, ROS production may be involved in SeMet toxicity in yeast cells.

Conclusion

Because of its ease of manipulation and amenability to genetic modifications, studies using *S. cerevisiae* have significantly contributed to our understanding of the mechanisms that drive the toxicity of several Se compounds and shed light on the metabolic pathways that protect cells against these compounds. These studies have unambiguously demonstrated that the mode of action of Se is compound specific. Inorganic Se species that are metabolized into hydrogen selenide induce DNA damage. In contrast, selenoamino acids disrupt protein homeostasis by triggering protein aggregation. Several studies in animal or human cells have shown that selenite induces ROS-dependent DNA strand breaks and/or base oxidation that lead to cell death by apoptosis or necrosis (for review see Letavayová et al. 2006a). These results, therefore, support the notion that conclusions drawn from yeast research are relevant to higher eukaryotes. Likewise, SeCystine treatment was shown to induce the unfolded protein response in human cancer cells (Wallenberg et al. 2014) or increased proteasome activity and levels of ubiquitinated proteins in a plant (Dimkovikj et al. 2015) (for review see Lazard et al. 2017). Thus, in these organisms as in yeast, selenoamino acids are likely to induce protein damages. The power of yeast genetics may still be exploited in the future to dissect the molecular mechanisms involved in the toxicity of other Se compounds of clinical interest but whose biological mechanisms remain poorly understood, such as methylselenol or its precursors (methylselenocysteine, methylseleninic acid, or demethyldiselenide). Information gathered in yeast could again be helpful to guide research aiming at understanding the response of human cells to these compounds in a cancer preventive or therapeutic goal.

Acknowledgments The authors gratefully acknowledge Prof. Sylvain Blanquet for his contribution and constant interest and encouragements over many years.

References

Arnaudguilhem C, Bierla K, Ouerdane L, Preud'homme H, Yiannikouris A, Lobinski R. Selenium metabolomics in yeast using complementary reversed-phase/hydrophilic ion interaction (HILIC) liquid chromatography-electrospray hybrid quadrupole trap/Orbitrap mass spectrometry. Anal Chim Acta. 2012;757:26–38.

Balasubramanian B, Pogozelski WK, Tullius TD. DNA strand breaking by the hydroxyl radical is governed by the accessible surface areas of the hydrogen atoms of the DNA backbone. Proc Natl Acad Sci U S A. 1998;95:9738–43.

Bierla K, Bianga J, Ouerdane L, Szpunar J, Yiannikouris A, Lobinski R. A comparative study of the Se/S substitution in methionine and cysteine in Se-enriched yeast using an inductively coupled plasma mass spectrometry (ICP MS)-assisted proteomics approach. J Proteome. 2013;87:26–39.

Birrell GW, Brown JA, Wu HI, Giaever G, Chu AM, Davis RW, Brown JM. Transcriptional response of *Saccharomyces cerevisiae* to DNA-damaging agents does not identify the genes that protect against these agents. Proc Natl Acad Sci U S A. 2002;99:8778–83.

Björnstedt M, Kumar S, Björkhem L, Spyrou G, Holmgren A. Selenium and the thioredoxin and glutaredoxin systems. Biomed Environ Sci. 1997;10:271–9.

Böck A, Forchhammer K, Heider J, Baron C. Selenoprotein synthesis: an expansion of the genetic code. Trends Biochem Sci. 1991;16:463–7.

Bockhorn J, Balar B, He D, Seitomer E, Copeland PR, Kinzy TG. Genome-wide screen of *Saccharomyces cerevisiae* null allele strains identifies genes involved in selenomethionine resistance. Proc Natl Acad Sci U S A. 2008;105:17682–7.

Boiteux S, Guillet M. Abasic sites in DNA: repair and biological consequences in *Saccharomyces cerevisiae*. DNA Repair (Amst). 2004;3:1–12.

Botstein D, Fink GR. Yeast: an experimental organism for 21st century biology. Genetics. 2011;189:695–704.

Brozmanová J, Mániková D, Vlcková V, Chovanec M. Selenium: a double-edged sword for defense and offence in cancer. Arch Toxicol. 2010;84:919–38.

Chalissery J, Jalal D, Al-Natour Z, Hassan AH. Repair of oxidative DNA damage in *Saccharomyces cerevisiae*. DNA Repair (Amst). 2017;51:2–13.

Chaudiere J, Courtin O, Leclaire J. Glutathione oxidase activity of selenocystamine: a mechanistic study. Arch Biochem Biophys. 1992;296:328–36.

Cherest H, Davidian JC, Thomas D, Benes V, Ansorge W, Surdin-Kerjan Y. Molecular characterization of two high affinity sulfate transporters in *Saccharomyces cerevisiae*. Genetics. 1997;145:627–35.

Colombani F, Cherest H, de Robichon-Szulmajster H. Biochemical and regulatory effects of methionine analogues in *Saccharomyces cerevisiae*. J Bacteriol. 1975;122:375–84.

Cupp-Sutton K, Ashby M. Biological chemistry of hydrogen selenide. Antioxidants. 2016;5:42.

Dimkovikj A, Fisher B, Hutchison K, Van Hoewyk D. Stuck between a ROS and a hard place: analysis of the ubiquitin proteasome pathway in selenocysteine treated *Brassica napus* reveals different toxicities during selenium assimilation. J Plant Physiol. 2015;181:50–4.

Dolinski K, Botstein D. Orthology and functional conservation in eukaryotes. Annu Rev Genet. 2007;41:465–507.

Foiani M, Pellicioli A, Lopes M, Lucca C, Ferrari M, Liberi G, Muzi Falconi M, Plevani P. DNA damage checkpoints and DNA replication controls in *Saccharomyces cerevisiae*. Mutat Res. 2000;451:187–96.

Ganther HE. Selenotrisulfides. Formation by the reaction of thiols with selenious acid. Biochemistry. 1968;7:2898–905.

Ganther HE. Reduction of the selenotrisulfide derivative of glutathione to a persulfide analog by glutathione reductase. Biochemistry. 1971;10:4089–98.

Garberg P, Hogberg J. The role of hypoxia in selenium metabolism. Biochem Pharmacol. 1987;36:1377–9.

Garberg P, Stahl A, Warholm M, Hogberg J. Studies of the role of DNA fragmentation in selenium toxicity. Biochem Pharmacol. 1988;37:3401–6.

Gharieb MM, Gadd GM. The kinetics of ^{75}[Se]-selenite uptake by *Saccharomyces cerevisiae* and the vacuolization response to high concentrations. Mycol Res. 2004;108:1415–22.

Herrero E, Wellinger RE. Yeast as a model system to study metabolic impact of selenium compounds. Microb Cell. 2015;2:139–49.

Hsieh HS, Ganther HE. Acid-volatile selenium formation catalyzed by glutathione reductase. Biochemistry. 1975;14:1632–6.

Izquierdo A, Casas C, Herrero E. Selenite-induced cell death in Saccharomyces cerevisiae: protective role of glutaredoxins. Microbiology. 2010;156:2608–20.

Jablonska E, Vinceti M. Selenium and human health: Witnessing a copernican revolution? J Environ Sci Health C Environ Carcinog Ecotoxicol Rev. 2015;33:328–68.

Kachroo AH, Laurent JM, Yellman CM, Meyer AG, Wilke CO, Evolution MEM. Systematic humanization of yeast genes reveals conserved functions and genetic modularity. Science. 2015;348:921–5.

Kitahara J, Seko Y, Imura N. Possible involvement of active oxygen species in selenite toxicity in isolated rat hepatocytes. Arch Toxicol. 1993;67:497–501.

Kitajima T, Chiba Y. Selenomethionine metabolism and its toxicity in yeast. Biomol Concepts. 2013;4:611–6.

Kitajima T, Chiba Y, Jigami Y. Mutation of high-affinity methionine permease contributes to selenomethionyl protein production in *Saccharomyces cerevisiae*. Appl Environ Microbiol. 2010;76:6351–9.

Kitajima T, Jigami Y, Chiba Y. Cytotoxic mechanism of selenomethionine in yeast. J Biol Chem. 2012;287:10032–8.

Kolas NK, Durocher D. DNA repair: DNA polymerase zeta and Rev1 break in. Curr Biol. 2006;16:R296–9.

Krogh BO, Symington LS. Recombination proteins in yeast. Annu Rev Genet. 2004;38:233–71.

Kumar S, Björnstedt M, Holmgren A. Selenite is a substrate for calf thymus thioredoxin reductase and thioredoxin and elicits a large non-stoichiometric oxidation of NADPH in the presence of oxygen. Eur J Biochem. 1992;207:435–9.

Lazard M, Blanquet S, Fisicaro P, Labarraque G, Plateau P. Uptake of selenite by *Saccharomyces cerevisiae* involves the high and low affinity orthophosphate transporters. J Biol Chem. 2010;285:32029–37.

Lazard M, Ha-Duong NT, Mounie S, Perrin R, Plateau P, Blanquet S. Selenodiglutathione uptake by the *Saccharomyces cerevisiae* vacuolar ATP-binding cassette transporter Ycf1p. FEBS J. 2011;278:4112–21.

Lazard M, Dauplais M, Blanquet S, Plateau P. Trans-sulfuration pathway seleno-amino acids are mediators of selenomethionine toxicity in *Saccharomyces cerevisiae*. J Biol Chem. 2015;290:10741–50.

Lazard M, Dauplais M, Blanquet S, Plateau P. Recent advances in the mechanism of selenoamino acids toxicity in eukaryotic cells. Biomol Concepts. 2017;8:93–104.

Letavayová L, Vlcková V, Brozmanová J. Selenium: from cancer prevention to DNA damage. Toxicology. 2006a;227:1–14.

Letavayová L, Markova E, Hermanska K, Vlckova V, Vlasakova D, Chovanec M, Brozmanova J. Relative contribution of homologous recombination and non-homologous end-joining to DNA double-strand break repair after oxidative stress in *Saccharomyces cerevisiae*. DNA Repair (Amst). 2006b;5:602–10.

Letavayová L, Vlasáková D, Spallholz JE, Brozmanová J, Chovanec M. Toxicity and mutagenicity of selenium compounds in *Saccharomyces cerevisiae*. Mutat Res. 2008a;638:1–10.

Letavayová L, Vlasáková D, Vlcková V, Brozmanová J, Chovanec M. Rad52 has a role in the repair of sodium selenite-induced DNA damage in Saccharomyces cerevisiae. Mutat Res. 2008b;652:198–203.

Lewinska A, Bartosz G. A role for yeast glutaredoxin genes in selenite-mediated oxidative stress. Fungal Genet Biol. 2008;45:1182–7.

Malkowski MG, Quartley E, Friedman AE, Babulski J, Kon Y, Wolfley J, Said M, Luft JR, Phizicky EM, DeTitta GT, Grayhack EJ. Blocking S-adenosylmethionine synthesis in yeast allows selenomethionine incorporation and multiwavelength anomalous dispersion phasing. Proc Natl Acad Sci U S A. 2007;104:6678–83.

Maniková D, Vlasáková D, Loduhová J, Letavayová L, Vigasová D, Krascsenitsová E, Vlcková V, Brozmanová J, Chovanec M. Investigations on the role of base excision repair and non-homologous end-joining pathways in sodium selenite-induced toxicity and mutagenicity in Saccharomyces cerevisiae. Mutagenesis. 2010;25:155–62.

Mániková D, Vlasáková D, Letavayová L, Klobucniková V, Griac P, Chovanec M. Selenium toxicity toward yeast as assessed by microarray analysis and deletion mutant library screen: a role for DNA repair. Chem Res Toxicol. 2012;25:1598–608.

McDermott JR, Rosen BP, Liu Z. Jen1p: a high affinity selenite transporter in yeast. Mol Biol Cell. 2010;21:3934–41.

Misra S, Boylan M, Selvam A, Spallholz JE, Björnstedt M. Redox-active selenium compounds—from toxicity and cell death to cancer treatment. Nutrients. 2015;7:3536–56.

Nakamuro K, Yoshikawa K, Sayato Y, Kurata H, Tonomura M. Studies on selenium-related compounds. V. Cytogenetic effect and reactivity with DNA. Mutat Res. 1976;40:177–84.

Painter EP. The chemistry and toxicity of selenium compounds, with special reference to the selenium problem. Chem Rev. 1941;28:179–213.

Perez-Sampietro M, Serra-Cardona A, Canadell D, Casas C, Arino J, Herrero E. The yeast Aft2 transcription factor determines selenite toxicity by controlling the low affinity phosphate transport system. Sci Rep. 2016;6:32836.

Peyroche G, Saveanu C, Dauplais M, Lazard M, Beuneu F, Decourty L, Malabat C, Jacquier A, Blanquet S, Plateau P. Sodium selenide toxicity is mediated by O_2-dependent DNA breaks. PLoS One. 2012;7:e36343.

Pinson B, Sagot I, Daignan-Fornier B. Identification of genes affecting selenite toxicity and resistance in Saccharomyces cerevisiae. Mol Microbiol. 2000;36:679–87.

Plateau P, Saveanu C, Lestini R, Dauplais M, Decourty L, Jacquier A, Blanquet S, Lazard M. Exposure to selenomethionine causes selenocysteine misincorporation and protein aggregation in *Saccharomyces cerevisiae*. Sci Rep. 2017;7:44761.

Prakash S, Johnson RE, Prakash L. Eukaryotic translesion synthesis DNA polymerases: specificity of structure and function. Annu Rev Biochem. 2005;74:317–53.

Preud'homme H, Far J, Gil-Casal S, Lobinski R. Large-scale identification of selenium metabolites by online size-exclusion-reversed phase liquid chromatography with combined inductively coupled plasma (ICP-MS) and electrospray ionization linear trap-Orbitrap mass spectrometry (ESI-MS[n]). Metallomics. 2012;4:422–32.

Rao Y, McCooeye M, Windust A, Bramanti E, D'Ulivo A, Mester Z. Mapping of selenium metabolic pathway in yeast by liquid chromatography-Orbitrap mass spectrometry. Anal Chem. 2010;82:8121–30.

Rattray AJ, Strathern JN. Error-prone DNA polymerases: when making a mistake is the only way to get ahead. Annu Rev Genet. 2003;37:31–66.

Salin H, Fardeau V, Piccini E, Lelandais G, Tanty V, Lemoine S, Jacq C, Devaux F. Structure and properties of transcriptional networks driving selenite stress response in yeasts. BMC Genomics. 2008;9:333.

Seitomer E, Balar B, He D, Copeland PR, Kinzy TG. Analysis of *Saccharomyces cerevisiae* null allele strains identifies a larger role for DNA damage versus oxidative stress pathways in growth inhibition by selenium. Mol Nutr Food Res. 2008;52:1305–15.

Seko Y, Imura N. Active oxygen generation as a possible mechanism of selenium toxicity. Biomed Environ Sci. 1997;10:333–9.

Tarze A, Dauplais M, Grigoras I, Lazard M, Ha-Duong NT, Barbier F, Blanquet S, Plateau P. Extracellular production of hydrogen selenide accounts for thiol-assisted toxicity of selenite against *Saccharomyces cerevisiae*. J Biol Chem. 2007;282:8759–67.

Thomas D, Surdin-Kerjan Y. Metabolism of sulfur amino acids in *Saccharomyces cerevisiae*. Microbiol Mol Biol Rev. 1997;61:503–32.

Turanov AA, Xu XM, Carlson BA, Yoo MH, Gladyshev VN, Hatfield DL. Biosynthesis of selenocysteine, the 21st amino acid in the genetic code, and a novel pathway for cysteine biosynthesis. Adv Nutr. 2011;2:122–8.

Valdiglesias V, Pasaro E, Mendez J, Laffon B. In vitro evaluation of selenium genotoxic, cytotoxic, and protective effects: a review. Arch Toxicol. 2010;84:337–51.

Wallenberg M, Misra S, Wasik AM, Marzano C, Björnstedt M, Gandin V, Fernandes AP. Selenium induces a multi-targeted cell death process in addition to ROS formation. J Cell Mol Med. 2014;18:671–84.

Weekley CM, Harris HH. Which form is that? The importance of selenium speciation and metabolism in the prevention and treatment of disease. Chem Soc Rev. 2013;42:8870–94.

Whiting RF, Wei L, Stich HF. Unscheduled DNA synthesis and chromosome aberrations induced by inorganic and organic selenium compounds in the presence of glutathione. Mutat Res. 1980;78:159–69.

Chapter 5
Selenium Metabolism, Regulation, and Sex Differences in Mammals

Caroline Vindry, Théophile Ohlmann, and Laurent Chavatte

Abstract Selenium is an essential trace element in mammals, which is closely related to sulfur in respect of chemistry, catalysis, and metabolism. Selenium is often mentioned in the context of cancer, immunity, brain development, and cardiovascular physiology. Most of the beneficial effects of selenium are expected to come from the pool of selenoproteins, which are involved in redox biology and homeostasis. Many chemical species of selenium can enter the organism to be transformed into selenide, the central metabolite for selenoprotein synthesis. In this chapter, the various selenium species as well as the several metabolic pathways leading to selenide are described, and a particular highlight is given on sexual dimorphic regulation of selenium metabolism and selenoprotein expression.

Keywords Selenoproteins · Selenocysteine · Selenomethionine · Selenide · Glutathione peroxidase · SelenoP

Abbreviations

APOER2	Apolipoprotein E receptor-2 (also referred to as LRP2)
GPX	Glutathione peroxidase
GR	Glutathione reductase
GSH	Glutathione
H_2Se	Hydrogen selenide
LRP8	Megalin

C. Vindry · T. Ohlmann · L. Chavatte (✉)
Centre International de Recherche en Infectiologie, CIRI, Lyon, France

Inserm U1111, Lyon, France

CNRS, Ecole Normale Supérieure de Lyon, Université de Lyon 1, UMR5308, Lyon, France
e-mail: laurent.chavatte@ens-lyon.fr

© Springer International Publishing AG, part of Springer Nature 2018
B. Michalke (ed.), *Selenium*, Molecular and Integrative Toxicology,
https://doi.org/10.1007/978-3-319-95390-8_5

MSeA   Methylseleninic acid (also referred to as mathaneseleninic acid)
PLP   Pyridoxal 5′-phosphate
SCL   Selenocysteine ß-lyase (also referred to as Scly)
Sec   L-Selenocysteine, selenocysteine (also referred to as SeCys)
SELENOP   Selenoprotein P, SEPP1
SeMeSeCys   Selenomethyl-selenocysteine
SeMet   L-Selenomethionine, selenomethionine
TXN   Thioredoxin
TXNRD   Thioredoxin reductase

Introduction

Interest in selenium research has dramatically increased in the past few decades with the recent insights into nutrigenomics for human health, and more precisely the role of genetically encoded selenoproteins (Labunskyy et al. 2014; Hesketh 2008; Whanger 2004). Selenium is an essential trace element in mammals, which shares many similarities with its above neighbor element in the periodic table, the atom sulfur. Therefore, many aspects of selenium chemistry, reactivity, and metabolism are similar to those of sulfur. However, one key difference between these two elements is the insertion of selenium in a group of essential proteins, named selenoproteins in the form of a rare amino acid, the selenocysteine. These selenoproteins are thought to be responsible for most of the beneficial effects of selenium in mammals (Hatfield and Gladyshev 2002; Driscoll and Copeland 2003; Papp et al. 2007; Rayman 2012; Latrèche and Chavatte 2008). Selenocysteine is a structural and functional analog of cysteine, where selenium replaces sulfur. The presence of selenocysteine in the catalytic site of these enzymes confers a higher reactivity in redox reaction than cysteine (Labunskyy et al. 2014). Catalytically, selenocysteine is often considered as a super cysteine. In selenium metabolism, the selenide molecule is the central precursor, into which every seleno-compound should be metabolized in order to be used in the selenoprotein synthesis pathway (Cupp-Sutton and Ashby 2016). This chapter describes how selenium enters the body, and then the cell to be incorporated into selenoproteins, the excess of selenium being excreted in a less reactive chemical species. In this context, we also focus on the gender-specific aspects of these metabolic pathways that are emerging in the field of selenium biochemistry and physiology.

Chemical Forms and Levels of Selenium in Environment and Food Diet

Chemical Forms of Selenium Found in Living Organisms

Selenium has five stable isotopes (^{74}Se, ^{76}Se, ^{77}Se, ^{78}Se, and ^{80}Se) and is present in the environment in multiple chemical forms and at variable concentrations. Selenium can be found in the soil, the water, and to a much lesser extent in the air. In soils, the average content of selenium is 0.4 mg kg^{-1}, with high variation worldwide. Seleniferous regions with up to 1200 mg kg^{-1} have been mapped in the USA, Canada, Colombia, the UK, China, Russia, and India (Fordyce 2007). Seleniprive regions (<0.1 mg kg^{-1}) are localized in China, Finland, New Zealand, South-East of USA, and the UK. In fact, selenium importance as a trace element in human health has been evidenced in a seleniprive area of China named Keshan, which then provided the name to the disease. Strikingly, Keshan disease has been eradicated by selenium supplementation. In salt and freshwaters, inorganic selenium species are often found in the form of selenide, selenite, selenate, and elemental selenium (see Table 5.1 and Fig. 5.1) (Vesper et al. 2008). On the other hand, organic selenocompounds predominate in air, soil, and plants in the form of volatile molecules or selenoamino acids (Pyrzynska 2002). Food is the primary source of selenium intake for mammals, but only four molecules (selenocysteine, selenomethionine, selenite, and selenate) account for most of the bioavailable selenium in food intake. Importantly, the content of selenium found in the soil and water determines the concentration of selenium in the living organisms growing in these territories, and notably the components of human food chain, including microorganisms, plants, cereals, vegetables, fruits, farm animals, etc. While inorganic species are limited to oxidation stages of selenium (−II, 0, +IV, and +VI), the panel of organic species that occur in nature is very diverse (Bierla et al. 2016). Indeed, higher plants and yeast, which do not require selenium, metabolize it through the sulfur pathway. It follows that, in these organisms, virtually any sulfur-containing molecule can have its selenium analogs. In mammals, most of the selenium is present in the form of selenocysteine (in selenoproteins), selenomethionine, and inorganic selenium (selenate and selenite). Prevalent selenium species in nature are listed in Table 5.1 and Fig. 5.1. As a general rule for mammals, organic species of selenium are less toxic than inorganic forms (selenite or selenate). In addition to natural organic species of selenium, selenodrugs have been designed and synthesized, mostly for antioxidant and anticancer properties (Ramoutar and Brumaghim 2010). A growing interest has developed for chemotherapies of human cancers involving selenium-containing molecules, due to the improvement of selenium chemistry (Bartolini et al. 2017) and therefore the wide variety of selenocompounds available for in vitro and in vivo assays.

Ebselen is a synthetic selenocompound (see Table 5.1) that mimics many aspects of the activity of the GPX selenoprotein. It reduces hydroperoxides including hydrogen peroxide, phospholipid hydroperoxide, and cholesterol ester hydroperoxide. In addition to GPX-like activities, ebselen also reacts with many kinds of thiols (other than glutathione) and peroxynitrites (Sies 1993). This drug exhibits anti-inflammatory, antioxidant, and cytoprotective activities, and low toxicity. However, since selenium is not released from the molecule, ebselen is not metabolized in selenoproteins. Another selenocompound, namely methylseleninic acid (MSeA), has been proved to have anticancer properties and has the ability to enter the selenoprotein biosynthesis metabolism. It is hypothesized to be produced from MeSeSECYS, but has never been detected in mammalian samples. Synthetic MSeA is often used during in vivo and in vitro experiments (Ramoutar and Brumaghim 2010). Selenoneine is an interesting selenium analog of ergothioneine, an efficient antioxidant. Selenoneine and its selenium-methylated form have been

Table 5.1 Prevalent inorganic and organic selenium species found in the environment or synthetic

Selenium species	Synonyms	Chemical forms	Comments
Inorganic species			
Elemental selenium	[Se(0)]		Elemental Selenium occurs in non-soluble form after chemical or microbial reduction processes
Selenide	[Se(-II)]	H_2Se, HSe^-, Se^{2-}	Central component for selenoprotein synthesis
Selenate	[Se(+VI)]	$H_2SeO_4^0$, $HSeO_4^-$, SeO_4^{2-}	
Selenite	[Se (+IV)]	$H_2SeO_3^0$, $HSeO_3^-$, SeO_3^{2-}, SeO_2	
Selenophosphate		H_3PSeO_3, $H_2PSeO_3^-$, $HPSeO_3^{2-}$, $PSeO_3^{3-}$	
Organic species			
Dimethyl selenide	DMSe	$(CH_3)_2Se$	Volatile compound
Dimethyl diselenide	DMDSe	$(CH_3)_2Se_2$	Volatile compound
Trimethylselenonium cation		$(CH_3)_3Se^+$	Found in urine
Selenocyanate		$SeCN^-$	Found as a metabolite in human cell lines, and wastewater from petroleum refineries
Selenoneine	Selenoergothioneine	$C_9H_{15}N_3O_2Se$	
Methylselenol	MeSeH	CH_3Se	
1β-Methylseleno-N-acetyl-D-galactosamine	MeSe-β-GalNAc, Selenosugar	$C_9H_{17}NO_5Se$	Found in urine
Selenocysteine	SeCys, Sec,	$C_3H_7NO_2Se$	21st amino acid
Selenocystine	SecSec	$C_6H_{12}N_2O_4Se_2$	
Selenomethyl selenocysteine	SeMeSeCys	$C_4H_9NO_2Se$	
Selenomethionine	SeMet	$C_5H_{11}NO_2Se$	
Selenodiglutathione	GSSeSG	$C_{20}H_{32}N_6O_{12}S_2Se$	
γ-Glutamyl-Se-methylselenocysteine	γ-Glutamyl-Se-MeSeCys, GGSeMe	$C_9H_{16}N_2O_5Se$	
Selenohomolanthionine		$C_8H_{16}N_2O_4Se$	
Synthetic species and selenodrugs			
Ebselen		$C_{13}H_9NOSe$	
2-Hydroxy-4-methylselenobutanoic acid	HMSeBA, NutraSelen	$C_5H_{10}O_3Se$	
Methylseleninic acid	MSA, MeSeA	CH_4O_2Se	

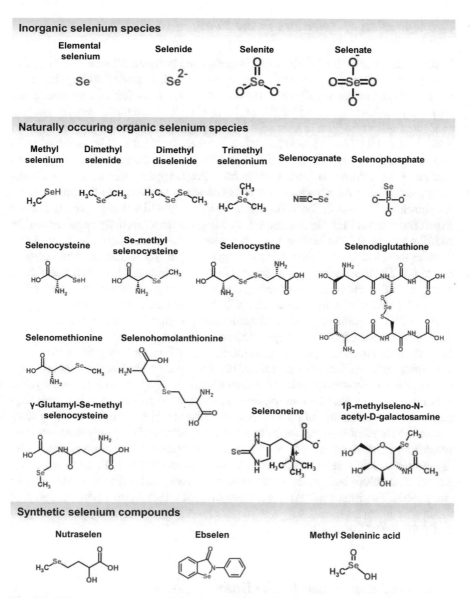

Fig. 5.1 Chemical structures of major selenium compounds found in nature or synthetically. Chemspider (http://www.chemspider.com/)

found in various human biological fluids. Selenoneine is the major selenium compound in the muscles and blood of ocean fish, such as tuna, mackerel, and swordfish (Klein et al. 2011; Yamashita and Yamashita 2010). How selenoneine is synthesized and whether it is efficiently metabolized into selenoproteins is a remaining issue.

Concentration of Selenium in the Food

Recommended daily intake for adults is comprised between 50 and 70 µg of selenium per day. Adverse effects could appear above the threshold of 500 µg/day, leading to selenosis and eventually death. On the other side, the effect of severe selenium deficiency appears below an intake of 12 µg/day. The chemical species and the concentration of selenium in terrestrial food depend on its concentration in soils and water where plants, cereals, and animals are grown. In general, selenium content in seafood is mostly replete. Table 5.2 illustrates a non-exhaustive list of selenium concentration in common foods from human diet. It appears that nowadays a well-balanced food diet from various origins is enough to fulfill the daily requirements. As shown in Table 5.2, the naturally most concentrated selenium foods are the Brazil nuts, several nuts being enough to complete an adult daily requirement. In addition to natural food, an important business market has emerged in the past few decades for selenium-enriched foods aiming at animal and human selenium supplementation. The most common supplement in the food industry is selenium-enriched yeast, which is obtained by growing *Saccharomyces cerevisiae* in a selenium-enriched medium (usually with selenite). To improve selenium accumulation (up to 3 mg of Se per gram of yeast) and favor incorporation in organic forms, sulfur-limited medium is often used. Depending on growing conditions and nutrient media used, the speciation of selenium in selenium-enriched yeast may greatly vary from one company to another (Bierla et al. 2016). Intervention studies for selenium supplementation in selected groups of volunteers often used selenium-enriched yeast, in comparison to a placebo control, over a period of several years. It has been suggested that the variability of the different outcomes from various intervention studies could be attributed to variability in selenium speciation in the selenium-enriched yeast from different companies. Whether the assimilation of selenium is affected by its speciation has been investigated for major components (Hoefig et al. 2011; Rebsch et al. 2006) but awaits further systematic analysis for less abundant organic compounds. An important issue remains to verify that these selenium-enriched foods are equivalent to naturally rich diet for human health benefits, and more generally for that of mammals.

Selenium Assimilation by the Body

Assimilation by the Digestive Tract

In addition to total concentration, the speciation of selenium in food intake is crucial to determine its bioavailability for the organism and also the upper limit uptake. In plants, as much as 90% of the selenium is present in the form of selenomethionine (randomly incorporated in proteins instead of methionine), while selenocysteine is predominant in animal source in the form of selenoproteins (Fig. 5.2). Inorganic

Table 5.2 Selenium content in selected food products and beverages, according to several authors (expressed relative to fresh weight)

Sample	Se content (ng/g)	References
Meat, chicken, fish and eggs		
Pork kidney	849–1543	Diaz-Alarcon et al. (1996)
Pork liver	256–800	Diaz-Alarcon et al. (1996)
Oyster (Australia)	770	Marro (1996)
Fish	153–686	Smrkolj et al. (2005)
Pork	144–450	USDoA (1999)
Salmon	270–368	Marro (1996)
Beef, steak (Australia)	80–200	Tinggi (1999)
Ham	200	Tinggi (1999)
Eggs	172.8	Pappa et al. (2006)
Beef (Slovenia)	33–155	Smrkolj et al. (2005)
Chicken breast	97–154	Smrkolj et al. (2005)
Rabbit	74–106	Diaz-Alarcon et al. (1996)
Lamb	27–30	Diaz-Alarcon et al. (1996)
Oyster (Australia)	0.7–14.2	Marro (1996)
Fruits, vegetables, cereals, and derivatives		
Brazil nuts	850–6860	Fairweather-Tait et al. (2011)
Bread	70.0–131.8	Pappa et al. (2006)
Grapes	40.0–76.0	Marro (1996)
Potato (Australia)	30.0–70.0	Marro (1996)
Pasta, boiled	35.6–50.0	Marro (1996)
Apple	30.0–50.0	Marro (1996)
Tomato	1.1–29.1	Smrkolj et al. (2005)
Lentils	28.0	USDoA (1999)
Lettuce	3.0–22.8	Marro (1996)
Rice (Italy)	20.1 ± 45.3	Panigati et al. (2007)
Rice (Greece)	19.1 ± 1.4	Pappa et al. (2006)
Garlic	13.4–13.7	Pappa et al. (2006)
Celery	9.3–14.2	Marro (1996)
Pasta	5.8 ± 0.2	Pappa et al. (2006)
Orange	5.00	Marro (1996)
Potato (Greece)	4.6 ± 1.4	Pappa et al. (2006)
Sharon fruit	3.9 ± 0.5	Pappa et al. (2006)
Mango	2.6 ± 0.6	Pappa et al. (2006)
Kiwi	1.4 ± 0.2	Pappa et al. (2006)
Milk and dairy products		
Ice cream	100.0 ± 40.0	Cabrera et al. (1996)
Gouda cheese	85.4 ± 10.0	Pappa et al. (2006)
Condensed milk (Spain)	75.0 ± 25.0	Cabrera et al. (1996)
Yoghurt (Spain)	50.0 ± 30.0	Cabrera et al. (1996)
Butter (Slovenia)	17.5–30.1	Smrkolj et al. (2005)

(continued)

Table 5.2 (continued)

Sample	Se content (ng/g)	References
Yoghurt (Greece)	21.9–26.9	Pappa et al. (2006)
Cow's milk (Greece)	13.1–21.9	Pappa et al. (2006)
Butter (Greece)	4.4–13.8	Pappa et al. (2006)
Cow's milk (Slovenia)	11.6–13.4	Smrkolj et al. (2005)
Yoghurt (Slovenia)	11.9–12.8	Smrkolj et al. (2005)
Miscellaneous		
Selenium yeast	3,000,000	Pedrero and Madrid (2009)
Sugar, raw	69.0	Marro (1996)
Cornflakes (Australia)	62.9	Marro (1996)
Chocolate	39.0	USDoA (1999)
Cornflakes (Greece)	19.7 ± 0.6	Pappa et al. (2006)
Olive oil	5.30	Marro (1996)
Tea infusion	5.00	Marro (1996)
Beer	5.00	Marro (1996)
Tap water	2.2 ± 0.7	Pappa et al. (2006)
Honey	1.7 ± 0.004	Pappa et al. (2006)
Olive oil	1.1 ± 0.6	Pappa et al. (2006)
Apple juice	0.7–5.1	Marro (1996)

Origin of the food is given when reported in various studies

species of selenium are mostly present in drinking water, depending on the soil where the groundwater is extracted. A larger intake in inorganic selenium often results from selenium supplements containing remaining amounts of non-assimilated selenite or selenate. Interestingly, the gut microbiota is influenced by the selenium levels in the food diet, which in turn modifies the metabolism of host selenium status and selenoproteome by sequestering or metabolizing selenium species (Kasaikina et al. 2011). It is clear that a better understanding of how microbiota influence the selenium metabolism of the host is needed.

The absorption of selenium from the food diet is a research field that has received little attention to date. It seems that the absorption of selenium from food is not homeostatic, and that this absorption is not a limiting factor for its bioavailability. The absorption of selenium occurs mainly in the lower part of the small intestine using species-specific mechanism that is often similar to their sulfur-containing analogs, as described in Fig. 5.2. The absorption of selenocysteine, selenomethionine, and selenate is highly efficient (70–90%) and seems to remain constant in the human population. Selenoamino acids follow the similar transcellular pathway as their sulfur analogs via the B^0 amino acid transporter, in which Na^+ is also co-transported. Selenate follows a paracellular pathway to cross the intestinal barrier and is then reduced into selenite (presumably similarly to sulfate reduction into sulfite). The absorption of selenite is less efficient (around 60%) and variable since it is stimulated by reduced glutathione in intestine, in order to form GSSeSG and be further assimilated by the gastrointestinal tract. The route for selenite through

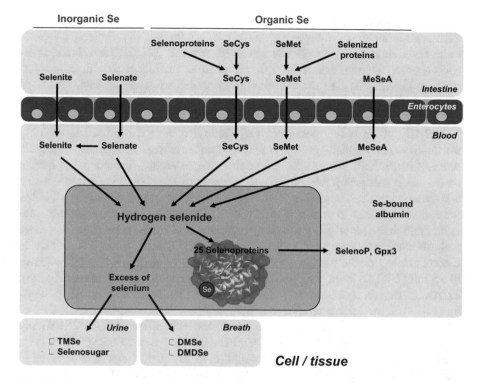

Fig. 5.2 Schematic of selenium intestinal absorption of predominant species

enterocytes remains elusive, and it is still unclear whether it follows a paracellular or a transcellular pathway.

Se in the Blood and Assimilation by Different Organs

In the blood, these organic and inorganic species will meet other selenocompounds, including SELENOP, GPX3, and Se-albumin which are predominant in plasma, with a ratio of 4:1:1, respectively (Callejon-Leblic et al. 2018). Very little is known about the speciation of selenium bound to albumin that could result from the binding of selenometabolites to cysteine-34 of albumin, via a Se-S bound. Indeed, this cysteine-34 is involved in the binding of many metabolites or drugs in human (Bal et al. 2013). It follows that half-life of these small selenium metabolites in the blood is rather short and will be taken up by the liver, other organs, and blood cells to synthesize selenoproteins. The excess or non-bioavailable forms of selenium will be eliminated in urine and through breathing (when volatile). Indeed, when radioactive ^{75}Se-selenite is injected to rat blood, it is rapidly assimilated by different organs and then found mostly in selenoproteins of high molecular weight (Suzuki et al. 2006a, b).

Upon a normal diet, tissue concentration of selenium in the human body follows a defined hierarchy (from highest levels to lowest): kidney, liver, spleen, pancreas, heart, brain, lung, bone, and skeletal muscle (Sonet et al. 2016). Kidney is an important organ in selenium metabolism, since it secretes the plasmatic glutathione peroxidase, GPX3, but also since it eliminates excess of selenium in the form of trimethylselenonium and selenosugar in urine (Ohta et al. 2009). The liver also plays an important role in selenium metabolism, since it produces and secretes SELENOP, which is the most abundant selenoprotein in the blood and the only selenoprotein that contains multiple selenocysteine residues in the primary sequence. Indeed, SELENOP accounts for 8% of the total selenium stocked in the human body (Read et al. 1990). Interestingly, the number of selenocysteine residues varies widely amongst selenoproteins, from 7 to 18 in vertebrates (Lobanov et al. 2009; Mariotti et al. 2012). Therefore, SELENOP is proposed to store and distribute selenium through the blood plasma to many organs, including the brain. There are three features that are conserved in vertebrates of SELENOP. From N-terminal to C-terminal end of the protein, these are a selenocysteine-containing thioredoxin-like motif (UXXC) known to interact with cysteine-containing substrates (N-term), a histidine-rich domain potentially interacting with many receptors including megalin (LRP2) in the middle region, and an apolipoprotein E receptor-2 (APORE2 or LRP8) binding domain in the C-term (Burk and Hill 2015). APOER2 is widely expressed in mammalian tissues and facilitates the uptake of SELENOP in various organs by endocytosis, mostly in brain and testis. Besides, megalin is involved in SELENOP uptake by the kidney. Therefore, the deletion of ApoER2 reduces selenium levels in testis and brain, but not in kidney. Additionally, the pinocytosis of SELENOP has been proposed for tissues devoid of APOER2 and megalin. Interestingly, the other plasmatic selenoprotein, GPX3, has never been demonstrated to transport selenium to any organ in mammals under adequate conditions.

Metabolism of Selenoprotein Synthesis in the Cell

Selenocysteine–tRNA[Ser]Sec Aminoacylation

A central RNA component of selenocysteine insertion machinery is the Sec-tRNA[Ser]Sec, which is the only tRNA governing by itself the expression of an entire family of proteins, namely the selenoproteome (Hatfield and Gladyshev 2002; Carlson et al. 2016). The Sec-tRNA[Ser]Sec is distinct from other cellular tRNAs regarding its size, aminoacylation, transcription, modification, and delivery to the ribosome. The aminoacylation of Sec-tRNA[Ser]Sec is particularly unique since it requires four enzymes instead of one for canonical tRNAs. Indeed, selenocysteine, in contrast to the 20 other genetically encoded amino acids, is not loaded as such onto its cognate tRNA but is instead co-synthesized directly on its tRNA. As illustrated in Fig. 5.3a, the tRNA[Ser]Sec is initially aminoacylated with Serine by the

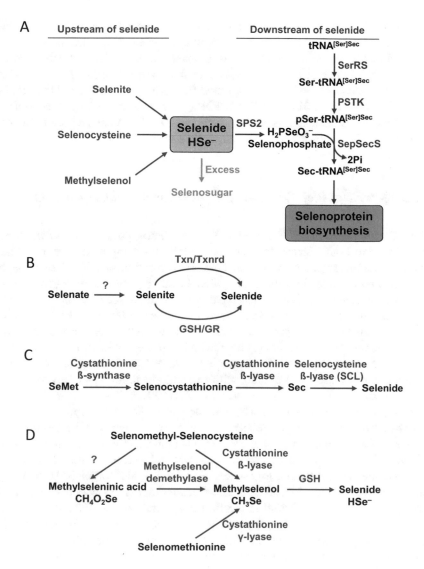

Fig. 5.3 Representation of the various metabolic pathways leading to selenoprotein synthesis

seryl-tRNA synthetase (SerRS) to generate the Ser-tRNA[Ser]Sec. An activation of the serine is performed by the phosphoseryl-tRNA kinase (PSKT) to form the pSer-tRNA[Ser]Sec. The Sec-tRNA[Ser]Sec is produced by the Sec synthase (SepSecS, also referred to as SLA/LP) using pSer-tRNA[Ser]Sec and selenophosphate as substrates. The only identified pathway to generate selenophosphate is from selenide via the selenophosphate 2 synthetase 2 (SEPHS2 or SPS2). Given this particular biosynthesis pathway, it is obvious that the levels of Sec-tRNA[Ser]Sec are highly dependent on selenium bioavailability in the cell. When selenium level is low, selenide is limited to produce fully mature selenocysteine-tRNA[Ser]Sec, which in turn will be limiting for selenoprotein synthesis. Another regulatory mechanism has been recently reported during selenium deficiency. It appears that Cys could substitute Sec in selenoproteins, since SEPHS2 could produce thiophosphate instead of selenophosphate. This phenomenon has been reported for TXNRD1 and TXNRD2 (Xu et al. 2010; Turanov et al. 2011) and SELENOP (Turanov et al. 2015). These findings reveal that, at least in mammal selenoprotein mRNAs, UGA can be decoded as stop, Sec, or Cys, the levels of which depend on Se bioavailability.

Hydrogen Selenide, the Central Precursor of Selenoproteins

The molecule selenide (H_2Se, or HSe^-) is the central point of the selenoprotein pathway from both organic and inorganic selenium compounds. Several details await further investigations in the interconversion reactions leading to selenide, but three metabolic routes have been identified so far to generate hydrogen selenide, namely from selenite, selenocysteine, and methylselenol; see Fig. 5.3.

Two metabolic pathways, at least, have been described to reduce selenite in selenide, as shown in Fig. 5.3b. Selenite can first be reduced by the thioredoxin (Txn)/ thioredoxin reductase (TXNRD) system, which is present ubiquitously in organism. An alternative pathway consists in a reaction of selenide with the glutathione (GSH)/ glutathione reductase (GR) system, with selenodiglutathione and glutathioselenol as intermediate molecules. The presence of TXN/TXNRD system or GSH/GR in virtually any cell lines explains why selenite is so efficient to supplement culture media at a nanomolar range. Selenate can also be metabolized for selenoprotein synthesis. The mechanism by which selenate is reduced into selenite in mammalian cells remains unclear (Fairweather-Tait et al. 2011). It seems that the TXN/TXNRD system alone is not sufficient for this reaction, but the addition of GSH to this system is sufficient to reduce selenate in selenite, although at a slow rate. Alternatively, the metabolic pathway of sulfite reduction into sulfate using ATP sulfurylase and ATP reductase has also been proposed. It turns out that selenate is as efficient as selenite to supplement culture medium, but this time at the micromolar range. Noteworthy, compared to selenite, the toxicity concentration of selenate is also shifted to higher concentration range.

A second route for selenide production originates from selenocysteine and selenomethionine, as illustrated in Fig. 5.3c. Selenocysteine ß-lyase (SCL) is a pyridoxal 5′-phosphate (PLP) enzyme that releases selenide from selenocysteine to yield alanine. Interestingly, mammalian SCL is uniquely dedicated to the reaction with selenocysteine since it does not accept the sulfur nor the oxygen analog, respectively, cysteine and serine, as substrates with any substantial activity. Instead, cysteine is inhibiting the SCL reaction with selenocysteine in vitro. The X-ray crystal structure of human SCL, confirmed by biochemical analyses, has deciphered the mechanism for the discrimination between selenium and sulfur that provides selenocysteine specificity in contrast to bacterial orthologs. In addition, it has been proposed that SCL and SEPHS2 interact to allow substrate channeling (Collins et al. 2012) from Sec to selenophosphate. In support of this hypothesis, in mammals the active site of SEPHS2 is occupied by a Sec residue that would presumably engage a Se-Se bound with the selenide released by the SCL enzyme. In this pathway, selenide would not be susceptible to react with other molecules. Selenomethionine can also be metabolized for selenoprotein synthesis. When present in the cell, selenomethionine can be converted in selenocysteine and therefore selenide, via the cystathionine ß-synthase and then cystathionine ß-lyase, which are shared with sulfur analog pathway. Similarly to selenite and selenate, selenocysteine and selenomethionine are similarly bioavailable compounds for selenoprotein synthesis but with different ranges of active concentration, when used to supplement culture media (Hoefig et al. 2011; Rebsch et al. 2006).

The last route identified to date for selenide generation is the release of selenium by a demethylation reaction of methylselenol (CH_3Se), catalyzed by the methylselenol demethylase as illustrated in Fig. 5.3d. Interestingly, several selenocompounds can generate methylselenol, and include selenomethyl-selenocysteine (SeMeSeCys), methylseleninic acid (MSeA), and selenomethionine. Selenomethyl-selenocysteine is converted to methylselenol by the cystathionine ß-lyase enzyme. Methylseleninic acid can be rapidly converted into methylselenol by reductant such as glutathione. Strikingly, selenomethionine metabolism can also be reduced in selenide via the methyl selenol pathway upon action of the cystathionine γ-lyase, as illustrated in Fig. 5.3.

Taken together, it is clear that the relative weight of these three different routes in the metabolic pathway leading to selenide depends on the selenium source available in the cell. Somehow, the cell line- or tissue-specific relative abundance of the components for each pathway determines the preference and efficiency of the selenium source used by the cell.

Selenoprotein Hierarchy

The human selenoproteome is encoded by 25 selenoprotein genes and is highly regulated by selenium bioavailability at the scale of organism, tissue, or cell lines. In response to selenium depletion or repletion, a prioritized regulation is induced that maintains the expression of essential selenoenzymes at the expense of others. This phenomenon is referred to as selenoprotein hierarchy. Several reports characterized this regulation for the different members of GPX family in various models of selenium fluctuation. Additionally it seems that the regulation of the selenoproteome in response to a variety of pathophysiological conditions and cellular stressors follows a different selenoprotein hierarchy. The repertoire of regulatory mechanisms responsible for selenoprotein hierarchy is getting more and more complex. However, it is now becoming clear that the insertion of selenocysteine during selenoprotein translation is the limiting stage that constitutes a regulatory checkpoint for selenoproteome expression. Several regulatory factors and pathways are currently under investigation and include selenoprotein mRNA-binding proteins, tRNA aminoacylation and modifications, and selenoprotein mRNA modifications (Bulteau and Chavatte 2015). In addition to this essential translation regulation network, a control of the transcriptional activity of selenoproteins can also occur in response to specific stimuli. Whether this selenoprotein hierarchy is also regulated by gender awaits further investigation. So far, the mRNA levels of two important recoding factors (EFSec and SECISBP2) are similar between males and females (Riese et al. 2006).

Sex Difference in Selenium Metabolism

Sex Differences in Selenoprotein Expression and Regulation

Males and females differ in several aspects of development, metabolism, and endocrine regulations that yield to variable predispositions to specific diseases, such as cancers, autoimmune disorders, inflammation, neurodegeneration, and allergy. Selenium is a typical micronutrient exhibiting a dimorphic aspect in relation to its metabolism and roles in health and disease. Therefore, special care should be given when designing or analyzing the results of clinical studies. The molecular bases of the gender-specific regulation of the metabolism of disease remain to be characterized. So far, only gender-specific phenotypic differences in selenium levels or selenoprotein expression were reported at mRNA or protein levels, without indications of their molecular mechanisms, except when organs are clearly different between males and females. Indeed, one obvious difference between males and females is the difference in the reproductive apparatus at the level of both organ anatomy and function. Selenium deficiency in human and rodents leads to male infertility (Schomburg 2016). In fact testis has high needs in selenium, since GPX4 is highly expressed and contributes to sperm architecture. It follows that APOER2 is highly expressed in testis to allow the uptake of SELENOP by Sertoli cells. In *apoER2$^{-/-}$* male mice, the selenium levels in testis are dramatically reduced compared to those of wild type, in a similar extent to that of *Selenop$^{-/-}$* male mice (Olson et al. 2007). These data confirmed the importance of APOER2/SELENOP system for the maintenance of selenium levels in testis, which is required for spermatogenesis and male fertility. In females, selenium is less concentrated in ovary and uterus and no direct link was observed between selenium levels and fertility. In accordance, the expression of APOER2 in ovary and uterus is not significant. Although selenium deficiency is not linked to female fertility, the needs for selenium seem to increase during pregnancy and lactation periods (Taylor et al. 2005).

Besides reproductive organs and fertility, the sexual dimorphic metabolism of selenium has been reported in blood serum and in several organs, notably liver, kidney, and pituitary gland (as reviewed in Schomburg 2016; Schomburg and Schweizer 2009). Upon adequate diet conditions, total selenium levels are similar between males and females (Riese et al. 2006). However, gender-specific distribution of selenium in blood serum appears in people or animals with similar global levels of selenium, especially between SELENOP, GPX3, and Se-albumin (Letsiou et al. 2014). Due to the unique mechanism of selenoprotein biosynthesis, and particularly translational control of their expression, special care should be given when analyzing selenoprotein mRNA levels. Sometimes, changes occur only at the protein levels with constant mRNA amounts (Bulteau and Chavatte 2015). This should be verified by western immunoblots and/or enzymatic activities when available. In the literature, northern blot analyses revealed different expression of SELENOP and DIO1, in liver and kidney, and of GPX3 in kidney, between male and female mice upon adequate diet. This is confirmed at protein levels by measuring DIO1 and GPX3 enzymatic activities (Riese et al. 2006; Schomburg et al. 2007; Ogawa et al. 1999). The gender dimorphic expression of DIO1 is exacerbated in Se-poor diet of animals. Whether the sex-specific difference in selenoprotein expression occurs at the transcriptional or translational level remains to be addressed. The removal of gonads has been performed in rodent animal models to analyze the impact of androgens and estrogens, after orchiectomy and ovariectomy, respectively. Interestingly, several dimorphic expressions of SELENOP, DIO1 and GPX3 are reduced after gonadectomies, suggesting a role for steroids in selenium metabolism and particularly selenoprotein regulation.

Sex-Dependent Phenotypes in Knockout Mice

As observed before, knockout mouse models have revealed powerful tools to demonstrate the sexual dimorphism of selenium metabolism. First, the targeted inactivation of the *Selenop* gene leads to reduced selenium levels in plasma, brain, testis, and kidney (Hill et al. 2003; Schomburg et al. 2003). *Selenop* $^{-/-}$ mice display neurological impairments, including cognitive, motor, and sensory symptoms that can be overcome by selenium supplementation in the diet, and which are exacerbated by dietary selenium restriction. In comparison, the targeted inactivation of the SLC gene, which is necessary for selenium metabolism from selenocysteine, and particularly useful to metabolized SELENOP, does not induce similar neurological dysfunctions, except when fed with a low-selenium diet. Only subtle gender differences could be observed between males and females, except that *Selenop* $^{-/-}$ male mice are sharply infertile. Interestingly, the transgenic mice lacking both genes (*Selenop* $^{-/-}$ *Scl* $^{-/-}$) show evidence that SCL and SELENOP work cooperatively to maintain selenoprotein function in the mammalian brain. The extent of neurological impairment is stronger with the double-knockout than in the single-*Selenop* $^{-/-}$ mice. The symptoms include reduced survival, impaired motor coordination, audiogenic seizures, and brainstem neurodegeneration even with selenium-supplemented diet (Pitts et al. 2015; Byrns et al. 2014). Interestingly, the symptoms are much stronger in males than in females. For example, in selenium-supplemented conditions, more than half of the males died before 14 weeks of age, while all females reached adulthood. As aforementionend, in males, testes are in competition with brain for selenium needs. To verify this statement in *Selenop* $^{-/-}$ *Scl*$^{-/-}$ double-knockout mice, prepubescent castration of males rescues most of the wild-type phenotype, therefore preventing behavioral deficits, attenuating neurodegeneration, and restoring brain selenoprotein levels (Pitts et al. 2015; Byrns et al. 2014). This particularly exceptional phenotype indicates a clear difference in brain selenium metabolism between males and females, and points out to a specific competition between testis and brain. This finding could have significant consequences in understanding the etiology of neurological development and neurodegenerative disease linked to selenium.

Concluding Remarks

Selenium metabolism in mammals follows in many aspects one of its close neighbors sulfur, with the noticeable exception of being incorporated in a specific group of protein, named selenoproteins. Although, as mentioned in this chapter, in very particular conditions, such as selenium deficiency, sulfur is also able to substitute selenium in selenoproteins. Most importantly, the essential and central metabolite of this pathway is selenide to which converges every known selenium metabolism pathway into selenoproteins. Additionally, many reports establish a dimorphic metabolism of selenium between males and females, both in animal and clinical data. Clearly, males appeared more dependent on selenium intake and more responsive to acute changes in selenium levels than females. It follows that analysis of selenoprotein regulation should take into consideration the sex of animal, population, and even cell line. In conclusion, this field remains largely unexplored and awaits further investigations to fully understand the sex-specific regulation of selenoprotein expression.

Acknowledgments This work was supported by the ENS de Lyon (Emerging project to LC), the CNRS (ATIP program to LC).

References

Bal W, Sokolowska M, Kurowska E, Faller P. Binding of transition metal ions to albumin: sites, affinities and rates. Biochim Biophys Acta. 2013;1830(12):5444–55.

Bartolini D, Sancineto L, Fabro de Bem A, Tew KD, Santi C, Radi R, Toquato P, Galli F. Selenocompounds in cancer therapy: an overview. Adv Cancer Res. 2017;136:259–302.

Bierla K, Szpunar J, Lobinski R. Biological selenium species and selenium speciation in biological samples. In: Hatfield DL, Schweizer U, Tsuji PA, Gladyshev VN, editors. Selenium: its molecular biology and role in human health. 4th ed. New York, NY: Springer Science+Business Media, LLC; 2016. p. 413–24. https://doi.org/10.1007/978-3-319-41283-2_35.

Bulteau A-L, Chavatte L. Update on selenoprotein biosynthesis. Antioxid Redox Signal. 2015;23(10):775–94.

Burk RF, Hill KE. Regulation of selenium metabolism and transport. Annu Rev Nutr. 2015;35:109–34.

Byrns CN, Pitts MW, Gilman CA, Hashimoto AC, Berry MJ. Mice lacking selenoprotein P and selenocysteine lyase exhibit severe neurological dysfunction, neurodegeneration, and audiogenic seizures. J Biol Chem. 2014;289(14):9662–74. doi:M113.540682 [pii]

Cabrera C, Lorenzo ML, De Mena C, Lopez MC. Chromium, copper, iron, manganese, selenium and zinc levels in dairy products: in vitro study of absorbable fractions. Int J Food Sci Nutr. 1996;47(4):331–9.

Callejon-Leblic B, Rodriguez-Moro G, Garcia-Barrera T, Gomez-Ariza JL. Simultaneous speciation of selenoproteins and selenometabolites in plasma and serum. Methods Mol Biol (Clifton, NJ). 2018;1661:163–75.

Carlson BA, Lee BJ, Tsuji PA, Tobe R, Park JM, Schweizer U, Gladyshev VN, Hatfield DL. Selenocysteine tRNA [Ser]Sec: from nonsense suppressor tRNA to the quintessential constituent in selenoprotein biosynthesis. In: Hatfield DL, Schweizer U, Tsuji PA, Gladyshev VN, editors. Selenium: its molecular biology and role in human health. 4th ed. New York, NY: Springer Science+Business Media, LLC; 2016. p. 3–12.

Collins R, Johansson A-L, Karlberg T, Markova N, van den Berg S, Olesen K, Hammarstrom M, Flores A, Schuler H, Schiavone LH, Brzezinski P, Arner ESJ, Hogbom M. Biochemical discrimination between selenium and sulfur 1: a single residue provides selenium specificity to human selenocysteine lyase. PLoS One. 2012;7(1):e30581.

Cupp-Sutton KA, Ashby MT. Biological chemistry of hydrogen selenide. Antioxidants (Basel). 2016;5(4):E42.

Diaz-Alarcon JP, Navarro-Alarcon M, Lopez-Garcia de la Serrana H, Lopez-Martinez MC. Determination of selenium in meat products by hydride generation atomic absorption spectrometry-selenium levels in meat, organ meats, and sausages in Spain. J Agric Food Chem. 1996;44(6):1494–7. https://doi.org/10.1021/jf9507021.

Driscoll DM, Copeland PR. Mechanism and regulation of selenoprotein synthesis. Annu Rev Nutr. 2003;23:17–40.

Fairweather-Tait SJ, Bao Y, Broadley MR, Collings R, Ford D, Hesketh JE, Hurst R. Selenium in human health and disease. Antioxid Redox Signal. 2011;14(7):1337–83.

Fordyce F. Selenium geochemistry and health. Ambio. 2007;36(1):94–7.

Hatfield DL, Gladyshev VN. How selenium has altered our understanding of the genetic code. Mol Cell Biol. 2002;22(11):3565–76.

Hesketh J. Nutrigenomics and selenium: gene expression patterns, physiological targets, and genetics. Annu Rev Nutr. 2008;28:157–77.

Hill KE, Zhou J, McMahan WJ, Motley AK, Atkins JF, Gesteland RF, Burk RF. Deletion of selenoprotein P alters distribution of selenium in the mouse. J Biol Chem. 2003;278(16):13640–6.

Hoefig CS, Renko K, Kohrle J, Birringer M, Schomburg L. Comparison of different selenocompounds with respect to nutritional value vs. toxicity using liver cells in culture. J Nutr Biochem. 2011;22(10):945–55. https://doi.org/10.1016/j.jnutbio.2010.08.006.

Kasaikina MV, Kravtsova MA, Lee BC, Seravalli J, Peterson DA, Walter J, Legge R, Benson AK, Hatfield DL, Gladyshev VN. Dietary selenium affects host selenoproteome expression by influencing the gut microbiota. FASEB J. 2011;25(7):2492–9.

Klein M, Ouerdane L, Bueno M, Pannier F. Identification in human urine and blood of a novel selenium metabolite, Se-methylselenoneine, a potential biomarker of metabolization in mammals of the naturally occurring selenoneine, by HPLC coupled to electrospray hybrid linear ion trap-orbital ion trap MS. Metallomics: Integr Biometal Sci. 2011;3(5):513–20.

Labunskyy VM, Hatfield DL, Gladyshev VN. Selenoproteins: molecular pathways and physiological roles. Physiol Rev. 2014;94(3):739–77. https://doi.org/10.1152/physrev.00039.2013.

Latrèche L, Chavatte L. Selenium incorporation into selenoproteins, implications in human health. Metal Ions Biol Med. 2008;X:731–7.

Letsiou S, Nomikos T, Panagiotakos DB, Pergantis SA, Fragopoulou E, Pitsavos C, Stefanadis C, Antonopoulou S. Gender-specific distribution of selenium to serum selenoproteins: associations with total selenium levels, age, smoking, body mass index, and physical activity. Biofactors. 2014;40(5):524–35.

Lobanov AV, Hatfield DL, Gladyshev VN. Eukaryotic selenoproteins and selenoproteomes. Biochim Biophys Acta. 2009;1790(11):1424–8. https://doi.org/10.1016/j.bbagen.2009.05.014.

Mariotti M, Ridge PG, Zhang Y, Lobanov AV, Pringle TH, Guigo R, Hatfield DL, Gladyshev VN. Composition and evolution of the vertebrate and mammalian selenoproteomes. PLoS One. 2012;7(3):e33066. https://doi.org/10.1371/journal.pone.0033066.

Marro N. The 1994 Australian market basket survey. Camberra: Australian Government Publishing Service; 1996.

Ogawa Y, Nishikawa M, Toyoda N, Yonemoto T, Gondou A, Inada M. Age- and sex-related changes in type-1 iodothyronine deiodinase messenger ribonucleic acid in rat liver and kidney. Horm Metab Res. 1999;31(5):295–9.

Ohta Y, Kobayashi Y, Konishi S, Hirano S. Speciation analysis of selenium metabolites in urine and breath by HPLC- and GC-inductively coupled plasma-MS after administration of seleno-methionine and methylselenocysteine to rats. Chem Res Toxicol. 2009;22(11):1795–801.

Olson GE, Winfrey VP, Nagdas SK, Hill KE, Burk RF. Apolipoprotein E receptor-2 (ApoER2) mediates selenium uptake from selenoprotein P by the mouse testis. J Biol Chem. 2007;282(16):12290–7.

Panigati M, Falciola L, Mussini P, Beretta G, Fancino RM. Determination of selenium in Italian rices by differential pulse cathodic stripping voltammetry. Food Chem. 2007;105:1091–8. https://doi.org/10.1016/j.foodchem.2007.02.002.

Papp LV, Lu J, Holmgren A, Khanna KK. From selenium to selenoproteins: synthesis, identity, and their role in human health. Antioxid Redox Signal. 2007;9(7):775–806.

Pappa EC, Pappas AC, Surai PF. Selenium content in selected foods from the Greek market and estimation of the daily intake. Sci Total Environ. 2006;372(1):100–8.

Pedrero Z, Madrid Y. Novel approaches for selenium speciation in foodstuffs and biological specimens: a review. Anal Chim Acta. 2009;634(2):135–52.

Pitts MW, Kremer PM, Hashimoto AC, Torres DJ, Byrns CN, Williams CS, Berry MJ. Competition between the brain and testes under selenium-compromised conditions: insight into sex differences in selenium metabolism and risk of neurodevelopmental disease. J Neurosci. 2015;35(46):15326–38.

Pyrzynska K. Determination of selenium species in environmental samples. Microchim Acta. 2002;140(1):55–62.

Ramoutar RR, Brumaghim JL. Antioxidant and anticancer properties and mechanisms of inorganic selenium, oxo-sulfur, and oxo-selenium compounds. Cell Biochem Biophys. 2010;58(1):1–23.

Rayman MP. Selenium and human health. Lancet. 2012;379(9822):1256–68.

Read R, Bellew T, Yang JG, Hill KE, Palmer IS, Burk RF. Selenium and amino acid composition of selenoprotein P, the major selenoprotein in rat serum. J Biol Chem. 1990;265(29):17899–905.

Rebsch CM, Penna FJ 3rd, Copeland PR. Selenoprotein expression is regulated at multiple levels in prostate cells. Cell Res. 2006;16(12):940–8.

Riese C, Michaelis M, Mentrup B, Gotz F, Kohrle J, Schweizer U, Schomburg L. Selenium-dependent pre- and posttranscriptional mechanisms are responsible for sexual dimorphic expression of selenoproteins in murine tissues. Endocrinology. 2006;147(12):5883–92.

Schomburg L. Sex-specifi c differences in biological effects and metabolism of selenium. In: Hatfield DLSU, Tsuji PA, Gladyshev VN, editors. Selenium: its molecular biology and role in human health. 4th ed. New York, NY: Springer Science+Business Media, LLC; 2016. p. 377–88.

Schomburg L, Schweizer U. Hierarchical regulation of selenoprotein expression and sex-specific effects of selenium. Biochim Biophys Acta. 2009;1790(11):1453–62.

Schomburg L, Schweizer U, Holtmann B, Flohe L, Sendtner M, Kohrle J. Gene disruption discloses role of selenoprotein P in selenium delivery to target tissues. Biochem J. 2003;370. (Pt 2:397–402.

Schomburg L, Riese C, Renko K, Schweizer U. Effect of age on sexually dimorphic selenoprotein expression in mice. Biol Chem. 2007;388(10):1035–41.

Sies H. Ebselen, a selenoorganic compound as glutathione peroxidase mimic. Free Radic Biol Med. 1993;14(3):313–23.

Smrkolj P, Pograjc L, Hlastan-Ribic C, Stibilj V. Selenium content in selected Slovenian foodstuffs and estimated daily intakes of selenium. Food Chem. 2005;90:691–7. https://doi.org/10.1016/j.foodchem.2004.04.028.

Sonet J, Bulteau A-L, Chavatte L. Selenium and selenoproteins in human health and diseases. In: Michalke B, editor. Metallomics: analytical techniques and speciation methods: Wiley-VCH Verlag GmbH & Co. KGaA; 2016. p. 364–81. https://doi.org/10.1002/9783527694907.ch13.

Suzuki KT, Somekawa L, Kurasaki K, Suzuki N. Simultaneous tracing of 76Se-selenite and 77Se-selenomethionine by absolute labeling and speciation. Toxicol Appl Pharmacol. 2006a;217(1):43–50.

Suzuki KT, Somekawa L, Suzuki N. Distribution and reuse of 76Se-selenosugar in selenium-deficient rats. Toxicol Appl Pharmacol. 2006b;216(2):303–8.

Taylor JB, Finley JW, Caton JS. Effect of the chemical form of supranutritional selenium on selenium load and selenoprotein activities in virgin, pregnant, and lactating rats. J Anim Sci. 2005;83(2):422–9.

Tinggi U. Determination of selenium in meat products by hydride generation atomic absorption spectrophotometry. J AOAC Int. 1999;82(2):364–7.

Turanov AA, Xu X-M, Carlson BA, Yoo M-H, Gladyshev VN, Hatfield DL. Biosynthesis of selenocysteine, the 21st amino acid in the genetic code, and a novel pathway for cysteine biosynthesis. Adv Nutr. 2011;2(2):122–8.

Turanov AA, Everley RA, Hybsier S, Renko K, Schomburg L, Gygi SP, Hatfield DL, Gladyshev VN. Regulation of selenocysteine content of human selenoprotein P by dietary selenium and insertion of cysteine in place of selenocysteine. PLoS One. 2015;10(10):e0140353.

USDA USDoA Nutrient database for standard reference release 13. Nutrient datalaboratory homepage on the World Wide Web. 1999. http://www.nalusdagov/fnic/foodcomp/Data/SR13/sr13html

Vesper DJ, Roy M, Rhoads CJ. Selenium distribution and mode of occurrence in the Kanawha Formation, southern West Virginia, U.S.A. Int J Coal Geol. 2008;73(3):237–49.

Whanger PD. Selenium and its relationship to cancer: an update. Br J Nutr. 2004;91(1):11–28.

Xu XM, Turanov AA, Carlson BA, Yoo MH, Everley RA, Nandakumar R, Sorokina I, Gygi SP, Gladyshev VN, Hatfield DL. Targeted insertion of cysteine by decoding UGA codons with mammalian selenocysteine machinery. Proc Natl Acad Sci U S A. 2010;107(50):21430–4.

Yamashita Y, Yamashita M. Identification of a novel selenium-containing compound, selenoneine, as the predominant chemical form of organic selenium in the blood of bluefin tuna. J Biol Chem. 2010;285(24):18134–8.

Part IV
The Role of Selenium within Redox Systems, Inflammation, and Thyroid Interaction

Chapter 6
Oxidative Stress, Selenium Redox Systems Including GPX/TXNRD Families

Irina Ingold and Marcus Conrad

Abstract A third of the mammalian selenoprotein repertoire accounts for the two main cellular redox systems in mammals, i.e., the glutathione- and thioredoxin-dependent systems. All three thioredoxin reductases contain selenocysteine as their penultimate amino acid and keep thioredoxins in their reduced, active state. Cytosolic thioredoxin reductase (TXNRD1) and mitochondrial thioredoxin reductase (TXNRD2) are directly involved in cell proliferation and cell protection of somatic cells, respectively, whereas thioredoxin-glutathione reductase (TXNRD3) contributes to sperm development. Five out of eight glutathione peroxidases (GPX) are selenoproteins in humans and are part of antioxidant network by keeping the levels of cellular peroxides in check. Among these, glutathione peroxidase 4 (GPX4) is unusual as it confers a moonlighting and essential function in sperm development because of its promiscuity towards reducing substrates. Moreover, due to its unique activity to efficiently reduce phospholipid hydroperoxides, GPX4 has emerged as one of the most important selenoproteins in mammals. In fact, we and others found that GPX4 is the key regulator of a recently described form of regulated necrotic cell death, called ferroptosis. Hence, this chapter aims at illuminating the importance of the main mammalian antioxidant systems in health and disease.

Keywords Cancer · Cardiomyopathy · Cardiovascular system · Embryogenesis · Ferroptosis · Neurodegeneration · Redox signaling

Introduction

Oxidative stress, a cellular condition defined by an excessive amount of electrophiles in cells, is in most cases considered the result of an increased level of reactive oxygen species (ROS) in cells. These include superoxide anion (O_2^-), hydrogen peroxide (H_2O_2), and other hydroperoxides (ROOH) and hydroxyl radicals (OH·), which

I. Ingold · M. Conrad (✉)
Helmholtz Zentrum München, Institute of Developmental Genetics, Neuherberg, Germany
e-mail: marcus.conrad@helmholtz-muenchen.de

© Springer International Publishing AG, part of Springer Nature 2018
B. Michalke (ed.), *Selenium*, Molecular and Integrative Toxicology,
https://doi.org/10.1007/978-3-319-95390-8_6

all constitute partly reduced forms of molecular oxygen (O_2) (Sies et al. 2017). Due to their electrophilic nature towards biological targets, such as DNA, proteins, and lipids, these molecules have often been associated with cellular dysfunction and cell death (Cross et al. 1987). In fact, oxidative stress has been linked to a myriad of pathological conditions including cancer (Trachootham et al. 2009), tissue ischemia/ reperfusion injury (IRI), and neurodegenerative disease (Andersen 2004; Shukla et al. 2011).

Although ROS have been solely viewed as harmful and damaging agents to biological molecules for a long time, it has become apparent within the past years that the non-radical species H_2O_2 and possibly other ROOH can act as important signaling molecules regulating various biological processes within the cell (Finkel 2011). In this regard, peroxides were identified as important mediators in growth factor signaling (Conrad et al. 2010), hypoxic signal transduction (Chandel et al. 1998), autophagy (Scherz-Shouval et al. 2007), immune response, and stem cell differentiation and proliferation (Holmstrom and Finkel 2014).

Hence, it is evident that the cellular level of peroxides must be tightly regulated in order to allow for physiological signaling while keeping their potentially harmful effects as little as possible. In this respect, a well-balanced regulation of the intracellular redox homeostasis by cellular antioxidant systems is essential for proper redox-dependent signaling and cellular purposes.

Intrinsic Sources of ROS and Their Immediate Effects on Cellular Targets

As a consequence of aerobic metabolism, there are a number of distinct sites within the cell contributing to the generation of substantial amounts of partially reduced forms of O_2. Complexes I, II, and III of the mitochondrial respiratory chain and the family of NADPH-dependent oxidases (NOXs) present the main intrinsic sources for O_2^- generation (Brandes et al. 2014; Quinlan et al. 2012). O_2^- is formed by a one-electron reduction of molecular O_2, which becomes readily converted to H_2O_2 by the enzymatic activity of superoxide dismutases (SOD) or by spontaneous disproportionation. There are two SODs, which are localized either in the cytosol and the mitochondrial intermembrane space (SOD1/CuZn-SOD) or in the mitochondrial matrix (SOD2/Mn-SOD). Since O_2^- is not able to diffuse through lipid membranes, it is kept in the compartment where it is generated and is converted to H_2O_2 by the respective SOD to prevent O_2^- accumulation.

Besides being formed as a product of O_2^-, H_2O_2 can also arise as a direct metabolic by-product at various cellular processes, including oxidative protein folding in the endoplasmic reticulum, β-oxidation of long fatty acids, and peroxisomal oxidation (Lodhi and Semenkovich 2014). Its ability to penetrate lipid membranes (facilitated by aquaporins) provides an advantage for H_2O_2 regarding its function as intracellular signaling molecule (Bienert and Chaumont 2014). This involves either the direct oxidation of critical cysteine residues of redox-sensitive target proteins or indirectly via professional thiol peroxidases, such as peroxiredoxins (PRX) or glutaredoxins (GRX) (Stocker et al. 2017). For instance, H_2O_2 first oxidizes PRX2, which then transmits the oxidative signal to a redox-sensitive protein, as exemplified for the transcription factor STAT3 (Sobotta et al. 2015). Regarding the mechanism of direct oxidation, H_2O_2 oxidizes redox-sensitive cysteine residues in target proteins leading to sulfenic acid formation. Sulfenic acid residues may then form inter- or intramolecular disulfide bonds with neighboring cysteine residues or sulfenylamides with nearby amino groups, thereby altering their activity, function, and/or stability. Sulfenic and sulfinic acid formation as well as protein disulfides and sulfenylamides are reversible cysteine modifications, which can be resolved by respective antioxidant systems in the cell. By contrast, sustained levels of ROS/H_2O_2 promote further oxidation steps leading to the formation of irreversible oxidation of redox-active cysteine residues like sulfonic acid. Well-studied examples of redox-sensitive proteins include phosphatases, such as protein tyrosine phosphatases 1B (PTPB1), receptor tyrosine kinases (RTK), and transcription factors, such as nuclear factor-κ B (NFκB) (Finkel 2011). Beyond this, certain transcription factors can also be indirectly modulated by H_2O_2 signaling as their activity depends on the redox state of interacting partners as reported for hypoxia-inducible factor (HIF), NFκB (Schreck et al. 1991) and nuclear factor (erythroid-derived 2)-like 2 (NFE2L2, Nrf2) (Taguchi et al. 2011).

Another common type of ROS molecules are lipid hydroperoxides (LOOH) and hydroxyl radicals (HO˙). HO˙ is formed from H_2O_2 in the presence of transition metals (Fe^{2+} and Cu^{2+}) via the Fenton reaction and is probably the most reactive and toxic species towards cellular macromolecules. Iron-driven formation of HO˙ induces and promotes lipid peroxidation in biological membranes including alkyl (R˙), alkoxyl (RO˙), and peroxyl radicals (ROO˙), which can all propagate autoxidation reactions leading to deleterious lipid modifications. In this context, iron-dependent lipid peroxidation is regarded the critical event in a recently recognized form of regulated necrotic cell death, named ferroptosis (Dixon et al. 2012). The induction of ferroptotic cell death has been associated with a number of pathological conditions, such as cancer, neurodegenerative disease, and tissue ischemia/reperfusion injury (IRI) (Angeli et al. 2017; Conrad et al. 2016a, b; Stockwell et al. 2017). Due to the importance of the selenoperoxidase GPX4 in this cell death paradigm, a separate section within this chapter is dedicated under "Involvement of GPXs in a myriad of (patho)physiological contexts".

Antioxidative Systems in Mammals

The intracellular antioxidative system consists of nonenzymatic antioxidant compounds and a large number of redox-active enzymes, which vary in their functions and intracellular localization. In contrast to enzymatic antioxidants, nonenzymatic compounds including the well-known vitamin C and E, ß-carotenes, and coenzyme Q10 may become radicals themselves after reacting with ROS molecules. Therefore, nonenzymatic antioxidative micronutrients and vitamines rather function as interception of radical chain reactions, which get either directly or indirectly regenerated by enzymatic systems.

The most abundant nonenzymatic antioxidant in the cell is the thiol-containing, water-soluble tripeptide glutathione (GSH). GSH is synthesized from cysteine, glutamate, and glycine in two steps by the enzyme γ-glutamylcysteine synthetase (γ-GCS) yielding γ-glutamylcysteine and by the enzyme glutathione synthetase producing GSH. The main source of cysteine utilized for GSH synthesis in vitro is extracellular cystine (i.e., oxidized cysteine) imported via the system Xc⁻ (i.e., cystine/glutamate antiporter) and reduced by TXNRD1 and GSH to cysteine in the cell (Mandal et al. 2010b). Besides its role in GSH S-transferase-mediated detoxification processes by GSH conjugation with toxic compounds, its actual antioxidant function relies on its role to serve as a reductant of the GSH-dependent enzymes, namely glutathione peroxidases (GPX) (see Sect. 6.5) and GRX. The protein family of GRX, present in different subcellular compartments, acts as reductant of protein disulfides, similar to the TXN-dependent system, but uses GSH as electron donor instead (Holmgren and Aslund 1995). Oxidized diglutathione (GSSG) in turn is reduced by glutathione reductase (GSR) at the expense of NADPH/H⁺.

Besides SODs and catalases, which reduce H_2O_2 to H_2O in peroxisomes, the family of thioredoxin-dependent peroxidases, called peroxiredoxins (PRX), consists of six distinct members. PRXs are localized in distinct subcellular compartments where they catalyze the reduction of H_2O_2 and different organic hydroperoxides by catalytically active, peroxidative cysteines in their active site. While PRX1–5 are dithiol PRXs that interact with TXNs, the monothiol PRX6 interacts with GSH/GST (Rhee et al. 2001; Seo et al. 2000). Furthermore, PRXs are able to modulate the activity of proteins by direct binding as exemplified for PRX2 (Sobotta et al. 2015). Oxidized mitochondrial and cytosolic PRXs are generally reduced by members of the thioredoxin-dependent systems (Fig. 6.1).

Unlike the aforementioned antioxidant systems, all three mammalian thioredoxin reductases (TXNRD) and some members of the glutathione peroxidases (GPX) family of enzymes contain the 21st amino acid selenocysteine (Sec). In these selenoenzymes, Sec constitutes the catalytically active site. Due to its physicochemical properties, Sec is regarded as a better redox catalyst in scavenging peroxides than in Cys-containing redox enzymes (Reich and Hondal 2016). At physiological pH Se is present in its ionized form due to a lower pKa (= 5.4) than thiols, which makes it a better nucleophile. In its oxidized, selenenic acid form Se is a better electrophile than sulfenic acid protecting it from overoxidation. Since the focus of this book chapter is to highlight the importance of both families of proteins—glutathione peroxidases and thioredoxin reductases—in the control of redox regulation and oxidative stress, the following sections will provide basic mechanistic details of these enzymes and their implication in pathological contexts in mice and man.

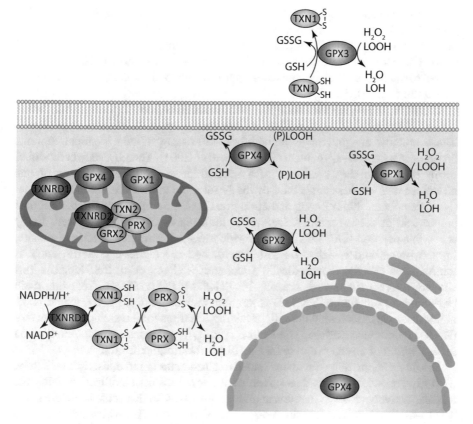

Fig. 6.1 Subcellular localization of selenoproteins of the mammalian antioxidative network. The two main selenium-containing antioxidative systems—glutathione peroxidases (GPX) and thioredoxin reductases (TXNRD)—are present in most cellular compartments to maintain cellular redox homeostasis. In the cytosol, H_2O_2 and other hydroperoxides are kept in check by GPX1, GPX2, and TXNRD1 via thioredoxin-1 (TXN1) and peroxiredoxins (PRXs). GPX4 is expressed in three different forms and is localized to the nucleus, mitochondria, and cytosol. While the nuclear and mitochondrial transcripts of GPX4 are solely expressed in sperm cells, cytosolic GPX4 and GPX1 are (besides the cytosol) also enriched in the intermembrane space of mitochondria in somatic cells via a yet-unrecognized mechanism. Cytosolic GPX4 reduces complex lipid hydroperoxides and is strongly associated with lipid membranes. GPX3 is an extracellular protein associated with membranous structures. TXNRD2 is located in the mitochondrial matrix and responsible for mitochondrial redox control via thioredoxin-2 (TXN2) and PRX

Structural Aspects and Cellular Functions of Thioredoxin Reductases (TXNRD)

The protein family of thioredoxin reductases (TXNRD) in mammals consists of three proteins encoded by three individual genes, which show different subcellular localization and tissue expression. TXNRD1 is mainly present in the cytosol and nucleus (Gladyshev et al. 1996; Zhong et al. 1998), whereas TXNRD2 is mainly present in the mitochondrial matrix (Biterova et al. 2005) (Fig. 6.1). While both proteins are ubiquitously expressed, the third member of this family, TXNRD3 (thioredoxin glutathione reductase), is a testis-specific one (Sun et al. 2001) involved in the formation of disulfide bonds of sperm mitochondrial capsules of maturing sperm (Su et al. 2005).

TXNRDs belong to the family of oxidoreductases containing an FAD- and a NADPH-binding domain as well as an interface domain (Sandalova et al. 2001). These proteins are present as homodimers consisting of two identical subunits arranged in a head-to-tail manner (Sandalova et al. 2001). Thereby, each homodimer forms two active sites consisting of a selenothiol of the C-terminal site of one monomer with an adjacent dithiol of the N-terminal site of the second monomer (Sandalova et al. 2001; Zhong and Holmgren 2000). Sec presents the penultimate amino acid at the C-terminus. Due to its high reactivity and its exposed, freely accessible position, TXNRDs display a wide range of substrates including selenite, lipid hydroperoxides, dehydroascorbic acid, and redox-active proteins, such as thioredoxins (TXN), protein-disulfide isomerases (Papp et al. 2007), and a less studied thioredoxin-related protein 14 (TRP14) (Woo 2004). Yet, the main physiological function of TXNRD is the reduction of oxidized TXN, which is the major disulfide reductase in the cell, providing electrons to ribonucleotide reductase (RNR), methionine sulfoxide reductase, PRXs, phosphatases, and transcription factors with redox-sensitive cysteines (Lillig and Holmgren 2007).

Due to its interaction with redox-sensitive phosphatases and transcription factors, the TXN-dependent system does not only act as a reductant of oxidized proteins, but it is also actively involved in redox signaling processes. In this context, TXNRD via TXN was shown to regulate the redox state of certain PTPs, which are known to become reversibly oxidized upon growth factor receptor-stimulated ROS formation via NADPH oxidase. Oxidation of the active site Cys of PTPs transiently inhibits their phosphatase activity, thereby leaving receptor tyrosine kinases in a more active state and leading to a net increase in downstream growth factor signaling. For instance, the TXN-dependent system was recently shown to reactivate oxidized PTPB1, thereby affecting platelet-derived growth factor β (PDGF-β) receptor tyrosine kinase signaling (Dagnell et al. 2013). In the context of transcription factor regulation, TXN1 was reported to translocate from the cytosol to the nucleus upon increased oxidative stress (Hirota et al. 1999), where it regulates the activity of various transcription factors. By modifying critical cysteine residues, TXN1 also helps to enhance DNA binding of transcription factors such as nuclear factor-κ B (NFκB) (Hirota et al. 1999), Nrf2, hypoxia-inducible factor 1 (HIF1) (Carrero et al. 2000; Ema et al. 1999), tumor suppressor p53 (Merrill et al. 1999), and activator protein 1 (AP-1) (Hirota et al. 1999). Taken together, by controlling the redox state of TXN, TXNRDs themselves are involved in the regulation of most cellular process, such as proliferation, antioxidant defense, and cell death.

The Contribution of TXNRDs to (Patho)Physiological Conditions

In order to understand the role of TXNRDs in embryonic development and adult physiology, various conditional knockout approaches targeting TXNRD1 and TXNRD2 in distinct tissues have been reported (Table 6.1). These studies showed that both proteins are essential for mammalian embryonic development, albeit at different embryonic stages. The systemic deletion of *Txnrd1* causes early embryonic death between E7.5 and E9.5 with embryos presenting generalized developmental retardation with the exception of the heart (Bondareva et al. 2007; Jakupoglu et al. 2005). The systemic loss of *Txnrd2* is associated with perturbed heart development and strongly impaired hematopoiesis of mutant embryos due to dysfunctional mitochondrial redox homeostasis causing lethality around E13.5 (Conrad et al. 2004). Studies using cardiac tissue-specific (± tamoxifen-inducible) deletion of *Txnrd2* pinpointed to a pivotal role for this enzyme not only for the newborn heart (Conrad et al. 2004), but also for protection against the deleterious effects of transient IRI in an experimental model of cardiac infarction in mice (Horstkotte et al. 2011). TXNRD1, however, does not play any apparent role in cardiac development or in adult heart tissue under physiological conditions and in response to experimental cardiac IRI (Horstkotte et al. 2011; Jakupoglu et al. 2005). An important role for TXNRD2 in maintaining mitochondrial integrity and energy

Table 6.1 Systemic knockout mouse models for redox-active selenoenzymes

Gene	Phenotype	Ref.
Txnrd1	Embryonic lethality between E7.5 and E9.5 due to overall maldevelopment and severe growth retardation	Bondareva et al. (2007), Jakupoglu et al. (2005)
Txnrd2	Embryonic lethality at E13.5 due to impaired heart development and impaired hematopoiesis	Conrad et al. (2004)
Gpx1	Fully viable but increased sensitivity towards experimentally induced oxidative stress	Esworthy et al. (2000), Ho et al. (1997)
Gpx2	Fully viable but increased sensitivity towards experimentally induced oxidative stress	Esworthy et al. (2001)
Gpx1/Gpx2	Viable but spontaneous development of intestinal inflammation and cancer	Esworthy et al. (2001)
Gpx3	Fully viable but increased thrombosis due to platelet activation	Jin et al. (2011)
Gpx4	Embryonic lethality at the gastrulation stage (E7.5)	Imai et al. (2003), Seiler et al. (2008), Yant et al. (2003)
Nuclear Gpx4 (*nGpx4$^{-/-}$*)	Fully viable but aberrant chromatin condensation due to decreased protamine oxidation	Conrad et al. (2005), Puglisi et al. (2012)
Mitochondrial Gpx4 (*mGpx4$^{-/-}$*)	Fully viable but male infertility due to perturbed mitochondrial capsule formation and decreased stability of the spermatozoan midpiece	Schneider et al. (2009)

metabolism also in the aging heart was reported recently (Kiermayer et al. 2015). Ageing cardio-specific knockout mice presented ventricular concentric hypertrophy, mitochondrial degeneration, and an accumulation of autophagic bodies as also evidenced by a p62 accumulation. The identification of the first missense mutations in the human *TXNRD2* gene in patients suffering from dilated cardiomyopathy further underpins the outstanding relevance of TXNRD2 in cardioprotection of the human heart (Sibbing et al. 2011).

Perturbed mitochondrial redox homeostasis as a consequence of *Txnrd2* loss does not only severely affect cardiac function, but also impairs tumor growth and tumor-related vascularization in transformed *Txnrd2⁻ᐟ⁻* fibroblasts by stabilizing prolyl hydroxylase 2, thereby preventing the transcription of hypoxia-inducible factor 1-α (HIF-1α) target genes (Hellfritsch et al. 2015). Besides cardiac tissue and tumor growth, TXNRD2 plays various roles in the endothelial compartment. Specifically, a pro-thrombotic and pro-inflammatory vascular phenotype, manifested as intravascular cellular deposits in arterioles, as well as microthrombi in glomerular capillaries, was shown in mice specifically lacking TXNRD2 in endothelium (Kirsch et al. 2016). Enhanced leukocyte migration into inflamed tissue and reduced flow-dependent vasodilation of arteries were also found in these knockout mice indicating insufficient nitric oxide signaling.

Unlike in cardiac tissue, TXNRD1 is of utmost importance for the developing cerebellum (Soerensen et al. 2008). Strong proliferation defects of granule cell precursors in the external granular layer underlie massive cerebellar hypoplasia and a severely perturbed Bergmann glial network of brain-specific *Txnrd1* knockout mice. As neuron-specific deletion of TXNRD1 does not affect cerebellar development, it is clear that these effects must be inflicted by impaired proliferation of granule cell precursors. Although not yet proven in the murine *Txnrd1* knockout model, a loss-of-function mutation in the TXNRD1 protein in patients causes genetically generalized epilepsy (Kudin et al. 2017). The Pro190Leu mutation detected in patients impairs the protein turnover rate and protein expression level leading to reduced protein activity indicating that increased oxidative stress triggers epilepsy development. Interestingly, *Txnrd2* deletion in the brain does not cause any obvious pathological phenotype in mice (Soerensen et al. 2008), although a patient carrying a loss-of-function mutation of mitochondrial thioredoxin (*TXN2*) was reported to suffer from severe neuropathological defects, such as epilepsy and cerebellar atrophy (Holzerova et al. 2016). Hence, it seems that in the cerebellum TXN2 is a viable substrate of TXNRD1.

Due to its function to maintain redox homeostasis in cells and to regulate the activity of different transcription factors, TXNRD1 confers an ambivalent role in cancer development, acting as both a promoting and a preventing factor. On the one hand TXNRD1 prevents tumor formation by maintaining redox balance and decreasing mutations in the DNA; on the other hand as a direct target of Nrf2 TXNRD1 is frequently overexpressed in many cancer and cancer cell lines protecting them from oxidative stress-induced cell death and enabling fast proliferation (Lu and Holmgren 2009). In the latter, TXNRD1 via TXN1 provides electrons to RNR, which is essential for the reduction of ribonucleotides to deoxyribonucleotides, the building blocks of DNA. By this, the TXNRD1/TXN1 system is directly involved in DNA synthesis, which was already highlighted by the brain-specific deletion of *Txnrd1* causing massive cerebellar hypoplasia (Soerensen et al. 2008). On the contrary, a hepatocyte-specific deletion of *Txnrd1* demonstrated increased hepatocarcinogenesis under chemically induced conditions in TXNRD1-deficient mice (Carlson et al. 2012). At the same time knockout livers displayed increased resistance towards acetaminophen-induced hepatotoxicity mediated by enhanced Nrf2 activation and upregulation of Nrf2 target genes including those involved in GSH synthesis and utilization (Patterson et al. 2013).

Functional Redundancies Between the TXN- and the GSH-Dependent Systems

The TXN-dependent system represented by TXN, TXNRD, and PRX on the one side and the GSH-dependent system made up of the GSH biosynthesis and GSH recycling machinery, as well as GSH-utilizing enzymes, such as GPX, glutaredoxins (GRX), and GSH-S-transferases (GST), on the other side were considered initially to entail entirely independent redox systems in mammalian cells. Although the two antioxidative systems were regarded for many decades to act in parallel rather than having overlapping functions, mouse- and cell-based studies performed within the last 15 years taught us the opposite as there are apparent widespread redundancies and cross talks between both systems (Table 6.2).

Some of the earliest key findings in this context are the identification of glutathionylated TXN (Casagrande et al. 2002), and a highly increased sensitivity of *Txnrd2*$^{-/-}$ cells towards GSH deprivation-induced cell death triggered by the γ-GCS inhibitor L-buthionine sulfoximine (BSO) (Conrad et al. 2004). Very similar findings were also obtained for *Txnrd1*$^{-/-}$ cells (Mandal et al. 2010a; Mandal et al. 2010b). Only the combined inhibition and deletion of the GSH biosynthesis and TXNRD1 was sufficient to elicit cell death in c-myc- and H-ras^{v12}-transformed fibroblasts in cells and in tumor-bearing mice (Mandal et al. 2010a). While GSH deprivation-induced cell death in *Txnrd2*$^{-/-}$ cells could be rescued by N-acetyl-cysteine (NAC) (Conrad et al. 2004), or increased cystine uptake mediated by forced system Xc$^-$ expression (Mandal et al. 2010b), these approaches did not hold true for *Txnrd1*$^{-/-}$ cells. Therefore, TXNRD1 seems to be indeed required for cystine reduction as proposed by Arne Holmgren already four decades ago (Holmgren 1977). Notably, a series of GSH-relevant enzymes were found to be overexpressed in *Txnrd1*$^{-/-}$ cells including glutamate-cysteine ligase, catalytic subunit (GCLC), glutamate-cysteine ligase, modifier subunit (GCLM), glutathione reductase (GSR), and various GSTs, all cognate target genes of Nrf2 (Mandal et al. 2010a). Elevated expression of glutaredoxin-2 (GRX2), which is present in the mitochondrial matrix, was described for TXNRD2 null cells (Hellfritsch et al. 2015).

Table 6.2 Redundancies between the GSH- and TXN-dependent systems

First genetic target/ treatment	Second treatment/genetic target	Major phenotype	Ref.
$Txnrd2^{-/-}$	BSO	Increased sensitivity and cell death in primary fibroblasts, which can be rescued by NAC	Conrad et al. (2004)
$Txnrd1^{-/-}$	BSO	Increased sensitivity and lethality of (tumor) cells in vitro; impaired tumor growth in vivo	Mandal et al. (2010a)
$Txnrd2^{-/-}$	BSO and system Xc^-overexpression	System Xc^- overexpression rescues BSO-induced cell death in $Txnrd2^{-/-}$ cells	Mandal et al. (2010b)
$Txnrd1^{-/-}$	BSO and system Xc^-overexpression	System Xc^- overexpression fails to rescue BSO-induced cell death in $Txnrd1^{-/-}$ cells	Mandal et al. (2010b)
$Txnrd1^{-/-}$	$Grs^{-/-}$	No phenotype observed	Eriksson et al. (2015)
$Txnrd2^{-/-}$	BSO	Reduction in tumor growth of transformed fibroblasts	Hellfritsch et al. (2015)
BSO	Auranofin/sulfasalazine	Increased cell death in malignant tumors in vitro; reduced tumor growth in a xenograft model	Harris et al. (2015)
$Txnrd1^{-/-}$	$Grs^{-/-}, Txn1^{-/-}$	Increased cell death compensated by hyperproliferation of hepatocytes	Prigge et al. (2017)

The concept of extensive redundant functions of both systems was underpinned by in vivo studies, showing that the genetic loss of *Txnrd1* in combination with *Grs* in hepatocytes allowed normal hepatocellular function as long as the de novo GSH biosynthesis and the conversion of methionine to cysteine are sustained (Eriksson et al. 2015). Maintenance of the hepatocellular redox homeostasis is thus achieved by electron transfer from the GSH/GRX system to TXN1 (Prigge et al. 2017). It is noteworthy that even upon the combined deletion of *Txnrd1, Grs* and *Txn1* cysteine provided by the transsulfuration pathway from methionine is sufficient to allow GSH synthesis, thereby maintaining the activity of intracellular disulfide reductase system. Hepatocellular death only occurred upon increased oxidative stress imposed by IRI. This was counteracted by increased proliferation in liver resulting in a hyperproliferation of hepatocytes (Prigge et al. 2017). Similarly, Harris and colleagues showed that only the simultaneous inhibition of the GSH and the TXN system by targeting GCLM, system Xc^-, and TXNRD1 allowed rising intracellular ROS to a level sufficient to trigger cell death in malignant tumors (Harris et al. 2015). This is highly similar to what we showed before for TXNRD1-deficient tumor cells deprived of intracellular GSH (Mandal et al. 2010a). Hence, one can conclude that effective anticancer treatment based on targeting the cellular antioxidant systems can perhaps only be achieved if both the GSH- and TXN-dependent systems are concomitantly impaired/inhibited.

Selenium-Containing Glutathione Peroxidases

Within the GSH-dependent system, only certain members of the glutathione peroxidase (GPX) family of proteins are selenocysteine-containing enzymes. There are eight designated GPX members in rodents and man (Brigelius-Flohe and Maiorino 2013). Four of them are selenoproteins (i.e., GPX1–4), whereas GPX5, GPX7, and GPX8 are cysteine-containing ones. GPX6 is somewhat different as it is a cysteine-containing homolog in rodents, while it is a selenoenzyme in human. GPX5 is expressed in epididymis and contributes to sperm maturation. GPX7 and GPX8 are the next related ones to GPX4 and are localized in the endoplasmic reticulum where they have been associated with processes, such as oxidative protein folding, calcium regulation, and HIF regulation. Since this book is dedicated to Sec-containing proteins, GPX5, GPX7, and GPX8 will not be further discussed here.

The protein family of GPX presents another essential stronghold against prooxidants such as H_2O_2 and a wide variety of organic hydroperoxides (Labunskyy et al. 2014). By keeping intracellular hydroperoxide levels in check, GPXs contribute to a number of cellular processes, such as detoxification, cell signaling, and oxidative protein folding (Brigelius-Flohe and Flohe 2017). During detoxification of H_2O_2 and other hydroperoxides to water and their corresponding alcohols, respectively, the active-site selenolate is oxidized yielding selenenic acid. Reduction of the active site is accomplished by two GSH molecules with a glutathionylated intermediate step. As two molecules of GSH are required for GPX reduction, a diglutathione (GSSG) is formed which is recovered by GSR at the expense of NADPH/H+. However, not all GPXs use GSH as substrate as 2-cysteine-containing GPX enzymes prefer thioredoxins and other thiol oxidoreductase instead (Koh et al. 2007).

The catalytically active site of all GPXs was first considered to consist of a triad, which is highly conserved within the GPX family even in Cys-containing homologs (Maiorino et al. 1995; Schlecker et al. 2007). Yet this paradigm was reconsidered showing that the catalytic site is in fact a tetrad consisting of Sec, glutamine (Gln), tryptophan (Trp), and asparagine (Asn) that accounts for the catalytic efficiency of this protein family (Tosatto et al. 2008). The only exception so far is mammalian GXP8 (Toppo et al. 2008) and two plant GPXs (Toppo et al. 2009). Although GPXs share overlapping substrate specificities, they are not uniformly expressed across tissues and organs (Brigelius-Flohe 1999). Among the selenium-containing GPXs, GPX1-3 and GPX6 are homotetrameric proteins acting in the aqueous phase (Flohe et al. 1971; Ladenstein et al. 1979; Ren et al. 1997; Scheerer et al. 2007). In contrast, GPX4 is monomeric and has a unique surface structure which allows its association with lipid bilayers in order to efficiently reduce peroxides in membranous compartments (Cozza et al. 2017).

Physiological Functions of GPXs

Glutathione Peroxidase 1 (GPX1)

The first described GPX enzyme and actually the first identified selenoprotein is GPX1 (Flohe et al. 1973; Mills 1957; Rotruck et al. 1973). GPX1 is a ubiquitously expressed cytosolic protein (Fig. 6.1) with high abundancy in liver, kidney, and red blood cells. Like the other homotetrameric GPX, GPX1 does not reduce complex lipid hydroperoxides but instead acts on H_2O_2 and free fatty acid hydroperoxides (Tan et al. 1984). GPX1 plays an important role in regulating redox homeostasis in liver, and as the only member expressed in erythrocytes it protects red blood cells from oxidative stress by efficiently scavenging H_2O_2.

Glutathione Peroxidase 2 (GPX2)

GPX2 is mainly expressed in the epithelium of the gastrointestinal tract (Chu et al. 1993). Like GPX1 it is a homotetrameric protein and shares kinetic and substrate characteristics with GPX1 (Fig. 6.1). With a cognate antioxidant response element (ARE) in its promotor site, GPX2 is a target gene of the Nrf2-ARE pathway (Banning et al. 2005), with increased expression upon oxidative stress (Brigelius-Flohe and Kipp 2012). GPX2 expression is also subject to Wnt regulation (Kipp et al. 2007; Kipp et al. 2012), the latter being involved in a myriad of cellular processes particularly during embryogenesis (e.g., body axis patterning, cell fate specification, cell proliferation, and migration) and cell proliferation and tissue regeneration. Its localization to the crypt bases of the intestinal epithelium, which is the site of proliferating stem cells in the gut, indicates that GPX2 contributes to the continuous self-renewal of the intestinal epithelium cells by regulating mucosal homeostasis (Brigelius-Flohe and Maiorino 2013).

Glutathione Peroxidase 3 (GPX3)

GPX3 is an extracellular protein that is synthesized in the kidney, namely the renal proximal tubule cells, and secreted into the plasma (Whitin et al. 2002), where it represents the major GPX isoform (Olson et al. 2010). Upon secretion from renal cells, GPX3 is transported via the plasma to other tissues, where it was found to associate with membranes of intestinal epithelium, bronchi, and type II pneumocytes (Burk et al. 2011). Besides this, GPX3 is expressed in the early stage of the placenta, where it is required for the reduction of H_2O_2 during the process of decidualization (Xu et al. 2014). The only other tissue known so far expressing GPX3 is the epididymis. Here, GPX3 is secreted into its lumen where spermatozoa undergo their final maturation steps. Besides GSH GPX3 may also use alternative reducing substrates, such as TXN and GRX (Fig. 6.1) (Bjornstedt et al. 1994; Maiorino et al. 2007).

Glutathione Peroxidase 4 (GPX4)

GPX4 (initially also called "phospholipid hydroperoxide glutathione peroxidase," PHGPX) was initially purified from pig liver and was characterized as lipid peroxidation-inhibiting enzyme by Ursini et al. (1982). As part of the GPX family, GPX4 shares some common features with other members of the family but clearly differs in terms of structural, biochemical, and functional traits. Unlike other selenium-containing GPX isoforms, GPX4 is monomeric, thereby enabling the reduction of complex peroxides in lipids in lipoprotein particles, including phospholipid hydroperoxides (PLOOH) and cholesterol hydroperoxides (Fig. 6.1). Additionally, GPX4 is able to reduce small-molecule peroxides, such as H_2O_2, tert-butyl-hydroperoxide and free fatty acid hydroperoxides.

Like for its oxidizing substrates, GPX4 is also promiscuous towards its electron source. In addition to GSH it works well with small-molecular-weight thiols (Roveri et al. 1994; Ursini et al. 1995), such as cysteine, and even protein thiols under limiting GSH conditions, as physiologically evident during sperm maturation (Conrad et al. 2015; Maiorino et al. 2005; Ursini et al. 1999). Thereby, the enzyme converts to a protein thiol peroxidase and introduces disulfide bridges into sperm proteins, particularly in the sperm midpiece and in nucleus.

Due to alternative transcription initiation, the *Gpx4* gene gives rise to three different isoforms referred to as mitochondrial, nuclear, and cytosolic (also named "short form") GPX4 (Brigelius-Flohe et al. 1994; Moreno et al. 2003) (Fig. 6.1). Cytosolic GPX4 is ubiquitously expressed and particularly high in kidney, brain, and testis. GPX4 is the only GPX member essential for embryogenesis and animal survival (Liang et al. 2009). Moreover, it is now well accepted that the cytosolic isoform of GPX4 is the master regulator of a recently described form of regulated necrotic cell death, named ferroptosis (Friedmann Angeli et al. 2014; Yang et al. 2014). Since iron-dependent lipid peroxidation is the key event in this cell death pathway, impairment of GPX4 function will ultimately have a direct impact on sparking this kind of death process.

Unlike cytosolic GPX4, the mitochondrial and nuclear isoforms are almost exclusively expressed in different spermatogenic cells and confer specific functions here (Conrad et al. 2005; Puglisi et al. 2012; Schneider et al. 2009). By oxidizing and thus polymerizing mitochondrial capsular proteins mitochondrial GPX4 contributes to the formation of the so-called mitochondrial capsule, thereby ensuring full stability and rigidity of the spermatozoan midpiece (Maiorino et al. 2005; Schneider et al. 2009). The same function is taken over by the nuclear isoform of GPX4, and only the target proteins are protamines, small nuclear cysteine-rich proteins that replace the majority of histones during spermiogenesis. Introduction of disulfide bridges into these proteins leads to tightly packed male chromatin (Conrad et al. 2005). Isoform-specific knockout of both isoforms is fully compatible with life, while mitochondrial *Gpx4*$^{-/-}$ males are infertile (Schneider et al. 2009) (Table 6.1).

Glutathione Peroxidase 6 (GPX6)

Homotetrameric GPX6 is a selenium-containing enzyme in humans but a cysteine-containing one in rodents (Kryukov et al. 2003). Its expression is confined to the Bowman's gland of the olfactory bulb, where it is believed to be involved in metabolizing odorants (Dear et al. 1991). Despite its rather confined expression in the olfactory system, a recent synthetic lethal screen identified GPX6 as a modulator of mutant huntingtin toxicity, and its forced expression in the striatum of R6/2 Huntington's disease model improved motor behavior deficits (Shema et al. 2015). Yet future studies are required to assign additional functions to this enzyme.

Involvement of GPXs in a Myriad of (Patho)Physiological Contexts

Glutathione Peroxidase 1 (GPX1)

Early knockout studies performed with *Gpx1* and *Gpx2* showed that both selenoenzymes are dispensable for mouse development and survival under normal housing conditions (Esworthy et al. 2000; Ho et al. 1997) (Table 6.1). Only in response to oxidative stress inflicted by UV light (Walshe et al. 2007), γ-irradiation (Esworthy et al. 2000), or intoxication with chemical compounds, such as paraquat (Cheng et al. 1998) and diquat (Fu et al. 1999), *Gpx1* KO mice proved to be more sensitive than their wild-type siblings, strongly suggesting that GPX1 plays an important antioxidant function in mice (Conrad and Schweizer 2017).

Besides its "classical" antioxidant role, GPX1 has been linked to proper insulin signaling. While mice overexpressing GPX1 suffer from diabetes mellitus type 2 and obesity due to increased insulin resistance, hyperglycemia, and hyperinsulinemia (McClung et al. 2004), the knockout of *Gpx1* is associated with decreased pancreatic β-cell mass, increased insulin sensitivity, and a resistance to high-fat diet-induced obesity, resembling the phenotype of diabetes mellitus type 1 (Loh et al. 2009). Since GPX1 is a prime scavenger of cellular H_2O_2, both phenotypes are regarded to be the consequence of perturbed PTP signaling. In case of GPX1 overexpression, reduced levels of cellular H_2O_2 lead to a net increase of PTP activity and consequently decreased insulin receptor phosphorylation and protein kinase B activation, ultimately causing reduced insulin signaling (McClung et al. 2004). In case of *Gpx1* knockout, increased H_2O_2 levels lead to increased steady-state PTP and PTEN oxidation and hence phosphatase inactivation, thereby resulting in elevated PI3K/Akt signaling and augmented insulin sensitivity (Loh et al. 2009).

Glutathione Peroxidase 2 (GPX2)

As aforementioned, *Gpx2* knockout mice are viable and animals are fertile under non-stressed conditions (Esworthy et al. 2001). Even though transgenic mice with a combined knockout for *Gpx1* and *Gpx2* are viable, double-mutant animals develop spontaneous intestinal inflammation and cancer (Chu et al. 2004). With regard to cancer development, GPX2 seems to play a janus-like role by either preventing or promoting tumorigenesis in a fashion similar to TXNRD1. As GPX2 is a direct target of Nrf2, it supports the notion that it plays indeed a protective role during cancer development. On the other hand, augmented activation of the Nrf2-ARE pathway may protect existing cancer cells from oxidative stress-induced injury. Another typical characteristic of colon cancer is the presence of an activated Wnt signaling pathway known to promote cell proliferation and migration. Accordingly, knockdown of *Gpx2* in human and rat cancer significantly impairs tumor growth (Yan and Chen 2006).

Glutathione Peroxidase 3 (GPX3)

The targeted deletion of *Gpx3* in mice is well compatible with the development and survival of these mice (Olson et al. 2010). Nevertheless, loss of *Gpx3* is associated with reduced bleeding times and augmented platelet activation. *Gpx3* knockout animals suffer from increased thromboembolic events due to enhanced platelet activation (Jin et al. 2011) and as a result develop larger brain infarcts in an animal stroke model. Treatment of *Gpx3* null mice with azoxymethane/dextran sodium sulfate revealed its tumor-suppressing function in colon consistent with the localization of GPX3 on the basolateral surface of the basement membrane of colon (Barrett et al. 2013).

Glutathione Peroxidase 4 (GPX4)

By far more is known about this particular member of the GPX family of proteins. A number of systemic knockout approaches for *Gpx4* established the essential role of GPX4 during early embryonic development (Imai et al. 2003; Liang et al. 2009; Seiler et al. 2008; Yant et al. 2003). An elegant study performed by the Ran laboratory eventually showed that it is the cytosolic isoform, which is essential for embryogenesis and adult survival of mice (Liang et al. 2009). This is in line with knockout studies, where the nuclear and mitochondrial isoforms were individually targeted, demonstrating that loss of both forms does not impact embryogenesis and survival of adult mice (Conrad et al. 2005; Schneider et al. 2009).

Being the only enzyme able to efficiently detoxify complex hydroperoxides in membranous compartments, GPX4 activity is required to prevent lipid peroxidation-induced cell death both in vivo and in cell culture (Seiler et al. 2008). Notably, the constitutive knockout of the GSH-synthesizing enzyme *Gclc* causes the same early embryonic lethal phenotype as the knockout of *Gpx4* (Shi et al. 2000), indicating that GPX4 might be also (one of) the most relevant GSH-dependent enzymes in mammals.

Since the systemic knockout of *Gpx4* is embryonically lethal, a series of conditional knockout approaches using Cre/loxP technology have been performed in the last 10 years to unravel the role of GPX4 in different tissues and disease contexts (Angeli et al. 2017; Conrad and Schweizer 2016). These investigations demonstrated a strong cyto-protective function of GPX4 in neurons of different brain regions including hippocampus, cortex and cerebellum (Hambright et al. 2017; Seiler et al. 2008; Wirth et al. 2010, 2014), motor neurons (Chen et al. 2015), photoreceptor cells (Ueta et al. 2012), hepatocytes (Carlson et al. 2016), renal tubular cells (Friedmann Angeli et al. 2014), and endothelium (Wortmann et al. 2013). The findings that GPX4 regulates ferroptotic cell death in cancer (Yang et al. 2014) and the in vivo proof that *Gpx4* deletion triggers ferroptosis (Friedmann Angeli et al. 2014) have sparked overwhelming interest in this field of research.

GPX4 and Its Role in Ferroptosis

For many years apoptosis was considered the only form of regulated cell death, whereas all other forms of cell death were regarded being accidental and necrotic. Only when it was discovered that tumor necrosis factor α (TNFα) is able to induce a form of non-apoptotic, regulated necrotic cell death, termed necroptosis (Laster et al. 1988), this paradigm was overhauled. Since then, numerous novel forms of regulated cell death have been discovered including entosis, parthanatos, netosis, cyclophilin D (CypD)-dependent necrosis, and ferroptosis. Of particular interest is ferroptosis as it is subject to obligate control by GPX4 (Yang et al. 2014). Yet, long before GPX4 was shown to be involved in the ferroptotic process, numerous mouse- (Imai et al. 2003; Liang et al. 2009; Yant et al. 2003) and cell-based (Seiler et al. 2008) studies assigned a cell-protective role for GPX4. In fact, early studies from our laboratory showed that the inducible loss of *Gpx4* causes cell death in a caspase-independent manner involving 12/15 lipoxygenase (Seiler et al. 2008). Parallel studies performed in the Stockwell Laboratory led to the identification of the small-molecule cell death inducers erastin and (1S, 3R)-RSL3, which target two key nodes of the ferroptotic pathway, i.e., system Xc$^-$ and GPX4, respectively (Conrad et al. 2016a, b). These compounds were particularly efficient in killing tumor cells expressing oncogenic Ras (Dolma et al. 2003; Yang and Stockwell 2008). This cell death was eventually coined ferroptosis when it was shown that it is entirely different from known forms of cell death and that it involves iron-dependent lipid peroxidation (Dixon et al. 2012). Hallmarks of ferroptotic cell death are loss of expression/ deletion of GPX4, GSH depletion causing impaired GPX4 activity, and deleterious lipid peroxidation due to impaired GPX4 activity (Stockwell et al. 2017). Since its discovery, ferroptosis—and consequently GPX4—has gained incredible attention as ferroptosis is considered at the root cause of a number of diseases, including tissue IRI (Friedmann Angeli et al. 2014; Gao et al. 2015; Linkermann et al. 2014), neurodegeneration (Cardoso et al. 2017; Chen et al. 2015; Hambright et al. 2017; Seiler et al. 2008; Wirth et al. 2010; 2014), immunity (Matsushita et al. 2015), and liver failure (Sun et al. 2016). In the context of cancer, targeting ferroptosis and GPX4 might offer unprecedented opportunities for the effective killing of malignant cells (Jiang et al. 2015). In fact, after showing that GPX4 is at the heart of ferroptotic cancer cell death (Yang et al. 2014) more recent studies have implied the GSH-GPX4 axis to be the Achilles heel in high-mesenchymal-state cancer cells (Viswanathan et al. 2017), and in so-called chemotherapeutic-resistant "persister" cancer cells (Hangauer et al. 2017).

Conclusion

Selenocysteine-containing enzymes of the GPX and TXNRD family of proteins are central players of cellular redox control in mammals, as evidenced by a series of knockout studies performed throughout the last two decades. These studies have underpinned that these systems are essentially involved in the majority of cellular processes, ranging from oxidative stress protection, cell proliferation, cell differentiation, as well as tissue development and protection. Notably, many of the phenotypes triggered by the (conditional) knockout of specific selenoproteins phenocopy the pathology of diseases long known to be associated with severe selenium deficiency, such as Kashin-Beck and Keshan disease. Beyond this, by controlling cellular peroxide levels these systems also contribute to receptor tyrosine kinase signaling, including insulin and PDGFß receptor signaling. Additionally, GPX4 has been identified as the key regulator of ferroptosis. As this kind of cell death is considered to contribute to a number of pathological conditions, future studies will help to further underscore the importance of selenium and proper GPX4 functioning in disease contexts including organ transplantation, pathogen defense, and neuronal loss in certain neurodegenerative diseases like amyotrophic lateral sclerosis and dementia.

References

Andersen JK. Oxidative stress in neurodegeneration: cause or consequence? Nat Med. 2004;10(Suppl):S18–25.

Angeli JPF, Shah R, Pratt DA, Conrad M. Ferroptosis inhibition: mechanisms and opportunities. Trends Pharmacol Sci. 2017;38:489–98.

Banning A, Deubel S, Kluth D, Zhou Z, Brigelius-Flohe R. The GI-GPx gene is a target for Nrf2. Mol Cell Biol. 2005;25:4914–23.

Barrett CW, Ning W, Chen X, Smith JJ, Washington MK, Hill KE, Coburn LA, Peek RM, Chaturvedi R, Wilson KT, et al. Tumor suppressor function of the plasma glutathione peroxidase gpx3 in colitis-associated carcinoma. Cancer Res. 2013;73:1245–55.

Bienert GP, Chaumont F. Aquaporin-facilitated transmembrane diffusion of hydrogen peroxide. Biochim Biophys Acta. 2014;1840:1596–604.

Biterova EI, Turanov AA, Gladyshev VN, Barycki JJ. Crystal structures of oxidized and reduced mitochondrial thioredoxin reductase provide molecular details of the reaction mechanism. Proc Natl Acad Sci U S A. 2005;102:15018–23.

Bjornstedt M, Xue J, Huang W, Akesson B, Holmgren A. The thioredoxin and glutaredoxin systems are efficient electron donors to human plasma glutathione peroxidase. J Biol Chem. 1994;269:29382–4.

Bondareva AA, Capecchi MR, Iverson SV, Li Y, Lopez NI, Lucas O, Merrill GF, Prigge JR, Siders AM, Wakamiya M, et al. Effects of thioredoxin reductase-1 deletion on embryogenesis and transcriptome. Free Radic Biol Med. 2007;43:911–23.

Brandes RP, Weissmann N, Schroder K. Nox family NADPH oxidases: molecular mechanisms of activation. Free Radic Biol Med. 2014;76:208–26.

Brigelius-Flohe R. Tissue-specific functions of individual glutathione peroxidases. Free Radic Biol Med. 1999;27:951–65.

Brigelius-Flohe R, Flohe L. Selenium and redox signaling. Arch Biochem Biophys. 2017;617:48–59.

Brigelius-Flohe R, Kipp AP. Physiological functions of GPx2 and its role in inflammation-triggered carcinogenesis. Ann N Y Acad Sci. 2012;1259:19–25.

Brigelius-Flohe R, Maiorino M. Glutathione peroxidases. Biochim Biophys Acta. 2013;1830:3289–303.

Brigelius-Flohe R, Aumann KD, Blocker H, Gross G, Kiess M, Kloppel KD, Maiorino M, Roveri A, Schuckelt R, Usani F, et al. Phospholipid-hydroperoxide glutathione peroxidase. Genomic DNA, cDNA, and deduced amino acid sequence. J Biol Chem. 1994;269:7342–8.

Burk RF, Olson GE, Winfrey VP, Hill KE, Yin D. Glutathione peroxidase-3 produced by the kidney binds to a population of basement membranes in the gastrointestinal tract and in other tissues. Am J Physiol Gastrointest Liver Physiol. 2011;301:G32–8.

Cardoso BR, Hare DJ, Bush AI, Roberts BR. Glutathione peroxidase 4: a new player in neurodegeneration? Mol Psychiatry. 2017;22:328–35.

Carlson BA, Yoo MH, Tobe R, Mueller C, Naranjo-Suarez S, Hoffmann VJ, Gladyshev VN, Hatfield DL. Thioredoxin reductase 1 protects against chemically induced hepatocarcinogenesis via control of cellular redox homeostasis. Carcinogenesis. 2012;33:1806–13.

Carlson BA, Tobe R, Yefremova E, Tsuji PA, Hoffmann VJ, Schweizer U, Gladyshev VN, Hatfield DL, Conrad M. Glutathione peroxidase 4 and vitamin E cooperatively prevent hepatocellular degeneration. Redox Biol. 2016;9:22–31.

Carrero P, Okamoto K, Coumailleau P, O'Brien S, Tanaka H, Poellinger L. Redox-regulated recruitment of the transcriptional coactivators CREB-binding protein and SRC-1 to hypoxia-inducible factor 1alpha. Mol Cell Biol. 2000;20:402–15.

Casagrande S, Bonetto V, Fratelli M, Gianazza E, Eberini I, Massignan T, Salmona M, Chang G, Holmgren A, Ghezzi P. Glutathionylation of human thioredoxin: a possible crosstalk between the glutathione and thioredoxin systems. Proc Natl Acad Sci U S A. 2002;99:9745–9.

Chandel NS, Maltepe E, Goldwasser E, Mathieu CE, Simon MC, Schumacker PT. Mitochondrial reactive oxygen species trigger hypoxia-induced transcription. Proc Natl Acad Sci U S A. 1998;95:11715–20.

Chen L, Hambright WS, Na R, Ran Q. Ablation of the ferroptosis inhibitor glutathione peroxidase 4 in neurons results in rapid motor neuron degeneration and paralysis. J Biol Chem. 2015;290:28097–106.

Cheng WH, Ho YS, Valentine BA, Ross DA, Combs GF Jr, Lei XG. Cellular glutathione peroxidase is the mediator of body selenium to protect against paraquat lethality in transgenic mice. J Nutr. 1998;128:1070–6.

Chu FF, Doroshow JH, Esworthy RS. Expression, characterization, and tissue distribution of a new cellular selenium-dependent glutathione peroxidase, GSHPx-GI. J Biol Chem. 1993;268:2571–6.

Chu FF, Esworthy RS, Chu PG, Longmate JA, Huycke MM, Wilczynski S, Doroshow JH. Bacteria-induced intestinal cancer in mice with disrupted Gpx1 and Gpx2 genes. Cancer Res. 2004;64:962–8.

Conrad M, Jakupoglu C, Moreno SG, Lippl S, Banjac A, Schneider M, Beck H, Hatzopoulos AK, Just U, Sinowatz F, et al. Essential role for mitochondrial thioredoxin reductase in hematopoiesis, heart development, and heart function. Mol Cell Biol. 2004;24:9414–23.

Conrad M, Moreno SG, Sinowatz F, Ursini F, Kolle S, Roveri A, Brielmeier M, Wurst W, Maiorino M, Bornkamm GW. The nuclear form of phospholipid hydroperoxide glutathione peroxidase is a protein thiol peroxidase contributing to sperm chromatin stability. Mol Cell Biol. 2005;25:7637–44.

Conrad M, Sandin A, Forster H, Seiler A, Frijhoff J, Dagnell M, Bornkamm GW, Radmark O, Hooft van Huijsduijnen R, Aspenstrom P, et al. 12/15-lipoxygenase-derived lipid peroxides control receptor tyrosine kinase signaling through oxidation of protein tyrosine phosphatases. Proc Natl Acad Sci U S A. 2010;107:15774–9.

Conrad M, Ingold I, Buday K, Kobayashi S, Angeli JP. ROS, thiols and thiol-regulating systems in male gametogenesis. Biochim Biophys Acta. 2015;1850:1566–74.

Conrad M, Schweizer U. Mouse models that target individual selenoproteins. In: Hatfield DL, Schweizer U, Tsuji PA, Gladyshev VN, editors. Selenium: its molecular biology and role in human health. Cham: Springer International Publishing; 2016. p. 567–8.

Conrad M, Angeli JP, Vandenabeele P, Stockwell BR. Regulated necrosis: disease relevance and therapeutic opportunities. Nat Rev Drug Discov. 2016a;15:348–66.

Conrad M, Friedmann Angeli JP, Proneth B. Glutathione peroxidase 4 and ferroptosis. In: Hatfield DL, Schweizer U, Tsuji PA, Gladyshev VN, editors. Selenium: its molecular biology and role in human health. 4th ed. Cham: Springer; 2016b.

Cozza G, Rossetto M, Bosello-Travain V, Maiorino M, Roveri A, Toppo S, Zaccarin M, Zennaro L, Ursini F. Glutathione peroxidase 4-catalyzed reduction of lipid hydroperoxides in membranes: The polar head of membrane phospholipids binds the enzyme and addresses the fatty acid hydroperoxide group toward the redox center. Free Radic Biol Med. 2017;112:1–11.

Cross CE, Halliwell B, Borish ET, Pryor WA, Ames BN, Saul RL, McCord JM, Harman D. Oxygen radicals and human disease. Ann Intern Med. 1987;107:526–45.

Dagnell M, Frijhoff J, Pader I, Augsten M, Boivin B, Xu J, Mandal PK, Tonks NK, Hellberg C, Conrad M, et al. Selective activation of oxidized PTP1B by the thioredoxin system modulates PDGF-beta receptor tyrosine kinase signaling. Proc Natl Acad Sci U S A. 2013;110:13398–403.

Dear TN, Campbell K, Rabbitts TH. Molecular cloning of putative odorant-binding and odorant-metabolizing proteins. Biochemistry. 1991;30:10376–82.

Dixon SJ, Lemberg KM, Lamprecht MR, Skouta R, Zaitsev EM, Gleason CE, Patel DN, Bauer AJ, Cantley AM, Yang WS, et al. Ferroptosis: an iron-dependent form of nonapoptotic cell death. Cell. 2012;149:1060–72.

Dolma S, Lessnick SL, Hahn WC, Stockwell BR. Identification of genotype-selective antitumor agents using synthetic lethal chemical screening in engineered human tumor cells. Cancer Cell. 2003;3:285–96.

Ema M, Hirota K, Mimura J, Abe H, Yodoi J, Sogawa K, Poellinger L, Fujii-Kuriyama Y. Molecular mechanisms of transcription activation by HLF and HIF1alpha in response to hypoxia: their stabilization and redox signal-induced interaction with CBP/p300. EMBO J. 1999;18:1905–14.

Eriksson S, Prigge JR, Talago EA, Arner ES, Schmidt EE. Dietary methionine can sustain cytosolic redox homeostasis in the mouse liver. Nat Commun. 2015;6:6479.

Esworthy RS, Mann JR, Sam M, Chu FF. Low glutathione peroxidase activity in Gpx1 knockout mice protects jejunum crypts from gamma-irradiation damage. Am J Physiol Gastrointest Liver Physiol. 2000;279:G426–36.

Esworthy RS, Aranda R, Martin MG, Doroshow JH, Binder SW, Chu FF. Mice with combined disruption of Gpx1 and Gpx2 genes have colitis. Am J Physiol Gastrointest Liver Physiol. 2001;281:G848–55.

Finkel T. Signal transduction by reactive oxygen species. J Cell Biol. 2011;194:7–15.

Flohe L, Eisele B, Wendel A. Glutathion peroxidase. I. Isolation and determinations of molecular weight. Hoppe Seylers Z Physiol Chem. 1971;352:151–8.

Flohe L, Gunzler WA, Schock HH. Glutathione peroxidase: a selenoenzyme. FEBS Lett. 1973;32:132–4.

Friedmann Angeli JP, Schneider M, Proneth B, Tyurina YY, Tyurin VA, Hammond VJ, Herbach N, Aichler M, Walch A, Eggenhofer E, et al. Inactivation of the ferroptosis regulator Gpx4 triggers acute renal failure in mice. Nat Cell Biol. 2014;16:1180–91.

Fu Y, Cheng WH, Porres JM, Ross DA, Lei XG. Knockout of cellular glutathione peroxidase gene renders mice susceptible to diquat-induced oxidative stress. Free Radic Biol Med. 1999;27:605–11.

Gao M, Monian P, Quadri N, Ramasamy R, Jiang X. Glutaminolysis and transferrin regulate ferroptosis. Mol Cell. 2015;59:298–308.

Gladyshev VN, Jeang KT, Stadtman TC. Selenocysteine, identified as the penultimate C-terminal residue in human T-cell thioredoxin reductase, corresponds to TGA in the human placental gene. Proc Natl Acad Sci U S A. 1996;93:6146–51.

Hambright WS, Fonseca RS, Chen L, Na R, Ran Q. Ablation of ferroptosis regulator glutathione peroxidase 4 in forebrain neurons promotes cognitive impairment and neurodegeneration. Redox Biol. 2017;12:8–17.

Hangauer MJ, Viswanathan VS, Ryan MJ, Bole D, Eaton JK, Matov A, Galeas J, Dhruv HD, Berens ME, Schreiber SL, et al. Drug-tolerant persister cancer cells are vulnerable to GPX4 inhibition. Nature. 2017;551:247–50.

Harris IS, Treloar AE, Inoue S, Sasaki M, Gorrini C, Lee KC, Yung KY, Brenner D, Knobbe-Thomsen CB, Cox MA, et al. Glutathione and thioredoxin antioxidant pathways synergize to drive cancer initiation and progression. Cancer Cell. 2015;27:211–22.

Hellfritsch J, Kirsch J, Schneider M, Fluege T, Wortmann M, Frijhoff J, Dagnell M, Fey T, Esposito I, Kolle P, et al. Knockout of mitochondrial thioredoxin reductase stabilizes prolyl hydroxylase 2 and inhibits tumor growth and tumor-derived angiogenesis. Antioxid Redox Signal. 2015;22:938–50.

Hirota K, Murata M, Sachi Y, Nakamura H, Takeuchi J, Mori K, Yodoi J. Distinct roles of thioredoxin in the cytoplasm and in the nucleus. A two-step mechanism of redox regulation of transcription factor NF-kappaB. J Biol Chem. 1999;274:27891–7.

Ho YS, Magnenat JL, Bronson RT, Cao J, Gargano M, Sugawara M, Funk CD. Mice deficient in cellular glutathione peroxidase develop normally and show no increased sensitivity to hyperoxia. J Biol Chem. 1997;272:16644–51.

Holmgren A. Bovine thioredoxin system. Purification of thioredoxin reductase from calf liver and thymus and studies of its function in disulfide reduction. J Biol Chem. 1977;252:4600–6.

Holmgren A, Aslund F. Glutaredoxin Methods Enzymol. 1995;252:283–92.

Holmstrom KM, Finkel T. Cellular mechanisms and physiological consequences of redox-dependent signalling. Nat Rev Mol Cell Biol. 2014;15:411–21.

Holzerova E, Danhauser K, Haack TB, Kremer LS, Melcher M, Ingold I, Kobayashi S, Terrile C, Wolf P, Schaper J, et al. Human thioredoxin 2 deficiency impairs mitochondrial redox homeostasis and causes early-onset neurodegeneration. Brain. 2016;139:346–54.

Horstkotte J, Perisic T, Schneider M, Lange P, Schroeder M, Kiermayer C, Hinkel R, Ziegler T, Mandal PK, David R, et al. Mitochondrial thioredoxin reductase is essential for early postischemic myocardial protection. Circulation. 2011;124:2892–902.

Imai H, Hirao F, Sakamoto T, Sekine K, Mizukura Y, Saito M, Kitamoto T, Hayasaka M, Hanaoka K, Nakagawa Y. Early embryonic lethality caused by targeted disruption of the mouse PHGPx gene. Biochem Biophys Res Commun. 2003;305:278–86.

Jakupoglu C, Przemeck GK, Schneider M, Moreno SG, Mayr N, Hatzopoulos AK, de Angelis MH, Wurst W, Bornkamm GW, Brielmeier M, et al. Cytoplasmic thioredoxin reductase is essential for embryogenesis but dispensable for cardiac development. Mol Cell Biol. 2005;25:1980–8.

Jiang L, Kon N, Li T, Wang SJ, Su T, Hibshoosh H, Baer R, Gu W. Ferroptosis as a p53-mediated activity during tumour suppression. Nature. 2015;520:57–62.

Jin RC, Mahoney CE, Coleman Anderson L, Ottaviano F, Croce K, Leopold JA, Zhang YY, Tang SS, Handy DE, Loscalzo J. Glutathione peroxidase-3 deficiency promotes platelet-dependent thrombosis in vivo. Circulation. 2011;123:1963–73.

Kiermayer C, Northrup E, Schrewe A, Walch A, de Angelis MH, Schoensiegel F, Zischka H, Prehn C, Adamski J, Bekeredjian R, et al. Heart-Specific knockout of the mitochondrial thioredoxin reductase (Txnrd2) induces metabolic and contractile dysfunction in the aging myocardium. J Am Heart Assoc. 2015;4:e002153.

Kipp A, Banning A, Brigelius-Flohe R. Activation of the glutathione peroxidase 2 (GPx2) promoter by beta-catenin. Biol Chem. 2007;388:1027–33.

Kipp AP, Muller MF, Goken EM, Deubel S, Brigelius-Flohe R. The selenoproteins GPx2, TrxR2 and TrxR3 are regulated by Wnt signalling in the intestinal epithelium. Biochim Biophys Acta. 2012;1820:1588–96.

Kirsch J, Schneider H, Pagel JI, Rehberg M, Singer M, Hellfritsch J, Chillo O, Schubert KM, Qiu J, Pogoda K, et al. Endothelial Dysfunction, and A Prothrombotic, Proinflammatory Phenotype Is Caused by Loss of Mitochondrial Thioredoxin Reductase in Endothelium. Arterioscler Thromb Vasc Biol. 2016;

Koh CS, Didierjean C, Navrot N, Panjikar S, Mulliert G, Rouhier N, Jacquot JP, Aubry A, Shawkataly O, Corbier C. Crystal structures of a poplar thioredoxin peroxidase that exhibits the structure of glutathione peroxidases: insights into redox-driven conformational changes. J Mol Biol. 2007;370:512–29.

Kryukov GV, Castellano S, Novoselov SV, Lobanov AV, Zehtab O, Guigo R, Gladyshev VN. Characterization of mammalian selenoproteomes. Science. 2003;300:1439–43.

Kudin AP, Baron G, Zsurka G, Hampel KG, Elger CE, Grote A, Weber Y, Lerche H, Thiele H, Nurnberg P, et al. Homozygous mutation in TXNRD1 is associated with genetic generalized epilepsy. Free Radic Biol Med. 2017;106:270–7.

Labunskyy VM, Hatfield DL, Gladyshev VN. Selenoproteins: molecular pathways and physiological roles. Physiol Rev. 2014;94:739–77.

Ladenstein R, Epp O, Bartels K, Jones A, Huber R, Wendel A. Structure analysis and molecular model of the selenoenzyme glutathione peroxidase at 2.8 A resolution. J Mol Biol. 1979;134:199–218.

Laster SM, Wood JG, Gooding LR. Tumor necrosis factor can induce both apoptic and necrotic forms of cell lysis. J Immunol. 1988;141:2629–34.

Liang H, Yoo SE, Na R, Walter CA, Richardson A, Ran Q. Short form glutathione peroxidase 4 is the essential isoform required for survival and somatic mitochondrial functions. J Biol Chem. 2009;284:30836–44.

Lillig CH, Holmgren A. Thioredoxin and related molecules--from biology to health and disease. Antioxid Redox Signal. 2007;9:25–47.

Linkermann A, Skouta R, Himmerkus N, Mulay SR, Dewitz C, De Zen F, Prokai A, Zuchtriegel G, Krombach F, Welz PS, et al. Synchronized renal tubular cell death involves ferroptosis. Proc Natl Acad Sci U S A. 2014;111:16836–41.

Lodhi IJ, Semenkovich CF. Peroxisomes: a nexus for lipid metabolism and cellular signaling. Cell Metab. 2014;19:380–92.

Loh K, Deng H, Fukushima A, Cai X, Boivin B, Galic S, Bruce C, Shields BJ, Skiba B, Ooms LM, et al. Reactive oxygen species enhance insulin sensitivity. Cell Metab. 2009;10:260–72.

Lu J, Holmgren A. Selenoproteins J Biol Chem. 2009;284:723–7.

Maiorino M, Aumann KD, Brigelius-Flohe R, Doria D, van den Heuvel J, McCarthy J, Roveri A, Ursini F, Flohe L. Probing the presumed catalytic triad of selenium-containing peroxidases by mutational analysis of phospholipid hydroperoxide glutathione peroxidase (PHGPx). Biol Chem Hoppe Seyler. 1995;376:651–60.

Maiorino M, Roveri A, Benazzi L, Bosello V, Mauri P, Toppo S, Tosatto SC, Ursini F. Functional interaction of phospholipid hydroperoxide glutathione peroxidase with sperm mitochondrion-associated cysteine-rich protein discloses the adjacent cysteine motif as a new substrate of the selenoperoxidase. J Biol Chem. 2005;280:38395–402.

Maiorino M, Ursini F, Bosello V, Toppo S, Tosatto SC, Mauri P, Becker K, Roveri A, Bulato C, Benazzi L, et al. The thioredoxin specificity of Drosophila GPx: a paradigm for a peroxiredoxin-like mechanism of many glutathione peroxidases. J Mol Biol. 2007;365:1033–46.

Mandal PK, Schneider M, Kolle P, Kuhlencordt P, Forster H, Beck H, Bornkamm GW, Conrad M. Loss of thioredoxin reductase 1 renders tumors highly susceptible to pharmacologic glutathione deprivation. Cancer Res. 2010a;70:9505–14.

Mandal PK, Seiler A, Perisic T, Kolle P, Banjac Canak A, Forster H, Weiss N, Kremmer E, Lieberman MW, Bannai S, et al. System x(c)- and thioredoxin reductase 1 cooperatively rescue glutathione deficiency. J Biol Chem. 2010b;285:22244–53.

Matsushita M, Freigang S, Schneider C, Conrad M, Bornkamm GW, Kopf M. T cell lipid peroxidation induces ferroptosis and prevents immunity to infection. J Exp Med. 2015;212:555–68.

McClung JP, Roneker CA, Mu W, Lisk DJ, Langlais P, Liu F, Lei XG. Development of insulin resistance and obesity in mice overexpressing cellular glutathione peroxidase. Proc Natl Acad Sci U S A. 2004;101:8852–7.

Merrill GF, Dowell P, Pearson GD. The human p53 negative regulatory domain mediates inhibition of reporter gene transactivation in yeast lacking thioredoxin reductase. Cancer Res. 1999;59:3175–9.

Mills GC. Hemoglobin catabolism. I. Glutathione peroxidase, an erythrocyte enzyme which protects hemoglobin from oxidative breakdown. J Biol Chem. 1957;229:189–97.

Moreno SG, Laux G, Brielmeier M, Bornkamm GW, Conrad M. Testis-specific expression of the nuclear form of phospholipid hydroperoxide glutathione peroxidase (PHGPx). Biol Chem. 2003;384:635–43.

Olson GE, Whitin JC, Hill KE, Winfrey VP, Motley AK, Austin LM, Deal J, Cohen HJ, Burk RF. Extracellular glutathione peroxidase (Gpx3) binds specifically to basement membranes of mouse renal cortex tubule cells. Am J Physiol Renal Physiol. 2010;298:F1244–53.

Papp LV, Lu J, Holmgren A, Khanna KK. From selenium to selenoproteins: synthesis, identity, and their role in human health. Antioxid Redox Signal. 2007;9:775–806.

Patterson AD, Carlson BA, Li F, Bonzo JA, Yoo MH, Krausz KW, Conrad M, Chen C, Gonzalez FJ, Hatfield DL. Disruption of thioredoxin reductase 1 protects mice from acute acetaminophen-induced hepatotoxicity through enhanced NRF2 activity. Chem Res Toxicol. 2013;26:1088–96.

Prigge JR, Coppo L, Martin SS, Ogata F, Miller CG, Bruschwein MD, Orlicky DJ, Shearn CT, Kundert JA, Lytchier J, et al. Hepatocyte Hyperproliferation upon Liver-Specific Co-disruption of Thioredoxin-1, Thioredoxin Reductase-1, and Glutathione Reductase. Cell Rep. 2017;19:2771–81.

Puglisi R, Maccari I, Pipolo S, Conrad M, Mangia F, Boitani C. The nuclear form of glutathione peroxidase 4 is associated with sperm nuclear matrix and is required for proper paternal chromatin decondensation at fertilization. J Cell Physiol. 2012;227:1420–7.

Quinlan CL, Treberg JR, Perevoshchikova IV, Orr AL, Brand MD. Native rates of superoxide production from multiple sites in isolated mitochondria measured using endogenous reporters. Free Radic Biol Med. 2012;53:1807–17.

Reich HJ, Hondal RJ. Why nature chose selenium. ACS Chem Biol. 2016;11:821–41.

Ren B, Huang W, Akesson B, Ladenstein R. The crystal structure of seleno-glutathione peroxidase from human plasma at 2.9 A resolution. J Mol Biol. 1997;268:869–85.

Rhee SG, Kang SW, Chang TS, Jeong W, Kim K. Peroxiredoxin, a novel family of peroxidases. IUBMB Life. 2001;52:35–41.

Rotruck JT, Pope AL, Ganther HE, Swanson AB, Hafeman DG, Hoekstra WG. Selenium: biochemical role as a component of glutathione peroxidase. Science. 1973;179:588–90.

Roveri A, Maiorino M, Nisii C, Ursini F. Purification and characterization of phospholipid hydroperoxide glutathione peroxidase from rat testis mitochondrial membranes. Biochim Biophys Acta. 1994;1208:211–21.

Sandalova T, Zhong L, Lindqvist Y, Holmgren A, Schneider G. Three-dimensional structure of a mammalian thioredoxin reductase: implications for mechanism and evolution of a selenocysteine-dependent enzyme. Proc Natl Acad Sci U S A. 2001;98:9533–8.

Scheerer P, Borchert A, Krauss N, Wessner H, Gerth C, Hohne W, Kuhn H. Structural basis for catalytic activity and enzyme polymerization of phospholipid hydroperoxide glutathione peroxidase-4 (GPx4). Biochemistry. 2007;46:9041–9.

Scherz-Shouval R, Shvets E, Fass E, Shorer H, Gil L, Elazar Z. Reactive oxygen species are essential for autophagy and specifically regulate the activity of Atg4. EMBO J. 2007;26:1749–60.

Schlecker T, Comini MA, Melchers J, Ruppert T, Krauth-Siegel RL. Catalytic mechanism of the glutathione peroxidase-type tryparedoxin peroxidase of Trypanosoma brucei. Biochem J. 2007;405:445–54.

Schneider M, Forster H, Boersma A, Seiler A, Wehnes H, Sinowatz F, Neumuller C, Deutsch MJ, Walch A, Hrabe de Angelis M, et al. Mitochondrial glutathione peroxidase 4 disruption causes male infertility. FASEB J. 2009;23:3233–42.

Schreck R, Rieber P, Baeuerle PA. Reactive oxygen intermediates as apparently widely used messengers in the activation of the NF-kappa B transcription factor and HIV-1. EMBO J. 1991;10:2247–58.

See RB, Awosika OO, Cambria RP, Conrad MF, Lancaster RT, Patel VI, Chitilian HV, Kumar S, Simon MV. Extended Motor Evoked Potentials Monitoring Helps Prevent Delayed Paraplegia After Aortic Surgery. Ann Neurol. 2016;79:636–45.

Seiler A, Schneider M, Forster H, Roth S, Wirth EK, Culmsee C, Plesnila N, Kremmer E, Radmark O, Wurst W, et al. Glutathione peroxidase 4 senses and translates oxidative stress into 12/15-lipoxygenase dependent- and AIF-mediated cell death. Cell Metab. 2008;8:237–48.

Seo MS, Kang SW, Kim K, Baines IC, Lee TH, Rhee SG. Identification of a new type of mammalian peroxiredoxin that forms an intramolecular disulfide as a reaction intermediate. J Biol Chem. 2000;275:20346–54.

Shema R, Kulicke R, Cowley GS, Stein R, Root DE, Heiman M. Synthetic lethal screening in the mammalian central nervous system identifies Gpx6 as a modulator of Huntington's disease. Proc Natl Acad Sci U S A. 2015;112:268–72.

Shi ZZ, Osei-Frimpong J, Kala G, Kala SV, Barrios RJ, Habib GM, Lukin DJ, Danney CM, Matzuk MM, Lieberman MW. Glutathione synthesis is essential for mouse development but not for cell growth in culture. Proc Natl Acad Sci U S A. 2000;97:5101–6.

Shukla V, Mishra SK, Pant HC. Oxidative stress in neurodegeneration. Adv Pharm Sci. 2011;2011:572634.

Sibbing D, Pfeufer A, Perisic T, Mannes AM, Fritz-Wolf K, Unwin S, Sinner MF, Gieger C, Gloeckner CJ, Wichmann HE, et al. Mutations in the mitochondrial thioredoxin reductase gene TXNRD2 cause dilated cardiomyopathy. Eur Heart J. 2011;32:1121–33.

Sies H, Berndt C, Jones DP. Oxidative Stress. Annu Rev Biochem. 2017;86:715–48.

Sobotta MC, Liou W, Stocker S, Talwar D, Oehler M, Ruppert T, Scharf AN, Dick TP. Peroxiredoxin-2 and STAT3 form a redox relay for H2O2 signaling. Nat Chem Biol. 2015;11:64–70.

Soerensen J, Jakupoglu C, Beck H, Forster H, Schmidt J, Schmahl W, Schweizer U, Conrad M, Brielmeier M. The role of thioredoxin reductases in brain development. PLoS One. 2008;3:e1813.

Stocker, S., Van Laer, K., Mijuskovic, A., and Dick, T.P. (2017). The conundrum of hydrogen peroxide signaling and the emerging role of peroxiredoxins as redox relay hubs. Antioxid Redox Signal.

Stockwell BR, Friedmann Angeli JP, Bayir H, Bush AI, Conrad M, Dixon SJ, Fulda S, Gascon S, Hatzios SK, Kagan VE, et al. Ferroptosis: a regulated cell death nexus linking metabolism, redox biology, and disease. Cell. 2017;171:273–85.

Su D, Novoselov SV, Sun QA, Moustafa ME, Zhou Y, Oko R, Hatfield DL, Gladyshev VN. Mammalian selenoprotein thioredoxin-glutathione reductase. Roles in disulfide bond formation and sperm maturation J Biol Chem. 2005;280:26491–8.

Sun QA, Kirnarsky L, Sherman S, Gladyshev VN. Selenoprotein oxidoreductase with specificity for thioredoxin and glutathione systems. Proc Natl Acad Sci U S A. 2001;98:3673–8.

Sun X, Ou Z, Chen R, Niu X, Chen D, Kang R, Tang D. Activation of the p62-Keap1-NRF2 pathway protects against ferroptosis in hepatocellular carcinoma cells. Hepatology. 2016;63:173–84.

Taguchi K, Motohashi H, Yamamoto M. Molecular mechanisms of the Keap1-Nrf2 pathway in stress response and cancer evolution. Genes Cells. 2011;16:123–40.

Tan KH, Meyer DJ, Belin J, Ketterer B. Inhibition of microsomal lipid peroxidation by glutathione and glutathione transferases B and AA. Role of endogenous phospholipase A2. Biochem J. 1984;220:243–52.

Toppo S, Vanin S, Bosello V, Tosatto SC. Evolutionary and structural insights into the multifaceted glutathione peroxidase (Gpx) superfamily. Antioxid Redox Signal. 2008;10:1501–14.

Toppo S, Flohe L, Ursini F, Vanin S, Maiorino M. Catalytic mechanisms and specificities of glutathione peroxidases: variations of a basic scheme. Biochim Biophys Acta. 2009;1790:1486–500.

Tosatto SC, Bosello V, Fogolari F, Mauri P, Roveri A, Toppo S, Flohe L, Ursini F, Maiorino M. The catalytic site of glutathione peroxidases. Antioxid Redox Signal. 2008;10:1515–26.

Trachootham D, Alexandre J, Huang P. Targeting cancer cells by ROS-mediated mechanisms: a radical therapeutic approach? Nat Rev Drug Discov. 2009;8:579–91.

Ueta T, Inoue T, Furukawa T, Tamaki Y, Nakagawa Y, Imai H, Yanagi Y. Glutathione peroxidase 4 is required for maturation of photoreceptor cells. J Biol Chem. 2012;287:7675–82.

Ursini F, Maiorino M, Valente M, Ferri L, Gregolin C. Purification from pig liver of a protein which protects liposomes and biomembranes from peroxidative degradation and exhibits glutathione peroxidase activity on phosphatidylcholine hydroperoxides. Biochim Biophys Acta. 1982;710:197–211.

Ursini F, Maiorino M, Brigelius-Flohe R, Aumann KD, Roveri A, Schomburg D, Flohe L. Diversity of glutathione peroxidases. Methods Enzymol. 1995;252:38–53.

Ursini F, Heim S, Kiess M, Maiorino M, Roveri A, Wissing J, Flohe L. Dual function of the selenoprotein PHGPx during sperm maturation. Science. 1999;285:1393–6.

Viswanathan VS, Ryan MJ, Dhruv HD, Gill S, Eichhoff OM, Seashore-Ludlow B, Kaffenberger SD, Eaton JK, Shimada K, Aguirre AJ, et al. Dependency of a therapy-resistant state of cancer cells on a lipid peroxidase pathway. Nature. 2017;547:453–7.

Walshe J, Serewko-Auret MM, Teakle N, Cameron S, Minto K, Smith L, Burcham PC, Russell T, Strutton G, Griffin A, et al. Inactivation of glutathione peroxidase activity contributes to UV-induced squamous cell carcinoma formation. Cancer Res. 2007;67:4751–8.

Whitin JC, Bhamre S, Tham DM, Cohen HJ. Extracellular glutathione peroxidase is secreted basolaterally by human renal proximal tubule cells. Am J Physiol Renal Physiol. 2002;283:F20–8.

Wirth EK, Conrad M, Winterer J, Wozny C, Carlson BA, Roth S, Schmitz D, Bornkamm GW, Coppola V, Tessarollo L, et al. Neuronal selenoprotein expression is required for interneuron development and prevents seizures and neurodegeneration. FASEB J. 2010;24:844–52.

Wirth EK, Bharathi BS, Hatfield D, Conrad M, Brielmeier M, Schweizer U. Cerebellar hypoplasia in mice lacking selenoprotein biosynthesis in neurons. Biol Trace Elem Res. 2014;158:203–10.

Woo JR, Kim SJ, Jeong W, Cho YH, Lee SC, Chung YJ, Rhee SG, Ryu SE. Structural basis of cellular redox regulation by human TRP14. J Biol Chem. 2004;279(46):48120–5. Epub 2004 Sep 7.

Wortmann M, Schneider M, Pircher J, Hellfritsch J, Aichler M, Vegi N, Kolle P, Kuhlencordt P, Walch A, Pohl U, et al. Combined deficiency in glutathione peroxidase 4 and vitamin e causes multiorgan thrombus formation and early death in mice. Circ Res. 2013;113:408–17.

Xu X, Leng JY, Gao F, Zhao ZA, Deng WB, Liang XH, Zhang YJ, Zhang ZR, Li M, Sha AG, et al. Differential expression and anti-oxidant function of glutathione peroxidase 3 in mouse uterus during decidualization. FEBS Lett. 2014;588:1580–9.

Yan W, Chen X. GPX2, a direct target of p63, inhibits oxidative stress-induced apoptosis in a p53-dependent manner. J Biol Chem. 2006;281:7856–62.

Yang WS, Stockwell BR. Synthetic lethal screening identifies compounds activating iron-dependent, nonapoptotic cell death in oncogenic-RAS-harboring cancer cells. Chem Biol. 2008;15:234–45.

Yang WS, Sriramaratnam R, Welsch ME, Shimada K, Skouta R, Viswanathan VS, Cheah JH, Clemons PA, Shamji AF, Clish CB, et al. Regulation of ferroptotic cancer cell death by GPX4. Cell. 2014;156:317–31.

Yant LJ, Ran Q, Rao L, Van Remmen H, Shibatani T, Belter JG, Motta L, Richardson A, Prolla TA. The selenoprotein GPX4 is essential for mouse development and protects from radiation and oxidative damage insults. Free Radic Biol Med. 2003;34:496–502.

Zhong L, Holmgren A. Essential role of selenium in the catalytic activities of mammalian thioredoxin reductase revealed by characterization of recombinant enzymes with selenocysteine mutations. J Biol Chem. 2000;275:18121–8.

Zhong L, Arner ES, Ljung J, Aslund F, Holmgren A. Rat and calf thioredoxin reductase are homologous to glutathione reductase with a carboxyl-terminal elongation containing a conserved catalytically active penultimate selenocysteine residue. J Biol Chem. 1998;273:8581–91.

Chapter 7
Selenium and Inflammatory Mediators

Solveigh C. Koeberle and Anna P. Kipp

Abstract The essential role of selenium during inflammatory processes and immune response has been established in various studies. Optimizing the expression of selenoproteins with antioxidant properties helps to maintain the levels of redox-active compounds (e.g., hydroperoxides) under control, both within inflammatory cells and in the extracellular milieu. In concert with other mediators, these redox-active compounds are needed to attract immune cells and to establish a proper immune response, which includes the activation of transcription factors such as NF-κB. This way, selenium and selenoproteins are involved in mediating cytokine production with subsequent effects on activation, proliferation, and differentiation of immune cell types. Besides that, the eicosanoid network, which comprises key mediators of inflammation, is extremely well orchestrated and regulated at different levels by selenium and selenoproteins. This chapter focusses on how selenium and selenoproteins influence the production of inflammatory mediators and thus fine-tune the immune response.

Keywords Eicosanoid network · Cyclopentenone prostaglandins · Cytokines · Redox regulation · Cyclooxygenases · Lipoxygenases · Macrophage polarization · T-cell populations

Introduction

To defend against pathogens from outside, multicellular organisms have developed a complex network of specialized cells, the immune system, which can be divided into two main parts. The innate immune response works nonspecifically but very quickly whereas the adaptive immune system requires more time after infection but has a high specificity towards particular pathogens. Cells of the innate response

S. C. Koeberle · A. P. Kipp (✉)
Department of Molecular Nutritional Physiology, Institute of Nutritional Sciences, Friedrich Schiller University Jena, Jena, Germany
e-mail: anna.kipp@uni-jena.de

© Springer International Publishing AG, part of Springer Nature 2018
B. Michalke (ed.), *Selenium*, Molecular and Integrative Toxicology,
https://doi.org/10.1007/978-3-319-95390-8_7

include phagocytic (neutrophils, monocytes, and macrophages), inflammatory (basophils, mast cells, and eosinophils), and natural killer cells whereas the adaptive response involves B and T cells. During the immune response, immune cells produce an inflammatory milieu in the affected region to attract additional cells to coordinately expand the immune reaction. The inflammatory milieu is created by excreted mediators including cytokines, chemokines, complement, eicosanoids, as well as reactive oxygen species (ROS, e.g., H_2O_2). Those mediators tightly influence each other and are highly coordinated to orchestrate the proper spatiotemporal immune response followed by a subsequent second, anti-inflammatory phase of pathogen removal and wound healing resulting in regeneration of tissue homeostasis (Medzhitov 2008; Griffiths et al. 2017; Fullerton and Gilroy 2016).

Cytokines are low-molecular-weight proteins that mediate the communication between different cells or act in an autocrine way. During the immune response, most cytokines are induced by the transcription factor nuclear factor kappa-light-chain enhancer of activated B cells (NF-κB), which is pivotal for coordinating both the innate and adaptive defense system (overview in (Zhang et al. 2017)). Each cytokine interacts with a specific receptor on the surface of cells leading to an up- or downregulation of genes, most commonly of other cytokines and/or the eicosanoid network. Eicosanoid signaling is critical in mediating inflammatory processes and affects also both innate and adaptive immune responses (Kim and Luster 2007; Harizi and Gualde 2005). Eicosanoid biosynthesis is activated by receptor-mediated agonists (e.g., immune complexes, factors of the complement system, interleukins), microorganisms (viruses, bacteria, fungi), phagocytosed particles (e.g., zymosan), and changes in the redox environment (hyperoxia, ozone) (Brock and Peters-Golden 2007). In the initial phase of inflammation, mainly pro-inflammatory prostaglandins and leukotrienes are formed whereas during later stages synthesis switches towards anti-inflammatory and pro-resolving mediators (Serhan et al. 2008; Serhan 2014). Tight timing of this switch is essential for the successful initiation and resolution of inflammation. Eicosanoid biosynthesis is regulated either by changing the expression of the generating enzymes cyclooxygenase (COX), lipoxygenase (LOX), prostaglandin E synthase (PGES), and prostaglandin D synthase (PGDS) or by mediating their enzyme activity. The latter can be achieved by modulating the cellular hydroperoxide tone, oxidation state of iron, feedback loops, and availability of cofactors, amongst other glutathione (GSH) (Brock and Peters-Golden 2007). All of them have been described to be altered by selenium (Se) or selenoproteins. In particular, selenoproteins have been suggested to play a key role in switching the eicosanoid pathway towards the resolution of inflammation.

The level of reactive species is typically increased in inflamed tissue being generated in high amounts during the oxidative burst to kill pathogens (Lei et al. 2015). ROS comprise superoxide ($O_2^{\cdot-}$), hydrogen peroxide (H_2O_2), and hydroxyl radicals ($^\cdot OH$). The NADPH oxidase NOX2 is located in the phagosome membrane where it reduces oxygen to superoxide, which is transported into the phagosome lumen (Babior 1995). Superoxide itself but also subsequently formed H_2O_2 and hypochlorous acid are needed to kill the ingested microorganisms. However, they are potentially toxic for the host cells (phagocytes, macrophages) themselves and, if secreted, also for the surrounding tissue. Therefore, the levels of reactive molecules need to be tightly controlled in inflammatory areas to protect from subsequent oxidative stress which is mainly achieved by antioxidant enzymes. Selenoproteins such as glutathione peroxidases (GPXs) and thioredoxin reductases (TXNRDs) are part of this antioxidant defense by reducing hydroperoxides including H_2O_2. Thus, GPXs and TXNRDs can be regarded as off-switch signal by counterbalancing the production of ROS (Forman and Torres 2001) which concomitantly prevents oxidative stress and chronic inflammation (Tan et al. 2016). Especially macrophages are prone to oxidative damage which results in impaired macrophage function and viability and, in consequence, in diminished immune function (Lei et al. 2015; Forman and Torres 2001).

Besides being important for oxidative burst, H_2O_2 acts as a specific signaling molecule which modulates redox-sensitive signaling cascades (see Chap. 6). By reversible protein oxidation, H_2O_2 impacts protein expression, activity, stability and subcellular localization (Lei et al. 2015). Mechanistically, the thiol group of cysteine residues reacts with the peroxide O-O bond in a nucleophilic attack, thereby forming sulfenic acid (R-SOH) which subsequently reacts with an additional cysteine residue to form a more stable disulfide bridge (S-S). This process is fully reversible involving the thioredoxin (TRX) and GSH/glutaredoxin (GRX) systems and thus indirectly also the selenoproteins TXNRDs and GPXs (Lei et al. 2015). Besides that, TXNRDs and GPXs can also limit the availability of H_2O_2 and this way fine-tune the redox signaling response (Simeoni and Bogeski 2015). NF-κB, a master regulator of the immune response, was the first mammalian transcription factor shown to be redox regulated (Staal et al. 1990). Similarly, other transcription factors like activator protein-1 (AP-1), hypoxia-inducible factor 1α (HIF-1α), signal transducer and activator of transcription (STAT), and peroxisome proliferator-activated receptors (PPARs) can be regulated via redox modification of susceptible cysteine residues (Lei et al. 2015). All of them exert their function in inflammation and immunity by upregulating the expression of pro-inflammatory mediators comprising cytokines, adhesion molecules, chemokines, and growth factors. Although not always investigated in the context of the immune system and inflammation, Se and selenoproteins have been shown to affect NF-κB (Kipp et al. 2012; Zhu et al. 2016; Jozsef and Filep 2003; Matthews et al. 1992), AP-1 (Jozsef and Filep 2003; Spyrou et al. 1995; Handel et al. 1995), HIF-1α (Huang et al. 2012a; Sinha et al. 2012; Naranjo-Suarez et al. 2012; Naranjo-Suarez et al. 2013), Nrf2 (Müller et al. 2010), and PPAR (Gandhi et al. 2011; Nelson et al. 2016) dependent transcription. Besides transcription factors, also the activity of phosphatases and proteinases can be regulated by reversible redox-dependent cysteine modification, thereby switching on or off signaling pathways (Lei et al. 2015). Thus, basal H_2O_2 levels are needed as a prerequisite for the proper functioning of the immune response, but need to be limited by selenoproteins to induce the resolution of inflammation.

However, when Se is supplied at higher concentrations than those needed to maximize the selenoprotein expression, excessive Se, usually in the form of selenite, can also have prooxidant effects (Lee and Wan 2002; Spallholz 1997; Stewart et al. 1999). This can be explained by the depletion of cellular GSH and the generation of superoxide anions (Lee and Jeong 2012). Thus, depending on the concentration range and chemical form, Se can either have anti- or prooxidant effects. This will be discussed in the context of how changes in the Se status impact two important groups of inflammatory mediators such as eicosanoids and cytokines which in turn modulate immune cell differentiation and proliferation.

The Eicosanoid Network

Eicosanoids comprise members of potent bioactive lipid mediators. They are oxygenated metabolites derived from arachidonic acid (AA) upon release from the cell membrane by phospholipase A2 (PLA2) (Dennis et al. 2011; Leslie 2015) and can be divided into the prostaglandins (PGs), leukotrienes (LTs), and lipoxins (LXs). Eicosanoids are synthesized in many cell types via distinct, cell-specific enzymatic pathways (Fig. 7.1) (Brock and Peters-Golden 2007). The rate-limiting

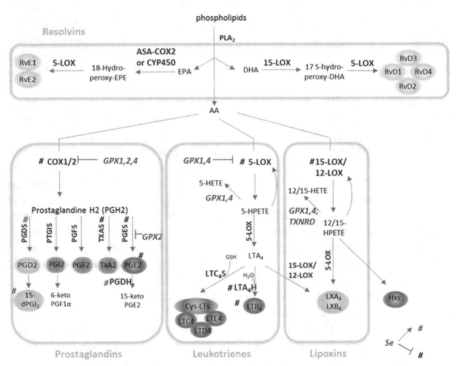

Fig. 7.1 Effects of Se and selenoproteins on the eicosanoid network. Expression of various enzymes of the prostaglandin and leukotriene synthesis is regulated by Se and selenoproteins modulating the amounts of pro-inflammatory (red circles) and anti-inflammatory (blue circles) mediators. Some mediators can have both pro- and anti-inflammatory effects (yellow circles). Additionally, enzyme activity of COXs and LOXs is regulated by GPXs. Further details are described in the text. *AA* arachidonic acid, *ASA-COX2* aspirin-acetylated COX-2, *CYP450* cytochrome P450, *EPA* eicosapentaenoic acid, *DHA* docosahexaenoic acid, *18-hydroperoxy-EPE* 18-hydroperoxy eicosapentaenoic acid, *GPX* glutathione peroxidase, *Hxs* hepoxilins, *LT* leukotriene, *LTA4H* leukotriene A4 hydrolase, *LTC4S* leukotriene C4 synthase, *LOX* lipoxygenase, *LX* lipoxin, *PLA2* phospholipase A2, *PG* prostaglandin, *PGDS* prostaglandin D synthase, *PTGIS* prostacyclin synthase, *PGFS* prostaglandin F synthase, *PGES* prostaglandin E synthase, *Rv* resolvin, *TXAS* thromboxane synthase, *TXNRD* thioredoxin reductase

step in PG synthesis is the production of prostaglandin H_2 (PGH_2) by prostaglandin synthase (PGHS), better known as COX. This reaction includes two steps: during the cyclooxygenase reaction, the reactive peroxide PGG_2 is formed which is subsequently reduced in a peroxidase reaction to form PGH_2 by the consumption of two molecules GSH. There are two isoforms, COX-1 and COX-2. While COX-1 is constitutively expressed in most tissues, COX-2 expression is induced by, e.g., cytokines or lipopolysaccharides (LPS) to enhance prostanoid synthesis (Brock and Peters-Golden 2007). PGH_2 is subsequently converted into various prostaglandins by specific PG synthases such as the microsomal prostaglandin E synthase 1 (mPGES-1) to form pro-inflammatory PGE_2. The synthesis of anti-inflammatory PGD_2 is catalyzed by PGDS followed by the nonenzymatic metabolism, into the downstream products PGJ_2, Δ^{12}-PGJ_2, and 15d-$\Delta^{12,14}$-PGJ_2 (Fig. 7.1). The leukotriene synthesis depends on 5-LOX. Similar to COX, 5-LOX has two catalytic functions. In a first step, molecular oxygen is inserted by the dioxygenase activity to form the instable 5-hydroperoxyeicosatetraenoic acid (5-HPETE) which can be converted to LTA_4 by the LTA_4 synthase activity of 5-LOX (Fig. 7.1). LTA_4 formed by 5-LOX is subsequently coupled to GSH to form inflammatory cysteinyl-leukotriene by LTC_4 synthase (LTC_4S) or converted to the inflammatory LTB_4 by LTA_4 hydrolase. In line with 5-LOX, 15-LOX/12-LOX forms 12/15-HETEs which can subsequently undergo isomerization to form the pro-inflammatory hepoxilins (Hxs).

Recently, so-called specialized pro-resolving mediators (SPMs) have been described which have potent immunomodulatory and anti-inflammatory effects (Serhan 2014; Freire and Van Dyke 2000). SPMs include lipoxins and resolvins whose synthesis involves both 5-LOX and 15-LOX/12-LOX (Basil and Levy 2016). The resolvin synthesis is based on eicosapentaenoic acid (EPA) and docosahexaenoic acid (DHA) instead of AA. For the synthesis of the E series of resolvins, EPA is converted into 18-hydroperoxy-eicosapentaenoic acid (18-hydroperoxy-EPE) by aspirin-acetylated (ASA)-COX2 or by cytochrome P450 enzymes (CYP450) which is subsequently converted to resolvins of the E-series by 5-LOX. Synthesis of resolvins from the D series involves 15-LOX which is followed by the 5-LOX reaction (Fig. 7.1).

Se and the Eicosanoid Network

The best investigated effect of the cellular Se status on the eicosanoid pathway is the modulation of the highly orchestrated eicosanoid class switching from the production of pro-inflammatory towards the synthesis of anti-inflammatory mediators. In LPS-stimulated RAW264.7 macrophages, Se deficiency resulted in an upregulation of COX-2 expression, which was dependent on the activation of the NF-κB pathway. Simultaneously, the level of PGE_2 was increased (Zamamiri-Davis et al. 2002). This is in line with the finding that Se-deficient conditions enhanced COX-2 expression in both RAW264.7 macrophages and bone marrow-derived macrophages (BMDM) after LPS stimulation (Vunta et al. 2007). In a second study, the Se-induced inhibition of COX-2 expression not only was mediated by inhibition of NF-κB but also involved an activation of PPARγ enhanced by increased production of 15d-$\Delta^{12,14}$-PGJ$_2$ (Vunta et al. 2007). In addition, Se was shown to upregulate H-PGDS and to decrease mPGES1 expression in RAW264.7 and in BMDMs of Se-treated mice. Thereby, Se was able to switch the prostanoid synthesis from PGE$_2$ to Δ^{12}-PGJ$_2$ and 15d-$\Delta^{12,14}$-PGJ$_2$, so-called cyclopentenone prostaglandins (CyPGs) (Gandhi et al. 2011). Interestingly, this effect was dependent on the Se compound supplied. Only sodium selenite and methylseleninic acid (MSA) were able to change expression levels of the respective PG synthases, whereas selenomethionine (SeMet) and 1,4-phenylenebis(methylene)selenocyanate (pXSC) failed to do so. Using parthenolide, an inhibitor of NF-κB indicated that the selenite and MSA induced upregulation of H-PGDS and the downregulation of mPGES-1 and thromboxane A synthase (TXAS) appears to be mediated by NF-κB (Gandhi et al. 2011). It is well established that CyPGs have a wide range of effects including the suppression of pro-inflammatory pathways, like NF-κB, AP-1, and STATs, in macrophages (Ricote et al. 1998). The NF-κB pathway can be impaired by CyPGs via the inhibition of IκB kinase-2 (IKK2). Because of their electrophilic nature, CyPGs are able to form covalent Michael adducts with a reactive cysteine thiol in the active site of IKK2 leading to its inhibition. Thus, IκB cannot be phosphorylated and degraded, thereby constantly binding and inhibiting NF-κB (Brigelius-Flohé and Flohé 2017). As already described above, a Se-induced increase in 15d-$\Delta^{12,14}$-PGJ$_2$ also activated PPARüFE; (Vunta et al. 2007). PPARüFE; activation is important to attenuate the oxidative burst (Johann et al. 2006), which would accordingly be enhanced by increasing the Se status. Besides that, Se-induced changes in CyPGs modulated protein expression via epigenetic mechanisms through limiting histone acetylation caused by inhibition of histone acetyltransferase p300 (p300 HAT). This way, the LPS-mediated stimulation of COX-2 and tumor necrosis factor α (TNF-α) expression was strongly inhibited (Narayan et al. 2015). Another anti-inflammatory effect of Se might involve the Se-dependent upregulation of 15-prostaglandin dehydrogenase (15-PGDH), which metabolizes pro-inflammatory PGE$_2$ to the biologically inactive 13,14-dihydro-15-keto PGE$_2$ (Kaushal et al. 2014).

Also the leukotriene network has been shown to be modulated by Se. In a model of isoproterenol-induced myocardial infarction in rats, 5-LOX activity was inhibited and expression of leukotriene A4 hydrolase (LTA$_4$H) was decreased by selenite supplementation (8 µg/100 g body weight) (Mattmiller et al. 2013; Panicker et al. 2012). Thereby, the hydrolysis of LTA$_4$ to the more pro-inflammatory leukotriene LTB$_4$ was reduced in monocytes under stimulated conditions. A significant decrease in LOX activity was only observed in the Se-treated isoproterenol-stimulated group as compared to the control. LTA$_4$ might therefore be available for the biosynthesis of the more resolving lipoxins (LX) like LXA$_4$.

Taken together, Se is able to reduce the expression and activity of the pro-inflammatory enzymes COX-2, mPGES-1, LOX, and LTA$_4$H and to upregulate the anti-inflammatory enzymes PGDS and PGDH upon stimulation of the immune response. Thereby Se can shift the eicosanoid profile towards anti-inflammatory, pro-resolving lipid mediators, which may be one major determinant of the anti-inflammatory effects of dietary Se. This effect is most likely mediated through the regulation of NF-κB and PPARγ activity.

Selenoproteins and the Eicosanoid Network

There is increasing evidence that GPXs are part of the eicosanoid network regulating the activity of COXs and LOXs by affecting the balance of hydroperoxide-generating and hydroperoxide-consuming processes (Radmark et al. 2007; Kulmacz 2005). Accordingly, activity of 5-LOX is regulated by the peroxide tone of its product 5-hydroperoxyeicosatetraenic acid (5-HPETE) (Weitzel and Wendel 1993). GPX1 and GPX4 metabolize 5-HPETE to 5-HETE and thereby inhibit the production of newly formed 5-HPETE (Weitzel and Wendel 1993; Burkert et al. 2003). In a similar way, COX enzyme activity can be limited by GPX1 by reducing hydroperoxides that could otherwise enhance enzyme oxidation and activity (Cook and Lands 1976). A decreased COX activity was described in human endothelial cells (HUVEC) due to an accumulation of peroxides during diminished GPX1 activity because of limited Se supply (Hampel et al. 1989). In platelets isolated from GPX1 KO mice, less 12-HETE was produced at higher concentration of AA indicating that GPX1 is needed to reduce 12-HPETE to 12-HETE (Ho et al. 1997). However, effects on the activity of the corresponding enzyme (12-LOX) were not investigated. It can be speculated that 12-LOX activity might be decreased in a similar way as 5-LOX and COX activity. The co-localization of GPX2 and COX-2 in areas of inflammation suggests that COX-2 activity might be inhibited by GPX2 likewise through the downregulation of hydroperoxides (Banning et al. 2008a). Furthermore, a conditional knockout of GPX4 omitted inhibition of murine 12/15-LOX which resulted in AIF-induced cell death of MEFs (Seiler et al. 2008). Other oxygenases (COX, 5-LOX) were unaffected in this model. Besides GPXs, two additional selenoproteins have been described to be involved in the removal of hydroperoxides produced by 15-LOX. Both selenoprotein P (SELENOP) and TXNRD1 protected cells from lipid hydroperoxides generated by 15-LOX by reducing 15-HPETE to 15-HETE (Rock and Moos 2010; Bjornstedt et al. 1995).

Besides influencing the activity of enzymes from the eicosanoid network, selenoproteins also affect their expression. To study the overall effect of selenoproteins, a mouse model was generated with a depletion of the whole selenoproteome, lacking selenoprotein synthesis by a knockout of the gene encoding for selenocysteine tRNA (Trsp) (Bosl et al. 1997). Selenoprotein-deficient macrophages (Trsp$^{fl/fl}$ LysM^{Cre}) were characterized by increased expression of COX-2, 15-LOX-1, 15-LOX-2, and 5-LOX as well as the pro-inflammatory cytokine TNF-α. Level of the pro-resolving lipoxin LXA$_4$ was significantly reduced together with 9-oxoODE (Mattmiller et al. 2014). So far, this study provides unique systemic data on the impact of selenoproteins on SPM synthesis. Given that the synthesis of SPMs requires LOX activity and that selenoproteins tightly interact with the LOX pathway, it is likely that Se and selenoproteins might, at least in part, exert their anti-inflammatory effects through changes in the SPM profile. Even though this study provided convincing evidence that selenoproteins are important mediators of oxylipid profiles, the model system was not aiming for the identification of individual selenoproteins but only measured the overall effect. To address this point, expression levels of individual selenoproteins must be modulated. In HT-29 cells, a stable knockdown of GPX2 increased the expression of COX-2 as well as mPGES1 both under basal and interleukin 1β (IL-1β)-stimulated conditions. This effect was specific for GPX2, because depletion of GPX1 by Se deprivation did not affect COX-2 and mPGES-1 expression (Banning et al. 2008a). The increased expression of COX-2 resulted in an enhanced COX-2-mediated migration/invasion of GPX2 knockdown (KD) cells (Banning et al. 2008b).

Interaction of Prostaglandins with Selenoproteins

Selenoproteins harbor selenocysteine residues in their active center, which are very reactive and typically reveal a nucleophilic character. CyPGs are α,β-unsaturated ketones with strong electrophilic character. It is speculated that these reactive PGs are able to modify multiple redox-sensitive transcription factors including p53, NF-κB, Nrf2, and HIF-1α (Moos et al. 2003) but might also react with selenoproteins, thereby influencing their activity. So far, only data on the interaction of reactive PGs and the TXNRD-TRX system are available while the interaction with other selenoproteins has not been analyzed. It was shown that TXNRD and TRX interact with electrophilic products of both the prostaglandin and the leukotriene network. Like this, CyPGs of the A and J series notably PGA can covalently bind to TXNRD, thereby impairing its enzymatic function (Moos et al. 2003). The same effect was observed for 15-LOX-1 products (Yu et al. 2004). In contrast, metabolites of the 5-LOX pathway were poor inhibitors of TXNRD. Furthermore, also the substrate of TXNRD, TRX, was shown to interact with reactive PGs such as PGA and 15d-$\Delta^{12,14}$-PGJ$_2$ to form covalent TRX adducts (Moos et al. 2003; Shibata et al. 2003).

Interestingly, 15d-$\Delta^{12,14}$-PGJ$_2$ is also able to affect the expression of the selenoprotein GPX2. In CaCo2 cells, 15d-$\Delta^{12,14}$-PGJ$_2$ stimulation increased GPX2 promotor activity and both GPX2 mRNA and protein expression (Hiller et al. 2015). Most probably, this effect was mediated via activation of the transcription factor Nrf2.

Taken together, there is a tight interrelationship between Se/selenoproteins and the eicosanoid network. Not only Se/selenoproteins modulate the activity and expression of important enzymes of the eicosanoid pathway but products of the eicosanoid pathway are also able to directly interact with selenoproteins or influence their expression.

Shifts in Cell Populations of the Immune System

Effects of Se and Selenoproteins on Macrophages

Depending on their differentiation state, macrophages can reveal both pro- and anti-inflammatory properties. In a first phase after infection, INF-γ stimulates classically activated myeloid cells, the pro-inflammatory M1 macrophages, to ensure a fast removal of the pathogens. In a second response phase, IL-10 can counterbalance inflammation by inducing the anti-inflammatory M2 macrophages, thereby promoting proliferation and healing processes and restricting excessive inflammation. The two types of macrophages also differ with regard to their redox state and are therefore called oxidative (M1 macrophages) or reductive macrophages (M2 macrophages) with high and low amounts of GSH, respectively (Kidd 2003; Murata et al. 2002). Accordingly, the intracellular GSH status is an important mediator of macrophage differentiation into one of the two types (Kim et al. 2004). As GSH levels are discussed to be increased by Se (Lee and Wan 2002), one can speculate that this could affect the differentiation of macrophages in a Se-dependent manner.

Indeed, supplementation with Se significantly reduced the level of M1 markers (TNF-α, IL-1β) in LPS-treated macrophages while significantly increasing the M2 makers arginase-I (Arg-I), Fizz1, and mannose receptor C-type 1 after IL-4 treatment (Fig. 7.2) (Nelson et al. 2011). This was ascribed to the Se-dependent production of the anti-inflammatory prostaglandin Δ^{12}-PGJ$_2$ and its dehydration product 15d-$\Delta^{12,14}$-PGJ$_2$ with subsequent PPARγ activation (Nelson et al. 2016). Furthermore, inhibition of the M1 phenotype by Se clearly correlated with the effect of Se on enzymes of the eicosanoid network: M1 activation involves increased expression of COX-2, TXAS1, and leukotriene A4 hydrolase (Tan et al. 2016), which was inhibited by Se.

For individual selenoproteins, it has been supposed that GPXs are involved in the polarization of macrophages into the M1 or M2 type. In BMDM of GPX1 KO mice, the activity of the M2 marker Arg-I was significantly decreased after combined IL-4 and LPS treatment (Nelson et al. 2011). Also SELENOP has been recently connected to macrophage function. The major function of SELENOP is its transport ability of Se from the liver to peripheral tissues mainly to the brain and testis (Burk and Hill 2005). Besides that, SELENOP is discussed to have antioxidant properties (Bosschaerts et al. 2008). During the switch from M1 to M2 macrophages, expression of SELENOP was induced by IL-10. This upregulation limited the pathogenicity of African trypanosome infection. Vice versa, SELENOP KO mice were characterized by increased amounts of necrotic and apoptotic immune cells (Bosschaerts et al. 2008). During colitis, loss of SELENOP resulted in higher numbers of M2-polarized macrophages (Barrett et al. 2015).

Macrophages are important for the phagocytosis of microorganisms as well as dead and dying cells. The oxidative burst concomitantly kills engulfed pathogens but also clears apoptotic cells accumulating during wound-healing processes (Tan et al. 2016). In macrophages lacking the selenoproteome (Trsp$^{fl/fl}$LysM^{Cre}) basal

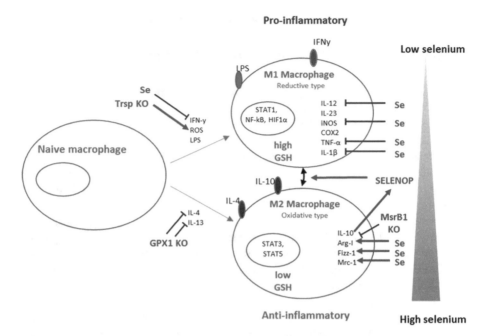

Fig. 7.2 Effects of Se and selenoproteins on macrophage polarization. Se is able to push polarization towards the anti-inflammatory M2 type by inhibiting the expression of various M1 genes whereas M2 genes are induced. M2 macrophages promote the resolution of inflammation, wound healing, and tissue remodeling. Vice versa, the knockout (KO) of either GPX1 or methionine sulfoxide reductase B1 (MsrB1) results in reduced expression of M2 cytokines shifting macrophages towards the M1 type which induces inflammation

levels of ROS were increased (Carlson et al. 2009). However, this did not impair macrophage function and immune response in different inflammation models such as LPS endotoxemia, acute edema formation with tetradecanoylphorbol-acetate (TPA), and zymosan-induced neutrophil infiltration (Carlson et al. 2010). However, these models all have in common that they focused on acute inflammation and did not investigate the resolution phase. Based on that, it can be speculated that selenoproteins are of ample importance during a rather late phase of inflammation. Evidence for this hypothesis is further supported by a study evaluating dextran-sodium sulfate (DSS)-induced colitis in mice with selenoprotein-deficient macrophages (Kaushal et al. 2014). In this model, transgenic mice were more prone to develop a colitis than wild-type mice. This effect was mainly attributed to the selenoprotein-dependent upregulation of 15-PGDH expression and subsequent degradation of PGE_2 resulting in anti-inflammatory and pro-resolving effects.

Another selenoprotein which is involved in regulating macrophage function is SELENOK (Verma et al. 2011). SELENOK is a transmembrane protein localized to ER which modulates proper protein folding and calcium flux in immune cells. Immune cells express high levels of SELENOK (Verma et al. 2011). Deletion of SELENOK in macrophages resulted in impaired oxidative burst mediated by immunoglobulin (Ig)G-dependent activation of the phagocytotic Fcγ receptor (FcγR) (Verma et al. 2011). However, here again, the phagocytosis itself was not affected (Verma et al. 2011). However, SELENOK was required for the efficient FcγR-mediated phagocytosis as demonstrated by less efficient engulfment of IgG-coated fluorescence beats by SELENOK KO macrophages (Norton et al. 2017).

Effects of Se and Selenoproteins on T Cells

T cells recognize foreign or altered substances on the surface of infected cells (MHC-I) or on antigen-presenting cells (APC) like macrophages, monocytes, and phagocytes (MHC-II) via the T-cell receptor and are then activated and differentiated. T cells can be divided into different categories including memory T cells, cytotoxic T (Tc) cells, T-helper (Th) cells, and T-regulatory cells (Treg, T-suppressor cells). Cytotoxic cells (CD8 receptor) destroy infected cells while memory T cells (either CD4 or CD8 receptor) can remember previously encountered pathogens. Thus, the next immune response works faster when the second contact to a pathogen takes place. Th cells (CD4 receptor) release cytokines, thereby attracting additional immune cells. In contrast, Treg cells protect from the uncontrolled reaction against body's own cells, thereby maintaining immunological tolerance. To do so, Treg cells inactivate Tc cells by secreting, e.g., IL-10 to prevent autoimmune diseases.

So far, effects of Se and selenoproteins on T cells have been studied with specific emphasis on Th cells whereas little is known about cytotoxic and memory T cells. Both intracellular and extracellular H_2O_2 produced by inflamed tissue (e.g., macrophages) and concomitant modulation of redox signaling affects T-cell activation and proliferation (Simeoni and Bogeski 2015). The latter has been demonstrated by the use of redox-modulating agents (GSH, iron chelators, butylated hydroxyanisole), which impaired IL-2 expression (Simeoni and Bogeski 2015). Indeed, increasing the Se supply (0.5–2 μM) upregulated GPX1 and TXNRD1 mRNA and total GPX activity in primary porcine T cells and concomitantly induced proliferation and IL-2 production. Interestingly, both effects were only observed after concanavalin A or T-cell receptor (TCR)-mediated T-cell activation whereas phytohemagglutinin-induced T-cell activation was not affected (Ren et al. 2012). Similar results were obtained for T cells isolated from mice fed with poor, adequate, or supraphysiological amounts of Se (Hoffmann et al. 2010). Increasing dietary Se enhanced T-cell proliferation, IL-2 and IL-2 receptor mRNA expression, as well as GSH levels. Addition of N-acetyl-cysteine (NAC) limited the Se-induced effects on proliferation. Another study with Trsp KO T cells (Trsp[fl/fl]Lck[Cre]) obtained similar results showing that selenoprotein expression is important for T-cell proliferation after TCR activation. In response to anti-CD28 and anti-CD3 antibodies, proliferation of selenoprotein-deficient T cells was dramatically decreased in comparison to wild-type cells (Shrimali et al. 2008). This effect was completely restored by NAC, indicating that the redox status of Trsp-deficient T cells was responsible for the impaired proliferation. Besides proliferation, Trsp KO T cells expressed less surface

IL-2 receptor upon TCR activation while IL-2 secretion was unchanged indicating that differentiation/maturation was disturbed (Shrimali et al. 2008). Inconsistent results were obtained for GPX1 KO T cells. In one study, GPX1-deficient T cells had a comparable phenotype as described for Trsp KO T cells. Basal H_2O_2 levels were already increased upon loss of GPX1; thus, levels could not be further upregulated after concanavalin stimulation. Subsequently, this resulted in an impaired T-cell response due to a general T-cell hyporesponsiveness (Lee et al. 2016). Interestingly, in another study deletion of GPX1 did not increase basal ROS level of T cells isolated from lymph nodes and spleen but only TCR-stimulated H_2O_2 levels, thereby increasing IL-2 production and proliferation (Won et al. 2010). Based on that, it appears to be of high relevance for the immune response at which exact time point GPX1 expression is repressed and how long GPX1 levels are maintained at low levels. As described for macrophages already, SELENOK is also very important for T-cell function (Verma et al. 2011). SELENOK-deficient T cells have an impaired calcium flux in response to TCR activation resulting in partially decreased T-cell proliferation. Similarly, chemokine-stimulated (RANTES, SDF-1) migration was decreased in SELENOK-deficient T cells. Mechanistically, SELENOK is part of a complex responsible for IP3 receptor palmitoylation which is a critical regulator of calcium flux in immune cells (Fredericks et al. 2014).

During immune response, CD4$^+$ T cells are activated and differentiated into different subtypes, including Th1, Th2, Th17, and Treg (Huang et al. 2012b). Depending on the pathogen faced, CD4$^+$ cells can be differentiated into Th1 and Th2 cells (Kidd 2003). While intracellular pathogens like viruses activate Th1 cells and stimulate cellular immune response, extracellular organisms activate Th2 cells and humoral immunity by increasing antibody production (Kidd 2003). Herein, the cytokine milieu plays an important role. IL-12 secreted by macrophages induces Th1 differentiation, whereas IL-2 and IL-7 stimulate Th2-cell differentiation. In a positive feedback loop, INF-γ released by Th1 cells and IL-4 secreted by Th2 cells stimulate Th1 and Th2 cell responses, respectively. Interestingly, the KO of GPX1 shifted differentiation of Th cells towards the Th1 phenotypes (Huang et al. 2012b) and attenuated differentiation into Th17 cells (Won et al. 2010).

Cytokine Networks

Cytokines are important mediators for the communication of immune cells. The cytokine milieu is very critical for both polarization of macrophages into M1 or M2 phenotype and differentiation of Th cells into Th1 or Th2 cells. TNF-α and IL-1β strongly stimulate M1 macrophages while IL-10 and IL-4 are essential for M2 macrophage activation. Interferon (IFN)-γ is the major stimulus for Th1 differentiation while IL-10 activates Th2 immune response. Expression of cytokines is mainly regulated by STATs but also by NF-κB, both of which are known to be redox sensitive (Lei et al. 2015).

Se and the Cytokine Network

Se has a wide range of effects on cytokine profiles in different models (Fig. 7.3). In RAW264.7 macrophages infected with *S. aureus*, Se supplementation (selenite, 1–2 μM) downregulated mRNA expression of TNF-α, IL-1β, and IL-6 (Bi et al. 2016). This was ascribed to the inhibition of the NF-κB and MAP kinase (ERK, JNK, p38) pathway. In a model of DSS-induced colitis in mice, Se given as Se-enriched Spirulina Platensis (0.12 ± 0.01 ppm Se) reduced the inflammatory response, inflammatory cell infiltration, and pathological damage (Zhu et al. 2016). Concomitantly, NF-κB activation and release of the pro-inflammatory cytokines TNF-α, IL-6, and monocyte chemoattractant protein-1 (MCP-1) were reduced by Se while secretion of IL-10 was markedly increased. In erythrocytes of male but not female mice, Se was able to decrease cytokine release (TNF-α, MCP-1, and IL-6) after injection of LPS (Stoedter et al. 2010). This was ascribed to sex-specific differences in SELENOS expression in response to LPS stimulation.

In studies investigating basal levels of cytokines without any stimulation, different Se-mediated effects on the cytokine profile were obtained (Fig. 7.3). In chicken bursa isolated from Se-deficient (0.033 mg/kg diet) and Se-adequate (0.15 mg/kg diet, enriched with selenite) animals, expression levels of IL-1β, IL-2, IL-6, IL-8, IL-10, IL-17, IFN-α, IFN-β, and IFN-γ were significantly increased while TNF-α was significantly decreased upon adequate Se supply (Khoso et al. 2015). In line with this, Se supplementation of chicken (0.2 mg selenite/kg diet) changed the level of all ten cytokines investigated in erythrocytes compared to chicken fed a Se-deficient diet (0.008 mg/kg diet) (Luan et al. 2016). Levels of IL-2, IL-4, IL-8, IL-10, IL-12β, TGF-β4, and IFN-γ increased with Se while expression

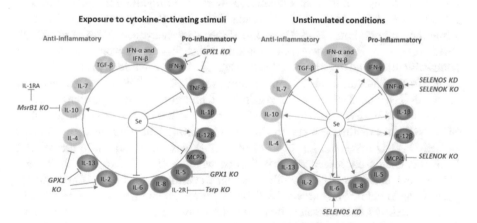

Fig. 7.3 Effects of Se and selenoproteins on the cytokine network. After treatment with cytokine-inducing stimuli, Se mainly exerts an inhibitory effect on pro-inflammatory cytokines. Under basal conditions, Se stimulates expression of anti-inflammatory cytokines but levels of various pro-inflammatory cytokines are increased as well. Red circles, inflammatory cytokines; blue circles, anti-inflammatory cytokines; red/blue circles, cytokines with pro- and anti-inflammatory properties

of IL-1γ, IL-6, and IL-7 decreased. Similar results were obtained in a study with mice on Se-poor (0 ppm selenite) and Se-adequate (0.1 ppm selenite) diets. Adequate level of Se increased IFN-regulated pro-inflammatory cytokine expression (Tsuji et al. 2015). Seven cytokines (IFN-γ, IL-6, IL-1β, IL-10, IL-12p70, Cxcl1 (KC/GRO), or TNF-α) were analyzed in serum out of which only IFN-γ and IL-6 were increased. In another study with rats, selenite (i.p. treatment with 0.2 mg/kg body weight) did not change basal levels of IL-6, IL-10, and TNF-α; however the treatment could prevent the mercury-induced decrease of these pro-inflammatory cytokines. High levels of Se were furthermore able to increase the IL-2 response by increasing both levels of IL-2 and IL-2 receptor (Hoffmann et al. 2010).

Selenoproteins and the Cytokine Network

Recently, the selenoprotein methionine sulfoxide reductase B1 (MsrB1) has been shown to control immune response by promoting anti-inflammatory cytokine expression in macrophages (Lee et al. 2017). After LPS stimulation, MsrB1 expression was highly increased. A knockout of MsrB1 resulted in significantly decreased plasma levels of the anti-inflammatory cytokines IL-10 (Figs. 7.2 and 7.3) and IL-1 receptor antagonist (RA) while production of the pro-inflammatory cytokines TNF-α, IL-6, and IL-1β was unaffected (Lee et al. 2017). This was associated with an increased inflammatory response and increased severity of inflammation. Interestingly, loss of GPX1 inhibited the expression of pro-inflammatory cytokines TNF-α, IL-2, and IFN-γ in a concanavalin-induced T-cell-mediated model of liver disease as described above (Lee et al. 2016). This was ascribed to changes in the redox balance. However, during allergen-induced airway inflammation, GPX1 deficiency increased IFN-γ and IL-2 expression in Th cells while the Th2 cytokines IL-4, IL-5, and IL-13 were decreased (Won et al. 2010). SELENOS is an ER-resident selenoprotein which has been proposed to protect against ER stress and to be involved in the degradation of misfolded proteins (Huang et al. 2012b; Stoedter et al. 2010). Knockdown of SELENOS increased levels of excreted IL-6 and TNF-α in the medium of phorbol myristate acetate (PMA)-stimulated RAW264.7 macrophages (Curran et al. 2005). Also the ER-localized SELENOK has distinct effects on the cytokine profile: In viral mimetic infected SELENOK KO mice, the serum level of TNF-α was increased while the MCP-1 level was decreased compared to WT mice whereas IL-6, IL-10, IL-12p70, and IFN-γ were not detectable in both genotypes (Verma et al. 2011). Interestingly, performing knockdown studies of SELENOK revealed that the exact time point of reduced SELENOK expression mediated the cytokine profile in a different way (Fan et al. 2017). After 24-h incubation of primary myoblast with SELENOK siRNA, levels of IL-1β, IL-6, IL-7, IL-8, IL-17, and IFN-γ were increased, while after 72 h only IL-6, IL-7, and IL-8 were increased. At this later time point, IL-1β, IL-17, and IFN-γ were significantly decreased (Fan et al. 2017).

Taken together, under challenged conditions, Se decreases the production of pro-inflammatory cytokines while under unstimulated conditions in particular the level of anti-inflammatory cytokines is increased by Se. In case of macrophages, Se shifts the cytokine milieu rather towards anti-inflammatory M2 cytokines. However, expression of Th-cell cytokines is balanced and increased for both phenotypes indicating that Se promotes Th-cell response depending on the pathogen faced.

Concluding Remarks

The importance of Se during inflammation and immunity has been verified in many studies. However, underlying mechanisms have just started being investigated in more detail. New methods established during the last years will help, e.g., to more precisely decipher the role of Se and selenoproteins during redox signaling. It should be furthermore kept in mind that inflammation is not per se an undesirable reaction but fulfills important functions in the body. The close interrelation and interdependence of GPXs with the eicosanoid network indicate a key function of this selenoprotein family in keeping the fragile balance between the necessary inflammatory response and an accurate switch off of this process. New lipidomic approaches detecting complete profiles of prostaglandins, leukotrienes, as well as pro-resolving lipid mediators such as lipoxins and resolvins will enable to specify the role of selenoproteins on eicosanoid profiles. Given that Se and selenoproteins are involved in (1) eicosanoid class switching towards the more anti-inflammatory CyPGs, (2) suppression of anti-inflammatory cytokine secretion, and (3) polarization of macrophages towards the rather anti-inflammatory M2 type, it is more and more becoming obvious that selenoproteins exert key functions in resolving inflammation, thereby preventing it to become chronic. In all these settings, the exact timing of induction and counter-regulation of both selenoproteins and inflammatory mediators is of ample importance.

References

Babior BM. The respiratory burst oxidase. Curr Opin Hematol. 1995;2:55–60.
Banning A, Florian S, Deubel S, Thalmann S, Muller-Schmehl K, Jacobasch G, Brigelius-Flohé R. Gpx2 counteracts pge2 production by dampening cox-2 and mpges-1 expression in human colon cancer cells. Antioxid Redox Signal. 2008a;10:1491–500.
Banning A, Kipp A, Schmitmeier S, Lowinger M, Florian S, Krehl S, Thalmann S, Thierbach R, Steinberg P, Brigelius-Flohé R. Glutathione peroxidase 2 inhibits cyclooxygenase-2-mediated migration and invasion of ht-29 adenocarcinoma cells but supports their growth as tumors in nude mice. Cancer Res. 2008b;68:9746–53.
Barrett CW, Reddy VK, Short SP, Motley AK, Lintel MK, Bradley AM, Freeman T, Vallance J, Ning W, Parang B, Poindexter SV, Fingleton B, Chen X, Washington MK, Wilson KT, Shroyer NF, Hill KE, Burk RF, Williams CS. Selenoprotein p influences colitis-induced tumorigenesis by mediating stemness and oxidative damage. J Clin Invest. 2015;125:2646–60.

Basil MC, Levy BD. Specialized pro-resolving mediators: endogenous regulators of infection and inflammation. Nat Rev Immunol. 2016;16:51–67.

Bi CL, Wang H, Wang YJ, Sun J, Dong JS, Meng X, Li JJ. Selenium inhibits staphylococcus aureus-induced inflammation by suppressing the activation of the nf-kappab and mapk signalling pathways in raw264.7 macrophages. Eur J Pharmacol. 2016;780:159–65.

Bjornstedt M, Hamberg M, Kumar S, Xue J, Holmgren A. Human thioredoxin reductase directly reduces lipid hydroperoxides by nadph and selenocystine strongly stimulates the reaction via catalytically generated selenols. J Biol Chem. 1995;270:11761–4.

Bosl MR, Takaku K, Oshima M, Nishimura S, Taketo MM. Early embryonic lethality caused by targeted disruption of the mouse selenocysteine trna gene (trsp). Proc Natl Acad Sci U S A. 1997;94:5531–4.

Bosschaerts T, Guilliams M, Noel W, Herin M, Burk RF, Hill KE, Brys L, Raes G, Ghassabeh GH, De Baetselier P, Beschin A. Alternatively activated myeloid cells limit pathogenicity associated with african trypanosomiasis through the il-10 inducible gene selenoprotein p. J Immunol. 2008;180:6168–75.

Brigelius-Flohé R, Flohé L. Selenium and redox signaling. Arch Biochem Biophys. 2017;617:48–59.

Brock TG, Peters-Golden M. Activation and regulation of cellular eicosanoid biosynthesis. ScientificWorldJournal. 2007;7:1273–84.

Burk RF, Hill KE. Selenoprotein p: an extracellular protein with unique physical characteristics and a role in selenium homeostasis. Annu Rev Nutr. 2005;25:215–35.

Burkert E, Arnold C, Hammarberg T, Radmark O, Steinhilber D, Werz O. The c2-like beta-barrel domain mediates the ca2+−dependent resistance of 5-lipoxygenase activity against inhibition by glutathione peroxidase-1. J Biol Chem. 2003;278:42846–53.

Carlson BA, Yoo MH, Sano Y, Sengupta A, Kim JY, Irons R, Gladyshev VN, Hatfield DL, Park JM. Selenoproteins regulate macrophage invasiveness and extracellular matrix-related gene expression. BMC Immunol. 2009;10:57.

Carlson BA, Yoo MH, Shrimali RK, Irons R, Gladyshev VN, Hatfield DL, Park JM. Role of selenium-containing proteins in t-cell and macrophage function. Proc Nutr Soc. 2010;69:300–10.

Cook HW, Lands WE. Mechanism for suppression of cellular biosynthesis of prostaglandins. Nature. 1976;260:630–2.

Curran JE, Jowett JB, Elliott KS, Gao Y, Gluschenko K, Wang J, Abel Azim DM, Cai G, Mahaney MC, Comuzzie AG, Dyer TD, Walder KR, Zimmet P, Maccluer JW, Collier GR, Kissebah AH, Blangero J. Genetic variation in selenoprotein s influences inflammatory response. Nat Genet. 2005;37:1234–41.

Dennis EA, Cao J, Hsu YH, Magrioti V, Kokotos G. Phospholipase a2 enzymes: physical structure, biological function, disease implication, chemical inhibition, and therapeutic intervention. Chem Rev. 2011;111:6130–85.

Fan R, Yao H, Cao C, Zhao X, Khalid A, Zhao J, Zhang Z, Xu S. Gene silencing of selenoprotein k induces inflammatory response and activates heat shock proteins expression in chicken myoblasts. Biol Trace Elem Res. 2017;180(1):135–45.

Forman HJ, Torres M. Redox signaling in macrophages. Mol Asp Med. 2001;22:189–216.

Fredericks GJ, Hoffmann FW, Rose AH, Osterheld HJ, Hess FM, Mercier F, Hoffmann PR. Stable expression and function of the inositol 1,4,5-triphosphate receptor requires palmitoylation by a dhhc6/selenoprotein k complex. Proc Natl Acad Sci U S A. 2014;111:16478–83.

Freire MO, Van Dyke TE. Natural resolution of inflammation. Periodontol. 2000;63(2013):149–64.

Fullerton JN, Gilroy DW. Resolution of inflammation: a new therapeutic frontier. Nat Rev Drug Discov. 2016;15:551–67.

Gandhi UH, Kaushal N, Ravindra KC, Hegde S, Nelson SM, Narayan V, Vunta H, Paulson RF, Prabhu KS. Selenoprotein-dependent up-regulation of hematopoietic prostaglandin d2 synthase in macrophages is mediated through the activation of peroxisome proliferator-activated receptor (ppar) gamma. J Biol Chem. 2011;286:27471–82.

Griffiths HR, Gao D, Pararasa C. Redox regulation in metabolic programming and inflammation. Redox Biol. 2017;12:50–7.

Hampel G, Watanabe K, Weksler BB, Jaffe EA. Selenium deficiency inhibits prostacyclin release and enhances production of platelet activating factor by human endothelial cells. Biochim Biophys Acta. 1989;1006:151–8.

Handel ML, Watts CK, Defazio A, Day RO, Sutherland RL. Inhibition of ap-1 binding and transcription by gold and selenium involving conserved cysteine residues in jun and fos. Proc Natl Acad Sci U S A. 1995;92:4497–501.

Harizi H, Gualde N. The impact of eicosanoids on the crosstalk between innate and adaptive immunity: the key roles of dendritic cells. Tissue Antigens. 2005;65:507–14.

Hiller F, Besselt K, Deubel S, Brigelius-Flohé R, Kipp AP. Gpx2 induction is mediated through stat transcription factors during acute colitis. Inflamm Bowel Dis. 2015;21:2078–89.

Ho YS, Magnenat JL, Bronson RT, Cao J, Gargano M, Sugawara M, Funk CD. Mice deficient in cellular glutathione peroxidase develop normally and show no increased sensitivity to hyperoxia. J Biol Chem. 1997;272:16644–51.

Hoffmann FW, Hashimoto AC, Shafer LA, Dow S, Berry MJ, Hoffmann PR. Dietary selenium modulates activation and differentiation of cd4+ t cells in mice through a mechanism involving cellular free thiols. J Nutr. 2010;140:1155–61.

Huang C, Ding G, Gu C, Zhou J, Kuang M, Ji Y, He Y, Kondo T, Fan J. Decreased selenium-binding protein 1 enhances glutathione peroxidase 1 activity and downregulates hif-1alpha to promote hepatocellular carcinoma invasiveness. Clin Cancer Res. 2012a;18:3042–53.

Huang Z, Rose AH, Hoffmann PR. The role of selenium in inflammation and immunity: from molecular mechanisms to therapeutic opportunities. Antioxid Redox Signal. 2012b;16:705–43.

Johann AM, Von Knethen A, Lindemann D, Brune B. Recognition of apoptotic cells by macrophages activates the peroxisome proliferator-activated receptor-gamma and attenuates the oxidative burst. Cell Death Differ. 2006;13:1533–40.

Jozsef L, Filep JG. Selenium-containing compounds attenuate peroxynitrite-mediated nf-kappab and ap-1 activation and interleukin-8 gene and protein expression in human leukocytes. Free Radic Biol Med. 2003;35:1018–27.

Kaushal N, Kudva AK, Patterson AD, Chiaro C, Kennett MJ, Desai D, Amin S, Carlson BA, Cantorna MT, Prabhu KS. Crucial role of macrophage selenoproteins in experimental colitis. J Immunol. 2014;193:3683–92.

Khoso PA, Yang Z, Liu C, Li S. Selenoproteins and heat shock proteins play important roles in immunosuppression in the bursa of fabricius of chickens with selenium deficiency. Cell Stress Chaperones. 2015;20:967–78.

Kidd P. Th1/th2 balance: the hypothesis, its limitations, and implications for health and disease. Altern Med Rev. 2003;8:223–46.

Kim N, Luster AD. Regulation of immune cells by eicosanoid receptors. ScientificWorldJournal. 2007;7:1307–28.

Kim JM, Kim H, Kwon SB, Lee SY, Chung SC, Jeong DW, Min BM. Intracellular glutathione status regulates mouse bone marrow monocyte-derived macrophage differentiation and phagocytic activity. Biochem Biophys Res Commun. 2004;325:101–8.

Kipp AP, Banning A, Van Schothorst EM, Meplan C, Coort SL, Evelo CT, Keijer J, Hesketh J, Brigelius-Flohé R. Marginal selenium deficiency down-regulates inflammation-related genes in splenic leukocytes of the mouse. J Nutr Biochem. 2012;23:1170–7.

Kulmacz RJ. Regulation of cyclooxygenase catalysis by hydroperoxides. Biochem Biophys Res Commun. 2005;338:25–33.

Lee KH, Jeong D. Bimodal actions of selenium essential for antioxidant and toxic pro-oxidant activities: the selenium paradox (review). Mol Med Rep. 2012;5:299–304.

Lee CY, Wan JM. Immunoregulatory and antioxidant performance of alpha-tocopherol and selenium on human lymphocytes. Biol Trace Elem Res. 2002;86:123–36.

Lee DH, Son DJ, Park MH, Yoon DY, Han SB, Hong JT. Glutathione peroxidase 1 deficiency attenuates concanavalin a-induced hepatic injury by modulation of t-cell activation. Cell Death Dis. 2016;7:e2208.

Lee BC, Lee SG, Choo MK, Kim JH, Lee HM, Kim S, Fomenko DE, Kim HY, Park JM, Gladyshev VN. Selenoprotein msrb1 promotes anti-inflammatory cytokine gene expression in macrophages and controls immune response in vivo. Sci Rep. 2017;7:5119.

Lei Y, Wang K, Deng L, Chen Y, Nice EC, Huang C. Redox regulation of inflammation: old elements, a new story. Med Res Rev. 2015;35:306–40.

Leslie CC. Cytosolic phospholipase a(2): physiological function and role in disease. J Lipid Res. 2015;56:1386–402.

Luan Y, Zhao J, Yao H, Zhao X, Fan R, Zhao W, Zhang Z, Xu S. Selenium deficiency influences the mrna expression of selenoproteins and cytokines in chicken erythrocytes. Biol Trace Elem Res. 2016;171:427–36.

Matthews JR, Wakasugi N, Virelizier JL, Yodoi J, Hay RT. Thioredoxin regulates the DNA binding activity of nf-kappa b by reduction of a disulphide bond involving cysteine 62. Nucleic Acids Res. 1992;20:3821–30.

Mattmiller SA, Carlson BA, Sordillo LM. Regulation of inflammation by selenium and selenoproteins: impact on eicosanoid biosynthesis. J Nutr Sci. 2013;2:e28.

Mattmiller SA, Carlson BA, Gandy JC, Sordillo LM. Reduced macrophage selenoprotein expression alters oxidized lipid metabolite biosynthesis from arachidonic and linoleic acid. J Nutr Biochem. 2014;25:647–54.

Medzhitov R. Origin and physiological roles of inflammation. Nature. 2008;454:428–35.

Moos PJ, Edes K, Cassidy P, Massuda E, Fitzpatrick FA. Electrophilic prostaglandins and lipid aldehydes repress redox-sensitive transcription factors p53 and hypoxia-inducible factor by impairing the selenoprotein thioredoxin reductase. J Biol Chem. 2003;278:745–50.

Müller M, Banning A, Brigelius-Flohé R, Kipp A. Nrf2 target genes are induced under marginal selenium-deficiency. Genes Nutr. 2010;5:297–307.

Murata Y, Shimamura T, Hamuro J. The polarization of t(h)1/t(h)2 balance is dependent on the intracellular thiol redox status of macrophages due to the distinctive cytokine production. Int Immunol. 2002;14:201–12.

Naranjo-Suarez S, Carlson BA, Tsuji PA, Yoo MH, Gladyshev VN, Hatfield DL. Hif-independent regulation of thioredoxin reductase 1 contributes to the high levels of reactive oxygen species induced by hypoxia. PLoS One. 2012;7:e30470.

Naranjo-Suarez S, Carlson BA, Tobe R, Yoo MH, Tsuji PA, Gladyshev VN, Hatfield DL. Regulation of hif-1alpha activity by overexpression of thioredoxin is independent of thioredoxin reductase status. Mol Cells. 2013;36:151–7.

Narayan V, Ravindra KC, Liao C, Kaushal N, Carlson BA, Prabhu KS. Epigenetic regulation of inflammatory gene expression in macrophages by selenium. J Nutr Biochem. 2015;26:138–45.

Nelson SM, Lei X, Prabhu KS. Selenium levels affect the il-4-induced expression of alternative activation markers in murine macrophages. J Nutr. 2011;141:1754–61.

Nelson SM, Shay AE, James JL, Carlson BA, Urban JF Jr, Prabhu KS. Selenoprotein expression in macrophages is critical for optimal clearance of parasitic helminth nippostrongylus brasiliensis. J Biol Chem. 2016;291:2787–98.

Norton RL, Fredericks GJ, Huang Z, Fay JD, Hoffmann FW, Hoffmann PR. Selenoprotein k regulation of palmitoylation and calpain cleavage of asap2 is required for efficient fcgammar-mediated phagocytosis. J Leukoc Biol. 2017;101:439–48.

Panicker S, Swathy SS, John F, M I. Impact of selenium on the leukotriene b4 synthesis pathway during isoproterenol-induced myocardial infarction in experimental rats. Inflammation. 2012;35:74–80.

Radmark O, Werz O, Steinhilber D, Samuelsson B. 5-lipoxygenase: regulation of expression and enzyme activity. Trends Biochem Sci. 2007;32:332–41.

Ren F, Chen X, Hesketh J, Gan F, Huang K. Selenium promotes t-cell response to tcr-stimulation and cona, but not pha in primary porcine splenocytes. PLoS One. 2012;7:e35375.

Ricote M, Li AC, Willson TM, Kelly CJ, Glass CK. The peroxisome proliferator-activated receptor-gamma is a negative regulator of macrophage activation. Nature. 1998;391:79–82.

Rock C, Moos PJ. Selenoprotein p protects cells from lipid hydroperoxides generated by 15-lox-1. Prostaglandins Leukot Essent Fatty Acids. 2010;83:203–10.

Seiler A, Schneider M, Forster H, Roth S, Wirth EK, Culmsee C, Plesnila N, Kremmer E, Radmark O, Wurst W, Bornkamm GW, Schweizer U. & Conrad, M.Glutathione peroxidase 4 senses and translates oxidative stress into 12/15-lipoxygenase dependent- and aif-mediated cell death. Cell Metab. 2008;8:237–48.

Serhan CN. Pro-resolving lipid mediators are leads for resolution physiology. Nature. 2014;510:92–101.

Serhan CN, Chiang N, Van Dyke TE. Resolving inflammation: dual anti-inflammatory and pro-resolution lipid mediators. Nat Rev Immunol. 2008;8:349–61.

Shibata T, Yamada T, Ishii T, Kumazawa S, Nakamura H, Masutani H, Yodoi J, Uchida K. Thioredoxin as a molecular target of cyclopentenone prostaglandins. J Biol Chem. 2003;278:26046–54.

Shrimali RK, Irons RD, Carlson BA, Sano Y, Gladyshev VN, Park JM, Hatfield DL. Selenoproteins mediate t cell immunity through an antioxidant mechanism. J Biol Chem. 2008;283:20181–5.

Simeoni L, Bogeski I. Redox regulation of t-cell receptor signaling. Biol Chem. 2015;396:555–68.

Sinha I, Null K, Wolter W, Suckow MA, King T, Pinto JT, Sinha R. Methylseleninic acid downregulates hypoxia-inducible factor-1alpha in invasive prostate cancer. Int J Cancer. 2012;130:1430–9.

Spallholz JE. Free radical generation by selenium compounds and their prooxidant toxicity. Biomed Environ Sci. 1997;10:260–70.

Spyrou G, Bjornstedt M, Kumar S, Holmgren A. Ap-1 DNA-binding activity is inhibited by selenite and selenodiglutathione. FEBS Lett. 1995;368:59–63.

Staal FJ, Roederer M, Herzenberg LA, Herzenberg LA. Intracellular thiols regulate activation of nuclear factor kappa b and transcription of human immunodeficiency virus. Proc Natl Acad Sci U S A. 1990;87:9943–7.

Stewart MS, Spallholz JE, Neldner KH, Pence BC. Selenium compounds have disparate abilities to impose oxidative stress and induce apoptosis. Free Radic Biol Med. 1999;26:42–8.

Stoedter M, Renko K, Hog A, Schomburg L. Selenium controls the sex-specific immune response and selenoprotein expression during the acute-phase response in mice. Biochem J. 2010;429:43–51.

Tan HY, Wang N, Li S, Hong M, Wang X, Feng Y. The reactive oxygen species in macrophage polarization: reflecting its dual role in progression and treatment of human diseases. Oxidative Med Cell Longev. 2016;2016:2795090.

Tsuji PA, Carlson BA, Anderson CB, Seifried HE, Hatfield DL, Howard MT. Dietary selenium levels affect selenoprotein expression and support the interferon-gamma and il-6 immune response pathways in mice. Nutrients. 2015;7:6529–49.

Verma S, Hoffmann FW, Kumar M, Huang Z, Roe K, Nguyen-Wu E, Hashimoto AS, Hoffmann PR. Selenoprotein k knockout mice exhibit deficient calcium flux in immune cells and impaired immune responses. J Immunol. 2011;186:2127–37.

Vunta H, Davis F, Palempalli UD, Bhat D, Arner RJ, Thompson JT, Peterson DG, Reddy CC, Prabhu KS. The anti-inflammatory effects of selenium are mediated through 15-deoxy-delta12,14-prostaglandin j2 in macrophages. J Biol Chem. 2007;282:17964–73.

Weitzel F, Wendel A. Selenoenzymes regulate the activity of leukocyte 5-lipoxygenase via the peroxide tone. J Biol Chem. 1993;268:6288–92.

Won HY, Sohn JH, Min HJ, Lee K, Woo HA, Ho YS, Park JW, Rhee SG, Hwang ES. Glutathione peroxidase 1 deficiency attenuates allergen-induced airway inflammation by suppressing th2 and th17 cell development. Antioxid Redox Signal. 2010;13:575–87.

Yu MK, Moos PJ, Cassidy P, Wade M, Fitzpatrick FA. Conditional expression of 15-lipoxygenase-1 inhibits the selenoenzyme thioredoxin reductase: modulation of selenoproteins by lipoxygenase enzymes. J Biol Chem. 2004;279:28028–35.

Zamamiri-Davis F, Lu Y, Thompson JT, Prabhu KS, Reddy PV, Sordillo LM, Reddy CC. Nuclear factor-kappab mediates over-expression of cyclooxygenase-2 during activation of raw 264.7 macrophages in selenium deficiency. Free Radic Biol Med. 2002;32:890–7.

Zhang Q, Lenardo MJ, Baltimore D. 30 years of nf-kappab: a blossoming of relevance to human pathobiology. Cell. 2017;168:37–57.

Zhu C, Ling Q, Cai Z, Wang Y, Zhang Y, Hoffmann PR, Zheng W, Zhou T, Huang Z. Selenium-containing phycocyanin from se-enriched spirulina platensis reduces inflammation in dextran sulfate sodium-induced colitis by inhibiting nf-kappab activation. J Agric Food Chem. 2016;64:5060–70.

Chapter 8
Selenium and Thyroid Function

Mara Ventura, Miguel Melo, and Francisco Carrilho

Abstract Selenium is an essential trace element embedded in several proteins. Most of the known selenoproteins are found in the thyroid gland and this is the organ with the highest amount of selenium per gram of tissue. Selenium levels in the body depend on the characteristics of the population and its diet, geographic area, and soil composition. In the thyroid, selenium is required for protection from oxidative damage and for the metabolism of thyroid hormones. The literature suggests that selenium intake is associated with autoimmune thyroid disorders and selenium supplementation in those patients is associated with a reduction in antithyroid antibody levels, improved thyroid ultrasound features, and improved quality of life. Selenium supplementation in Graves' ophthalmopathy is associated with an improved quality of life, less eye involvement, and delayed orbitopathy progression. Supplementation with the organic form is more effective, and benefits in immunological mechanisms have been observed in patients with autoimmune thyroiditis.

Keywords Selenium · Thyroid dysfunction · Selenoproteins · Autoimmune thyroid disease · Hashimoto thyroiditis · Graves' disease · Graves' orbitopathy

M. Ventura · F. Carrilho
Department of Endocrinology, Diabetes and Metabolism, Centro Hospitalar e Universitário de Coimbra, Coimbra, Portugal

M. Melo (✉)
Department of Endocrinology, Diabetes and Metabolism, Centro Hospitalar e Universitário de Coimbra, Coimbra, Portugal

Faculty of Medicine, University of Coimbra, Coimbra, Portugal

Instituto de Investigação e Inovação em Saúde (I3S), Porto, Portugal

Institute of Pathology and Immunology of the University of Porto, Porto, Portugal

Introduction

Selenium is a micronutrient first described in 1817 by the physician Jons Jacob Berzelius (Duntas and Benvenga 2015). Selenium levels in the body are dependent on the population's characteristics and its diet and geographical area (mainly on the soil composition): while soils of central Asian regions and most European countries are generally poor in selenium, no such deficiencies are observed in other parts of the world (Schomburg and Kohrle 2008). This micronutrient has been studied over the last years, and scientific reports have revealed its crucial role in the maintenance of immune-endocrine function, metabolism, and cellular homeostasis. The thyroid gland has the highest selenium concentration of all tissues, incorporated into selenoproteins (Rayman 2012). Some of these selenoproteins have an important antioxidant activity, contributing to the antioxidant defense in the thyroid by removing oxygen free radicals generated during the production of thyroid hormones. Being incorporated into iodothyronine deiodinases, selenium plays also an essential role in the metabolism of thyroid hormones.

Selenium Intake, Availability, and Metabolism

Selenium can be available both in organic compounds (selenomethionine and selenocysteine) and in inorganic compounds (selenite and selenate) (Duntas and Benvenga 2015). The organic form seems to be more efficiently absorbed in the small intestine and, as so, is the formulation preferred for supplementation or treatment (Thiry et al. 2013). Selenomethionine is found in vegetable sources (especially cereals), selenium yeast, and other selenium supplements (Duntas and Benvenga 2015). Selenium is incorporated into body proteins in place of methionine; therefore, supplements containing selenomethionine have more bioavailable selenium. In turn, selenocysteine, a selenium analogue of the amino acid cysteine, is found essentially in animal foods. The inorganic forms (selenate and selenite) are the components of dietary supplements and are present only in small quantities in foodstuffs.

Even though the daily intake of selenium in a lot of countries does not reach the recommended levels, the opposite spectrum—excess of selenium in the body with toxic effects—can also occur in rare occasions. Selenium toxicity, known as selenosis, generally arises when this micronutrient's concentrations exceed 400 µg per day, and can be acute or chronic (Goyens et al. 1987). This rare situation was mainly reported by epidemiological studies in populations living in areas with high selenium concentration in the soil and can result from acute poisoning or prolonged exposure to high levels of selenium (Agency for Toxic Substances and Disease Registry (ATSDR) 2003). Selenium toxicity symptoms include nausea, vomiting, abdominal pain, diarrhea, fatigue, arthralgia, hair loss, discoloration or brittleness of the nails, peripheral neuropathy, and the characteristic smell of garlic in sweat and breath. Nail changes are the most common sign of chronic selenium poisoning and the absence of characteristic nail changes suggests the lack of chronic poisoning (Dharmasena 2014).

Selenium Homeostasis and the Thyroid Gland

The first clinical data establishing a link between selenium and thyroid function were collected in Zaire (Democratic Republic of the Congo) because of myxedematous endemic cretinism, a condition characterized by a deficit of iodine and selenium, hypothyroidism, myxedema, developmental problems, and intellectual disability (Goyens et al. 1987). From that moment, more studies were performed to investigate the role of this micronutrient in the thyroid. In fact, it was found that selenium deficiency decreases the synthesis of thyroid hormones, as it decreases the function of selenoproteins, in particular iodothyronine deiodinases (DIOs) that convert T4 to T3. This decreased production of thyroid hormones leads to the stimulation of the hypothalamic-pituitary axis, increasing TSH production which in turn stimulates the DIOs to convert T4–T3 (Kohrle 1990). This results in hydrogen peroxide production that accumulates in thyroid parenchyma, as it is not adequately removed by less active glutathione peroxidases (GPX), and causes thyrocyte damage with subsequent fibrosis.

The Selenoproteins

The thyroid gland is characterized by a high tissue concentration of selenium (0.2–2 µg/g), being the organ with the highest amount of selenium per gram of tissue, because it contains most of the selenoproteins (Duntas and Benvenga 2015; Dickson and Tomlinson 1967). Selenoproteins are a group of proteins coded by the triplet UGA that is a stop codon. Dietary intake of selenium may modify the readout of the genetic code, affecting the synthesis and expression of selenoproteins (Duntas and Benvenga 2015). Selenium, being incorporated into selenoproteins, contributes to the antioxidant defense in the thyroid, by removing oxygen free radicals generated during the production of thyroid hormones (Schomburg 2011; Saranac et al. 2011). Being incorporated into iodothyronine deiodinases, selenium plays also an essential role in the metabolism of thyroid hormones (Duntas and Benvenga 2015). So far, about 25 selenoproteins were described (Dharmasena 2014). Selenoproteins with a major role in thyroid homeostasis are presented in Table 8.1.

The main selenoproteins that affect thyroid function are glutathione peroxidases (GPXs), thioredoxin reductases (TXNRDs), and iodothyronine deiodinases (DIOs) (Santos et al. 2014). Glutathione peroxidases are responsible for glandular protection, as they remove the excess of oxygen free radicals produced during thyroid hormone synthesis (Negro 2008). TXNRDs sustain the oxidation-reduction systems

Table 8.1 Main groups of selenoproteins found in the thyroid gland and their function (Duntas and Benvenga 2015; Rayman 2012; Ventura et al. 2017)

Iodothyronine deiodinase	DIO	Production of active thyroid hormone T3, reverse T3 (rT3) and T2
Type I DIO	DIO1	Conversion of T4 to T3
Type II DIO	DIO2	Local production (intracellular) of T3 from T4
Type III DIO	DIO3	Production of rT3 from T4, and T2 from T3
Glutathione peroxidase	GPX	Catalyzes the reduction of H_2O_2 and protects against oxidative stress
Cytosolic GPX 1	GPX1	Antioxidative defense
Gastrointestinal GPX 2	GPX2	Antiapoptotic function in colon crypts; maintenance of intestinal mucosal integrity
Extracellular GPX 3	GPX3	Antioxidant in extracellular fluid; thyroid protection from hydrogen peroxide in thyrocytes and follicular lumen
Phospholipid GPX 4	GPX4	Reduces the phospholipid hydroperoxides; regulates apoptosis
Thioredoxin reductase	TXNRD	Oxidoreductase activity having NADPH as a cofactor
TXNRD cytosolic	TXNRD1	Main antioxidant at the cellular level
TXNRD mitochondrial	TXNRD2	Regulates cell proliferation

within the body and regulate some transcription and cell growth factors. The DIOs control the thyroid hormone turnover and catalyze the conversion of T4 to its biologically active form, T3, through the removal of an iodine atom from the external ring (Kohrle et al. 2005) and inactivate thyroid hormones through the conversion of T4 to reverse T3 (rT3) by the removal of an iodine atom of the inner ring. Selenoprotein P is the source of more than 50% of plasmatic selenium and, therefore, it constitutes the main transporter and distributor of this micronutrient, being able to carry between 10 and 17 selenocysteine moieties (Schweizer et al. 2005). It is produced by hepatocytes and has an essential role in selenium homeostasis, since it ensures selenium retention in the body and promotes its distribution to the liver and extrahepatic tissues, including its transportation to the brain in conditions associated with nutrient deficit (Hill et al. 2012). There seems to exist a hierarchy among different selenoproteins with respect to selenium supply and resynthesis in the case of selenium deprivation: DIO1 is preferentially supplied, allowing conversion of T4 to its biologically active hormone T3 even in deprivation situations, but other selenoproteins, like GPX1, are dependent on high selenium supply (Schomburg et al. 2006). A second hierarchy is observed respecting selenium concentration in different tissues when there is selenium deficiency: endocrine organs and the brain are preferentially supplied whereas serum, liver, kidney, and muscles readily lose their selenium stores (Schomburg et al. 2006). These features seem to demonstrate that a moderate to transient selenium deficiency caused by insufficient nutritional supply or impaired uptake dose not result in adverse health effects. The thyroid gland may be able to accumulate, retain, and recycle selenium efficiently, even in the absence of selenoprotein P (Schomburg et al. 2006). Even though thyroid is one of the endocrine organs preferentially supplied, selenium deficiency impairs thyroid hormone metabolism essentially because the antioxidant thyroid defense is compromised, and thyroid metabolism is disturbed within the thyroid gland and systemically (Schomburg et al. 2006).

Selenium and Thyroid Disease

Selenium and Autoimmune Thyroiditis

Selenium deficiency has proved an impact on humoral and cellular aspects of the immune system (Duntas and Benvenga 2015). Several studies have focused on the importance of selenium in thyroid function and autoimmune processes, aiming at understanding if supplementation of organic and inorganic selenium compounds may have an impact on the evolution of thyroid disease (Table 8.2).

In fact, the effect of selenium supplementation on the evolution of Hashimoto's thyroiditis, a condition characterized by the presence of antithyroperoxidase and antithyroglobulin antibodies (TPOAb and TgAb, respectively), has been addressed in several publications. Gärtner et al. (2002) conducted a study that evaluated the effect of supplementing diet with 200 µg sodium selenite per day during 90 days on the level of TPOAb and TgAb in patients with autoimmune thyroiditis; 70 patients with autoimmune thyroiditis under therapy with levothyroxine and with high levels of TPOAb and/or TgAb were evaluated. Patients were divided into two groups: one group that was supplemented with sodium selenite and the other group that just kept therapy with levothyroxine. At the end of the study, the concentration of TPOAb decreased by 36% in the group treated with selenium (*versus* 12% in the placebo group) and in 9 of 36 patients (25%), TPOAb completely normalized; during this period, thyroid echogenicity also improved. In this trial, patients receiving selenium supplementation reported better well-being compared with the placebo group. Forty-seven patients from the initial 70 patients agreed to continue the follow-up for 6 more months (Gärtner and Gasnier 2003) and those who were continuously supplemented with 200 µg/day of sodium selenite demonstrated a final 44% statistically significant reduction on TPOAb concentrations ($p = 0.004$). The group of patients who discontinued supplementation presented a subsequent increase in TPOAb and those who started 200 µg/day of sodium selenite supplementation demonstrated a 46% decrease in TPOAb after 6 months of follow-up. On the other hand, Duntas et al. (2003) conducted a randomized placebo-controlled prospective study including 65 patients with autoimmune thyroiditis, aged between 22 and 61 years old, that were under treatment with levothyroxine and were divided into two groups: one group received 200 µg selenomethionine per day and the other received placebo. The aim of this study was to assess the effects of selenium treatment on patients with autoimmune thyroiditis through the impact on the level of TPOAb and TgAb after 3 and 6 months. In the group supplemented with selenomethionine, the

Table 8.2 Randomized clinical trials on the effect of selenium supplementation on antithyroperoxidase antibody (TPOAb) concentration

Ref.	Patients	Daily supplementation	On levothyroxine treatment at baseline	Follow-up	TPOAb	Country
Karanikas et al. (2008)	36 adults	200 µg Sodium selenite	Yes	3 months	No effect	Austria
Bonfig et al. (2010)	49 children	200 µg Sodium selenite	Yes	1 year	No effect	Germany
Eskes et al. (2014)	61 adults	200 µg Sodium selenite	No	6 months	No effect	The Netherlands
Gärtner et al. (2002, Gärtner and Gasnier (2003)	70 adults	200 µg Sodium selenite	Yes	3 and 6 months	Reduction of 36% and 44%, respectively	Germany
Nacamulli et al. (2010)	76 adults	80 µg Sodium selenite	No	1 year	Reduction of 30%	Italy
Negro et al. (2007)	77 pregnant women, TPOAb +	200 µg Selenomethionine during pregnancy and postpartum	Yes (19%)	1 year	Reduction of 62% (pregnancy) and 48% (postpartum)	Italy
Mao et al. (2016)	230 pregnant women, 25 TPOAb+	60 µg Selenium-yeast per day	No	35 weeks	No effect	UK
Duntas et al. (2003)	65 adults	200 µg Selenomethionine	Yes	6 months	Reduction of 56%	Greece
Mazokopakis et al. (2007)	80 adults	200 µg Selenomethionine	Yes (33/80)	6 months	Reduction of 11%	Greece
Turker et al. (2006)	88 adults	200 µg Selenomethionine	Yes	3 months	Reduction of 26%	Turkey
Esposito et al. (2017)	76	166 µg Selenomethionine	No	6 months	No effect	Italy

level of TPOAb decreased by 46% at 3 months and 56% at 6 months, compared to a decrease of only 21% and 27%, respectively, at 3 and 6 months, in the group under single therapy with thyroxine. Nevertheless, there was no statistically significant difference in the level of TPOAb or in the concentration of TSH, free T4, and T3 between the two groups (Duntas et al. 2003). Mazokopakis et al. (2007) conducted a prospective study including 80 women with known autoimmune thyroiditis, 41% under levothyroxine therapy, followed for 1 year and aimed to evaluate the effects of 200 µg/day selenomethionine supplementation on TPOAb levels. An 11% reduction of TPOAb levels after 6 months of selenium supplementation was observed. After the first 6 months, the group was divided: 40 patients continued selenium for 6 more months and the remaining patients stopped this treatment. In the first group, an overall 21% reduction of TPOAb was observed after 12 months of supplementation (by 13% during the first 6-month period and by 8% during the second 6-month period). On the other hand, cessation of selenium supplementation at 6 months resulted in a 4.8% increase on TPOAb levels. Turker et al. (2006) evaluated the effects of long-term (9 months) treatment with variable doses of selenomethionine (100/200 µg per day) on autoimmune thyroiditis, particularly on the concentration of TPOAb and TgAb. Eighty-eight female patients with autoimmune thyroiditis under therapy with thyroxine were randomized into two groups according to their age and initial TSH and TPOAb serum levels and followed for 9 months: 48 patients received 200 µg selenomethionine per day and the remaining 40 patients received placebo. After the first 3 months, the first group was divided: 20 patients received 200 µg selenomethionine per day over 6 more months and the other 20 patients received 100 µg selenomethionine per day for 3 months. Twelve patients from the last group continued the study until 9 months and received 200 µg selenomethionine per day. After the first 3 months of selenium supplementation, a 26.2% decrease on TPOAb levels was observed. In the group that continued selenium supplementation for 9 months, a decrease in serum levels of TPOAb until 6 months of treatment was observed, after which the values tended to level off (23.7% at 6 months, and 3.6% at 9 months). As so, it seems that the suppression rate decreases with time. In the group in which selenium dosage was reduced to 100 µg per day a 38% increase on TPOAb levels was observed, suggesting an inefficacy of the low dose. However, this same group of patients received again supplementation with 200 µg selenomethionine per day for 3 more months and a 30% reduction of TPOAb levels was observed. The authors concluded that replacement with selenomethionine suppresses serum concentrations of TPOAb, but the suppression required doses greater than 100 µg/day to maximize glutathione peroxidase activity. Thereby, the authors demonstrated that the oral administration of 200 µg/day of selenomethionine reduces effectively serum levels of TPOAb. Nacamulli et al. (2010) conducted a prospective study involving 76 patients with autoimmune thyroiditis with normal or slightly elevated TSH levels and normal free T4 levels, which were not under levothyroxine treatment, and aimed to investigate whether physiological doses of selenium influence the natural course of autoimmune thyroiditis. Forty-six patients received supplementation with physiological doses of selenium (80 µg/day of sodium selenite) for 12 months, and a reduction of the thyroid echogenicity and

TPOAb and TgAb levels was observed, without affecting significantly the concentration of TSH or T4 (Mazokopakis et al. 2007). Esposito et al. (2017) performed a randomized placebo-controlled prospective study with 76 euthyroid untreated patients with autoimmune thyroiditis: 38 patients received 166 μg/day selenomethionine and the remaining 38 patients received placebo during 6 months. The authors aimed to evaluate the short-term effect of selenium supplementation on the thyroid function (evaluated through the level of TSH, thyroid hormones, thyroid peroxidase antibodies, thyroglobulin antibodies, and thyroid echogenicity). The authors also measure CXCL10 levels to evaluate the possibility of a modulation of the autoimmune mechanism by selenomethionine. After 6 months of study, the authors concluded that TSH, the levels of thyroid hormones and TPOAb, thyroid echogenicity, and CXCL10 concentration did not show a statistically significant difference between the control and the supplemented group. In fact, they observed an increase in FT3 levels after 3 and 6 months and a decrease in FT4 levels after 3 months in the group supplemented with selenium compared to baseline levels; in the placebo group, the authors observed a decrease in FT3 after 3 and 6 months when compared to baseline.

Selenium and Autoimmune Thyroiditis in Pregnancy

Several studies demonstrate that pregnant women with positive TPOAb are prone to develop postpartum thyroid dysfunction and permanent hypothyroidism (Negro et al. 2007). In pregnancy, supplementation of selenium appears to influence thyroid function and may be beneficial. Mao et al. (2016) conducted a double-blind, randomized, placebo-controlled study that enrolled 230 pregnant women without known autoimmune thyroid disease and aimed to evaluate the effect of 60 μg/day selenium-yeast supplementation or placebo yeast on TPOAb levels. At baseline, 25 (11%) women were TPOAb positive. The authors concluded that selenium supplementation was not associated with an additional benefit on TPOAb compared to placebo, though it tended to affect thyroid function in this group of patients. In fact, in TPOAb-positive women supplemented with selenium, free T4 levels (FT4) fell with more extent in the selenium group. Negro et al. (2007) recruited 2143 pregnant women with autoimmune thyroiditis in euthyroidism without levothyroxine therapy and evaluated whether selenium supplementation, during and after pregnancy, influenced thyroid function. Of the 2143 women selected, 169 were positive for thyroid peroxidase antibodies (TPOAb+) and were randomly divided into two groups: 77 pregnant women received 200 μg/day selenomethionine and 74 received placebo. Either selenomethionine or placebo was started after 12 weeks of gestation. The two groups had similar TSH levels at baseline and 19.4% of patients in the group on selenomethionine started levothyroxine therapy during the follow-up *versus* 21.6% of patients on placebo, because they have either low free T4 levels or high TSH values. The authors found that, in the group supplemented with 200 μg/day of selenomethionine during pregnancy and postpartum, a decrease in the progression of autoimmune thyroiditis was observed. During pregnancy, the group supplemented with selenomethionine presented a greater reduction in TPOAb levels compared to those receiving placebo (62.4% *vs.* 43.9%, *p* < 0.01) and improved thyroid echogenicity. The first group also demonstrated decreased incidence of thyroid dysfunction in the postpartum period, and decreased permanent hypothyroidism (Esposito et al. 2017). It must be noted that the number of women with positive TPOAb in Negro et al. study (2007) is higher compared to Mao et al. study (2016) (151 *vs.* 25 patients), which increases the chance of finding an effect, and in the latter study the selenium dosage given was lower than the selenium dose given in the first study, which may also had affected the results.

Even though it is known that selenium supplementation may benefit people with proved low status and that people with adequate or high status could be adversely affected (Rayman 2012), in most of these studies the authors did not measure selenium concentration prior to, during, or after supplementation. Furthermore, the most frequent primary outcome measurement was thyroid antibody levels, so at the moment, there is no recommendation for selenium supplementation in patients with autoimmune thyroiditis.

Currently, some clinical trials are being performed and may provide some answers to these still open questions. The CATALYST trial ("The chronic autoimmune thyroiditis quality of life selenium trial") is an ongoing investigator-initiated randomized, blinded, multicenter clinical trial that enrolled 472 patients with autoimmune thyroiditis treated with levothyroxine (LT4). Their primary outcome is thyroid-related quality of life, evaluating the effect of 200 μg selenium-enriched yeast *versus* placebo supplementation during 12 months. Secondary objectives are to evaluate the effect of selenium supplementation *versus* placebo on TPOAb concentration, LT4 dosage, serum T3/T4 ratio, plasma selenium concentration, and immunological and oxidative stress biomarkers. In this trial, unlike other studies about this issue, plasma selenium concentrations will be measured periodically to assess selenium intake. This is also the first study that will evaluate selenium's mechanisms of action in autoimmune thyroiditis and the effect of selenium supplementation on LT4 dosage. According to the study protocol, this trial is scheduled to finish in 2018 (Winther et al. 2014).

Selenium, Thyroid Volume, and Thyroid Nodules

Other studies have also evaluated the connection between thyroid volume and selenium concentration (Rasmussen et al. 2011; Derumeaux et al. 2003; Wu et al. 2015).

Many of them were small studies and operator dependent, but they seem to suggest that there is an inverse relationship between the concentration of selenium in the plasma or urine and the thyroid volume or its hypoechogenicity. Rasmussen et al. (2011) conducted a cross-sectional study in Denmark including 805 patients and aimed to evaluate the association between serum selenium concentration and thyroid volume and risk for thyroid enlargement in an area with mild iodine deficiency, before and after iodine supplementation was introduced. In the 654 woman included, low serum selenium concentration was associated with a larger thyroid volume, a higher risk for enlarged thyroid gland, and with development of thyroid nodules. On the other hand, in the 151 men included, there was no association between thyroid volume and serum selenium concentration. Derumeaux et al. (2003) conducted a cross-sectional study including 1900 participants to investigate the relationship between selenium status and thyroid volume and echostructure. They founded that selenium status and thyroid volume were inversely associated in women and observed a protective effect of selenium against goiter and thyroid tissue damage. Regarding the sample size, one of the most impressive epidemiological studies in this area was conducted by Wu et al. (2015). This is a cross-sectional observational study, including 6152 participants selected by stratified cluster sampling: 3038 were defined as adequate-selenium county participants and 3114 were defined as low-selenium county, with a median difference in the selenium concentration between the groups of almost twofold. The authors aimed at evaluating if the prevalence of thyroid disease differed in two areas of China that were similar except for very different soil/crop selenium concentrations. Participants completed demographic and dietary questionnaires and underwent ultrasound thyroid evaluation and serum samples were obtained to assess selenium status and thyroid function. The authors concluded that the prevalence of thyroid diseases (hypothyroidism, subclinical hypothyroidism, autoimmune thyroiditis, and an enlarged thyroid) was significantly lower in the adequate-selenium county than in the low-selenium county.

Most of the studies about this issue seem to demonstrate that selenium deficiency is associated with higher prevalence of thyroid disease; however, further data are needed to assess if selenium can be protective against multinodular goiter and autoimmune thyroiditis.

Selenium and Graves' Disease

Scientific evidence demonstrated that oxidative stress plays a major role on Graves' disease (Vrca et al. 2004). Studies about the effect of antioxidants in the treatment of Graves' disease are scarce. Vrca et al. (2004) performed an investigation including 57 patients with newly diagnosed Graves' disease, treated with methimazole, and aimed to determine the effect of supplementation with a fixed combination of antioxidants (vitamins C and E, beta-carotene, and selenium) on the speed of attaining euthyroidism. This study was conducted in Croatia, a country where nutritional Se levels are among the lowest in Europe. The patients were randomized into two groups: 29 received a daily capsule of a fixed combination of pharmacological antioxidants (6 mg beta-carotene, 200 mg vitamin C, 36 mg vitamin E, and 60 μg selenium) and the remaining 28 patients took only methimazole in the same dosage as the first group. The results of this study showed that patients who received supplementation with antioxidants in addition to therapy with methimazole attained euthyroidism faster than the group treated with methimazole only. Another study by Wang et al. (2016) enrolled 41 patients with recurrent Graves' disease under treatment with methimazole. The authors aimed to evaluate the efficacy of selenium supplementation therapy on recurrent Graves' disease. Twenty-one patients received additional selenium supplementation for 6 months. The authors founded that, at 2 months of supplementation, both FT4 and FT3 decreased more and TSH level increased more in the selenium group than in the control group. The TSH receptor antibodies' (TRAb) level was significantly lower in the selenium group and the proportion of patients with normal TRAb level at the final follow-up visit was also significantly higher in the selenium group. This study suggests that antioxidants administered together with antithyroid drugs may lead to a faster control of clinical manifestations and a faster normalization of thyroid function. Another randomized clinical trial by Leo et al. (2017) including 30 newly diagnosed hyperthyroid Graves' disease patients assigned to treatment with methimazole or methimazole and selenium was performed to assess the impact of selenium on clinical and biochemical control of hyperthyroidism at 90 days. This study was performed in a selenium-sufficient population and failed to show an adjuvant role of selenium in the short-term control of hyperthyroidism. Recently, Kahaly et al. (2017) performed a double-blind, placebo-controlled, randomized, prospective clinical trial including 70 untreated hyperthyroid patients with Graves' disease and aimed to assess the safety and efficacy of adding-on selenium to medical treatment on clinical course, serological parameters, and response and recurrence rates of Graves' disease. All patients received methimazole at the beginning of the study and were randomized in a two-harm design: 35 patients received sodium-selenite 300 µg/day and 35 patients received placebo for 24 weeks. The authors concluded that selenium supplementation in the form of sodium-selenite showed no obvious advantage to methimazole therapy alone in terms of response rate, decreased serum thyroid antibodies, and relapse rate. Adverse events occurred in both groups and were partly disease related.

Another prospective study was performed in Scandinavia (Calissendorff et al. 2015) and included 38 patients with initially untreated Graves' disease thyrotoxicosis that started receiving block and replace therapy with methimazole and levothyroxine and were then randomized to receive either 200 µg selenized-yeast per day or placebo. The objective was to investigate if selenium supplementation for 36 weeks could change the immune mechanisms, hormone levels, and/or depression and anxiety. The authors concluded that FT4 decreased more and TSH increased more in the selenium-treated group. Regarding symptom ratings, depression, or anxiety, no differences were found between the two groups.

These contradictory results between studies may have several explanations. First, we think that a direct comparison of the results of the different studies cannot be made because of the differences in the selenium compound used, its dosage, and time of supplementation chosen. To add to this, baseline selenium status of the patients was only evaluated in a few studies, and selenium supplementation may have different effects depending upon the baseline status of the patients.

The ongoing GRASS trial (GRAves' disease Selenium Supplementation trial) (Watt et al. 2013) is an investigator-initiated, randomized, blinded, multicenter clinical trial including 492 patients with Graves' hyperthyroidism, treated with antithyroid drugs, which were randomized to receive 200 µg daily of selenium-enriched yeast over the 24–30 months' intervention period or placebo. The aim of this trial is to investigate if selenium addition to antithyroid drugs will lead to a decrease in antithyroid drug treatment failures, faster remission of the disease, and improved quality of life. The GRASS and CATALYST trials are being performed by the same group of investigators and both expected to be completed in 2018.

Selenium and Graves' Orbitopathy

Graves' orbitopathy is a potentially sight-threatening ocular disease with a close clinical relationship with hyperthyroidism, suggesting a single underlying systemic process with variable expression in different organs. In fact, the characteristic Graves' disease oxidative stress and the increased generation of oxygen free radicals might play a role in the pathogenesis of Graves's ophthalmopathy (Marcocci et al. 2011). Nearly half of the patients with Graves' disease have symptoms of Graves' orbitopathy, which include upper eyelid retraction, edema, proptosis, and erythema of the periorbital tissues and conjunctivae, the most common clinical feature, and dry and gritty ocular sensation, photophobia, excessive tearing, double vision, and a pressure sensation behind the eyes (Bahn 2010). In this regard, the importance of selenium supplementation in patients with Graves' orbitopathy has been under investigation. Marcocci et al. (2011) carried out a randomized, double-blind, placebo-controlled trial to determine the effect of selenium or pentoxifylline in 152 patients with mild Graves' orbitopathy. The patients were given sodium selenite 100 μg twice daily, pentoxifylline 600 mg twice daily, or placebo twice daily for 6 months. After this 6-month period, the treatment was withdrawn and the patients were followed for 6 more months. The authors aimed to evaluate if selenium supplementation has any impact on overall ophthalmic assessment and quality of life. They found that treatment with selenium, but not with pentoxifylline, was associated with improved quality of life, less eye involvement, and delayed progression of Graves' orbitopathy at 6 months. After 6 months without selenium, pentoxifylline, or placebo supplementation, patients were reassessed and the results obtained in the first assessment were confirmed. Indeed, a recommendation for selenium supplementation in mild orbitopathy cases was incorporated into the recent guidelines from the European Group On Graves' Orbitopathy (EUGOGO) (Bartalena et al. 2016). In order to clarify the cellular mechanisms by which selenium may act, Dottore et al. (2017) performed a study including six patients with Graves' orbitopathy and six controls, from which they collected and established primary orbital fibroblast culture. Cells were treated with hydrogen peroxide (H_2O_2) to induce oxidative stress, after preincubation with selenium in the form of selenocysteine. The authors founded that incubation of H_2O_2-treated fibroblasts with selenocysteine was followed by an increase in glutathione-peroxidase activity and a blockade of the increase in TNFα and IFNγ, two endogenous cytokines involved in response to oxidative stress and Graves' orbitopathy pathogenesis. This effect of selenium was observed both in fibroblasts from Graves' orbitopathy patients and control group, suggesting that fibroblasts are susceptible to oxidative stress and to protection by selenocysteine regardless of the underlying conditions and/or of their genetic background.

These studies show that selenium supplementation may be clinically relevant in patients with Graves' orbitopathy, notably in the mild forms. Furthermore, selenium seems to have a direct action in orbital fibroblasts, presumably the major target of the immune system in Graves' orbitopathy.

Selenium and Thyroid Cancer

The overproduction of free radicals and the consequent increase in oxidative stress leading to irreversible cellular damage may drive genomic instability events and somatic mutations that are associated with cancer pathophysiology (Metere et al. 2018; Young et al. 2010). Cells that regulate the redox status by balancing the generation of free radicals with their elimination by antioxidant systems are essential to prevent DNA damage, one of the earlier events on cancer pathogenesis. One of the studies showing the involvement of oxidative stress in thyroid cancer was performed by Metere et al. (2018); the authors evaluated 20 samples of healthy thyroid tissue and thyroid tumor collected for analysis after total thyroidectomy, and analyzed the expression of two selenium antioxidant molecules, glutathione peroxidase and thioredoxin reductase, in thyroid cancer cells. They found a decreased expression of glutathione peroxidase and thioredoxin reductase in thyroid cancer cells compared to healthy cells; they also found an increase of free radicals in tumor tissue, whose concentrations were significantly higher than the ones found in healthy thyroid tissue. A wide array of minerals, vitamins, and minor compounds are involved in these antioxidant systems; selenoproteins seem to have a critical role in the balance of redox systems and several studies evaluated the relationship between selenium levels in serum, plasma, or urine and cancer (Patrick 2004). Overall, lower selenium levels have been associated with increased cancer diagnoses. Baltaci et al. (2017) aimed to examine the changes in the serum levels of trace elements, including selenium, before and after thyroidectomy in 30 thyroid cancer patients compared to 20 control patients. They found a significantly lower serum selenium level preoperatively and postoperatively in male and female thyroid cancer patients than in the control group patients. Concerning thyroid pathology, Shen et al. (2015) performed a meta-analysis comprising 8 articles and 1291 subjects, to clarify the association of selenium, copper, and magnesium levels with thyroid cancer. The authors concluded that thyroid cancer patients had lower serum selenium and magnesium levels and higher copper levels when compared with healthy controls. Jonklaas et al. (2013) performed a study with 65 euthyroid patients who were scheduled for thyroidectomy for thyroid cancer, suspicion of thyroid cancer, or nodular disease. The authors concluded that although selenium concentrations were not significantly lower in patients with thyroid cancer, serum selenium concentrations were inversely correlated with thyroid cancer stage. Although the specific mechanisms are not yet fully understood, it seems that the antioxidant properties of selenoenzymes are relevant in carcinogenesis and tumor progression. A few studies have examined the relationship between selenium and cancer metastasis and have evaluated the potential of selenium as an antiangiogenesis or anti-metastasis agent (Chen et al. 2013). Although further research needs to be performed specifically on thyroid cancer metastasis, selenium seems to affect cancer cell migration and invasion, inhibit angiogenesis, and promote vascular maturation. In the future, selenium may have a potential application in cancer metastasis prevention or treatment.

Conclusions

Selenium is an essential trace element. The maintenance of a physiological concentration of selenium (selenostasis) through a balanced diet or via supplementation is a prerequisite not only to prevent thyroid disease but also to maintain overall health. Selenium takes part in activation and deactivation of thyroid hormones and plays an important role in thyroid protection against oxidative damage. For that reason, the supplementation of this micronutrient in autoimmune thyroiditis patients with confirmed deficiency may be useful, although further studies are needed to clearly recommend this therapy. In Hashimoto thyroiditis, selenium supplementation seems to potentiate the activity of selenoproteins, thereby decreasing local inflammatory reactions, decreasing TPOAb, and improving thyroid parenchyma's morphology. In patients with Graves' disease, selenium treatment could help to promote euthyroidism, but its main clinical use at the present time is on mild-to-moderate Graves' orbitopathy, a situation in which selenium supplementation is recommended. Different formulations of selenium are available, and the organic formula (selenomethionine) seems to be preferable due to its increased bioavailability.

References

Agency for Toxic Substances and Disease Registry (ATSDR). Toxicologic profile for selenium. Atlanta, GA: US Department of Health and Human Services, Public Health Service; 2003.
Bahn RS. Graves' ophthalmopathy. N Engl J Med. 2010;362(8):726–38.
Baltaci AK, Dundar TK, Aksoy F, Mogulkoc R. Changes in the serum levels of trace elements before and after the operation in thyroid cancer patients. Biol Trace Elem Res. 2017;175(1):57–64.
Bartalena L, Baldeschi L, Boboridis K, Eckstein A, Kahaly GJ, Marcocci C, Perros P, Salvi M, Wiersinga WM. The European Thyroid Association/European Group on Graves' Orbitopathy Guidelines for the Management of Graves' Orbitopathy. Eur Thyroid J 2016. European Group on Graves O. 2016;5(1):9–26.
Bonfig W, Gartner R, Schmidt H. Selenium supplementation does not decrease thyroid peroxidase antibody concentration in children and adolescents with autoimmune thyroiditis. ScientificWorldJournal. 2010;10:990–6.
Calissendorff J, Mikulski E, Larsen EH, Moller M. A prospective investigation of Graves' disease and selenium (Se): thyroid hormones, auto-antibodies and self-rated symptoms. Eur Thyroid J. 2015;4(2):93–8.

Chen YC, Prabhu KS, Mastro AM. Is selenium a potential treatment for cancer metastasis? Nutrients. 2013;5(4):1149–68.

Derumeaux H, Valeix P, Castetbon K, Bensimon M, Boutron-Ruault MC, Arnaud J, Hercberg S. Association of selenium with thyroid volume and echostructure in 35- to 60-year-old French adults. Eur J Endocrinol. 2003;148(3):309–15.

Dharmasena A. Selenium supplementation in thyroid associated ophthalmopathy: an update. Int J Ophthalmol. 2014;7(2):365–75.

Dickson RC, Tomlinson RH. Selenium in blood and human tissues. Clin Chim Acta. 1967;16(2):311–21.

Duntas LH, Benvenga S. Selenium (Se): an element for life. Endocrine. 2015;48(3):756–75.

Duntas LH, Mantzou E, Koutras DA. Effects of a six month treatment with selenomethionine in patients with autoimmune thyroiditis. Eur J Endocrinol. 2003;148(4):389–93.

Eskes SA, Endert E, Fliers E, Birnie E, Hollenbach B, Schomburg L, Kohrle J, Wiersinga WM. Selenite supplementation in euthyroid subjects with thyroid peroxidase antibodies. Clin Endocrinol. 2014;80(3):444–51.

Esposito D, Rotondi M, Accardo G, Vallone G, Conzo G, Docimo G, Selvaggi F, Cappelli C, Chiovato L, Giugliano D, Pasquali D. Influence of short-term selenium supplementation on the natural course of Hashimoto's thyroiditis: clinical results of a blinded placebo-controlled randomized prospective trial. J Endocrinol Invest. 2017;40(1):83–9.

Gärtner R, Gasnier BC. Selenium in the treatment of autoimmune thyroiditis. Biofactors. 2003;19(3–4):165–70.

Gärtner R, Gasnier BC, Dietrich JW, Krebs B, Angstwurm MW. Selenium supplementation in patients with autoimmune thyroiditis decreases thyroid peroxidase antibodies concentrations. J Clin Endocrinol Metab. 2002;87(4):1687–91.

Goyens P, Golstein J, Nsombola B, Vis H, Dumont JE. Selenium deficiency as a possible factor in the pathogenesis of myxoedematous endemic cretinism. Acta Endocrinol. 1987;114(4):497–502.

Hill KE, Wu S, Motley AK, Stevenson TD, Winfrey VP, Capecchi MR, Atkins JF, Burk RF. Production of selenoprotein P (Sepp1) by hepatocytes is central to selenium homeostasis. J Biol Chem. 2012;287(48):40414–24.

Jonklaas J, Danielsen M, Wang H. A pilot study of serum selenium, vitamin D, and thyrotropin concentrations in patients with thyroid cancer. Thyroid. 2013;23(9):1079–86.

Kahaly GJ, Riedl M, Konig J, Diana T, Schomburg L. Double-blind, placebo-controlled, randomized trial of selenium in Graves hyperthyroidism. J Clin Endocrinol Metab. 2017;102(11):4333–41.

Karanikas G, Schuetz M, Kontur S, Duan H, Kommata S, Schoen R, Antoni A, Kletter K, Dudczak R, Willheim M. No immunological benefit of selenium in consecutive patients with autoimmune thyroiditis. Thyroid. 2008;18(1):7–12.

Kohrle J. Thyrotropin (TSH) action on thyroid hormone deiodination and secretion: one aspect of thyrotropin regulation of thyroid cell biology. Horm Metab Res Suppl. 1990;23:18–28.

Kohrle J, Jakob F, Contempre B, Dumont JE. Selenium, the thyroid, and the endocrine system. Endocr Rev. 2005;26(7):944–84.

Leo M, Bartalena L, Rotondo Dottore G, Piantanida E, Premoli P, Ionni I, Di Cera M, Masiello E, Sassi L, Tanda ML, et al. Effects of selenium on short-term control of hyperthyroidism due to Graves' disease treated with methimazole: results of a randomized clinical trial. J Endocrinol Invest. 2017;40(3):281–7.

Mao J, Pop VJ, Bath SC, Vader HL, Redman CW, Rayman MP. Effect of low-dose selenium on thyroid autoimmunity and thyroid function in UK pregnant women with mild-to-moderate iodine deficiency. Eur J Nutr. 2016;55(1):55–61.

Marcocci C, Kahaly GJ, Krassas GE, Bartalena L, Prummel M, Stahl M, Altea MA, Nardi M, Pitz S, Boboridis K, et al. Selenium and the course of mild Graves' orbitopathy. N Engl J Med. 2011;364(20):1920–31.

Mazokopakis EE, Papadakis JA, Papadomanolaki MG, Batistakis AG, Giannakopoulos TG, Protopapadakis EE, Ganotakis ES. Effects of 12 months treatment with L-selenomethionine on serum anti-TPO Levels in Patients with Hashimoto's thyroiditis. Thyroid. 2007;17(7):609–12.

Metere A, Frezzotti F, Graves CE, Vergine M, De Luca A, Pietraforte D, Giacomelli L. A possible role for selenoprotein glutathione peroxidase (GPx1) and thioredoxin reductases (TrxR1) in thyroid cancer: our experience in thyroid surgery. Cancer Cell Int. 2018;18:7.

Nacamulli D, Mian C, Petricca D, Lazzarotto F, Barollo S, Pozza D, Masiero S, Faggian D, Plebani M, Girelli ME, et al. Influence of physiological dietary selenium supplementation on the natural course of autoimmune thyroiditis. Clin Endocrinol. 2010;73(4):535–9.

Negro R. Selenium and thyroid autoimmunity. Biologics. 2008;2(2):265–73.

Negro R, Greco G, Mangieri T, Pezzarossa A, Dazzi D, Hassan H. The influence of selenium supplementation on postpartum thyroid status in pregnant women with thyroid peroxidase autoantibodies. J Clin Endocrinol Metab. 2007;92(4):1263–8.

Patrick L. Selenium biochemistry and cancer: a review of the literature. Altern Med Rev. 2004;9(3):239–58.

Rasmussen LB, Schomburg L, Kohrle J, Pedersen IB, Hollenbach B, Hog A, Ovesen L, Perrild H, Laurberg P. Selenium status, thyroid volume, and multiple nodule formation in an area with mild iodine deficiency. Eur J Endocrinol. 2011;164(4):585–90.

Rayman MP. Selenium and human health. Lancet. 2012;379(9822):1256–68.

Rotondo Dottore G, Leo M, Casini G, Latrofa F, Cestari L, Sellari-Franceschini S, Nardi M, Vitti P, Marcocci C, Marino M. Antioxidant actions of selenium in orbital fibroblasts: a basis for the effects of selenium in Graves' orbitopathy. Thyroid. 2017;27(2):271–8.

Santos LR, Duraes C, Mendes A, Prazeres H, Alvelos MI, Moreira CS, Canedo P, Esteves C, Neves C, Carvalho D, et al. A polymorphism in the promoter region of the selenoprotein S gene (SEPS1) contributes to Hashimoto's thyroiditis susceptibility. J Clin Endocrinol Metab. 2014;99(4):E719–23.

Saranac L, Zivanovic S, Bjelakovic B, Stamenkovic H, Novak M, Kamenov B. Why is the thyroid so prone to autoimmune disease? Horm Res Paediatr. 2011;75(3):157–65.

Schomburg L. Selenium, selenoproteins and the thyroid gland: interactions in health and disease. Nat Rev Endocrinol. 2011;8(3):160–71.

Schomburg L, Kohrle J. On the importance of selenium and iodine metabolism for thyroid hormone biosynthesis and human health. Mol Nutr Food Res. 2008;52(11):1235–46.

Schomburg L, Riese C, Michaelis M, Griebert E, Klein MO, Sapin R, Schweizer U, Kohrle J. Synthesis and metabolism of thyroid hormones is preferentially maintained in selenium-deficient transgenic mice. Endocrinology. 2006;147(3):1306–13.

Schweizer U, Streckfuss F, Pelt P, Carlson BA, Hatfield DL, Kohrle J, Schomburg L. Hepatically derived selenoprotein P is a key factor for kidney but not for brain selenium supply. Biochem J. 2005;386(Pt 2):221–6.

Shen F, Cai WS, Li JL, Feng Z, Cao J, Xu B. The association between serum levels of selenium, copper, and magnesium with thyroid cancer: a meta-analysis. Biol Trace Elem Res. 2015;167(2):225–35.

Thiry C, Ruttens A, Pussemier L, Schneider YJ. An in vitro investigation of species-dependent intestinal transport of selenium and the impact of this process on selenium bioavailability. Br J Nutr. 2013;109(12):2126–34.

Turker O, Kumanlioglu K, Karapolat I, Dogan I. Selenium treatment in autoimmune thyroiditis: 9-month follow-up with variable doses. J Endocrinol. 2006;190(1):151–6.

Ventura M, Melo M, Carrilho F. Selenium and thyroid disease: from pathophysiology to treatment. Int J Endocrinol. 2017;2017:1297658.

Vrca VB, Skreb F, Cepelak I, Romic Z, Mayer L. Supplementation with antioxidants in the treatment of Graves' disease; the effect on glutathione peroxidase activity and concentration of selenium. Clin Chim Acta. 2004;341(1–2):55–63.

Wang L, Wang B, Chen SR, Hou X, Wang XF, Zhao SH, Song JQ, Wang YG. Effect of selenium supplementation on recurrent hyperthyroidism caused by Graves' disease: a prospective pilot study. Horm Metab Res. 2016;48(9):559–64.

Watt T, Cramon P, Bjorner JB, Bonnema SJ, Feldt-Rasmussen U, Gluud C, Gram J, Hansen JL, Hegedus L, Knudsen N, et al. Selenium supplementation for patients with Graves' hyperthyroidism (the GRASS trial): study protocol for a randomized controlled trial. Trials. 2013;14:119.

Winther KH, Watt T, Bjorner JB, Cramon P, Feldt-Rasmussen U, Gluud C, Gram J, Groenvold M, Hegedus L, Knudsen N, et al. The chronic autoimmune thyroiditis quality of life selenium trial (CATALYST): study protocol for a randomized controlled trial. Trials. 2014;15:115.

Wu Q, Rayman MP, Lv H, Schomburg L, Cui B, Gao C, Chen P, Zhuang G, Zhang Z, Peng X, et al. Low population selenium status is associated with increased prevalence of thyroid disease. J Clin Endocrinol Metab. 2015;100(11):4037–47.

Young O, Crotty T, O'Connell R, O'Sullivan J, Curran AJ. Levels of oxidative damage and lipid peroxidation in thyroid neoplasia. Head Neck. 2010;32(6):750–6.

Part V
The Role of Selenium in Neurodevelopment and Neurological Disorders

Chapter 9
Selenium and Neurodevelopment

Noelia Fradejas-Villar and Ulrich Schweizer

Abstract Brain is a privileged organ regarding selenium accumulation and metabolism. The discovery of a neurological phenotype in selenoprotein P knockout mouse provided a new perspective on the function of selenoproteins in brain. Since then, genetic studies in mice have revealed that some selenoproteins are indispensable to normal brain function. Neurodegeneration of GABAergic interneurons (PV+ neurons and Purkinje cells in cerebellum) was observed in *Trsp* and *Secisbp2* knockout mice. *Gpx4* knockout mice showed a similar phenotype, which could indicate that Gpx4 is necessary for maintenance or development of GABAergic interneurons. Similarly, SelT has a protective role for dopaminergic neurons and Txnrd1 is involved in radial glia development.

Progress of genome sequencing methods allowed to uncover inborn errors in selenoproteins or their biosynthetic factors, which lead to developmental and degenerative diseases in humans. Thus, mutations in *SEPSECS* gene lead to pontocerebellar hypoplasia type 2D, a neurodegenerative disease. Sedaghatian disease is caused by *GPX4* mutations. Some of these patients show malformations of the central nervous system. A homozygous mutation in the *TXNRD1* causes generalized epilepsy. Hearing loss and impaired movement coordination were symptoms found in patients suffering from SECISBP2 syndrome.

This chapter highlights neurological diseases and phenotypes detected in mouse and patients with impaired selenoprotein expression in the brain. Similarities and differences between mouse models and human disease are discussed.

Keywords SelenoP · GABAergic interneurons · Sedaghatian · PCH2D

N. Fradejas-Villar · U. Schweizer (✉)
Institut für Biochemie und Molekularbiologie,
Rheinische Friedrich-Wilhelms-Universität Bonn, Bonn, Germany
e-mail: uschweiz@uni-bonn.de

177

Selenium Deficiency and Neurological Disorders

Selenium Levels in Brain

Selenium status differs among tissues and organs. In animals fed an adequate selenium diet, selenium levels in brain were significantly lower than in other organs. However, selenium status in brain was conserved even under selenium-deficient conditions. Animals fed with low-selenium diets maintained brain selenium levels at the expense of other organs, like liver and kidney, which were depleted of this micronutrient (Kuhbacher et al. 2009). Therefore, the brain is privileged regarding selenium accumulation and metabolism.

Human Brain Phenotypes Related to Low Selenium Level

Selenium protects the brain from oxidative stress through selenoproteins. This family of proteins contain selenium in the form of the amino acid selenocysteine (Sec). Several selenoproteins, which are involved in antioxidant defense, are expressed in brain. Three features render the brain vulnerable to oxidative stress: its high rate of oxygen consumption, the high content of polyunsaturated fatty acids which are susceptible to lipid peroxidation, and the high content of redox-active transition metals (Steinbrenner and Sies 2013). Many studies have determined the relationship between increased oxidative stress and brain diseases. Reduced plasma and brain selenium levels and deregulation of selenoprotein expression and activities have been observed in patients suffering from neurological disorders, including Alzheimer disease (AD), multiple sclerosis, Parkinson's disease (PD), brain ischemia, and epilepsy (de Wilde et al. 2017; Dominiak et al. 2016). However, available data on selenium status in patients of AD and PD are inconclusive. Besides, selenium supplementation clinical studies for the treatment and prevention of AD and PD are inconsistent (de Wilde et al. 2017; Dominiak et al. 2016). Selenium supplementation has been effective in the treatment of intractable seizures associated with low selenium status (Ramaekers et al. 1994).

In the same way, two human diseases have been associated with selenium deficiency, which can be alleviated by selenium supplementation. These are Keshan disease and Kashin-Beck disease. They are endemic in geographic areas low in soil selenium. In both cases, affected individuals do not show any brain phenotype (Wrobel et al. 2016). This fact could be an indication that brain selenium levels are maintained even under selenium-deficient conditions. Patients with myxedematous endemic cretinism present mental retardation (Wrobel et al. 2016). Despite its relation to low selenium levels, it is believed to depend on thyroid hormone deficiency caused by concomitant deficiency of iodine (Vanderpas et al. 1990).

Three studies conducted with elder people associated low selenium levels with decreased motor coordination and impaired cognitive functions (Berr et al. 2012; Gao et al. 2007; Shahar et al. 2010).

Several clinical studies, which relate selenium status during pregnancy and neurophysiological development in infants, have been conducted. However, conclusions were not consistent probably because selenium content was measured in different kinds of samples. Some studies measured selenium content in plasma or serum while others used erythrocytes or urine. In addition, infant selenium status was measured at different time points after birth and maternal selenium status is variable during pregnancy (Amoros et al. 2018).

Impaired Selenium Transport to the Brain Impacts Brain Function

Selenium is contained in the diet as inorganic and organic compounds. The latter is predominantly selenomethionine. Inorganic and organic selenocompounds are absorbed in the small intestine by anion transporters and methionine transporters, respectively. They reach the liver *via* portal vein, where they are converted into selenocysteine and incorporated into selenoproteins (Krol et al. 2012). Liver produces the highest amount of the selenium-rich glycoprotein, selenoprotein P (Selenop according to the new nomenclature (Gladyshev et al. 2016)), which is secreted into blood. Selenop contains various selenocysteine residues (ten in humans) mostly concentrated in its C-terminal domain. Selenop represents more than 50% of plasma selenium (Burk and Hill 2009). For that reason, it was early on proposed as selenium transport protein.

The function of Selenop as selenium supplier was demonstrated by *Selenop* knockout mice (Hill et al. 2003; Schomburg et al. 2003). Selenium levels of these mice were drastically reduced in plasma, brain, testis, and kidney, whereas they were elevated in liver and urine (Hill et al. 2003; Schomburg et al. 2003). Therefore, Selenop is transported through the blood to target tissues, including brain, testis, and kidneys.

Besides, the excess of selenium, which accumulates in the liver of these mice due to the lack of Selenop production, is incorporated in selenocompounds, which are excreted by the urine (Burk and Hill 2009).

Moreover, since testis and brain are important target tissues of Selenop, abrogation of this selenoprotein in mice caused ataxia, seizures, and male infertility when they were fed a regular lab chow (Schomburg et al. 2003). This phenotype was aggravated by selenium deficiency. *Selenop*-deficient mice fed at low selenium diet developed severe motor impairment (spasticity and progressive paralysis) and died within few weeks (Hill et al. 2003). When selenium-sufficient diet started after mice had developed neurological abnormalities, selenium supplementation improved neurological defects but it did not reverse the brain damage (Hill et al. 2004;

Schweizer and Schomburg 2006). A closer look to the axons of brain stems and cervical spinal cords showed dystrophy and degeneration independent of the selenium intake (Valentine et al. 2005).

Accordingly to *Selenop* knockout mouse, testis and brain selenium levels of liver-specific *Selenop*-deficient mice dropped significantly (Hill et al. 2012; Schweizer et al. 2005). These mice also developed a neurological defect when were fed a low-selenium diet. Mice with a deletion of the C-terminal domain (Sec-rich domain) showed the same phenotype as *Selenop* knockout mice (Hill et al. 2007). On the contrary, the phenotype was rescued by liver-specific expression of human SELENOP (Renko et al. 2008). All these results support that liver Selenop is the main selenium source for brain and testis.

In addition to liver, brain is able to produce Selenop. *Selenop*-deficient mice rescued with hepatic human *SELENOP* and liver-specific *Selenop* knockout mice developed a neurological phenotype only under selenium-deficient conditions (Hill et al. 2012; Renko et al. 2008). These mice are deficient in brain Selenop. However, liver-specific tRNA[Ser]Sec knockout mice, which produce brain Selenop, maintained brain selenium levels and they did not develop any neurological anomaly (Schweizer et al. 2005). This fact supports the idea that brain selenium retention depends on brain Selenop, which could serve as storage of selenium in brain under selenium-deficient conditions. Moreover, Selenop could also have a protective function in the brain, since it has been shown that the N-terminal domain of Selenop has peroxidase activity (Kurokawa et al. 2014).

It is difficult to envision that a glycoprotein as selenoprotein P traverses the blood–brain barrier by diffusion. The identification of ApoER2/*Lrp8* (apolipoprotein E receptor 2) as a Selenop receptor was an important step forward (Burk et al. 2007; Olson et al. 2007). ApoER2/*Lrp8* is a member of the lipoprotein receptor family which was first identified in Sertoli cells in testis. *ApoER2*-deficient mice showed the same reduced testis selenium levels and sperm defects as *Selenop* knockout mice (Olson et al. 2007). ApoER2/*Lrp8* is also expressed in brain, especially in neurons. *ApoER2*-deficient mice also reproduced the *Selenop* knockout mice phenotype when fed with a low-selenium diet (Burk et al. 2007). An interaction between ApoER2/*Lrp8* and Selenop at the blood–brain barrier and the choroid plexus was demonstrated (Burk et al. 2014). Moreover, megalin/*Lrp2*, which was identified as a Selenop receptor in kidney, is also expressed in the blood–brain barrier (Chiu-Ugalde et al. 2010; Olson et al. 2008). *Megalin* knockout mice die prenatally on a pure C57Bl/6 genetic background, but *megalin*-deficient mice carrying a stop mutation on a mixed CD1 genetic background survive into adulthood. These *megalin*-mutant mice fed at selenium-deficient diet showed an impairment of movement coordination, reminiscent of the *Selenop* knockout phenotype (Chiu-Ugalde et al. 2010). Recently, it was published that Selenop must be in an oxidized state for uptake (Shetty et al. 2017). It is also not clear how other selenocompounds can be taken up directly by the brain cells. Neurological phenotype was retarded in male *Selenop*-deficient mice, which were castrated before sexual maturation (Pitts et al. 2015). It was concluded that selenium in these mice is redistributed to brain, probably as a different selenocompound since these mice do not express Selenop.

Accordingly, brain selenium levels *of Selenop*-deficient mice, which were selenium supplemented (Hill et al. 2003), were similar as wild-type mice fed with the same diet. Therefore, brain can take up selenium from other selenocompounds than Selenop and probably uses another mechanism.

Once Selenop is inside the brain cells, it has to be processed in order to use selenocysteine (Sec) for the production of selenoproteins. Lysosomes could be involved in the initial Selenop processing (Kurokawa et al. 2012). Moreover, it was believed that Sec residues of Selenop were metabolized by selenocysteine lyase (Scly) (Pitts et al. 2015). Hence, *Scly*-deficient mice would show a similar phenotype as *Selenop* knockout mice. However, these mice showed only a reduced selenoprotein expression but not the characteristic Selenop phenotype (Raman et al. 2012). The neurological phenotype was aggravated in combination with *Selenop* deletion (Byrns et al. 2014).

Brain Phenotypes Explained Through Selenoprotein-Deficient Mouse Models

Most selenoproteins are expressed in brain, especially in neurons (Zhang et al. 2008). Although, their expression can be upregulated in astrocytes after brain damage (Fradejas et al. 2011). Selenoproteins protect the brain from oxidative stress; therefore, it is logical to reason that disruption of them would lead to neurological anomalies.

Global Selenoprotein Deficiency Mouse Models

tRNA$^{[Ser]Sec}$

Selenocysteine (Sec) insertion into selenoproteins depends only on one tRNA, tRNA$^{[Ser]Sec}$. tRNA$^{[Ser]Sec}$ gene (*Trsp*) is encoded by a single copy gene; therefore deletion of *Trsp* gene abrogates the total selenoprotein expression when targeted in a specific tissue. *Trsp*-deficient mice are embryonic lethal; hence conditional mouse models are needed (Carlson et al. 2009a).

Neuron-specific ablation of *Trsp* gene (Tα1-Cre) in mice led to loss of neuronal selenoprotein expression and their corresponding selenoprotein activities. At postnatal day 8, mice developed seizures and died after 12 days (Wirth et al. 2010). Mice with specific deficiency of *Trsp* gene in cortical and hippocampal neurons (CamK-Cre) showed a milder neurological phenotype than the previously mentioned, and died at postnatal days 13–15. Neurodegeneration and astrogliosis were evident in these mice (Wirth et al. 2010). The most remarkable finding was the complete absence of cortical and hippocampal parvalbumin-positive (PV+) interneurons in these *Trsp* knockout mice. However, other GABAergic interneurons, somatostatin-14-, neuropeptide Y-, and calretinin-expressing cells, developed normally. Similarly, neuron-specific *Gpx4*-deficient mice showed a total lack of PV+ neurons (Wirth et al. 2010). Therefore, development of PV+ interneurons depends on Gpx4. Moreover, selenium and vitamin E deprivation reduced PV+ interneurons in culture. Therefore, PV+ interneurons are sensitive to lipid peroxides, the main substrate of the Gpx4 enzyme.

Conditional inactivation of *Trsp* gene in cerebellum led to loss of Purkinje cells (also PV+ GABAergic neurons) and reduced number of granule cells, which produced cerebellar hypoplasia. Accordingly, mice failed to coordinate their movements properly. Inactivation of *Gpx4* gene in cerebellum reproduced the same phenotype: loss of Purkinje cells and other kinds of cerebellar interneurons like basket and stellate cells were greatly reduced (Wirth et al. 2014).

Trsp knockout mice were complemented with a *Trsp* transgene lacking the STAF-binding site, a transcription activating factor which controls *Trsp* expression. *Trsp* is expressed in these mice in different amounts depending on the tissue. Brain selenoprotein expression was reduced, especially Gpx1 and Gpx4. Neurodegeneration and astrogliosis were evident in these mice as well as lack of PV+ interneurons in cerebral cortex and hippocampus. These mice were hyperexcitable and resembled the *Selenop*-deficient mice (Carlson et al. 2009b).

Specific deletion of hypothalamic *Trsp* gene led to type 2 diabetes in mice. And counteracting the oxidative stress by activation of Nrf2 in the hypothalamus could rescue the onset of diabetes (Yagishita et al. 2017).

Secisbp2

Selenocysteine insertion sequence (SECIS)-binding protein 2 (Secisbp2) binds to the SECIS elements located in the 3'UTR of the selenoprotein mRNAs and it is involved in UGA recoding as selenocysteine. Inactivation of *Secisbp2* is embryonic lethal in mice. Hepatocyte-specific deletion of *Secisbp2* reduced selenoprotein expression although to a lesser extent than *Trsp* knockout in hepatocytes (Seeher et al. 2014a).

Selenoprotein expression was impaired in neuron-specific *Secisbp2*-deficient mice as well as Gpx and Txnrd activities. Similar to the hepatocyte-specific *Secisbp2*-deleted mouse, neuron-specific *Secisbp2*-deficient mice showed a milder phenotype compared with neuron-specific *Trsp* knockout mice. *Secisbp2*-deficient mice survived longer (beyond postnatal day 16), showed a higher selenoprotein expression, and PV+ neurons were detectable, but reduced in numbers. A reduction of GABAergic interneurons was confirmed by *in situ* hybridization against glutamate decarboxylase, the GABA-producing enzyme. Neurodegeneration of GABAergic neurons in *Secisbp2*-deficient mice probably represents a degenerative process, since astrogliosis was observed. The movement of these mice resembles the *Selenop*-deficient mice movement phenotype. Since the *Secisbp2* deletion in these mice was not targeted to cerebellar neurons, a dysfunction of the basal ganglia was suspected. GABAergic neurons, PV+ neurons, and cholinergic neurons were reduced in the striatum of these mice. Hence, different kinds of striatal neurons also depend on selenoprotein expression (Seeher et al. 2014b).

Recently, a *Secisbp2*-deficient inducible mouse model has been described. These mice reproduce the thyroid phenotype characteristic of human SECISBP2 syndrome. As expected, selenoprotein expression and Gpx activity were reduced in the cerebrum of these mice (Fu et al. 2017).

Specific Selenoprotein Deficiency

Gpx4

Ablation of *Gpx4* caused embryonic lethality between E7.5 and E8 (Yant et al. 2003), indicating that Gpx4 is indispensable for mouse development. Several neuron-specific Gpx4 mouse models have been reported. Specific ablation of Gpx4 in hippocampal and cortex neurons (CamK-Cre) caused neurodegeneration, specifically of parvalbumin-positive neurons, and it was accompanied by astrogliosis. These mice suffered from seizures and had to be sacrificed at postnatal day 13 (Seiler et al. 2008). This phenotype resembles the one of *Trsp*-deficient neurons expressing CamK-Cre (Wirth et al. 2010). In the same way, *Trsp* deficiency controlled by Tα1-Cre expression in brain led to the same cerebellar phenotype than *Gpx4*-deficient mice using the same Cre driver (Wirth et al. 2014). Similarly, a systemic inducible Gpx4-deficient mouse showed hippocampal neuronal loss and increased astrogliosis (Yoo et al. 2012). Specific deletion of *Gpx4* in photoreceptors produced their degeneration (Ueta et al. 2012). In another neuron-specific mouse model, Gpx4 ablation caused neurodegeneration of motor neurons and paralysis (Chen et al. 2015). The most plausible cause of neuron death was ferroptosis, a recently described form of cell death. Treatment with vitamin E or anti-ferroptotic drugs alleviated neurodegeneration in these mice (Chen et al. 2015) and in another mouse model, where Gpx4 was conditionally deleted in forebrain neurons (Hambright et al. 2017). Deletion of Gpx4 in dopaminergic neurons made mice more anxious and showed a decreased locomotor activity when DJ-1, an antioxidant enzyme, was also deleted (Schriever et al. 2017). In conclusion, Gpx4 is necessary for neuronal survival probably because it protects neurons from ferroptosis.

Thioredoxin Reductases

Thioredoxin reductases (Txnrd) are flavin-containing NADPH-dependent oxidoreductases, which restore oxidized thioredoxin (Txn) to its reduced state. Both cooperate together providing reducing equivalents to many reactions (Kiermayer et al. 2007).

Three different Txnrd isoenzymes exist in mammals: Txnrd1 is the cytosolic isoform, Txnrd2 is the mitochondrial isoform, and Txnrd3 is mostly found in testis (Kiermayer et al. 2007).

Both *Txnrd1* knockout and *Txnrd2* knockout mice were embryonic lethal (Conrad et al. 2004; Jakupoglu et al. 2005). Whereas neural specific *Txnrd2* knockout mice did not show an evident brain phenotype (Conrad et al. 2004), neural specific *Txnrd1* knockout mice developed ataxia and tremor (Soerensen et al. 2008). The latter mice showed cerebellar hypoplasia, produced by decreased proliferation of granule cell precursors. Moreover, anterior cerebellar layer organization was disordered, Purkinje cells were delocalized, and Bergmann glia fibers were shortened. However, neuron-specific *Txnrd1* knockout mice did not show any of these anatomical anomalies (Soerensen et al. 2008). This fact indicates that Txnrd1 and Txnrd2 are dispensable to neurons but Txnrd1 could be involved in radial glia development, which in turn supports migration of cerebellar granule neurons.

Deiodinases

These three enzymes (named Dio1-3) eliminate iodide from thyroid hormones and their metabolites. The thyroid gland mostly secretes the inactive prohormone T4 (3,3′,5,5′-tetraiodothyronine, thyroxine) which is converted into the active T3 (3,3′,5-triiodothyronine) by the action of Dio2 or inactivated to rT3 (reverse 3,3′,5′-triiodothyronine) by Dio3 (Mendoza and Hollenberg 2017).

Dio1 knockout mouse did not show any evident phenotype, only gain of weight and increased levels of rT3 (Schneider et al. 2006). *Dio2* knockout mouse showed pituitary resistance to thyroid hormone (Schneider et al. 2001) and delayed cochlear development (Ng et al. 2004), which produces an auditory deficit. *Dio3* knockout mice suffered auditory defects, due to premature cochlear differentiation (Ng et al. 2009). Moreover, developmental defects in photoreceptors of the retina were reported in these mice (Ng et al. 2010). Therefore, auditory and visual systems depend on deiodinases.

Selenoprotein T

Selenoprotein T (Selenot) is a thioredoxin-like selenoprotein, which is located in the endoplasmic reticulum. It is regulated in the endocrine pancreas by pituitary adenylate cyclase-activating polypeptide (PACAP) and involved in glucose homeostasis (Prevost et al. 2013). *Selenot* gene disruption leads to embryonic lethality. Brain-specific *Selenot*-deficient mice developed parkinsonism phenotype when treated with 1-methyl-4-phenyl-1,2,3,6-tetrahydropyridine (MPTP) or rotenone. According to the parkinsonism phenotype, nigrostriatal tyrosine hydroxylase activity and dopamine levels dropped. Moreover, dopaminergic neurons from wild-type mice treated with MPTP overexpress Selenot, consistent with the high levels of

SELENOT found in PD patients (Boukhzar et al. 2016). Therefore, Selenot appears to play a role in protection of dopaminergic neurons.

Human Diseases Affecting the Central Nervous System that Are Related to Selenoprotein Deficiency

An early indication that selenium or selenoproteins might be important for human brain function came from two cases of intractable childhood epilepsy. The patients showed hair depigmentation and bone anomalies that were compatible with their low plasma selenium levels. Selenium supplementation was effective in normalizing plasma selenium levels and controlling the seizures, while the phenotypes returned upon discontinuation of selenium supplementation (Ramaekers et al. 1994). While the molecular genetic reason for the disorder was never elucidated, several selenoprotein-deficient mouse models generated shortly afterwards suffered from seizures. In recent years, several molecular genetic causes of neurodegeneration and/or epilepsy have been identified (Schweizer and Fradejas-Villar 2016).

Pontocerebellar Hypoplasia Type 2D (PCH2D) (Mutations in Selenocysteine Synthase)

This severe early-onset neurodegenerative disease was first discovered in non-consanguineous families of Iraqi or Moroccan origin. Patients suffer from severe spasticity, profound mental retardation, and progressive microcephaly. Myoclonic or generalized tonic-clonic seizures and progressive brain atrophy were also observed. The patients do not survive beyond 12 years. The syndrome was thus initially named progressive cerebello cerebral atrophy (Agamy et al. 2010). Two mutations in *SEPSECS* (*O*-phosphoseryl-tRNA:selenocysteinyl-tRNA synthase or selenocysteine synthase) gene were responsible of this phenotype. SEPSECS is a PLP (pyridoxal phosphate)-dependent enzyme, which catalyzes the final step of selenocysteine (Sec) biosynthesis using selenophosphate as selenium donor. The Iraqi mutation (p.Tyr334Cys) affects a conserved amino acid in the vicinity of the binding site of PLP; hence catalysis is supposed to be impaired. The Moroccan mutation (p.Ala239Thr) affects the binding of the enzyme to tRNA[Ser]Sec. Patients were homozygous (p.Tyr334Cys) or compound heterozygous for these missense mutations. Both mutations, but the human wild-type gene, failed to complement an *E. coli* strain, which lacks its endogenous selenocysteine synthase (Agamy et al. 2010). It is difficult to believe that these patients could survive without any SEPSECS activity, since knocking out tRNA[Ser]Sec or even some single selenoproteins is embryonic lethal in mouse models. Therefore, these patients likely conserve some SEPSECS residual activity.

After the discovery of the Iraqi and Moroccan mutations, several additional *SEPSECS* mutations have been reported in different populations. Two different mutations were found in a Finnish population, Thr325Ser and Tyr429*. Patients were compound heterozygous for these mutations. Selenoprotein expression (GPX1, GPX4, TXNRD1, and TXNRD2) was reduced in brain and SEPSECS protein was increased. Moreover, Thr325Ser showed some SEPSECS activity in the complementation assay described previously, but Tyr429* activity was undetectable. A special feature of these patients was elevated blood and CSF lactate, which might be related to mitochondrial dysfunction. However, respiratory chain complexes and subunits were analyzed from patient brain, but no indication of mitochondrial anomaly was found (Anttonen et al. 2015). Conversely, another patient showed a mild secondary mitochondrial myopathy and optic nerve atrophy. It is remarkable that this patient's point mutation occurs in the same amino acid as the Iraqi mutation (p.Tyr334His) (Pavlidou et al. 2016). Recently, other mutations have been reported in patients from Japanese origin. Both patients carry p.Asn119Ser mutation, but one of them in combination with p.Arg26Profs* and the other in combination with p.Arg156Gln. These patients present with a milder phenotype than the previous patients. They are able to speak words and walk, although with difficulties. They showed late-onset cerebellar atrophy, which appeared at 9 years for one of the patients and at 21 for the other. Both patients developed spasticity and ataxia, but no seizures (Iwama et al. 2016).

Spondylometaphyseal Chondrodysplasia of Sedaghatian Type (GPX4 *Mutations*)

When Sedaghatian described this syndrome, he did not know that mutations in the *GPX4* gene were the cause of the disease. He described an autosomal recessive skeletal disorder characterized by severe metaphyseal chondrodysplasia, mild platyspondyly, and rhizomelic shortness of the limbs. Patients showed low plasma calcium, high phosphorus, and high alkaline phosphatase levels attributed to a renal defect. They died prematurely by cardiorespiratory failure. *Postmortem* analysis exhibited pulmonary, renal, and adrenal hemorrhage, and subendocardial myocarditis and myocardial necrosis (Sedaghatian 1980). Since then, a total of 18 patients have been reported with Sedaghatian disease. For some patients, malformations of the central nervous system were reported, like simplified gyral pattern, hypogenesis of corpus callosum, and severe cerebellar hypoplasia (Aygun et al. 2012). Myoclonic seizures were also reported. Recently, mutations which impair the splicing of *GPX4* (c.587+5G>A) and (c.588-8_588-4del) and a nonsense mutation (p.Tyr127*) were identified in patients with Sedaghatian disease (Smith et al. 2014).

Gpx4-deficient mice are embryonic lethal. Conditional knockout of Gpx4 in neurons showed seizures (Seiler et al. 2008). Systemic inducible *Gpx4* knockout mice died because of kidney failure (Friedmann Angeli et al. 2014). Sedaghatian already suggested a renal defect in the first cases reported. No bone anomalies were reported in these mouse models. Vitamin E was able to support mouse *Gpx4*-deficient fibroblast in culture (Seiler et al. 2008) and liproxstatin-1, an inhibitor of ferroptosis, prolonged the survival of systemic inducible *Gpx4* knockout mice (Friedmann Angeli et al. 2014). Moreover, a recent publication showed that both molecules ameliorate neurodegeneration of forebrain neurons in an inducible *Gpx4* knockout mouse (Hambright et al. 2017).

Deficiencies in TXNRD Systems

In contrast with *Txnrd2* knockout mice (Conrad et al. 2004), which are embryonic lethal due to impaired hematopoiesis and heart function, a homozygous nonsense mutation in the *TXNRD2* gene (p.Y447X) produced isolated glucocorticoid deficiency in humans. Patients showed hyperpigmentation, low serum cortisol levels, and high plasma ACTH (Prasad et al. 2014). It is surprising that *TXNRD2* mutations caused such a mild phenotype, while a homozygous stop mutation in *TXN2*, its mitochondrial substrate, led to a severe neurodegenerative disorder in a child (Holzerova et al. 2016). It appears as if TXN2 can be reduced by another redox system in mitochondria, possibly related to the glutathione/glutaredoxin system. Moreover, two different heterozygous point mutations (p.Ala59Thr and p.Gly375Arg) in the Flavin adenine dinucleotide (FAD)-binding domain of TXNRD2 lead to dilated cardiomyopathy (Sibbing et al. 2011). This phenotype corresponds to the phenotype of cardiac-specific *Txnrd2* knockout mice.

Recently we reported a homozygous mutation in the *TXNRD1* gene (p. Pro190Leu) in a family with genetic generalized epilepsy (Kudin et al. 2017). TXNRD1 activity was reduced in patient fibroblasts and muscle biopsies. Mutant fibroblast showed a lower expression of TXNRD1. Assessment of in vitro kinetic properties of the mutant enzyme disclosed a decrease of the turnover rate. Therefore, the point mutation could render TXNRD1 prone to protein degradation and decrease the turnover rate due to a conformational instability.

SECISBP2 Syndrome

A number of patients have been described who carry different homozygous or compound heterozygous mutations in the *SECISBP2* gene. Visible symptoms of these patients are delayed longitudinal growth and delayed bone age. The key biochemical findings are abnormal thyroid function tests, characterized by high circulating thyroxine (T4), low or normal triiodothyronine (T3), elevated reverse T3 (rT3), and normal or elevated thyroid-stimulating hormone (TSH). There is consensus that these findings are related to reduced expression of thyroid hormone deiodinases

(Azevedo et al. 2010; Dumitrescu et al. 2005; Hamajima et al. 2012; Schoenmakers et al. 2010; Di Cosmo et al. 2009).

Some patients showed hearing loss, in agreement with impaired cochlear development due to DIO2 deficiency. Several patients also showed neurological and muscular disorders (Azevedo et al. 2010; Dumitrescu et al. 2005; Hamajima et al. 2012; Schoenmakers et al. 2010; Di Cosmo et al. 2009). The neurological phenotype cannot be attributed to a specific selenoprotein; probably several ones are playing a role. In the case of the muscle phenotype, lack of selenoprotein N could be responsible, since SECISBP2 patients showed a similar myopathy as the patients suffering from isolated *SEPN1* deficiency (Schweizer and Fradejas-Villar 2016).

tRNA[Ser]Sec Mutation

Recently, a patient with abdominal pain, fatigue, muscle weakness, thyroid dysfunction, and low plasma selenium was reported. These symptoms were similar to SECISBP2 syndrome patients. However, a homozygous point mutation (C65G) in the *TRNAU1* gene, which encodes the unique tRNA[Ser]Sec, was found in this patient. Housekeeping selenoproteins (TXNRD 1, GPX4) were preserved, but on the contrary biosynthesis of stress-related selenoproteins (GPX1 and SELENOW) was impaired. This is consistent with reduced tRNA[Ser]Sec levels and decreased 2'-*O* methylation at ribose 34, a tRNA[Ser]Sec modification which supports expression of stress-related selenoproteins. No neurological phenotype was reported for this patient (Schoenmakers et al. 2016).

References

Agamy O, et al. Mutations disrupting selenocysteine formation cause progressive cerebello-cerebral atrophy. Am J Hum Genet. 2010;87:538–44.

Amoros R, et al. Selenium status during pregnancy: Influential factors and effects on neuropsychological development among Spanish infants. Sci Total Environ. 2018;610–611:741–9.

Anttonen AK, et al. Selenoprotein biosynthesis defect causes progressive encephalopathy with elevated lactate. Neurology. 2015;85:306–15.

Aygun C, et al. Simplified gyral pattern with cerebellar hypoplasia in Sedaghatian type spondylometaphyseal dysplasia: a clinical report and review of the literature. Am J Med Genet A. 2012;158A:1400–5.

Azevedo MF, et al. Selenoprotein-related disease in a young girl caused by nonsense mutations in the SBP2 gene. J Clin Endocrinol Metab. 2010;95:4066–71.

Berr C, Arnaud J, Akbaraly TN. Selenium and cognitive impairment: a brief-review based on results from the EVA study. Biofactors. 2012;38:139–44.

Boukhzar L, et al. Selenoprotein T exerts an essential oxidoreductase activity that protects dopaminergic neurons in mouse models of Parkinson's disease. Antioxid Redox Signal. 2016;24:557–74.

Burk RF, Hill KE. Selenoprotein P-expression, functions, and roles in mammals. Biochim Biophys Acta. 2009;1790:1441–7.

Burk RF, et al. Deletion of apolipoprotein E receptor-2 in mice lowers brain selenium and causes severe neurological dysfunction and death when a low-selenium diet is fed. J Neurosci. 2007;27:6207–11.

Burk RF, et al. Selenoprotein P and apolipoprotein E receptor-2 interact at the blood-brain barrier and also within the brain to maintain an essential selenium pool that protects against neurodegeneration. FASEB J. 2014;28:3579–88.

Byrns CN, Pitts MW, Gilman CA, Hashimoto AC, Berry MJ. Mice lacking selenoprotein P and selenocysteine lyase exhibit severe neurological dysfunction, neurodegeneration, and audiogenic seizures. J Biol Chem. 2014;289:9662–74.

Carlson BA, Yoo MH, Tsuji PA, Gladyshev VN, Hatfield DL. Mouse models targeting selenocysteine tRNA expression for elucidating the role of selenoproteins in health and development. Molecules. 2009a;14:3509–27.

Carlson BA, et al. The selenocysteine tRNA STAF-binding region is essential for adequate selenocysteine tRNA status, selenoprotein expression and early age survival of mice. Biochem J. 2009b;418:61–71.

Chen L, Hambright WS, Na R, Ran Q. Ablation of the ferroptosis inhibitor glutathione peroxidase 4 in neurons results in rapid motor neuron degeneration and paralysis. J Biol Chem. 2015;290:28097–106.

Chiu-Ugalde J, et al. Mutation of megalin leads to urinary loss of selenoprotein P and selenium deficiency in serum, liver, kidneys and brain. Biochem J. 2010;431:103–11.

Conrad M, et al. Essential role for mitochondrial thioredoxin reductase in hematopoiesis, heart development, and heart function. Mol Cell Biol. 2004;24:9414–23.

Di Cosmo C, et al. Clinical and molecular characterization of a novel selenocysteine insertion sequence-binding protein 2 (SBP2) gene mutation (R128X). J Clin Endocrinol Metab. 2009;94:4003–9.

Dominiak A, Wilkaniec A, Wroczynski P, Adamczyk A. Selenium in the therapy of neurological diseases. Where is it Going? Curr Neuropharmacol. 2016;14:282–99.

Dumitrescu AM, et al. Mutations in SECISBP2 result in abnormal thyroid hormone metabolism. Nat Genet. 2005;37:1247–52.

Fradejas N, Serrano-Perez Mdel C, Tranque P, Calvo S. Selenoprotein S expression in reactive astrocytes following brain injury. Glia. 2011;59:959–72.

Friedmann Angeli JP, et al. Inactivation of the ferroptosis regulator Gpx4 triggers acute renal failure in mice. Nat Cell Biol. 2014;16:1180–91.

Fu J, Fujisawa H, Follman B, Liao XH, Dumitrescu AM. Thyroid hormone metabolism defects in a mouse model of SBP2 deficiency. Endocrinology. 2017;158(12):4317–30.

Gao S, et al. Selenium level and cognitive function in rural elderly Chinese. Am J Epidemiol. 2007;165:955–65.

Gladyshev VN, et al. Selenoprotein Gene Nomenclature. J Biol Chem. 2016;291:24036–40.

Hamajima T, Mushimoto Y, Kobayashi H, Saito Y, Onigata K. Novel compound heterozygous mutations in the SBP2 gene: characteristic clinical manifestations and the implications of GH and triiodothyronine in longitudinal bone growth and maturation. Eur J Endocrinol. 2012;166:757–64.

Hambright WS, Fonseca RS, Chen L, Na R, Ran Q. Ablation of ferroptosis regulator glutathione peroxidase 4 in forebrain neurons promotes cognitive impairment and neurodegeneration. Redox Biol. 2017;12:8–17.

Hill KE, et al. Deletion of selenoprotein P alters distribution of selenium in the mouse. J Biol Chem. 2003;278:13640–6.

Hill KE, Zhou J, McMahan WJ, Motley AK, Burk RF. Neurological dysfunction occurs in mice with targeted deletion of the selenoprotein P gene. J Nutr. 2004;134:157–61.

Hill KE, et al. The selenium-rich C-terminal domain of mouse selenoprotein P is necessary for the supply of selenium to brain and testis but not for the maintenance of whole body selenium. J Biol Chem. 2007;282:10972–80.

Hill KE, et al. Production of selenoprotein P (Sepp1) by hepatocytes is central to selenium homeo-stasis. J Biol Chem. 2012;287:40414–24.

Holzerova E, et al. Human thioredoxin 2 deficiency impairs mitochondrial redox homeostasis and causes early-onset neurodegeneration. Brain. 2016;139:346–54.

Iwama K, et al. Milder progressive cerebellar atrophy caused by biallelic SEPSECS mutations. J Hum Genet. 2016;61:527–31.

Jakupoglu C, et al. Cytoplasmic thioredoxin reductase is essential for embryogenesis but dispens-able for cardiac development. Mol Cell Biol. 2005;25:1980–8.

Kiermayer C, Michalke B, Schmidt J, Brielmeier M. Effect of selenium on thioredoxin reductase activity in Txnrd1 or Txnrd2 hemizygous mice. Biol Chem. 2007;388:1091–7.

Krol MB, Gromadzinska J, Wasowicz W. SeP, ApoER2 and megalin as necessary factors to main-tain Se homeostasis in mammals. J Trace Elem Med Biol. 2012;26:262–6.

Kudin AP, et al. Homozygous mutation in TXNRD1 is associated with genetic generalized epi-lepsy. Free Radic Biol Med. 2017;106:270–7.

Kuhbacher M, et al. The brain selenoproteome: priorities in the hierarchy and different levels of selenium homeostasis in the brain of selenium-deficient rats. J Neurochem. 2009;110:133–42.

Kurokawa S, Hill KE, McDonald WH, Burk RF. Long isoform mouse selenoprotein P (Sepp1) supplies rat myoblast L8 cells with selenium via endocytosis mediated by heparin binding properties and apolipoprotein E receptor-2 (ApoER2). J Biol Chem. 2012;287:28717–26.

Kurokawa S, et al. Sepp1(UF) forms are N-terminal selenoprotein P truncations that have peroxi-dase activity when coupled with thioredoxin reductase-1. Free Radic Biol Med. 2014;69:67–76.

Mendoza A, Hollenberg AN. New insights into thyroid hormone action. Pharmacol Ther. 2017;173:135–45.

Ng L, et al. Hearing loss and retarded cochlear development in mice lacking type 2 iodothyronine deiodinase. Proc Natl Acad Sci U S A. 2004;101:3474–9.

Ng L, et al. A protective role for type 3 deiodinase, a thyroid hormone-inactivating enzyme, in cochlear development and auditory function. Endocrinology. 2009;150:1952–60.

Ng L, et al. Type 3 deiodinase, a thyroid-hormone-inactivating enzyme, controls survival and mat-uration of cone photoreceptors. J Neurosci. 2010;30:3347–57.

Olson GE, Winfrey VP, Nagdas SK, Hill KE, Burk RF. Apolipoprotein E receptor-2 (ApoER2) mediates selenium uptake from selenoprotein P by the mouse testis. J Biol Chem. 2007;282:12290–7.

Olson GE, Winfrey VP, Hill KE, Burk RF. Megalin mediates selenoprotein P uptake by kidney proximal tubule epithelial cells. J Biol Chem. 2008;283:6854–60.

Pavlidou E, et al. Pontocerebellar hypoplasia type 2D and optic nerve atrophy further expand the spectrum associated with selenoprotein biosynthesis deficiency. Eur J Paediatr Neurol. 2016;20:483–8.

Pitts MW, et al. Competition between the brain and testes under selenium-compromised condi-tions: insight into sex differences in selenium metabolism and risk of neurodevelopmental dis-ease. J Neurosci. 2015;35:15326–38.

Prasad R, et al. Thioredoxin Reductase 2 (TXNRD2) mutation associated with familial glucocor-ticoid deficiency (FGD). J Clin Endocrinol Metab. 2014;99:E1556–63.

Prevost G, et al. The PACAP-regulated gene selenoprotein T is abundantly expressed in mouse and human beta-cells and its targeted inactivation impairs glucose tolerance. Endocrinology. 2013;154:3796–806.

Ramaekers VT, Calomme M, Vanden Berghe D, Makropoulos W. Selenium deficiency triggering intractable seizures. Neuropediatrics. 1994;25:217–23.

Raman AV, et al. Absence of selenoprotein P but not selenocysteine lyase results in severe neuro-logical dysfunction. Genes Brain Behav. 2012;11:601–13.

Renko K, et al. Hepatic selenoprotein P (SePP) expression restores selenium transport and prevents infertility and motor-incoordination in Sepp-knockout mice. Biochem J. 2008;409:741–9.

Schneider MJ, et al. Targeted disruption of the type 2 selenodeiodinase gene (DIO2) results in a phenotype of pituitary resistance to T4. Mol Endocrinol. 2001;15:2137–48.

Schneider MJ, et al. Targeted disruption of the type 1 selenodeiodinase gene (Dio1) results in marked changes in thyroid hormone economy in mice. Endocrinology. 2006;147:580–9.

Schoenmakers E, et al. Mutations in the selenocysteine insertion sequence-binding protein 2 gene lead to a multisystem selenoprotein deficiency disorder in humans. J Clin Invest. 2010;120:4220–35.

Schoenmakers E, et al. Mutation in human selenocysteine transfer RNA selectively disrupts selenoprotein synthesis. J Clin Invest. 2016;126:992–6.

Schomburg L, et al. Gene disruption discloses role of selenoprotein P in selenium delivery to target tissues. Biochem J. 2003;370:397–402.

Schriever SC, et al. Alterations in neuronal control of body weight and anxiety behavior by glutathione peroxidase 4 deficiency. Neuroscience. 2017;357:241–54.

Schweizer U, Fradejas-Villar N. Why 21? The significance of selenoproteins for human health revealed by inborn errors of metabolism. FASEB J. 2016;30:3669–81.

Schweizer U, Schomburg L. In: Hatfield DL, Berry MJ, Gladyshev VN, editors. Selenium: its molecular biology and role in human health. Boston, MA: Springer US; 2006. p. 233–48.

Schweizer U, et al. Hepatically derived selenoprotein P is a key factor for kidney but not for brain selenium supply. Biochem J. 2005;386:221–6.

Sedaghatian MR. Congenital lethal metaphyseal chondrodysplasia: a newly recognized complex autosomal recessive disorder. Am J Med Genet. 1980;6:269–74.

Seeher S, et al. Secisbp2 is essential for embryonic development and enhances selenoprotein expression. Antioxid Redox Signal. 2014a;21:835–49.

Seeher S, et al. Impaired selenoprotein expression in brain triggers striatal neuronal loss leading to co-ordination defects in mice. Biochem J. 2014b;462:67–75.

Seiler A, et al. Glutathione peroxidase 4 senses and translates oxidative stress into 12/15-lipoxygenase dependent- and AIF-mediated cell death. Cell Metab. 2008;8:237–48.

Shahar A, et al. Plasma selenium is positively related to performance in neurological tasks assessing coordination and motor speed. Mov Disord. 2010;25:1909–15.

Shetty S, Marsicano JR, Copeland PR. Uptake and utilization of selenium from selenoprotein P. Biol Trace Elem Res. 2018;181:54–61.

Sibbing D, et al. Mutations in the mitochondrial thioredoxin reductase gene TXNRD2 cause dilated cardiomyopathy. Eur Heart J. 2011;32:1121–33.

Smith AC, et al. Mutations in the enzyme glutathione peroxidase 4 cause Sedaghatian-type spondylometaphyseal dysplasia. J Med Genet. 2014;51:470–4.

Soerensen J, et al. The role of thioredoxin reductases in brain development. PLoS One. 2008;3:e1813.

Steinbrenner H, Sies H. Selenium homeostasis and antioxidant selenoproteins in brain: implications for disorders in the central nervous system. Arch Biochem Biophys. 2013;536:152–7.

Ueta T, et al. Glutathione peroxidase 4 is required for maturation of photoreceptor cells. J Biol Chem. 2012;287:7675–82.

Valentine WM, et al. Brainstem axonal degeneration in mice with deletion of selenoprotein p. Toxicol Pathol. 2005;33:570–6.

Vanderpas JB, et al. Iodine and selenium deficiency associated with cretinism in northern Zaire. Am J Clin Nutr. 1990;52:1087–93.

de Wilde MC, Vellas B, Girault E, Yavuz AC, Sijben JW. Lower brain and blood nutrient status in Alzheimer's disease: results from meta-analyses. Alzheimers Dement (N Y). 2017;3:416–31.

Wirth EK, et al. Neuronal selenoprotein expression is required for interneuron development and prevents seizures and neurodegeneration. FASEB J. 2010;24:844–52.

Wirth EK, et al. Cerebellar hypoplasia in mice lacking selenoprotein biosynthesis in neurons. Biol Trace Elem Res. 2014;158:203–10.

Wrobel JK, Power R, Toborek M. Biological activity of selenium: revisited. IUBMB Life. 2016;68:97–105.

Yagishita Y, et al. Nrf2 improves leptin and insulin resistance provoked by hypothalamic oxidative stress. Cell Rep. 2017;18:2030–44.

Yant LJ, et al. The selenoprotein GPX4 is essential for mouse development and protects from radiation and oxidative damage insults. Free Radic Biol Med. 2003;34:496–502.

Yoo SE, et al. Gpx4 ablation in adult mice results in a lethal phenotype accompanied by neuronal loss in brain. Free Radic Biol Med. 2012;52:1820–7.

Zhang Y, et al. Comparative analysis of selenocysteine machinery and selenoproteome gene expression in mouse brain identifies neurons as key functional sites of selenium in mammals. J Biol Chem. 2008;283:2427–38.

Chapter 10
Selenium and Autism Spectrum Disorder

Anatoly V. Skalny, Margarita G. Skalnaya, Geir Bjørklund,
Viktor A. Gritsenko, Jan Aaseth, and Alexey A. Tinkov

Abstract Autism spectrum disorder (ASD) represents a complex neurodevelopmental disorder, being associated with various metabolic abnormalities. Micronutrients, including selenium (Se), are frequently used for ASD management. However, their efficiency remains unclear. Moreover, data on the role of Se metabolism in ASD are insufficient and contradictory. Therefore, the objective of this chapter is to review the existing data on Se status of children with ASD. Current data demonstrate that Se intake varies in children with ASD from low to high values in comparison to the daily recommendations. Similarly, data on Se status in ASD are also contradictory. Of 16 studies reviewed, eight indicate decreased Se levels in samples from autistic children, whereas six demonstrate opposite changes. Correspondingly, two recent meta-analyses failed to reveal any significant

A. V. Skalny (✉)
Yaroslavl State University, Yaroslavl, Russia

Peoples' Friendship University of Russia (RUDN University), Moscow, Russia

All-Russian Research Institute of Medicinal and Aromatic Plants (VILAR), Moscow, Russia
e-mail: skalny3@microelements.ru

M. G. Skalnaya
Peoples' Friendship University of Russia (RUDN University), Moscow, Russia

G. Bjørklund
Council for Nutritional and Environmental Medicine, Mo i Rana, Norway

V. A. Gritsenko
Institute of Cellular and Intracellular Symbiosis, Russian Academy of Sciences, Orenburg, Russia

J. Aaseth
Innlandet Hospital Trust, Kongsvinger, Norway

Inland Norway University of Applied Sciences, Terningen Arena, Elverum, Norway

A. A. Tinkov
Yaroslavl State University, Yaroslavl, Russia

Peoples' Friendship University of Russia (RUDN University), Moscow, Russia

Institute of Cellular and Intracellular Symbiosis, Russian Academy of Sciences, Orenburg, Russia

© Springer International Publishing AG, part of Springer Nature 2018
B. Michalke (ed.), *Selenium*, Molecular and Integrative Toxicology,
https://doi.org/10.1007/978-3-319-95390-8_10

association between Se status and ASD. The activity of GPX in children with ASD is also highly variable from study to study. The observed difference in Se level in ASD patients may be related to different substrates used, as well as to specific features of the studied populations. However, the existing studies indicate involvement of Se imbalance in metabolic/psychometabolic disturbances in ASD. The mechanisms of a proposed Se neuroprotective effect in ASD may involve inhibition of oxidative stress, neuroinflammation, and microglia activation. In addition, synaptic dysfunction and gut-brain axis disturbances might be modified. However, further studies are required to highlight the mechanisms of the potential neuroprotective effects of Se in ASD as well as its efficiency in clinical trials.

Keywords Selenium · Autism · Glutathione peroxidase · Deficiency

Introduction

The number of children diagnosed with autism spectrum disorder (ASD) or related disorders has been growing exponentially. In the USA in 2006–2008, about one of six children had a developmental disability, which ranged from mild to serious (Boyle et al. 2011). ASD occurs in all ethnic, socioeconomic, and racial groups (Durkin et al. 2010). ASD is about 4.5 times more common in males (1 in 42) than in females (1 in 189) (Christensen et al. 2016). Studies have identified an average prevalence of ASD of 1–2% in the European, North American, and Asian populations (CDC 2016). However, the prevalence of ASD varies widely among different countries (CDC 2016; Charron 2017). In South Korea, it has been estimated that the prevalence of ASD is as high as 2.6% of the population of school-age children, which is equivalent to 1 in 38 children (Kim et al. 2011).

A study published by the Centers for Disease Control and Prevention (CDC) shows that 1 in every 68 children in the USA under the age of 8 has ASD (Christensen et al. 2016). The prevalence of the disorder in the USA has increased by 30% compared to data released in 2012, which indicated that 1 in every 88 children in the country would be within the autistic spectrum (CDC 2012). In the 1980s, this number was 1 in 2000 children (Gillberg and Wing 1999). In part, the increase in the prevalence of ASD may be explained due to improved diagnostics and greater awareness (Macedoni-Lukšič et al. 2015).

Older parents have a higher risk of getting children with ASD than younger parents (Durkin et al. 2008). Parents who have a child with ASD have a 2–18% possibility also getting a second child with the disorder (Sumi et al. 2006; Ozonoff et al. 2011).

ASD often occurs together with other psychiatric, developmental, neurologic genetic, or chromosomal diagnoses (Levy et al. 2010). However, genetic factors explain alone only about 37% of the ASD cases (Shaw et al. 2014). Research shows that different environmental, metabolic, nutritional, and immunological factors also may play a role in the development of ASD (Bjørklund et al. 2016; Crăciun et al. 2016; Matelski and Van de Water 2016). Moreover, it has been demonstrated that gene-environment interactions provide a significant contribution to ASD (Tordjman et al. 2014).

Due to complex etiology of the disease and a high number of pathways involved, multiple treatment strategies have been used for ASD management (Blenner et al. 2011). Various nutritional interventions are widely used as a treatment, often complementary to traditional medications (Geraghty et al. 2010). Micronutrients (vitamins and minerals) possess certain advantages as compared to the standard medication management (Mehl-Madrona et al. 2010). However, the most recent systematic review indicates insufficient evidence for the use of nutritional interventions in ASD (Sathe et al. 2017).

Selenium (Se), an essential trace element (Reich and Hondal 2016), is used in line with magnesium and calcium in children with ASD (Wong and Smith 2006). Certain studies demonstrate that Se may be recommended for autistic children (Robson 2013). A regular dose of Se recommended for use in autistic children (60 lb weight) is 80 µg/day (Adams 2007). The formulations of Autism Nutrition Research Center (ANRC) propose the use of 40 µg/day Se with 80% as selenomethionine and 20% as sodium selenite (Adams 2015). However, Se supplementation is graded as N category, indicating the absence of evidence-based guidelines (Rossignol 2009). Moreover, data on Se status of autistic children are contradictory.

Therefore, the objective of this chapter was to review the existing data on Se status of children with ASD, as assessed by Se intake, its levels in different substrates, and activity of selenoproteins (especially glutathione peroxidase (GPX)). The potential mechanisms of the protective effect of Se in ASD are briefly discussed.

Selenium Intake in Autistic Children

Multiple studies have demonstrated insufficient intake of various micronutrients (Herndon et al. 2009). However, data regarding Se intake are insufficient and contradictory. In particular, it has been demonstrated that Se intake in American autistic children appeared to be adequate (Lindsay et al. 2006). Similar findings were obtained during examination of children with ASD from Children's Hospital of Pittsburgh's Child Development Unit/Autism Center (86.67 vs. 98.75 µg/day, $p = 0.293$) (Johnson et al. 2008). Moreover, examination of children with ASD participating in the Autism Treatment Network (Arkansas, Cincinnati, Colorado, Pittsburgh, and Rochester) demonstrated excessive dietary consumption of Se as compared to the recommended values (Hyman et al. 2012).

At the same time, significantly lower Se intake was detected in American non-Hispanic boys with ASD as compared to the healthy controls (34.66 (29.36–39.96) µg/day vs. 43.29 (37.31–49.27) µg/day, $p = 0.019$). However, no significant association between Se intake and bone mineral density or other health indices was reported (Barnhill et al. 2017). In a cohort of Egyptian children with ASD, the Se intake was 12% lower than that in the healthy controls (7.3 ± 2.0 vs. 8.3 ± 2.3, $p = 0.004$) (Meguid et al. 2017).

Selenium Status in Autism Spectrum Disorder

The majority of studies have demonstrated significantly lower levels of Se in biological matrices of children with ASD compared to controls (Table 10.1). In particular, the prevalence of Se deficiency as assessed by hair Se levels was significantly higher in a Georgian ASD children group as compared to the controls (38% vs. 4%) (Tabatadze et al. 2015). It has also been demonstrated that hair Se levels in children with low-, medium-, and high-functioning autism were 83%, 41%, and 24% lower than the respective values in the control group. Similar differences were observed in nail Se levels, being 70%, 49%, and 18% lower in low-, medium-, and high-functioning autism groups as compared to the control values, respectively (Lakshmi Priya and Geetha 2011). These findings are in agreement with the earlier indications of decreased hair (Skalny 2013), plasma, and RBC (Yorbık et al. 2000) Se levels, although the absolute values were not accessible from the publications.

Red blood cell (RBC) Se levels were also found to be decreased by 15% ($p = 0.0006$) in a Canadian sample of autistic children as compared to the controls (Jory and McGinnis 2008). It has also been reported a significant ($p < 0.001$) decrease in RBC Se levels in ASD children as compared to the controls. Moreover, decreased Se levels were accompanied by an elevation of Hg and lead (Pb) levels in children with ASD (El-Ansary et al. 2017). Similarly, while cerebellar Se levels only slightly decreased in children with ASD, the Se/Hg ratio was characterized by a significant 42.9% decrease as compared to the control values (232.9 vs. 407.4) (Sajdel-Sulkowska et al. 2008), being in agreement with a proposed role of Hg-Se antagonism in modulating neurotoxicity. Plasma Se levels were also found to be significantly lower than those in the controls (Sezgin et al. 2010).

Some studies have demonstrated the absence of significant interaction between Se metabolism and ASD (Table 10.1). In particular, a study from Arizona involving 55 autistic and 44 neurotypical children aged 5–16 years demonstrated that the level of Se in whole blood and RBC was nearly similar between the groups (Adams et al. 2011). The results of meta-analysis also demonstrated the lack of association between hair Se levels and ASD (De Palma et al. 2012). Moreover, a recent meta-analysis demonstrated the absence of significant difference in both hair and RBC Se levels in ASD and control children (Saghazadeh et al. 2017). Correspondingly, only two of ten patients with attention-deficit/hyperactivity disorder (ADHD) and ASD were characterized by significantly reduced erythrocyte Se levels (Patel and Curtis 2007). Blaurock-Busch et al. (2011) demonstrated a nearly twofold lower hair Se values in autistic children, although the difference was not significant due to a high variability of data. Urinary Se was also found to be nearly similar between the ASD and control groups (Blaurock-Busch et al. 2011).

Despite a high number of studies demonstrating various indices and rates of Se deficiency in ASD, certain studies have demonstrated increased hair Se levels in autistic children (Lubkowska and Sobieraj 2009) (Table 10.1). Moreover, examination of 44 autistic children from Italy (Verona) demonstrated significantly increased hair Se levels in the autism group as compared to the respective control values by

Table 10.1 Serum levels in various substrates of children with ASD in comparison to the control values (sorted according to the publication date)

No.	Origin	Participants	Age, years	Sample	Change	Se levels	References
1	Canada	ASD Controls	3.90 ± 1.68 3.87 ± 1.06	RBC	↓	3.12 ± 0.54 μmol/L 3.67 ± 0.38 μmol/L	Jory and McGinnis (2008)
2	Poland	ASD Controls	4.8 ± 2.4	Hair	↑	0.33 ± 0.18 μg/g N.A.	Lubkowska and Sobieraj (2009)
3	Turkey	ASD Controls	N.S.	Plasma	↓	34.83 ± 7.14 μg/L 77.03 ± 18.84 μg/L	Sezgin et al. (2010)
4	USA	ASD Controls	5–16	Whole blood	↔	207 ± 28 μg/L 210 ± 20 μg/L	Adams et al. (2011)
		ASD Controls		RBC		0.24 ± 0.04 μg/g 0.23 ± 0.03 μg/g	
5	India	LFA MFA HFA	4–12	Hair	↓	0.57 ± 0.06 μg/g 1.98 ± 0.23 μg/g 2.55 ± 0.30 μg/g	Priya and Geetha (2011)
		Controls			↓	3.37 ± 0.40 μg/g	
		LFA MFA HFA Controls		Nails		5.70 ± 0.68 μg/g 1.73 ± 0.20 μg/g 2.93 ± 0.35 μg/g 4.67 ± 0.56 μg/g	
6	Saudi Arabia	ASD Controls	5.29 ± 1.9 6.25 ± 2.3	Hair	↔	0.80 ± 0.25 μg/g 0.36 ± 0.29 μg/g	Blaurock-Busch et al. (2011)
		ASD Controls		Urine		286.18 ± 236.75 μg/g creatinine 311.17 ± 254.15 μg/g creatinine	
7	Italy	ASD Controls	9 ± 4.05 8.4 ± 3.1	Hair	↑	0.90(0.60–1.17) μg/g 0.65(0.36–0.87) μg/g	De Palma et al. (2012)
8	Turkey	Controls Classic autism PDD-NOS	5.8 ± 2.5	RBC	↑	93.81 ± 32.1 μg/L 120.23 ± 45.1 μg/L 86.46 (57.76–157.70) μg/L	Kondolot et al. (2016)
9	Saudi Arabia	ASD Controls	3–12	RBC	↓	111.9 ± 15.1 μg/L 194.6 ± 26.7 μg/L	El-Ansary et al. (2017)
10	Russia	ASD Controls	2–9	Hair	↑	0.365 (0.315–0.424) μg/g 0.279 (0.201–0.362) μg/g	Skalny et al. (2017a)

(continued)

Table 10.1 (continued)

No.	Origin	Participants	Age, years	Sample	Change	Se levels	References
11	Russia	ASD Controls		Hair	↑	0.406 (0.343–0.460) μg/g 0.361 (0.269–0.410) μg/g	
			2–10	Serum	↔	0.081 (0.072–0.095) μg/L 0.087 (0.075–0.098) μg/L	Skalny et al. (2017b)
12	Russia	Control Childhood autism Atypical autism	6.4 ± 1.0 6.5 ± 1.1 6.7 ± 1.2	Serum	↓	0.087 ± 0.015 μg/L 0.079 ± 0.011 μg/L 0.076 ± 0.017 μg/L	Skalny et al. (2017c)

N.A. not accessible, *PDD-NOS* pervasive developmental disorder not otherwise specified, *LFA* low-functioning autism, *MFA* medium-functioning autism, *HFA* high-functioning autism

38%. However, logistic regression did not find a significant association between Se status and ASD (De Palma et al. 2012).

Our previous study also demonstrated a significant 31% ($p < 0.001$) increase in hair Se levels in children with ASD as compared to healthy controls. It has also been noted that age significantly affects Se metabolism in autistic children. In particular, no significant difference in hair Se levels was detected in ASD children aged 2–4 years (0.362 (0.306–0.407) μg/g vs. 0.319 (0.208–0.412) μg/g, $p = 0.205$). At the same time, in an elder group of autistic children hair Se levels were found to be 45% higher as compared to the control values (0.367 (0.315–0.447) μg/g vs. 0.253 (0.200–0.339) μg/g, $p < 0.001$) (Skalny et al. 2017a). Similarly, comparative analysis of hair Se levels in children with communication disorders and ASD demonstrated the significant disturbance of Se status in the elder group. In particular, children with communication disorders and ASD aged 5–8 years were characterized by a 97% and 77% increase in hair Se levels as compared to the respective control values (0.451 (0.347–0.676) μg/g and 0.406 (0.253–0.437) μg/g vs. 0.229 (0.191–0.304) μg/g) (Skalny et al. 2017d).

Further, we have assessed the relationship between hair and serum Se levels in children suffering from ASD (Skalny et al. 2017b). During the examination of 70 children with ASD aged 2–10 years and the respective number of age- and gender-matched controls it has been revealed that a significant 12% increase in hair Se levels ($p = 0.013$) was not accompanied by elevation of serum Se concentrations ($p = 0.385$). Further analysis demonstrated that age significantly affects the relationship between ASD status and Se status. In particular, younger autistic children (2–5 y.o.) were characterized by significantly lower serum Se levels (0.079 mg/L (0.069–0.088) vs. 0.090 (0.077–0.106), $p = 0.015$) but nearly similar hair Se levels as compared to the control values. Oppositely, elder patients' (6–10 y.o.) serum Se levels did not differ significantly from the control group, whereas hair Se content was characterized by 16% elevation as compared to that in healthy children (0.412 μg/g (0.361–0.486) vs. 0.354 (0.261–0.400), $p = 0.003$). The relationship between hair and serum Se levels was also ASD specific. In particular, no significant correlation between hair and serum Se levels was detected in a group of healthy controls

($r = -0.106; p = 0.420$), whereas children with ASD were characterized by a significant direct relationship between Se content in the assessed substrates ($r = 0.405$;
$p = 0.001$), being present in all age and gender groups (Skalny et al. 2017b). Taking
into account the observed direct relationship between hair and serum Se levels in
children with ASD as well as significantly higher hair Se and lower serum Se levels,
we propose that children with ASD are characterized by increased Se loss with hair
that is used as one of the excretory mechanisms (Pyrzyńska 2002).

Despite the presence of multiple studies of Se levels in different substrates in
ASD children, data on the effect of ASD speciation on Se metabolism (as well as
other trace elements) are insufficient. Therefore, we aimed at investigating the association between Se levels and ASD types according to ICD-10: childhood autism
(F84.0) and atypical autism (F84.1). It has been found that serum Se levels in children with childhood and atypical autism were 8% and 12% lower than those in the
control group (Skalny et al. 2017c). Based on ICP-DRC-MS analysis of hair from
35 children with childhood autism, 27 children with atypical autism, and 37 healthy
controls we have examined the relationship between ASD type and hair Se levels. It
has been found that children with childhood and atypical autism were characterized
by a 49% and 37% elevation of hair Se levels as compared to the control values.
Another study dealing with ASD types did not reveal any significant difference in
RBC Se levels between healthy children and those with pervasive developmental
disorder not otherwise specified (PDD-NOS) (Kondolot et al. 2016), a DSM-5 analog for atypical autism in ICD-10. At the same time, Se level in a group of classic
autism exceeded the control values by 28% (Kondolot et al. 2016).

Se Status and Psychiatric Symptoms in ASD Children

A limited number of studies demonstrated that Se status is not only altered in autistic
children but also associated with psychiatric symptoms and disease severity. In particular, both hair and nail Se levels were inversely associated with CARS values
($r = -0.913$ and $r = -0.891$, respectively) (Lakshmi Priya and Geetha 2011). It has
been noted that ASD children with sleep disorders have significantly lower hair Se
levels as compared to autistic children without sleep disorders (0.99 vs. 1.19 ppm)
(Adams et al. 2006). Lower hair Se levels in autistic children were negatively associated with adaptation to changes ($r = -0.303; p = 0.045$) (Blaurock-Busch et al. 2012).

Glutathione Peroxidase in Autism Spectrum Disorder

In parallel with altered Se imbalance in ASD, certain studies have assessed the potential interaction between ASD and selenoproteins with a special focus on GPX. In
particular, Geier et al. (2009) have estimated the prevalence of low GPX activity
(lower than the reference range) in children with ASD as 35.7% (Geier et al. 2009). A
significant ($p < 0.005$) reduction in GPX activity was observed in ASD children

(19.17 ± 1.16) as compared to the control values (24.81 ± 1.19) irrespectively of the age of examinees (<6 and >6 y.o.) (Meguid et al. 2011). Similar findings were obtained in a Hungarian study (László et al. 2013). Correspondingly, a study involving 45 autistic children and 41 controls from Turkey demonstrated significantly reduced both erythrocyte (28.72 ± 2.64 U/g Hb vs. 38.01 ± 5.03 U/g Hb) and plasma (0.27 ± 0.04 U/g Hb vs. 0.39 ± 0.08 U/g Hb) GPX activities in ASD (Yorbik et al. 2002).

It has also been noted that plasma GPX activity significantly ($p < 0.001$) decreased in children with mild-to-moderate autism (456.50 nmol/min/mL) and severe autism (381.00 nmol/min/mL) as compared to the healthy controls (589 nmol/min/mL). Moreover, GPX activity was related to neuronal autoimmunity, being higher in antineuronal positive children and those with a family history of autoimmunity (406.00 vs. 450.50) (Mostafa et al. 2010).

The results of meta-analysis demonstrated that low GPX activity was detected in 18% of children suffering from ASD (Frustaci et al. 2012). These findings are generally in agreement with the indication of reduced glutathione (GSH)/oxidized glutathione (GSSG) levels in the cerebellum (52.8%) and temporal cortex (60.8%) of children with ASD, being indicative of the altered GSSG reduction, being catalyzed by GPX (Chauhan et al. 2012). It has also been demonstrated that GSH-to-GSSG ratio is a significant negative predictor of glutamate-to-glutamine ratio in autistic children (El-Ansary 2016), being indicative of the potential role of GPX in neuroinflammation.

At the same time, certain studies did not corroborate to the observations of decreased GPX activity in ASD. In particular, Paşca et al. (2006) did not reveal any significant differences in serum GPX levels between ASD and neurotypical children (7.45 ± 0.65 vs. 7.75 ± 0.93 U/g Hb), whereas GPX activity was characterized by a significant negative correlation with homocysteine levels ($r = 0.769$, $p = 0.023$) (Paşca et al. 2006). At the same time, examination of 30 Saudi autistic children aged 3–15 years demonstrated significantly higher plasma GPX activity as compared to the control group (246.88 ± 99.93 vs. 143.85 ± 61.12 U/dL) (Al-Gadani et al. 2009). Correspondingly, Söğüt et al. (2003) also revealed significantly elevated plasma GPX activity in Turkish children with ASD as compared to healthy controls (40.9 ± 11.3 vs. 24.2 ± 6.3 U/L, $p < 0.0001$) (Söğüt et al. 2003).

It is also notable that examination of GCG repeat polymorphism of a human GPX1 polyalanine repeat (ALA5, ALA6, and ALA7) demonstrated that ALA6 allele might be protective against ASD (Ming et al. 2010).

Potential Targets of Protective Effects of Selenium in ASD

In general, reported effects of Se in the brain are predominantly mediated by its role in the SELENOProteins, especially the antioxidave enzymes, GPX, thioredoxin reductases (TXNRD) and selenoprotein P (SELENOP) (Steinbrenner and Sies 2013), and methionine sulfoxide reductase B (Scharpf et al. 2007). Therefore, reduced brain Se bioavailability results in increased susceptibility to oxidative stress, which may lead to neuronal dysfunction (Steinbrenner and Sies 2013). It is also notable that expression of SELENOProtein W gene in amygdala changed significantly in a rat model of valproic acid-induced autism (Oguchi-Katayama et al. 2013). At the same time, the GPX activity in various brain regions was relatively unaffected by intraventricular infusions of propionic acid in experimental autism model (MacFabe et al. 2008). And it is still unknown whether the deficiency of one or more selenoprotein(s) contributes to the brain damage in ASD (Raymond et al. 2014; Schweizer and Seeher 2015).

Oxidative stress has been reported to play a significant role in ASD (Chauhan and Chauhan 2006), linking together mitochondrial dysfunction, immune dysfunction, and inflammation (Rossignol and Frye 2014). Therefore, Se-mediated modulation of oxidative stress may be considered as the key mechanisms of the proposed neuroprotective effect of Se in ASD. In particular, it has been demonstrated that Se treatment alleviates oxidative stress through modulation of antioxidant activity and cytosolic Ca^{2+} influx in neuronal cells (Demirci et al. 2013). Correspondingly, Se deficiency was shown to be associated with brain protein oxidation (Moskovitz and Stadtman 2003). These data are in agreement with the mitigating role of Se in H_2O_2-induced oxidative stress and apoptosis. These effects were associated with Se-induced inhibition of activation of c-jun N-terminal protein kinase (JNK)/P38 mitogen-activated protein kinase (MAPK), and Akt pathways (Yeo and Kang 2007). These findings are generally in agreement with the redox methylation hypothesis of ASD (Deth et al. 2014).

As stated earlier, numerous pollutants including persistent organic pollutants (POPs) and heavy metal exposure appear to play a significant role in ASD development. It is reasonable that one of the protective effects of Se in ASD may be related to prevention of heavy metal toxicity (Sikarwar et al. 2015). In particular, it has been demonstrated that Se significantly reduces Pb (Wang et al. 2013) and mercury neurotoxicity (Choi et al. 2008; Bjørklund et al. 2017) that has been hypothesized to play a causative role in ASD development (Currenti 2010; Kern et al. 2016; Bjørklund et al. 2018). Certain indications of the antagonistic effects of Se and POPs exist (Twaroski et al. 2001; Ravoori et al. 2010), although it is unclear whether Se will be effective in alleviating the neurotoxicity of POPs.

Altered gut microbiota is also presumed to play a significant role in ASD pathogenesis (Li and Zhou 2016), resulting in alteration of the gut-brain axis (Mayer et al. 2014). Moreover, microbiota transfer therapy significantly improved ASD symptoms. In particular, fecal microbiota transplantation after a 2-week course of antibiotic treatment in autistic children aged 7–16 years resulted in increased *Bifidobacterium*, *Prevotella*, and *Desulfovibrio* population, being accompanied by a reduction of gastrointestinal and behavioral symptoms of ASD (Kang et al. 2017). Certain studies have demonstrated a significant interplay between Se metabolism and gut microbiota. In particular, it has been demonstrated that Se deficiency results in decreased Firmicutes, Actinobacteria, and Proteobacteria population, whereas Bacteroides, as well as Bacteroides-to-Firmicutes ratio, are increased under Se deprivation (Lu et al. 2015, 2016). Hypothetically, such changes in bacterial populations may be associated with LPS overproduction and translocation with further development of the inflammatory milieu. It has also been noted that high-Se treatment results in increased Bifidobacteria population (Taussig and Combs 2015). Moreover, under Se-deficient conditions gut microbiota may compete for Se with the host (Hrdina et al. 2009). Correspondingly, it has been demonstrated that gut microbiota significantly modifies the effect of Se on host selenoproteome expression (Kasaikina et al. 2011).

In line with the effects of Se on gut microbiota, Se may also significantly modify LPS-induced inflammatory pathways. In particular, Se was proposed to be protective against endotoxinemia, through modulation of p38 MAPK and NF-κB (Kim et al. 2004). Correspondingly, pretreatment of mice with organoselenium compound (3-((4-chlorophenyl)selanyl)-1-methyl-1H-indole) resulted in a reduction of LPS-induced neuroinflammation through reduction of IL-1β, IL-4, and IL-6 levels as well as oxidative stress in the hippocampus and prefrontal cortex (Casaril et al. 2017). Another Se donor, selol, also prevented LPS-induced increase of TNFa, IL-6, and IFN-y through upregulation of antioxidant enzymes, including the selenoproteins GPX and TXNRD (Dominiak et al. 2017). Selenium (as 5-chloroacetyl-2-amino-1,3-selenazoles) was also shown to reduce LPS-induced microglia activation via inhibition of NF-kB signaling (Nam et al. 2008). Selenium-induced inhibition of microglial activation was also demonstrated in a model of streptozotocin toxicity. In particular, p,p′-methoxy-diphenyl diselenide treatment inhibited microglia activation and astrogliosis, reduced neuronal apoptosis, as well as prevented dendrite and synapse damage (Pinton et al. 2013). It is also notable that Se-enriched products were shown to reduce intestinal permeability (Maseko et al. 2014), thus inhibiting LPS and bacterial translocation and reducing proinflammatory signaling.

Excitotoxicity is considered as one of the key mechanisms underlying neuronal dysfunction in ASD (Essa et al. 2013). It has been demonstrated that Se treatment prevents glutamate-induced cytotoxicity in neuronal HT22 cells. Moreover, Se ameliorated glutamate-induced upregulation of autophagy markers, Beclin 1 and LC3-II (Kumari et al. 2012). These data are in agreement with the earlier indication of the efficiency of ebselen in the prevention of glutamate-induced neuronal death and oxidative stress (Porciúncula et al. 2001). It has also been demonstrated that Se prevents apoptotic signaling and NF-κB activation in a model of quinolinate-induced excitotoxicity (Santamaría et al. 2003, 2005). It has been proposed that the protective effect of Se against quinolinate neurotoxicity is mediated through modulation of Txn/Txnrd system (Maldonado 2012). These findings are in agreement with the earlier observation by Savaskan et al. (2003) who reported that the neuroprotective effect of Se is mediated through inhibition of glutamate-induced NF-kB and AP-1 upregulation, whereas Se deficiency significantly increases susceptibility to glutamate-induced excitotoxicity (Savaskan et al. 2003). It has also been demonstrated that ebselen, but not diphenyl diselenide (PhSe)$_2$ or diphenyl ditelluride (PhTe)$_2$, treatment significantly inhibited glutamate release by brain synaptosomes (Nogueira et al. 2002).

Synaptic dysfunction was also shown to play a significant role in ASD pathogenesis (Bourgeron 2015). In turn, adequate nutritional Se supply is required for synaptic membrane synthesis (Cansev et al. 2017) due to Se-induced increase in Kennedy pathways' key enzyme activity (van Wijk et al. 2013). It has also been shown that SELENOP is essential for hippocampal synaptic function (Peters et al. 2006). It has been demonstrated that Se prevents negative effects of Pb exposure on synaptic morphology, resulting in increased synaptic active zone, higher thickness of post-synaptic density, as well as smaller synaptic cleft (Han et al. 2013). Similar findings were made in a model of fluoride toxicity, with postsynaptic density-93 (PSD-93) expression as the key factor for fluoride toxicity and Se neuroprotection (Qian et al. 2013). Moreover, Se treatment also resulted in a significant increase in the number of neurons and synapses in Pb-exposed animals (Han et al. 2014). It is also notable that Se-enriched yeast was also effective in the prevention of synaptic dysfunction in a murine model of Alzheimer's disease (Zhang et al. 2017).

Therefore, it is expected that Se may possess neuroprotective effects in ASD due to its inhibition of oxidative stress, neuroinflammation, microglia activation, excito-toxicity, synapse dysfunction, and gut-brain axis disturbance. However, further studies are required to highlight the mechanisms of the potential neuroprotective effects of Se in ASD as well as its efficiency in clinical trials.

Acknowledgments The current investigation is supported by the Russian Foundation for Basic Research within project № 18-315-00103.

Conflict of Interest The authors declare no conflict of interest.

References

Adams JB. Summary of biomedical treatments for autism. ARI Publication. 2007;40.
Adams JB. Vitamin/Mineral Supplements for Children and Adults with. Autism Vitam Miner. 2015;3(127):2376–1318. https://doi.org/10.4172/2376-1318.1000127.
Adams JB, Holloway CE, George F, Quig D. Analyses of toxic metals and essential minerals in the hair of Arizona children with autism and associated conditions, and their mothers. Boil Trace Elem Res. 2006;110(3):193–209. https://doi.org/10.1385/BTER:110:3:193.
Adams JB, Audhya T, McDonough-Means S, Rubin RA, Quig D, Geis E, Gehn E, Loresto M, Mitchell J, Atwood S, Barnhouse S. Nutritional and metabolic status of children with autism vs. neurotypical children, and the association with autism severity. Nutr Metab. 2011;8(1):34. https://doi.org/10.1186/1743-7075-8-34.
Al-Gadani Y, El-Ansary A, Attas O, Al-Ayadhi L. Metabolic biomarkers related to oxidative stress and antioxidant status in Saudi autistic children. Clin Biochem. 2009;42(10):1032–40. https://doi.org/10.1016/j.clinbiochem.2009.03.011.
Baio J, et al. Centers for Disease Control and Prevention. Prevalence of autism spectrum disorders: autism and developmental disabilities monitoring network, 14 sites, United States, 2008. MMWR Surveill Summ. 2012;61(3):1–19.
Barnhill K, Ramirez L, Gutierrez A, Richardson W, Marti CN, Potts A, Shearer R, Schutte C, Hewitson L. Bone mineral density in boys diagnosed with autism spectrum disorder: a case-control study. J Autism Dev Disord. 2017;47(11):3608–19. https://doi.org/10.1007/s10803-017-3277-z.
Bjørklund G, Saad K, Chirumbolo S, Kern JK, Geier DA, Geier MR, Urbina MA. Immune dysfunction and neuroinflammation in autism spectrum disorder. Acta Neurobiol Exp. 2016;76:257–68.
Bjørklund G, Aaseth J, Ajsuvakova OP, Nikonorov AA, Skalny AV, Skalnaya MG, Tinkov AA. Molecular interaction between mercury and selenium in neurotoxicity. Coord Chem Rev. 2017;332:30–37.

Bjørklund G, Skalny AV, Rahman MM, Dadar M, Yassa HA, Aaseth J, Skalnaya MG, Tinkov AA. Toxic metal (loid)-based pollutants and their possible role in autism spectrum disorder. Environ Res. 2018;166:234–50.

Blaurock-Busch E, Amin OR, Rabah T. Heavy metals and trace elements in hair and urine of a sample of arab children with autistic spectrum disorder. Maedica. 2011;6:247.

Blaurock-Busch E, Amin OR, Dessoki HH, Rabah T. Toxic metals and essential elements in hair and severity of symptoms among children with autism. Maedica. 2012;7(1):38.

Blenner S, Reddy A, Augustyn M. Diagnosis and management of autism in childhood. BMJ. 2011;343:d6238. https://doi.org/10.1136/bmj.d6238.

Bourgeron T. From the genetic architecture to synaptic plasticity in autism spectrum disorder. Nat Rev Neurosci. 2015;16(9):551–63. https://doi.org/10.1038/nrn3992.

Boyle CA, Boulet S, Schieve LA, Cohen RA, Blumberg SJ, Yeargin-Allsopp M, Visser S, Kogan MD. Trends in the prevalence of developmental disabilities in US children, 1997–2008. Pediatrics. 2011;127(6):1034–42. https://doi.org/10.1542/peds.2010-2989.

Cansev M, Turkyilmaz M, Sijben JW, Sevinc C, Broersen LM, van Wijk N. Synaptic membrane synthesis in rats depends on dietary sufficiency of vitamin C, vitamin E, and selenium: relevance for Alzheimer's disease. J Alzheimers Dis. 2017;59(1):301–11. https://doi.org/10.3233/JAD-170081.

Casaril AM, Domingues M, Fronza M, Vieira B, Begnini K, Lenardão EJ, Seixas FK, Collares T, Nogueira CW, Savegnago L. Antidepressant-like effect of a new selenium-containing compound is accompanied by a reduction of neuroinflammation and oxidative stress in lipopolysaccharide-challenged mice. J Psychopharmacol. 2017;31(9):1263–73. https://doi.org/10.1177/0269881117711713.

CDC. Summary of Autism Spectrum Disorder (ASD) Prevalence Studies 2016. https://www.cdc.gov/ncbddd/autism/documents/ASDPrevalenceDataTable2016.pdf. Accessed 17 Nov 2017.

Charron R. Autism Rates across the Developed World. 2017. https://www.focusforhealth.org/autism-rates-across-the-developed-world/. Accessed 17 Nov 2017.

Chauhan A, Chauhan V. Oxidative stress in autism. Pathophysiology. 2006;13(3):171–81. https://doi.org/10.1016/j.pathophys.2006.05.007.

Chauhan A, Audhya T, Chauhan V. Brain region-specific glutathione redox imbalance in autism. Neurochem Res. 2012;37(8):1681–9. https://doi.org/10.1007/s11064-012-0775-4.

Choi AL, Budtz-Jørgensen E, Jørgensen PJ, Steuerwald U, Debes F, Weihe P, Grandjean P. Selenium as a potential protective factor against mercury developmental neurotoxicity. Environ Res. 2008;107(1):45–52.

Christensen DL, Baio J, Van Naarden Braun K, Bilder D, Charles J, Constantino JN, Daniels J, Durkin MS, Fitzgerald RT, Kurzius-Spencer M, Lee LC, Pettygrove S, Robinson C, Schulz E, Wells C, Wingate MS, Zahorodny W, Yeargin-Allsopp M, Centers for Disease Control and Prevention (CDC). Prevalence and characteristics of autism spectrum disorder among children aged 8 years—Autism and developmental disabilities monitoring network, 11 Sites, United States, 2012. MMWR Surveill Summ. 2016;65(3):1–23. https://doi.org/10.15585/mmwr.ss6503a1.

Crăciun EC, Bjørklund G, Tinkov AA, Urbina MA, Skalny AV, Rad F, Dronca E. Evaluation of whole blood zinc and copper levels in children with autism spectrum disorder. Metab Brain Dis. 2016;31(4):887–90. https://doi.org/10.1007/s11011-016-9823-0.

Currenti SA. Understanding and determining the etiology of autism. Cell Mol Neurobiol. 2010;30(2):161–71.

De Palma G, Catalani S, Franco A, Brighenti M, Apostoli P. Lack of correlation between metallic elements analyzed in hair by ICP-MS and autism. J Autism Dev Disord. 2012;42(3):342–53. https://doi.org/10.1007/s10803-011-1245-6.

Demirci S, Kutluhan S, Nazıroğlu M, Uğuz AC, Yürekli VA, Demirci K. Effects of selenium and topiramate on cytosolic Ca2+ influx and oxidative stress in neuronal PC12 cells. Neurochem Res. 2013;38(1):90–7. https://doi.org/10.1007/s11064-012-0893-z.

Deth R, Trivedi MS, Hodgson NW, Muratore CR, Waly MI. Redox/methylation theory and autism. In: Comprehensive guide to autism. New York: Springer; 2014. p. 1389–410. https://doi.org/10.1007/978-1-4614-4788-7_78.

Dominiak A, Wilkaniec A, Jęśko H, Czapski GA, Lenkiewicz AM, Kurek E, Wroczyński P, Adamczyk A. Selol, an organic selenium donor, prevents lipopolysaccharide-induced oxidative stress and inflammatory reaction in the rat brain. Neurochem Int. 2017;108:66–77. https://doi.org/10.1016/j.neuint.2017.02.014.

Durkin MS, Maenner MJ, Newschaffer CJ, Lee LC, Cunniff CM, Daniels JL, Kirby RS, Leavitt L, Miller L, Zahorodny W, Schieve LA. Advanced parental age and the risk of autism spectrum disorder. Am J Epidemiol. 2008;168(11):1268–76. https://doi.org/10.1093/aje/kwn250.

Durkin MS, Maenner MJ, Meaney FJ, Levy SE, DiGuiseppi C, Nicholas JS, Kirby RS, Pinto-Martin JA, Schieve LA. Socioeconomic inequality in the prevalence of autism spectrum disorder: evidence from a U.S. cross-sectional study. PLoS One. 2010;5(7):e11551. https://doi.org/10.1371/journal.pone.0011551.

El-Ansary A. Data of multiple regressions analysis between selected biomarkers related to glutamate excitotoxicity and oxidative stress in Saudi autistic patients. Data Brief. 2016;7:111–6. https://doi.org/10.1016/j.dib.2016.02.025.

El-Ansary A, Bjørklund G, Tinkov AA, Skalny AV, Al Dera H. Relationship between selenium, lead, and mercury in red blood cells of Saudi autistic children. Metab Brain Dis. 2017;32(4):1073–80. https://doi.org/10.1007/s11011-017-9996-1.

Essa MM, Braidy N, Vijayan KR, Subash S, Guillemin GJ. Excitotoxicity in the pathogenesis of autism. Neurotox Res. 2013;23(4):393–400. https://doi.org/10.1007/s12640-012-9354-3.

Frustaci A, Neri M, Cesario A, Adams JB, Domenici E, Dalla Bernardina B, Bonassi S. Oxidative stress-related biomarkers in autism: systematic review and meta-analyses. Free Radical Bio Med. 2012;52(10):2128–41. https://doi.org/10.1016/j.freeradbiomed.2012.03.011.

Geier DA, Kern JK, Geier MA. A prospective study of oxidative stress biomarkers in autistic disorders. E-J Appl Phychol. 2009;5(1)

Geraghty ME, Bates-Wall J, Ratliff-Schaub K, Lane AE. Nutritional interventions and therapies in autism: a spectrum of what we know: Part 2. ICAN: Infant, Child, & Adolescent Nutrition. 2010;2(2):120–33. https://doi.org/10.1177/1941406410366848.

Gillberg C, Wing L. Autism: not an extremely rare disorder. Acta Psychiatr Scand. 1999;99:399–406. https://doi.org/10.1111/j.1600-0447.1999.tb00984.x.

Han XJ, Hu XX, Wei Q, Yu DE, Chen YL, Hu QS. Effect of lead and selenium on synaptic structural parameters in the hippocampus of Wistar rats. Chin J Health Lab Technol. 2013;13:012.

Han XJ, Xiao YM, Ai BM, Hu XX, Wei Q, Hu QS. Effects of organic selenium on lead-induced impairments of spatial learning and memory as well as synaptic structural plasticity in rats. Biol Pharm Bull. 2014;37(3):466–74. https://doi.org/10.1248/bpb.b13-00892.

Herndon AC, DiGuiseppi C, Johnson SL, Leiferman J, Reynolds A. Does nutritional intake differ between children with autism spectrum disorders and children with typical development? J Autism Dev Disord. 2009;39:212. https://doi.org/10.1007/s10803-008-0606-2.

Hrdina J, Banning A, Kipp A, Loh G, Blaut M, Brigelius-Flohé R. The gastrointestinal microbiota affects the selenium status and SELENOProtein expression in mice. J Nutr Biochem. 2009;20(8):638–48. https://doi.org/10.1016/j.jnutbio.2008.06.009.

Hyman SL, Stewart PA, Schmidt B, Lemcke N, Foley JT, Peck R, Clemons T, Reynolds A, Johnson C, Handen B, James SJ. Nutrient intake from food in children with autism. Pediatrics. 2012;130(Supplement 2):S145–53. https://doi.org/10.1542/peds.2012-0900L.

Johnson CR, Handen BL, Mayer-Costa M, Sacco K. Eating habits and dietary status in young children with autism. J Dev Phys Disabil. 2008;20(5):437–48. https://doi.org/10.1007/s10882-008-9111-y.

Jory J, McGinnis WR. Red-cell trace minerals in children with autism. Am J Biochem Biotechnol. 2008;4(2):101–4.

Kang DW, Adams JB, Gregory AC, Borody T, Chittick L, Fasano A, Khoruts A, Geis E, Maldonado J, McDonough-Means S, Pollard EL. Microbiota Transfer Therapy alters gut ecosystem and improves gastrointestinal and autism symptoms: an open-label study. Microbiome. 2017;5(1):10. https://doi.org/10.1186/s40168-016-0225-7.

Kasaikina MV, Kravtsova MA, Lee BC, Seravalli J, Peterson DA, Walter J, Legge R, Benson AK, Hatfield DL, Gladyshev VN. Dietary selenium affects host SELENOProteome expression by influencing the gut microbiota. FASEB J. 2011;25(7):2492–9. https://doi.org/10.1096/fj.11-181990.

Kern JK, Geier DA, Sykes LK, Haley BE, Geier MR. The relationship between mercury and autism: A comprehensive review and discussion. J Trace Elem Med Biol. 2016;37:8–24.

Kim SH, Johnson VJ, Shin TY, Sharma RP. Selenium attenuates lipopolysaccharide-induced oxidative stress responses through modulation of p38 MAPK and NF-κB signaling pathways. Exp Biol M. 2004;229(2):203–13. https://doi.org/10.1177/153537020422900209.

Kim YS, Leventhal BL, Koh YJ, Fombonne E, Laska E, Lim EC, Cheon KA, Kim SJ, Kim YK, Lee H, Song DH, Grinker RR. Prevalence of autism spectrum disorders in a total population sample. Am J Psychiatry. 2011;168(9):904–12. https://doi.org/10.1176/appi.ajp.2011.10101532.

Kondolot M, Ozmert EN, Ascı A, Erkekoglu P, Oztop DB, Gumus H, Kocer-Gumusel B, Yurdakok K. Plasma phthalate and bisphenol a levels and oxidant-antioxidant status in autistic children. Environ Toxicol Pharmacol. 2016;43:149–58. https://doi.org/10.1016/j.etap.2016.03.006.

Kumari S, Mehta SL, Li PA. Glutamate induces mitochondrial dynamic imbalance and autophagy activation: preventive effects of selenium. PLoS One. 2012;7(6):e39382. https://doi.org/10.1371/journal.pone.0039382.

László A, Novák Z, Szőllősi-Varga I, Hai DQ, Vetro A, Kovacs A. Blood lipid peroxidation, antioxidant enzyme activities and hemorheological changes in autistic children. Ideggyogy Szemle. 2013;66(1–2):23–8.

Levy SE, Giarelli E, Lee LC, Schieve LA, Kirby RS, Cunniff C, Nicholas J, Reaven J, Rice CE. Autism spectrum disorder and co-occurring developmental, psychiatric, and medical conditions among children in multiple populations of the United States. J Dev Behav Pediatr. 2010;31(4):267–75. https://doi.org/10.1097/DBP.0b013e3181d5d03b.

Li Q, Zhou JM. The microbiota–gut–brain axis and its potential therapeutic role in autism spectrum disorder. Neuroscience. 2016;324:131–9. https://doi.org/10.1016/j.neuroscience.2016.03.013.

Lindsay RL, Eugene Arnold L, Aman MG, Vitiello B, Posey DJ, McDougle CJ, Scahill L, Pachler M, McCracken JT, Tierney E, Bozzolo D. Dietary status and impact of risperidone on nutritional balance in children with autism: a pilot study. J Intellect Develop Disabil. 2006;31(4):204–9. https://doi.org/10.1080/13668250601006924.

Lu HY, Wu R, Cheng WH. Effect of Long-Term Dietary Selenium Deprivation and Aging on Gut Microbiota in Short Telomere Mice. FASEB J. 2015;29(1 Supplement):759–10.

Lu HY, Wu RT, Cheng WH. Sex Differences in the Responses of Gut Microbiome to Long-term Dietary Selenium Deprivation and Aging in Short Telomere Mice. FASEB J. 2016;30(1 Supplement):1170–9.

Lubkowska A, Sobieraj W. Concentrations of magnesium, calcium, iron, selenium, zinc and copper in the hair of autistic children. Trace Elem Electroly. 2009;26(2)

Macedoni-Lukšič M, Gosar D, Bjørklund G, Oražem J, Kodrič J, Lešnik-Musek P, Zupančič M, France-Štiglic A, Sešek-Briški A, Neubauer D, Osredkar J. Levels of metals in the blood and specific porphyrins in the urine in children with autism spectrum disorders. Biol Trace Elem Res. 2015;163(1–2):2–10. https://doi.org/10.1007/s12011-014-0121-6.

MacFabe DF, Rodríguez-Capote K, Hoffman JE, Franklin AE, Mohammad-Asef Y, Taylor A, Boon F, Cain DP, Kavaliers M, Possmayer F, Ossenkopp KP. A novel rodent model of autism: intraventricular infusions of propionic acid increase locomotor activity and induce neuroinflammation and oxidative stress in discrete regions of adult rat brain. Am J Biochem Biotechnol. 2008;4(2):146–66.

Maldonado PD. Pérez-De La Cruz V, Torres-Ramos M, Silva-Islas C, Lecona-Vargas R, Lugo-Huitrón R, Blanco-Ayala T, Ugalde-Muñiz P, Vázquez-Cervantes GI, Fortoul TI, Ali SF. Selenium-induced antioxidant protection recruits modulation of thioredoxin reductase during excitotoxic/pro-oxidant events in the rat striatum. Neurochem Int. 2012;61(2):195–206. https://doi.org/10.1016/j.neuint.2012.05.004.

Maseko T, Dunshea FR, Howell K, Cho HJ, Rivera LR, Furness JB, Ng K. Selenium-enriched Agaricus bisporus mushroom protects against increase in gut permeability ex vivo and up-regulates glutathione peroxidase 1 and 2 in hyperthermally-induced oxidative stress in rats. Nutrients. 2014;6(6):2478–92. https://doi.org/10.3390/nu6062478.

Matelski L, Van de Water J. Risk factors in autism: thinking outside the brain. J Autoimmun. 2016;67:1–7. https://doi.org/10.1016/j.jaut.2015.11.003.

Mayer EA, Padua D, Tillisch K. Altered brain-gut axis in autism: comorbidity or causative mechanisms? BioEssays. 2014;36(10):933–9. https://doi.org/10.1002/bies.201400075.

Meguid NA, Dardir AA, Abdel-Raouf ER, Hashish A. Evaluation of oxidative stress in autism: defective antioxidant enzymes and increased lipid peroxidation. Biol Trace Elem Res. 2011;143(1):58–65. https://doi.org/10.1007/s12011-010-8840-9.

Meguid NA, Anwar M, Bjørklund G, Hashish A, Chirumbolo S, Hemimi M, Sultan E. Dietary adequacy of Egyptian children with autism spectrum disorder compared to healthy developing children. Metab Brain Dis. 2017;32(2):607–15. https://doi.org/10.1007/s11011-016-9948-1.

Mehl-Madrona L, Leung B, Kennedy C, Paul S, Kaplan BJ. Micronutrients versus standard medication management in autism: a naturalistic case–control study. J Child Adol Psychop. 2010;20(2):95–103. https://doi.org/10.1089/cap.2009.0011.

Ming X, Johnson WG, Stenroos ES, Mars A, Lambert GH, Buyske S. Genetic variant of glutathione peroxidase 1 in autism. Brain Dev-Jpn. 2010;32(2):105–9. https://doi.org/10.1016/j.braindev.2008.12.017.

Moskovitz J, Stadtman ER. Selenium-deficient diet enhances protein oxidation and affects methionine sulfoxide reductase (MsrB) protein level in certain mouse tissues. Proc Natl Acad Sci. 2003;100(13):7486–90. https://doi.org/10.1073/pnas.1332607100.

Mostafa GA, El-Hadidi ES, Hewedi DH, Abdou MM. Oxidative stress in Egyptian children with autism: relation to autoimmunity. J Neuroimmunol. 2010;219(1):114–8. https://doi.org/10.1016/j.jneuroim.2009.12.003.

Nam KN, Koketsu M, Lee EH. 5-Chloroacetyl-2-amino-1, 3-selenazoles attenuate microglial inflammatory responses through NF-κB inhibition. Eur J Pharmacol. 2008;589(1):53–7. https://doi.org/10.1016/j.ejphar.2008.03.034.

Nogueira CW, Rotta LN, Zeni G, Souza DO, Rocha JB. Exposure to ebselen changes glutamate uptake and release by rat brain synaptosomes. Neurochem Res. 2002;27(4):283–8. https://doi.org/10.1023/A:1014903127672.

Oguchi-Katayama A, Monma A, Sekino Y, Moriguchi T, Sato K. Comparative gene expression analysis of the amygdala in autistic rat models produced by pre-and post-natal exposures to valproic acid. J Toxicol Sci. 2013;38(3):391–402. https://doi.org/10.2131/jts.38.391.

Ozonoff S, Young GS, Carter A, Messinger D, Yirmiya N, Zwaigenbaum L, Bryson S, Carver LJ, Constantino JN, Dobkins K, Hutman T, Iverson JM, Landa R, Rogers SJ, Sigman M, Stone WL. Recurrence risk for autism spectrum disorders: a baby siblings research consortium study. Pediatrics. 2011;128:e488–95. https://doi.org/10.1542/peds.2010-2825.

Paşca SP, Nemeş B, Vlase L, Gagyi CE, Dronca E, Miu AC, Dronca M. High levels of homocysteine and low serum paraoxonase 1 arylesterase activity in children with autism. Life Sci. 2006;78(19):2244–8. https://doi.org/10.1016/j.lfs.2005.09.040.

Patel K, Curtis LT. A comprehensive approach to treating autism and attention-deficit hyperactivity disorder: a prepilot study. J Altern Complement Med. 2007;13(10):1091–8. https://doi.org/10.1089/acm.2007.0611.

Peters MM, Hill KE, Burk RF, Weeber EJ. Altered hippocampus synaptic function in SELENOProtein P deficient mice. Mol Neurodegener. 2006;1(1):12. https://doi.org/10.1186/1750-1326-1-12.

Pinton S, Sampaio TB, Ramalho RM, Rodrigues CM, Nogueira CW. p, p′-Methoxyl-diphenyl diselenide prevents neurodegeneration and glial cell activation induced by streptozotocin in rats. J Alzheimers Dis. 2013;33(1):133–44. https://doi.org/10.3233/JAD-2012-121150.

Porciúncula LO, Rocha JB, Boeck CR, Vendite D, Souza DO. Ebselen prevents excitotoxicity provoked by glutamate in rat cerebellar granule neurons. Neurosci Lett. 2001;299(3):217–20. https://doi.org/10.1016/S0304-3940(01)01519-1.

Priya MD, Geetha A. Level of trace elements (copper, zinc, magnesium and selenium) and toxic elements (lead and mercury) in the hair and nail of children with autism. Biol Trace Elem Res. 2011;142(2):148–58. https://doi.org/10.1007/s12011-010-8766-2.

Pyrzyńska K. Determination of selenium species in environmental samples. Microchim Acta. 2002;140(1):55–62. https://doi.org/10.1007/s00604-001-0899-8.

Qian W, Miao K, Li T, Zhang Z. Effect of selenium on fluoride-induced changes in synaptic plasticity in rat hippocampus. Biol Trace Elem Res. 2013;155(2):253–60. https://doi.org/10.1007/s12011-013-9773-x.

Ravoori S, Srinivasan C, Pereg D, Robertson LW, Ayotte P, Gupta RC. Protective effects of selenium against DNA adduct formation in Inuit environmentally exposed to PCBs. Environ Int. 2010;36(8):980–86.

Raymond LJ, Deth RC, Ralston NV. Potential role of selenoenzymes and antioxidant metabolism in relation to autism etiology and pathology. Autism Res Treat. 2014;164938 https://doi.org/10.1155/2014/164938.

Reich HJ, Hondal RJ. Why nature chose selenium. ACS Chem Biol. 2016;11(4):821–41. https://doi.org/10.1021/acschembio.6b00031.

Robson B. A naturopathic approach to the treatment of children with autism spectrum disorder: combining clinical practicalities and theoretical strategies. Aust J Herb Med. 2013;25(4):172.

Rossignol DA. Novel and emerging treatments for autism spectrum disorders: a systematic review. Ann Clin Psychiatry. 2009;21(4):213–36.

Rossignol DA, Frye RE. Evidence linking oxidative stress, mitochondrial dysfunction, and inflammation in the brain of individuals with autism. Front Physiol. 2014;5 https://doi.org/10.3389/fphys.2014.00150.

Saghazadeh A, Ahangari N, Hendi K, Saleh F, Rezaei N. Status of essential elements in autism spectrum disorder: systematic review and meta-analysis. Rev Neurosci. 2017;28(7):783–809. https://doi.org/10.1515/revneuro-2017-0015.

Sajdel-Sulkowska EM, Lipinski B, Windom H, Audhya T, McGinnis W. Oxidative stress in autism: elevated cerebellar 3-nitrotyrosine levels. Am J Biochem Biotechnol. 2008;4:73–84.

Santamaría A, Salvatierra-Sánchez R, Vázquez-Román B, Santiago-López D, Villeda-Hernández J, Galván-Arzate S, Jiménez-Capdeville ME, SF A. Protective effects of the antioxidant selenium on quinolinic acid-induced neurotoxicity in rats: in vitro and in vivo studies. J Neurochem. 2003;86(2):479–88. https://doi.org/10.1046/j.1471-4159.2003.01857.x.

Santamaría A, Vázquez-Román B, González-Cortés C, Trejo-Solís M, Galván-Arzate S, Jara-Prado A, Guevara-Fonseca J, Ali SF. Selenium reduces the proapoptotic signaling associated to NF-κB pathway and stimulates glutathione peroxidase activity during excitotoxic damage produced by quinolinate in rat corpus striatum. Synapse. 2005;58(4):258–66. https://doi.org/10.1002/syn.20206.

Sathe N, Andrews JC, McPheeters ML, Warren ZE. Nutritional and dietary interventions for autism spectrum disorder: a systematic review. Pediatrics. 2017;139(6):e20170346. https://doi.org/10.1542/peds.2017-0346.

Savaskan NE, Bräuer AU, Kühbacher M, Eyüpoglu IY, Kyriakopoulos A, Ninnemann O, Behne D, Nitsch R. Selenium deficiency increases susceptibility to glutamate-induced excitotoxicity. FASEB J. 2003;17(1):112–4. https://doi.org/10.1096/fj.02-0067fje.

Scharpf M, Schweizer U, Arzberger T, Roggendorf W, Schomburg L, Köhrle J. Neuronal and ependymal expression of SELENOProtein P in the human brain. J Neural Transm. 2007;114(7):877–84. https://doi.org/10.1007/s00702-006-0617-0.

Schweizer U, Seeher S. SELENOProteins in Brain. In Selenium. 2015. (pp. 479–496).

Sezgin C, Kaya S, Keskin S. Comparison of blood toxic and plasma essential elements of the autistic Turkish infants. FEBS J. 2010;277:88.

Shaw CA, Sheth S, Li D, Tomljenovic L. Etiology of autism spectrum disorders: genes, environment, or both. OA Autism. 2014;2(2):11.

Sikarwar AS, Balakrishnan H, Tong SP, Vien KV, Yoong J, Hao KJ, Chin NS, Xuan KX, Jiayi L, Yee TK. A review of potential metal toxicity and mineral deficiency in autism. Int J Biochem Res Rev. 2015;7:1–12.

Skalny AV. Low Se and elevated hair Mn, Cd: a specific feature for autistic children? Trace Elem Med. 2013;14(4):84.

Skalny AV, Simashkova NV, Klyushnik TP, Grabeklis AR, Bjørklund G, Skalnaya MG, Nikonorov AA, Tinkov AA. Hair toxic and essential trace elements in children with autism spectrum disorder. Metab Brain Dis. 2017a;32(1):195–202. https://doi.org/10.1007/s11011-016-9899-6.

Skalny AV, Simashkova NV, Klyushnik TP, Grabeklis AR, Radysh IV, Skalnaya MG, Tinkov AA. Analysis of hair trace elements in children with autism spectrum disorders and communication disorders. Biol Trace Elem Res. 2017b;177(2):215–23. https://doi.org/10.1007/s12011-016-0878-x.

Skalny AV, Simashkova NV, Klyushnik TP, Grabeklis AR, Radysh IV, Skalnaya MG, Nikonorov AA, Tinkov AA. Assessment of serum trace elements and electrolytes in children with childhood and atypical autism. J Trace Elem Med Biol. 2017c;43:9–14. https://doi.org/10.1016/j.jtemb.2016.09.009.

Skalny AV, Simashkova NV, Skalnaya AA, Klyushnik TP, Bjørklund G, Skalnaya MG, Tinkov AA. Assessment of gender and age effects on serum and hair trace element levels in children with autism spectrum disorder. Metab Brain Dis. 2017d;32(5):1675–84. https://doi.org/10.1007/s11011-017-0056-7.

Söğüt S, Zoroğlu SS, Özyurt H, Yılmaz HR, Özuğurlu F, Sivaslı E, Yetkin Ö, Yanık M, Tutkun H, Savaş HA, Tarakçıoğlu M. Changes in nitric oxide levels and antioxidant enzyme activities may have a role in the pathophysiological mechanisms involved in autism. Clin Chim Acta. 2003;331(1):111–7. https://doi.org/10.1016/S0009-8981(03)00119-0.

Steinbrenner H, Sies H. Selenium homeostasis and antioxidant SELENOProteins in brain: implications for disorders in the central nervous system. Arch Biochem Biophys. 2013;536(2):152–7. https://doi.org/10.1016/j.abb.2013.02.021.

Sumi S, Taniai H, Miyachi T, Tanemura M. Sibling risk of pervasive developmental disorder estimated by means of an epidemiologic survey in Nagoya, Japan. J Hum Genet. 2006;51:518–22. https://doi.org/10.1007/s10038-006-0392-7.

Tabatadze T, Zhorzholiani L, Kherkheulidze M, Kandelaki E, Ivanashvili T. Hair heavy metal and essential trace element concentration in children with autism spectrum disorder. Georgian Med News. 2015;248:77–82.

Taussig D, Combs G Jr. Conditional Effect of Selenium on the Mammalian Hind Gut Microbiota. FASEB J. 2015;29(1 Supplement):759–2.

Tordjman S, Somogyi E, Coulon N, Kermarrec S, Cohen D, Bronsard G, Bonnot O, Weismann-Arcache C, Botbol M, Lauth B, Ginchat V. Gene× Environment interactions in autism spectrum disorders: role of epigenetic mechanisms. Fron Psychiatry. 2014;5 https://doi.org/10.3389/fpsyt.2014.00053.

Twaroski TP, O'Brien ML, Robertson LW. Effects of selected polychlorinated biphenyl (PCB) congeners on hepatic glutathione, glutathione-related enzymes, and selenium status: implications for oxidative stress☆ 1. Biochem pharm. 2001;62(3):273–81.

van Wijk N, Sijben J, de Wilde M, Groenendijk M, Broersen L, Kamphuis P. Enhanced neuronal membrane and synapse formation by nutritional membrane precursors and cofactors. Alzheimers Dement. 2013;9(4):P801–2. https://doi.org/10.1016/j.jalz.2013.05.1657.

Wang M, Fu H, Xiao Y, Ai B, Wei Q, Wang S, Liu T, Ye L, Hu, Q. Effects of low-level organic selenium on leadinduced alterations in neural cell adhesion molecules. Brain Res. 2013; 1530:76–81.

Wong HH, Smith RG. Patterns of complementary and alternative medical therapy use in children diagnosed with autism spectrum disorders. J Autism Dev Disord. 2006;36(7):901–9. https://doi.org/10.1007/s10803-006-0131-0.

Yeo JE, Kang SK. Selenium effectively inhibits ROS-mediated apoptotic neural precursor cell death in vitro and in vivo in traumatic brain injury. BBA-Mol Basis Dis. 2007;1772(11):1199–210. https://doi.org/10.1016/j.bbadis.2007.09.004.

Yorbık Ö, Sayal A, Akay C, Söhmen T. Investigation of antioxidant enzymes and related trace elements in the children with autistic disorder. Turk J Child Adolesc Mental Health. 2000;7:173–81. https://doi.org/10.1054/plef.2002.0439.

Yorbik O, Sayal A, Akay C, Akbiyik DI, Sohmen T. Investigation of antioxidant enzymes in children with autistic disorder. Prostag Leukotr Ess. 2002;67(5):341–3. https://doi.org/10.1054/plef.2002.0439.

Zhang Z, Wen L, Wu Q, Chen C, Zheng R, Liu Q, Ni J, Song GL. Long-term dietary supplementation with selenium-enriched yeast improves cognitive impairment, reverses synaptic deficits and mitigates tau pathology in a triple transgenic mouse model of Alzheimer's disease. J Agric Food Chem. 2017;65(24):4970–9. https://doi.org/10.1021/acs.jafc.7b01465.

Chapter 11
Selenium in Ischemic Stroke

Anatoly V. Skalny, Margarita G. Skalnaya, Lyudmila L. Klimenko,
Aksana N. Mazilina, and Alexey A. Tinkov

Abstract Selenium plays a significant role in brain physiology, whereas data on the role of selenium in stroke pathophysiology are inconsistent. The objective of this chapter is to review current findings on the role of selenium in ischemic stroke. The existing human data demonstrate that stroke is associated with significantly reduced Se levels as well as glutathione peroxidase activity. Oppositely, we have revealed significantly higher serum Se levels in stroke, being inversely associated with brain damage markers. However, Se supplementation trials in stroke patients provided inconsistent results. Experimental studies provided a significant contribution to potential neuroprotective effects in stroke. Se supplementation was shown to increase antioxidant enzyme activity, thus reducing reactive oxygen species (ROS) production and macromolecule oxidative damage. Se-induced prevention of mitochondrial dysfunction may also significantly contribute to reduced ROS production

A. V. Skalny (✉)
Peoples' Friendship University of Russia (RUDN University), Moscow, Russia

Yaroslavl State University, Yaroslavl, Russia

All-Russian Research Institute of Medicinal and Aromatic Plants (VILAR), Moscow, Russia
e-mail: skalny3@microelements.ru

M. G. Skalnaya
Peoples' Friendship University of Russia (RUDN University), Moscow, Russia

L. L. Klimenko
Institute of Chemical Physics of N. N. Semenov of the Russian Academy of Sciences,
Moscow, Russia

A. N. Mazilina
Institute of Chemical Physics of N. N. Semenov of the Russian Academy of Sciences,
Moscow, Russia

Clinical Hospital No 123 Federal Medical-Biological Agency of Russia, Moscow, Russia

A. A. Tinkov
Peoples' Friendship University of Russia (RUDN University), Moscow, Russia

Yaroslavl State University, Yaroslavl, Russia

Institute of Cellular and Intracellular Symbiosis, Russian Academy of Sciences,
Orenburg, Russia

and restoration of ATP levels. Se exposure was also shown to prevent NF-kB and AP-1 activation, thus reducing proinflammatory cytokine production and leukocyte infiltration. Reduce caspase 3 activation and apoptosis, as well as decreased autophagy, were observed under ischemic conditions in Se-treated animals. Se may also reduce adhesion molecule expression, as well as glutamate excitotoxicity, although these effects were not demonstrated in stroke models. The existing data demonstrate the neuroprotective potential of selenium in ischemic stroke. However, the majority of indications of the neuroprotective effect of selenium arise from experimental studies, whereas human data remain insufficient. Further clinical studies and especially placebo-controlled trials are strongly required to highlight the potential effects of selenium supplements in ischemic stroke management.

Keywords Selenium · Ischemia · Reperfusion · Brain · Stroke

Introduction

Stroke is the second-leading cause of death worldwide (WHO 2017). It is estimated that a total of 16.9 million people suffer from ischemic stroke annually with a global incidence of 258/100,000 (Béjot et al. 2016). Although stroke-related age-standardized incidence/prevalence, mortality, and disability-adjusted life years (DALYs) lost have been reduced during the last decades (Feigin et al. 2014), the absolute number of stroke patients has significantly increased (Feigin et al. 2015). Particularly, the number of stroke survivors has been doubled in a period of 1990–2010 reaching 33 million people, and is prognosed to increase to 77 million by 2030 (Béjot et al. 2016). Ischemic stroke was found to be more prevalent as compared to hemorrhagic stroke (Suwanwela and Poungvarin 2016).

Stroke is one of the leading causes of acquired disability in adults (Mendis 2013). Disability may be related to neurological complications including cognitive impairment (Sun et al. 2014), brain edema, epilepsy, delirium, sleep disorders, and headache (Balami et al. 2011), as well as medical (cardiac, pulmonary, gastrointestinal, genitourinary, vascular, and musculoskeletal) complications of stroke (Kumar et al. 2010). Poor outcome in stroke mediates high social and medical costs of stroke. For example, the total stroke costs in Ireland were € 489–€805 million in 2007 with a 2:1 ratio between direct and indirect costs (Smith et al. 2011). At the same time, disability status had a significant effect on stroke costs, resulting in $107,883 and $48,339 in disabling and non-disabling strokes, respectively (Mittmann et al. 2012). Being in agreement with a tendency to increased incidence of stroke, the total annual costs of stroke are projected to increase by 129% by 2030 in the USA (Ovbiagele et al. 2013).

Stroke pathophysiology includes multiple mechanisms mediating involvement of different systems. Ischemia triggers ischemic cascade resulting in reduced oxygen and energy, resulting in alteration of energy-dependent processes and cell death (both apoptosis and necrosis) promotion (Deb et al. 2010). Further mechanisms involved in ischemic stroke pathogenesis include oxidative stress due to mitochondrial dysfunction, activation of prooxidant enzymes in parallel with depletion of antioxidant system (Rodrigo et al. 2013), inflammation and neuroinflammation with overexpression of proinflammatory cytokines, adhesion molecules, activation of microglia, leukocyte infiltration (Jin et al. 2010), excitotoxicity (Szydlowska and Tymianski 2010) with underlying calcium overload due to glutamate-induced activation of Ca^{2+}-permeable NMDA receptors (Lai et al. 2014), and a number of other mechanisms including Toll-like receptors and notch- and adiponectin-receptor signaling (Woodruff et al. 2011). Understanding of the pathogenetic mechanisms involved in stroke development is essential for search of both novel markers of brain damage (Jickling and Sharp 2011) and targets for neuroprotection (Moretti et al. 2015).

Selenium is an essential metalloid playing a variety of functions through its structural role in different selenoproteins (Hatfield et al. 2014). Despite a low Se content, brain has high requirements in selenium due to its numerous functions (Steinbrenner and Sies 2013; Schweizer and Seeher 2015). Moreover, anatomical differences in brain selenium levels are indicative of different requirements and Se-related functional activity of brain regions (Ramos et al. 2015). Se and selenoproteins are modulators of brain functions (Schweizer et al. 2004a, b). In particular, appropriate selenoprotein expression is required for neuronal interaction (Wirth et al. 2010). Glutathione peroxidases (Gpx) and thioredoxin reductases (Txnrd) play a significant role in the maintenance of brain redox homeostasis (Schweizer et al. 2004a, b). SELENOP1, being secreted by astrocytes and taken up by neurons, plays a key role in brain Se homeostasis (Steinbrenner and Sies 2013). Other selenoproteins also play a significant role in brain biology (Schweizer et al. 2004a, b; Savaskan et al. 2012). In particular, it has been demonstrated that selenoprotein H positively regulates mitochondrial biogenesis (Li et al. 2015a, b, c). Selenium also plays a key role in heavy metals (e.g., mercury) detoxication, thus reducing their neurotoxicity (Oliveira et al. 2017; Bjørklund et al. 2017). Correspondingly, altered selenium metabolism and selenoprotein dysfunction are associated with a broad range of brain pathologies, including Alzheimer's disease, Parkinson's disease, Huntington's disease, epilepsy, and other disorders (Pillai et al. 2014). Thus, selenium was proposed as a potential neuroprotective agent (Bräuer and Savaskan 2004). At the same time, a growing body of data demonstrate that selenium may also possess neurotoxic effects at high exposure levels (Vinceti et al. 2014). However, data on the role of selenium and particular selenoproteins in stroke pathophysiology are inconsistent.

Therefore, the objective of this chapter is to review current experimental and clinical findings on the role of selenium in ischemic stroke. While discussing the mechanisms underlying potential effects of selenium in ischemic stroke we have aimed at the publications dealing with nervous tissue under ischemic conditions. However, the existing studies demonstrate the protective mechanisms of Se against ischemia/reperfusion damage in various tissues including ovary (Bozkurt et al. 2012), intestine (Kim et al. 2014), and especially heart (Venardos and Kaye 2007).

Human Studies of the Role of Se in Stroke

Multiple studies have demonstrated the association between selenium metabolism and stroke. Plasma levels of selenium and other antioxidants were found to be lower in ischemic stroke patients (Chang et al. 1998). Se levels were significantly reduced in ischemic stroke, whereas GPX activity was elevated in 1 day after stroke onset. Moreover, GPX activity was shown to be inversely associated with National Institutes of Health Stroke Scale scores on admission and after 7 days (Zimmermann et al. 2004). Moreover, lower Se levels in patients with ischemic stroke were also predictive of hyperhomocysteinemia (Angelova et al. 2008). Low Se levels in men were associated with higher stroke mortality (RR: 3.7 (95% Cl, 1.0–13.1)) (Virtamo et al. 1985). Similar data were obtained in the Netherlands (Kok et al. 1987). It is also notable that neonates with hypoxic ischemic encephalopathy were also characterized by significantly lower serum selenium levels. The latter also negatively correlated with ischemic encephalopathy severity and alkalosis, whereas a positive association was detected for Apgar scale values (El-Mazary et al. 2015).

At the same time, a 12-year follow-up study involving 13,887 adults demonstrated a nonlinear association between serum Se and stroke mortality. In particular, hazard ratios for stroke mortality in persons with tertile 2 and 3 selenium levels were 0.73 (95% CI, 0.41–1.30) and 1.23 (95% CI, 0.66–2.28), respectively (Bleys et al. 2008).

The results of the International Polar Year Inuit Health Survey 2007–2008 demonstrate that each 50 µg/L increase in blood selenium levels is associated with 38% lower risk of stroke in Canadian Inuit population. Similar relationship was detected for dietary selenium intake (Hu et al. 2017a, b). Moreover, high Se in parallel with low and high Hg levels in Canadian Inuits was associated with reduced stroke prevalence (OR = 0.54 (95%CI: 0.12, 2.51) and OR = 0.25 (95%CI: 0.09, 0.70)) (Hu et al. 2017a, b).

At the same time, no significant relationship between serum Se levels and stroke was observed in a 10-year follow-up study in Finland (Marniemi et al. 2005). Harboe-Gonçalves et al. (2007) also failed to detect any significant change in serum Se levels between stroke patients and healthy controls. Moreover, Se concentration was not associated with hyperhomocysteinemia (Harboe-Gonçalves et al. 2007). Similarly, no significant association between blood plasma selenium and stroke was observed in a recent meta-analysis (Zhang et al. 2016). No significant association between hair Se levels and incidence of cerebrovascular diseases in an adult Russian population was observed ($r = -0.124$; $p = 0.267$). However, after taking into consideration the level of mercury (correlation for Hg levels alone: $r = 0.227$; $p = 0.041$), the Se-to-Hg ratio was characterized by a significant negative relationship with the incidence of cerebrovascular diseases ($r = -0.312$; $p = 0.004$) in an adult population of 83 regions of Russia (Skalny et al. 2016).

It is notable that certain studies have demonstrated a significant association between Se exposure and stroke. In particular, a recent study demonstrated an association between environmental selenium exposure and increased stroke risk

(HR = 1.33 (95% CI: 1.09, 1.62)) (Merrill et al. 2017). These findings may be associated to an earlier demonstrated relationship between high Se exposure and increased total and LDL cholesterol (Laclaustra et al. 2010; Stranges et al. 2010; Ju et al. 2017), being the risk factor for ischemic stroke (Ohira et al. 2006).

Earlier, we have detected significantly increased serum Se levels in patients with transient ischemic attack (Klimenko et al. 2016) and acute ischemic stroke (Skalny et al. 2017a). Our findings corroborate to a recent study by Nahan et al. (2017) who demonstrated a significant increase in protein-bound Se levels in stroke patients (Nahan et al. 2017). A significant association between serum Se levels and inflammatory markers (C4 complement fragment) was revealed in stroke patients (Skalny et al. 2017a). However, serum Se was not associated with thyroid dysfunction in acute ischemic stroke (Skalny et al. 2017b). Notably, the results of principal component analysis (PCA) (R Core Team, Vienna, Austria) demonstrate that serum Se levels were specifically clustered in stroke patients and healthy controls in parallel with a number of laboratory stroke risk factors including hypercoagulation and inflammation (Fig. 11.1).

We have also assessed the relationship between circulating Se levels and brain damage markers including S100 (Saenger and Christenson 2010), NR2 antibodies (NR2Ab) (Weissman et al. 2011), and vascular endothelial growth factor (VEGF) (Matsuo et al. 2013) in multiple regression models (Table 11.1). The models also included the parameters of blood count, lipid profile, hemostasis, inflammation, and oxidative stress as independent predictors. It has been demonstrated that serum Se levels in stroke patients are significant negative predictors of brain damage marker values. It is also notable that the effect of Se on the assessed stroke markers is significant even after adjustment for other stroke risk factors (blood count, hemostasis, inflammation, oxidative stress). The tightest interaction with serum Se was observed for NR2Ab levels (NR2Ab > VEGF > S100), being in agreement with our earlier observation of the association between low serum Se and high NR2Ab in stroke patients (Klimenko et al. 2015). These findings demonstrate that despite a significant increase in serum Se levels in patients with acute ischemic stroke, it may possess neuroprotective effects.

Selenoprotein levels were also shown to be altered in ischemic stroke patients. In particular, it has been demonstrated that both selenium and selenoprotein P (SELENOP) were characterized by a significant reduction in stroke patients as compared to the control ones (Koyama et al. 2009).

However, more data are available on the association between selenoprotein polymorphisms and ischemic stroke risk. In particular, polymorphisms in the Gpx-3 gene promoter (haplotypes H1 and H2) are associated with significantly elevated ischemic stroke risk both in children and young adults (Voetsch et al. 2007). Polymorphisms of GPX3 may be considered as risk factors for arteriopathy ischemic stroke, but not for thromboembolic stroke or cerebral sinovenous thrombosis in a pediatric population (Nowak-Göttl et al. 2011). Notably, it has been demonstrated that C718T polymorphism in the 3′-untranslated region of the GPX4 significantly increases susceptibility to ischemic stroke in a population of hypertensives (Polonikov et al. 2012).

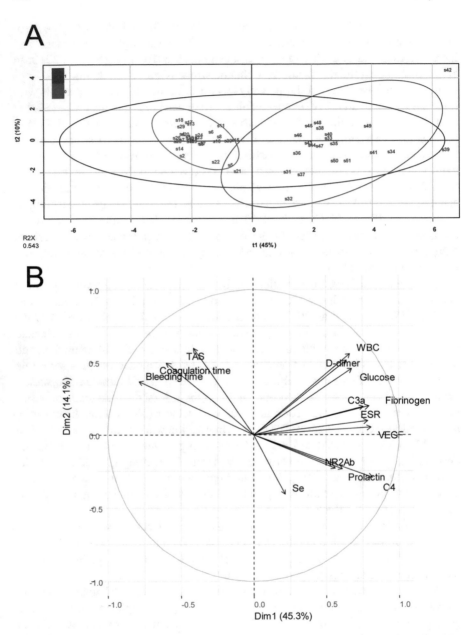

Fig. 11.1 Principal component analysis (PCA): (**a**) Clustering of patients with stroke and healthy subjects (x-score). The first two components explain 65% of dispersion, which shows the validity of a model; (**b**) contributions of variables into model (loading). Direction of the vector shows direction of shifting each point (patient) from one place to another (toward different class). The closer the arrows the bigger their correlations to each other. The length of the vector shows contribution into the model

Table 11.1 Multiple regression models for the association between serum selenium levels and other laboratory parameters and S100, NR2Ab, and VEGF as brain damage markers

Parameters	S100b		NR2Ab		VEGF	
	β	p	β	p	β	p
Hb, g/L	−0.025	0.889	−0.302	0.178	−0.185	0.136
RBC, 10^{12}/L	0.498	0.010[a]	0.561	0.018[a]	0.326	0.013[a]
PLT, 10^9/L	0.142	0.520	0.448	0.109	0.129	0.393
WBC, 10^9/L	−0.210	0.289	−0.220	0.368	0.198	0.146
ESR, mm/h	0.522	0.050[a]	−0.164	0.606	0.205	0.246
Bleeding time, s	−0.401	0.117	−0.755	0.021[a]	−0.420	0.019[a]
Coagulation time, s	−0.069	0.646	−0.186	0.320	−0.098	0.340
TC, mmol/L	0.299	0.143	0.462	0.071	0.023	0.865
TG, mmol/L	−0.162	0.326	−0.191	0.347	−0.001	0.993
LDL-C, mmol/L	0.029	0.885	−0.106	0.673	0.312	0.032[a]
HDL-C, mmol/L	0.063	0.678	−0.164	0.381	0.130	0.212
AI	0.064	0.656	0.096	0.587	0.037	0.703
Glucose, mmol/L	−0.139	0.371	0.012	0.951	−0.166	0.122
APPT, s	−0.376	0.127	−0.224	0.454	0.023	0.888
Fibrinogen, mg/dl	−0.058	0.726	0.091	0.659	−0.085	0.453
Soluble fibrin monomer, mg/dl	0.214	0.235	−0.062	0.779	−0.032	0.790
D-dimer, ng/mL	0.058	0.787	0.047	0.860	0.319	0.038[a]
C3a, g/L	0.109	0.671	0.376	0.242	−0.069	0.694
C4, g/L	−0.053	0.729	0.032	0.866	0.075	0.473
TAS, μmol/L	−0.025	0.889	−0.302	0.178	−0.185	0.136
Se, μg/L	−0.349	0.009[a]	−0.448	0.007[a]	−0.405	Spilt0.001[a]
Multiple R	0.895		0.829		0.951	
Adjusted R^2	0.604		0.399		0.817	
p for a model	<0.001[a]		0.020[a]		<0.001[a]	

[a]All models also included anthropometric parameters (age, gender, body weight, height, body mass index) as predictors

Certain studies demonstrated the association between selenoprotein S (SELENOS) polymorphisms and stroke. Particularly, SELENOS polymorphisms are associated with higher susceptibility to ischemic stroke both in men and women (Li et al. 2015a, b, c), corresponding to the earlier observation of the direct association between rs7178239 genetic variant of SEPS1 and increased stroke risk in women (HR: 3.35 (1.66–6.76)) and in general cohort of men and women (HR: 1.75 (1.17–2.64)) (Alanne et al. 2007). These data are in agreement with the indication of the role of SELENOS overexpression in astrocyte resistance to inflammation and endoplasmic reticulum stress (Fradejas et al. 2011), and cell survival in ischemic conditions (Fradejas et al. 2008). It has also been demonstrated that SELENOS expression is diminished in the ischemic core, whereas in the ischemic penumbra SELENOS expression is characterized by a significant increase in 3–7 days after reperfusion, being indicative of the protective role of SELENOS against inflammation (Liu et al. 2013).

Although certain cross-sectional and prospective studies have demonstrated the association between Se status markers and various disorders, data from supplementation studies are insufficient. In particular, no significant reduction in stroke (RR 0.99 (95% CI: 0.88, 1.11)) was observed in a 15-year follow-up study (Wei et al. 2004). Another 7.6-year follow-up Se supplementation trial (200 μg/day) also did not observe a significant impact of Se on stroke HR = 1.02, 95% CI: 0.63, 1.65 (Stranges et al. 2006). However, the results of the earlier ebselen supplementation trial demonstrated a significant improvement in stroke outcome as compared to placebo. Better outcome was registered only in patients who started ebselen treatment within, but not after, 24 h from stroke manifestation (Yamaguchi et al. 1998). Therefore, the existing human data on the interrelationship between selenium metabolism and stroke are insufficient.

Experimental Studies

Se Supplementation in Stroke

In contrast to the earlier noted insufficiency of human selenium supplementation data, experimental in vivo studies have demonstrated a significant neuroprotective effect of Se supplementation in animal stroke models. These findings are in agreement with the observation of significant decrease in brain Se content in a Mongolian gerbil model of ischemic stroke (Fang et al. 2013). In particular, it has also been demonstrated that Se treatment (diphenyl diselenide) reduced ischemia-reperfusion cerebral damage. Se pretreatment and treatment resulted in a significant reduction of ischemia-reperfusion-induced ROS production and Hsp70 expression and improved mitochondrial membrane potential both in cerebral cortex and hippocampus. Mitochondrial effects of Se also included amelioration of mitochondrial dehydrogenase, complex I, and antioxidant enzyme (Gpx, SOD) activity inhibition (Dobrachinski et al. 2014). Similar protective effect of Se was observed in the case of catalase (Ansari et al. 2004). It has also been demonstrated that Se treatment reduced inflammatory cytokine levels (IL-1β, IL-6, TNF-α, IFN-ɣ) associated with cerebral ischemia/reperfusion damage (Brüning et al. 2012). Correspondingly, Se treatment reduced ischemia/reperfusion-induced increase in proinflammatory cytokine expression and apoptosis in hippocampal and cortical cells, as well as increased nerve growth factor (NGF) (Özbal et al. 2008). These findings are at least partially in agreement with the observation by Wang et al. (2010) who revealed Na_2SeO_3-induced decrease in neuronal TNF-α and IL-1β expression and apoptosis, although no increase in NGF expression was detected (Wang et al. 2010).

Se pretreatment significantly reduced ischemia-induced increase in intracellular calcium in synaptosomes, HSP70 expression, and caspase 3 activity, being also accompanied by an improvement of ATP levels (Yousuf et al. 2007). These findings are in agreement with the observation of the protective effect of Se against hypoxia-induced apoptosis via Bcl2 upregulation (Sarada et al. 2008).

Diphenyl diselenide was also shown to reduce oxygen-glucose deprivation-induced reduction of cell viability and increase iNOS activity (Ghisleni et al. 2003). Se supplementation improved anti-ischemic effect of melatonin in a rat model of ischemic stroke through reduction of iNOS activity (Ahmad et al. 2011).

It has also been demonstrated that selenite pretreatment resulted in a significant decrease in brain damage area and reduced DNA oxidation in a murine model of cerebral ischemia, being associated with improved mitochondrial biogenesis (peroxisome proliferator-activated receptor-γ coactivator 1alpha (PGC-1α) and nuclear respiratory factor 1 (NRF1)) and reduced autophagia (Beclin 1 and microtubule-associated protein 1 light chain 3-II (LC3-II)) (Mehta et al. 2012). In turn, intraperitoneal Se injection was also shown to reduce cerebral vasospasm in rabbits (Kocaogullar et al. 2010).

Ebselen Supplementation in Stroke

Multiple studies have investigated the protective effect of ebselen, 2-phenyl-1, 2-benzisoselenazoL3 (2*H*)-one. Ebselen, a Gpx mimic, was proposed to be a potential therapy for cerebral ischemia (Parnham and Sies 2013), also being a potent inhibitor of lipoxygenases, NADPH oxidase, NO synthases, protein kinase C, and H+/K+-ATPase (Parnham and Sies 2000). A particular model of the ebselen mimicking Gpx was provided (Antony and Bayse 2011). Ebselen was shown to be a substrate for another selenoprotein, thioredoxin reductase (Txnrd) (Zhao and Holmgren 2002), mimicking dehydroascorbate reductase activity (Zhao and Holmgren 2004). It is also notable that ebselen is also capable of induction of phase 2 detoxication enzymes (Sakurai et al. 2006).

It has been demonstrated that ebselen treatment substantially reduced cortical ischemic damage, as well as both lipid and DNA peroxidation (Imai et al. 2003). These findings corroborate to the earlier data from the authors, who have demonstrated that ebselen protects both white and gray matter in cerebral ischemia (Imai et al. 2001). It is notable that ebselen significantly reduced the volume of ischemic damage in cerebral medisphere and cortex, but not caudate nucleus (Takasago et al. 1997). At the same time, the protective effects of ebselen are not related to the changes in blood pressure, body temperature, or blood gases (Dawson et al. 1995). Ebselen was found to be neuroprotective while given with thrombolytic tissue plasminogen activator in a rabbit model of embolic stroke in 60 min after embolism (Lapchak and Zivin 2003).

Being in agreement with the well-demonstrated antioxidant effect of ebselen (Azad and Tomar 2014), treatment with the agent was shown to effectively reduce neuronal damage and oxidative DNA damage as assessed by 8-hydroxy-2′-deoxyguanosine (8-OHdG) levels and 8-oxoguanine DNA glycosylase (OGG1) activity (He et al. 2007).

Ebselen treatment also prevented neurotoxicity through apoptosis reduction (Bcl-2, Bax), being the most potent neuroprotector (ebselen Spigt carvedilol >

3-methyl-1-phenyl-2-pyrazolin-5-one > vitamin E) (Yamagata et al. 2008). Moreover, ebselen treatment in 24 h after middle cerebral artery occlusion significantly prevented neuronal loss and gliosis in thalamus, through reduction of autophagy and apoptosis, as assessed by decreased LC3-II and Beclin-1 levels (Li et al. 2015a, b, c). Another possible pathway of antiapoptotic effect of Se may be related to the inhibition of the JNK and AP-1 pathways (Yoshizumi et al. 2002). Ebselen-dependent reduction of cytochrome c oxidase release from ischemic hemispheres and DNA fragmentation is also associated with reduced neuronal apoptosis (Namura et al. 2001).

It is also proposed that the neuroprotective effect of ebselen treatment may be at least partially mediated by inhibition of NO production and glutamate release (Koizumi et al. 2011). However, in stroke-prone animals ebselen treatment resulted in a significant increase in plasma NO levels, as well as eNOS expression in parallel with reduced intima-media thickness of the carotid artery, being indicative of the protective role of Se against endothelial damage and vascular remodeling (Sui et al. 2005).

At the same time, opposing data exist. The lack of efficiency of single-dose ebselen treatment in reduction of brain infarct volume was observed (Salom et al. 2004). Moreover, it has been noted that under ischemic conditions Ebselen treatment may significantly increase C6 glioma cell death especially in terms of GSH deficiency (Shi et al. 2006). It is also notable that ebselen treatment was shown to reduce the protective effect of ischemic preconditioning in a rat model of brain ischemia-reperfusion injury, being hypothetically associated with a reduction of ischemic preconditioning-induced oxidative stress (Puisieux et al. 2004).

The Role of Glutathione Peroxidase in Stroke

Glutathione peroxidase (GPX) is a family of antioxidant selenoproteins using reduced glutathione (GSH) as a cofactor (proton donor). It is also the most studied selenoprotein in the context of ischemic stroke and the role of selenium in its modulation.

Earlier studies demonstrated the effect of stroke on Gpx activity. In particular, brain GPx levels were also characterized by a significant decrease in GPx activity in ischemic brain regions (İşlekel et al. 1999). Both ischemic and peri-ischemic tissue Gpx activity was found to be insignificantly decreased after stroke. However, starting from 72 h after stroke the enzyme activity was found to be significantly increased as compared to the baseline (Mahadik et al. 1993). It has also been demonstrated that in infarcted human brain Gpx is detected in the cytoplasm of glia in the marginal area, as well as in macrophages of the ischemic core (Takizawa et al. 1994).

Modulation of GPx activity was also shown to mediate the effect of certain neuroprotective agents. It has been demonstrated that the neuroprotective effect of nerve growth factor (NGF) may be at least partially mediated by upregulation of antioxidant enzymes, as demonstrated by dose- and time-dependent NGF-induced increase in GPx mRNA expression in PC 12 cells (Sampath et al. 1994). Moreover, preconditioning to hyperoxia significantly increases glutathione peroxidase and other antioxidant enzyme activity as well as reduces ischemic damage in rats (decreased mortality and infarct volume) (Bigdeli 2009).

Interesting data were obtained from experimental studies with genetic modulation of GPx activity (knockout, overexpression). Earlier studies demonstrated significantly increased brain damage in animal models of stroke with decreased Gpx activity, being indicative of its essential role in neuroprotection. In particular, Gpx-1 knockout mouse brain resulted in a threefold increase of ischemia-reperfusion-induced infarction size, being accompanied by an earlier activation apoptosis as assessed by caspase-3 expression (Crack et al. 2001). Gpx1 provided neuroprotection in SOD1 transgenic mice (Crack et al. 2003). *Gpx1-/-* mice were also characterized by brain NF-κB upregulation. Moreover, NF-κB inhibitor pyrrolidinedithiocarbamate provided partial neuroprotection inpx1-/- mice, being indicative of the potential role of NF-κB activation in Gpx1 deficiency in ischemia-reperfusion (Crack et al. 2006). Deficiency of Gpx1 (*Gpx1-/-*) also resulted in a differential pattern of transcriptional regulation in response to ischemia-reperfusion injury as compared to the wild-type controls. In particular, a significant modulation of apoptotic (upregulation of *p53*, *Fas/FasL*), MAPK-signaling pathways (downregulation of the majority of genes, accompanied by *Dusp1* and *Dusp3* upregulation), oxidative stress response (downregulation of *Mt3*, *Hsp90b1*, *Mafg*, *Prkcb1*, *Mapk4*, upregulation of *Hspa1a*, *Naprt1*, *Hmox1*, *Maff*), ubiquitin–proteasome system (downregulation of *Psmd1*, *Uchl(3,5)*, *Usp(2,11)*), and immune response (*Cadm1*, *Foxp1*, *Socs5*, *Meis1*, *Pbx1* downregulation) was observed (Chen et al. 2011).

Correspondingly, increased Gpx activity (overexpression, transfection) was associated with amelioration of pathogenetic mechanisms involved in stroke pathogenesis. In particular, it has been demonstrated that Gpx1 overexpression reduced brain damage and edema in mice with ischemic stroke (Weisbrot-Lefkowitz et al. 1998). In a murine stroke model it has been demonstrated that overexpression of human glutathione peroxidase (hGPX1) significantly reduces astrocyte and microglia activation, as well as inflammatory infiltration (Ishibashi et al. 2002a). Correspondingly, hGPX1 overexpression in mice with ischemia-reperfusion brain injury significantly reduced MIP-1, MIP-1, MIP-2, IP-10, MCP-1, TNF-a, IL-6, and FasL expression in brain (Ishibashi et al. 2002b).

Gpx1 transfection to rat striatum prior to the ischemia onset significantly improved neuronal viability as well as decreased cytosolic translocation of cytochrome c. These changes were accompanied by reduced apoptosis as assessed by increased number of Bcl-2-positive cells, as well as reduced Bax and activated caspase-3 abundance (Hoehn et al. 2003).

At the same time, Gpx1 overexpression significantly reversed the protective effect of hypoxia preconditioning, hypothetically, through aberrant ERK activation (Autheman et al. 2012). This observation corresponds to a similar effect of ebselen supplementation (Puisieux et al. 2004), being indicative that the modulatory effect of ebselen on hypoxia preconditioning is mediated by GPx activation.

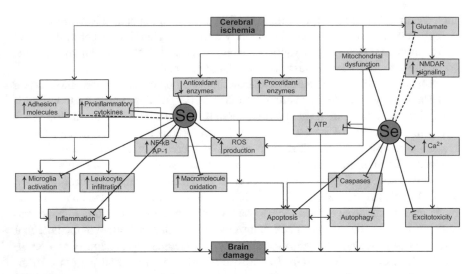

Fig. 11.2 The impact of selenium on the mechanisms of ischemic stroke pathogenesis. Continuous lines indicate the effect of Se on the highlighted mechanisms in brain tissue under ischemic conditions. Dotted lines indicate the data obtained from experiments with brain tissue without ischemia

The Summary of Selenium Neuroprotective Effects on Stroke

The reviewed studies demonstrate that Se may play a significant neuroprotective role in stroke (Fig. 11.2). Se-induced upregulation of selenoprotein (and especially Gpx) expression mediates the protective effects of Se treatment. Se supplementation was shown to increase antioxidant enzyme activity (Gpx, SOD, catalase), thus reducing ROS production and macromolecule oxidative damage including lipid peroxidation and DNA oxidation (8-OHdG, OGG1). Se-induced prevention of mitochondrial dysfunction (PGC-1α, NRF1) may also significantly contribute to reduced ROS production. Se exposure also prevents NF-kB and AP-1 activation, thus reducing proinflammatory cytokine production (TNF-α, IL-1β, IFN-y, MIP-1, MIP-1, MIP-2, IP-10, MCP-1, FasL), as well as leukocyte infiltration. Although the inhibitory effect of Se on adhesion molecules was not demonstrated in experimental stroke models, it has been shown that sodium selenite prevents TNF-a-induced ICAM-1, VCAM-1, and E-selectin expression in human umbilical vein endothelial cells (Zhang et al. 2002). It has been noted that Se treatment restores ATP levels, hypothetically by improvement of mitochondrial function. Se was shown to reduce caspase 3 activation and subsequent apoptosis (Bcl2, Bax, p53, Fas/FasL) under ischemic conditions, as well as decrease autophagy (Beclin1, LC3-II).

It has been demonstrated that selenium treatment prevents glutamate-induced neurotoxicity in HT22 neuronal cells (Ma et al. 2017), whereas Se deficiency increases susceptibility to glutamate excitotoxicity (Savaskan et al. 2003). Selenium (as ebselen) was also shown to modulate NMDA receptor through redox-modulatory site (Herin et al. 2001). Although these studies demonstrate the effect of selenium on excitotoxicity pathways without ischemia-reperfusion, one can suppose that similar protective mechanisms may be involved in stroke. These observations are in agreement with data indicating the reduction of intracellular Ca^{2+} levels in a model of stroke.

It is also notable that hypoxia also affects selenium metabolism, resulting in the observed differences in both selenium and selenoprotein levels in ischemic stroke patients. In particular, it has been demonstrated that hypoxia in hepatocytes decreases transcription of selenophosphate synthetase-2, phosphoseryl-tRNASerSec kinase, and selenocysteine lyase, being one of the key factors of selenoprotein biosynthesis. However, GPX4 was shown to be increased in response to hypoxia. These findings were accompanied by reduced SELENOP levels and Se export from hepatocytes, whereas Se treatment abolished these changes (Becker et al. 2014). This observation underlines a mutual interaction between Se metabolism and ischemia.

Therefore, the existing data demonstrate the neuroprotective potential of selenium in ischemic stroke. However, the majority of indications of the neuroprotective effect of selenium arise from experimental in vivo and in vitro studies, whereas human data remain insufficient and contradictory. Further clinical studies and especially placebo-controlled trials are strongly required to highlight the potential effects of selenium supplements in ischemic stroke management.

Acknowledgments The publication was prepared with the support of the RUDN University Program 5-100.

Conflict of Interest The authors declare no conflict of interest.

References

Ahmad A, Khan MM, Ishrat T, Khan MB, Khuwaja G, Raza SS, Shrivastava P, Islam F. Synergistic effect of selenium and melatonin on neuroprotection in cerebral ischemia in rats. Biol Trace Elem Res. 2011;139(1):81–96. https://doi.org/10.1007/s12011-010-8643-z.

Alanne M, Kristiansson K, Auro K, Silander K, Kuulasmaa K, Peltonen L, Salomaa V, Perola M. Variation in the selenoprotein S gene locus is associated with coronary heart disease and ischemic stroke in two independent Finnish cohorts. Hum Genet. 2007;122(3–4):355–65. https://doi.org/10.1007/s00439-007-0402-7.

Angelova EA, Atanassova PA, Chalakova NT, Dimitrov BD. Associations between serum selenium and total plasma homocysteine during the acute phase of ischaemic stroke. Eur Neurol. 2008;60(6):298–303. https://doi.org/10.1159/000157884.

Ansari MA, Ahmad AS, Ahmad M, Salim S, Yousuf S, Ishrat T, Islam F. Selenium protects cerebral ischemia in rat brain mitochondria. Biol Trace Elem Res. 2004;101(1):73–86. https://doi.org/10.1385/BTER:101:1:73.

Antony S, Bayse CA. Modeling the mechanism of the glutathione peroxidase mimic ebselen. Inorg Chem. 2011;50(23):12075–84. https://doi.org/10.1021/ic201603v.

Autheman D, Sheldon RA, Chaudhuri N, von Arx S, Siegenthaler C, Ferriero DM, Christen S. Glutathione peroxidase overexpression causes aberrant ERK activation in neonatal mouse cortex after hypoxic preconditioning. Pediatr Res. 2012;72(6):568–75. https://doi.org/10.1038/pr.2012.124.

Azad GK, Tomar RS. Ebselen, a promising antioxidant drug: mechanisms of action and targets of biological pathways. Mol Biol Rep. 2014;41(8):4865–79. https://doi.org/10.1007/s11033-014-3417-x.

Balami JS, Chen RL, Grunwald IQ, Buchan AM. Neurological complications of acute ischaemic stroke. Lancet Neurol. 2011;10(4):357–71. https://doi.org/10.1016/S1474-4422(10)70313-6.

Becker NP, Martitz J, Renko K, Stoedter M, Hybsier S, Cramer T, Schomburg L. Hypoxia reduces and redirects selenoprotein biosynthesis. Metallomics. 2014;6(5):1079–86. https://doi.org/10.1039/C4MT00004H.

Béjot Y, Daubail B, Giroud M. Epidemiology of stroke and transient ischemic attacks: Current knowledge and perspectives. Rev Neurol. 2016;172(1):59–68. https://doi.org/10.1016/j.neurol.2015.07.013.

Bigdeli MR. Preconditioning with prolonged normobaric hyperoxia induces ischemic tolerance partly by upregulation of antioxidant enzymes in rat brain tissue. Brain Res. 2009;1260:47–54. https://doi.org/10.1016/j.brainres.2008.12.065.

Bjørklund G, Aaseth J, Ajsuvakova OP, Nikonorov AA, Skalny AV, Skalnaya MG, Tinkov AA. Molecular interaction between mercury and selenium in neurotoxicity. Coord Chem Rev. 2017;332:30–7. https://doi.org/10.1016/j.ccr.2016.10.009.

Bleys J, Navas-Acien A, Guallar E. Serum selenium levels and all-cause, cancer, and cardiovascular mortality among US adults. Arch Intern Med. 2008;168(4):404–10. https://doi.org/10.1001/archinternmed.2007.74.

Bozkurt S, Arikan DC, Kurutas EB, Sayar H, Okumus M, Coskun A, Bakan V. Selenium has a protective effect on ischemia/reperfusion injury in a rat ovary model: biochemical and histopathologic evaluation. J Pediatr Surg. 2012;47(9):1735–41. https://doi.org/10.1016/j.jpedsurg.2012.03.053.

Bräuer AU, Savaskan NE. Molecular actions of selenium in the brain: neuroprotective mechanisms of an essential trace element. Rev Neurosci. 2004;15(1):19–32. https://doi.org/10.1515/REVNEURO.2004.15.1.19.

Brüning CA, Prigol M, Luchese C, Jesse CR, Duarte MM, Roman SS, Nogueira CW. Protective effect of diphenyl diselenide on ischemia and reperfusion-induced cerebral injury: involvement of oxidative stress and pro-inflammatory cytokines. Neurochem Res. 2012;37(10):2249–58. https://doi.org/10.1007/s11064-012-0853-7.

Chang CY, Lai YC, Cheng TJ, Lau MT, Hu ML. Plasma levels of antioxidant vitamins, selenium, total sulfhydryl groups and oxidative products in ischemic-stroke patients as compared to matched controls in Taiwan. Free Radic Res. 1998;281:15–24. https://doi.org/10.3109/10715769809097872.

Chen MJ, Wong CH, Peng ZF, Manikandan J, Melendez AJ, Tan TM, Crack PJ, Cheung NS. A global transcriptomic view of the multifaceted role of glutathione peroxidase-1 in cerebral ischemic–reperfusion injury. Free Radic Biol Med. 2011;50(6):736–48. https://doi.org/10.1016/j.freeradbiomed.2010.12.025.

Crack PJ, Taylor JM, Flentjar NJ, De Haan J, Hertzog P, Iannello RC, Kola I. Increased infarct size and exacerbated apoptosis in the glutathione peroxidase-1 (Gpx-1) knockout mouse brain in response to ischemia/reperfusion injury. J Neurochem. 2001;78(6):1389–99. https://doi.org/10.1046/j.1471-4159.2001.00535.x.

Crack PJ, Taylor JM, de Haan JB, Kola I, Hertzog P, Iannello RC. Glutathione peroxidase-1 contributes to the neuroprotection seen in the superoxide dismutase-1 transgenic mouse in response to ischemia/reperfusion injury. J Cerebr Blood F Met. 2003;23(1):19–22. https://doi.org/10.1097/01.WCB.0000035181.38851.71.

Crack PJ, Taylor JM, Ali U, Mansell A, Hertzog PJ. Potential contribution of NF-κB in neuronal cell death in the glutathione peroxidase-1 knockout mouse in response to ischemia-reperfusion injury. Stroke. 2006;37(6):1533–8. https://doi.org/10.1161/01.STR.0000221708.17159.64.

Dawson DA, Masayasu H, Graham DI, Macrae IM. The neuroprotective efficacy of ebselen (a glutathione peroxidase mimic) on brain damage induced by transient focal cerebral ischaemia in the rat. Neurosci Lett. 1995;185(1):65–9. https://doi.org/10.1016/0304-3940(94)11226-9.

Deb P, Sharma S, Hassan KM. Pathophysiologic mechanisms of acute ischemic stroke: An overview with emphasis on therapeutic significance beyond thrombolysis. Pathophysiology. 2010;17(3):197–218. https://doi.org/10.1016/j.pathophys.2009.12.001.

Dobrachinski F, da Silva MH, Tassi CL, de Carvalho NR, Dias GR, Golombieski RM, da Silva Loreto ÉL, da Rocha JB, Fighera MR, Soares FA. Neuroprotective effect of diphenyl diselenide in a experimental stroke model: maintenance of redox system in mitochondria of brain regions. Neurotox Res. 2014;26(4):317–30. https://doi.org/10.1007/s12640-014-9463-2.

El-Mazary AA, Abdel-Aziz RA, Mahmoud RA, El-Said MA, Mohammed NR. Correlations between maternal and neonatal serum selenium levels in full term neonates with hypoxic ischemic encephalopathy. Ital J Pediatr. 2015;41(1):83. https://doi.org/10.1186/s13052-015-0185-8.

Fang KM, Cheng FC, Huang YL, Chung SY, Jian ZY, Lin MC. Trace element, antioxidant activity, and lipid peroxidation levels in brain cortex of gerbils after cerebral ischemic injury. Biol Trace Elem Res. 2013;152(1):66–74. https://doi.org/10.1007/s12011-012-9596-1.

Feigin VL, Forouzanfar MH, Krishnamurthi R, Mensah GA, Connor M, Bennett DA, Moran AE, Sacco RL, Anderson L, Truelsen T, O'Donnell M. Global and regional burden of stroke during 1990–2010: findings from the Global Burden of Disease Study 2010. Lancet. 2014;383(9913):245–55. https://doi.org/10.1016/S0140-6736(13)61953-4.

Feigin VL, Mensah GA, Norrving B, Murray CJ, Roth GA. Atlas of the global burden of stroke (1990-2013): the GBD 2013 study. Neuroepidemiology. 2015;45(3):230–6. https://doi.org/10.1159/000441106.

Fradejas N, Pastor MD, Mora-Lee S, Tranque P, Calvo S. SEPS1 gene is activated during astrocyte ischemia and shows prominent antiapoptotic effects. J Mol Neurosci. 2008;35:259–65. https://doi.org/10.1007/s12031-008-9069-3.

Fradejas N, Del Carmen Serrano-Pérez M, Tranque P, Calvo S. Selenoprotein S expression in reactive astrocytes following brain injury. Glia. 2011;59(6):959–72. https://doi.org/10.1002/glia.21168.

Ghisleni G, Porciuncula LO, Cimarosti H, Rocha JB, Salbego CG, Souza DO. Diphenyl diselenide protects rat hippocampal slices submitted to oxygen–glucose deprivation and diminishes inducible nitric oxide synthase immunocontent. Brain Res. 2003;986(1):196–9. https://doi.org/10.1016/S0006-8993(03)03193-7.

Harboe-Gonçalves L, Vaz LS, Marcelo B. Assesment of homocysteine, vitamin E, selenium, copper, ceruloplasmin and ferritin levels in patients with ischemic stroke diagnosis. J Bras Patol Med Lab. 2007;43(1):9–15. https://doi.org/10.1590/S1676-24442007000100004.

Hatfield DL, Tsuji PA, Carlson BA, Gladyshev VN. Selenium and selenocysteine: roles in cancer, health, and development. Trends Biochem Sci. 2014;39(3):112–20. https://doi.org/10.1016/j.tibs.2013.12.007.

He M, Xing S, Yang B, Zhao L, Hua H, Liang Z, Zhou W, Zeng J, Pei Z. Ebselen attenuates oxidative DNA damage and enhances its repair activity in the thalamus after focal cortical infarction in hypertensive rats. Brain Res. 2007;1181:83–92. https://doi.org/10.1016/j.brainres.2007.08.072.

Herin GA, Du S, Aizenman E. The neuroprotective agent ebselen modifies NMDA receptor function via the redox modulatory site. J Neurochem. 2001;78(6):1307–14. https://doi.org/10.1046/j.1471-4159.2001.00517.x.

Hoehn B, Yenari MA, Sapolsky RM, Steinberg GK. Glutathione peroxidase overexpression inhibits cytochrome C release and proapoptotic mediators to protect neurons from experimental stroke. Stroke. 2003;34(10):2489–94. https://doi.org/10.1161/01.STR.0000091268.25816.19.

Hu XF, Eccles KM, Chan HM. High selenium exposure lowers the odds ratios for hypertension, stroke, and myocardial infarction associated with mercury exposure among Inuit in Canada. Environ Int. 2017a;102:200–6. https://doi.org/10.1016/j.envint.2017.03.002.

Hu XF, Sharin T, Chan HM. Dietary and blood selenium are inversely associated with the prevalence of stroke among Inuit in Canada. J Trace Elem Med Biol. 2017b;44:322. https://doi.org/10.1016/j.jtemb.2017.09.007.

Imai H, Masayasu H, Dewar D, Graham DI, Macrae IM. Ebselen protects both gray and white matter in a rodent model of focal cerebral ischemia. Stroke. 2001;32(9):2149–54. https://doi.org/10.1161/hs0901.095725.

Imai H, Graham DI, Masayasu H, Macrae IM. Antioxidant ebselen reduces oxidative damage in focal cerebral ischemia. Free Radical Bio Med. 2003;34(1):56–63. https://doi.org/10.1016/S0891-5849(02)01180-2.

Ishibashi N, Prokopenko O, Reuhl KR, Mirochnitchenko O. Inflammatory response and glutathione peroxidase in a model of stroke. J Immunal. 2002a;168(4):1926–33. https://doi.org/10.4049/jimmunol.168.4.1926.

Ishibashi N, Prokopenko O, Weisbrot-Lefkowitz M, Reuhl KR, Mirochnitchenko O. Glutathione peroxidase inhibits cell death and glial activation following experimental stroke. Mol Brain Res. 2002b;109(1):34–44. https://doi.org/10.1016/S0169-328X(02)00459-X.

Işlekel S, Işlekel H, Güner G, Özdamar N. Alterations in superoxide dismutase, glutathione peroxidase and catalase activities in experimental cerebral ischemia-reperfusion. Res Exp Med. 1999;199(3):167–76. https://doi.org/10.1007/s004330050121.

Jickling GC, Sharp FR. Blood biomarkers of ischemic stroke. Neurotherapeutics. 2011;8(3):349. https://doi.org/10.1007/s13311-011-0050-4.

Jin R, Yang G, Li G. Inflammatory mechanisms in ischemic stroke: role of inflammatory cells. J Leukoc Biol. 2010;87(5):779–89. https://doi.org/10.1189/jlb.1109766.

Ju W, Ji M, Li X, Li Z, Wu G, Fu X, Yang X, Gao X. Relationship between higher serum selenium level and adverse blood lipid profile. Clin Nutr. 2017; https://doi.org/10.1016/j.clnu.2017.08.025.

Kim Y, Kim DC, Cho ES, Ko SO, Kwon WY, Suh GJ, Shin HK. Antioxidant and anti-inflammatory effects of selenium in oral buccal mucosa and small intestinal mucosa during intestinal ischemia-reperfusion injury. J Inflamm. 2014;11(1):36. https://doi.org/10.1186/s12950-014-0036-1.

Klimenko LL, Skalny AV, Turna AA, Kuznetsova AV, Senko OV, Baskakov IS, Budanova MN, Savostina MS, Mazilina AN. The role of selenium in multifactorial etiopathogenesis of ischemic stroke. Trace Element Med. 2015;16(4):28–35. https://doi.org/10.19112/2413-6174-2015-16-4-28-35.

Klimenko LL, Skalny AV, Turna AA, Tinkov AA, Budanova MN, Baskakov IS, Savostina MS, Mazilina AN, Deev AI, Nikonorov AA. Serum trace element profiles, prolactin, and cortisol in transient ischemic attack patients. Biol Trace Elem Res. 2016;172(1):93–100. https://doi.org/10.1007/s12011-015-0586-y.

Kocaogullar Y, Ilik K, Esen H, Koc O, Guney O. Preventive effects of intraperitoneal selenium on cerebral vasospasm in experimental subarachnoid hemorrhage. J Neurosurg Anesthesiol. 2010;22(1):53–8. https://doi.org/10.1097/ANA.0b013e3181b26a63.

Koizumi H, Fujisawa H, Suehiro E, Shirao S, Suzuki M. Neuroprotective effects of ebselen following forebrain ischemia: involvement of glutamate and nitric oxide. Neurol Med-Chir. 2011;51(5):337–43. https://doi.org/10.2176/nmc.51.337.

Kok FJ, De Bruijn AM, Vermeeren R, Hofman A, Van Laar A, De Bruin M, Hermus RJ, Valkenburg HA. Serum selenium, vitamin antioxidants, and cardiovascular mortality: a 9-year follow-up study in the Netherlands. Am J Clin Nutr. 1987;45(2):462–8.

Koyama H, Abdulah R, Ohkubo T, Imai Y, Satoh H, Nagai K. Depressed serum selenoprotein P: possible new predicator of increased risk for cerebrovascular events. Nutr Res. 2009;29(2):94–9. https://doi.org/10.1016/j.nutres.2009.01.002.

Kumar S, Selim MH, Caplan LR. Medical complications after stroke. Lancet Neurol. 2010;9(1):105–18. https://doi.org/10.1016/S1474-4422(09)70266-2.

Laclaustra M, Stranges S, Navas-Acien A, Ordovas JM, Guallar E. Serum selenium and serum lipids in US adults: National Health and Nutrition Examination Survey (NHANES) 2003–2004. Atherosclerosis. 2010;210(2):643–8. https://doi.org/10.1016/j.atherosclerosis.2010.01.005.

Lai TW, Zhang S, Wang YT. Excitotoxicity and stroke: identifying novel targets for neuroprotection. Prog Neurobiol. 2014;115:157–88. https://doi.org/10.1016/j.pneurobio.2013.11.006.

Lapchak PA, Zivin JA. Ebselen, a seleno-organic antioxidant, is neuroprotective after embolic strokes in rabbits. Stroke. 2003;34(8):2013–8. https://doi.org/10.1161/01.STR.0000081223.74129.04.

Li PA, Mehta SL, Jing L. Selenoprotein H in neuronal cells. In: Selenium. 2015a; 497–515. doi:https://doi.org/10.1039/9781782622215-00497.

Li XX, Guan HJ, Liu JP, Guo YP, Yang Y, Niu YY, Yao LY, Yang YD, Yue HY, Meng LL, Cui XY. Association of selenoprotein S gene polymorphism with ischemic stroke in a Chinese case–control study. Blood Coagul Fibrinolysis. 2015b;26(2):131–5. https://doi.org/10.1097/MBC.0000000000000202.

Li Y, Zhang J, Chen L, Xing S, Li J, Zhang Y, Li C, Pei Z, Zeng J. Ebselen reduces autophagic activation and cell death in the ipsilateral thalamus following focal cerebral infarction. Neurosci Lett. 2015c;600:206–12. https://doi.org/10.1016/j.neulet.2015.06.024.

Liu LX, Zhou XY, Li CS, Liu LQ, Huang SY, Zhou SN. Selenoprotein S expression in the rat brain following focal cerebral ischemia. Neurol Sci. 2013;34(9):1671–8. https://doi.org/10.1007/s10072-013-1319-7.

Ma YM, Ibeanu G, Wang LY, Zhang JZ, Chang Y, Dong JD, Li PA, Jing L. Selenium suppresses glutamate-induced cell death and prevents mitochondrial morphological dynamic alterations in hippocampal HT22 neuronal cells. BMC Neurosci. 2017;18(1):15. https://doi.org/10.1186/s12868-017-0337-4.

Mahadik SP, Makar TK, Murthy JN, Ortiz A, Wakade CG, Karpiak SE. Temporal changes in superoxide dismutase, glutathione peroxidase, and catalase levels in primary and peri-ischemic tissue. Mol Chem Neuropathol. 1993;18(1–2):1–4. https://doi.org/10.1007/BF03160018.

Marniemi J, Alanen E, Impivaara O, Seppänen R, Hakala P, Rajala T, Rönnemaa T. Dietary and serum vitamins and minerals as predictors of myocardial infarction and stroke in elderly subjects. Nutr Metab Cardiovas. 2005;15(3):188–97. https://doi.org/10.1016/j.numecd.2005.01.001.

Matsuo R, Ago T, Kamouchi M, Kuroda J, Kuwashiro T, Hata J, Kitazono T. Clinical significance of plasma VEGF value in ischemic stroke-research for biomarkers in ischemic stroke (REBIOS) study. BMC Neurol. 2013;13(1):32.

Mehta SL, Kumari S, Mendelev N, Li PA. Selenium preserves mitochondrial function, stimulates mitochondrial biogenesis, and reduces infarct volume after focal cerebral ischemia. BMC Neurosci. 2012;13(1):79. https://doi.org/10.1186/1471-2202-13-79.

Mendis S. Stroke disability and rehabilitation of stroke: World Health Organization perspective. Int J Stroke. 2013;8(1):3–4.

Merrill PD, Ampah SB, He K, Rembert NJ, Brockman J, Kleindorfer D, McClure LA. Association between trace elements in the environment and stroke risk: the reasons for geographic and racial differences in stroke (REGARDS) study. J Trace Elem Med Biol. 2017;42:45–9. https://doi.org/10.1016/j.jtemb.2017.04.003.

Mittmann N, Seung SJ, Hill MD, Phillips SJ, Hachinski V, Coté R, Buck BH, Mackey A, Gladstone DJ, Howse DC, Shuaib A. Impact of disability status on ischemic stroke costs in Canada in the first year. Can J Neurol Sci. 2012;39(6):793–800. https://doi.org/10.1017/S0317167100015638.

Moretti A, Ferrari F, Villa RF. Neuroprotection for ischaemic stroke: current status and challenges. Pharmacol Therapeut. 2015;146:23–34. https://doi.org/10.1016/j.pharmthera.2014.09.003.

Nahan KS, Walsh KB, Adeoye O, Landero-Figueroa JA. The metal and metalloprotein profile of human plasma as biomarkers for stroke diagnosis. J Trace Elem Med Biol. 2017;42:81–91. https://doi.org/10.1016/j.jtemb.2017.04.004.

Namura S, Nagata I, Takami S, Masayasu H, Kikuchi H. Ebselen reduces cytochrome c release from mitochondria and subsequent DNA fragmentation after transient focal cerebral ischemia in mice. Stroke. 2001;32(8):1906–11. https://doi.org/10.1161/01.STR.32.8.1906.

Nowak-Göttl U, Fiedler B, Huge A, Niederstadt T, Thedieck S, Seehafer T, Stoll M. Plasma glutathione peroxidase in pediatric stroke families. J Tromb Haemost. 2011;9(1):33–8. https://doi.org/10.1111/j.1538-7836.2010.04103.x.

Ohira T, Shahar E, Chambless LE, Rosamond WD, Mosley TH, Folsom AR. Risk factors for ischemic stroke subtypes. Stroke. 2006;37(10):2493–8. https://doi.org/10.1161/01.STR.0000239694.19359.88.

Oliveira CS, Piccoli BC, Aschner M, Rocha JB. Chemical speciation of selenium and mercury as determinant of their neurotoxicity. In: Neurotoxicity of metals. Cham: Springer; 2017. p. 53–83. https://doi.org/10.1007/978-3-319-60189-2_4.

Ovbiagele B, Goldstein LB, Higashida RT, Howard VJ, Johnston SC, Khavjou OA, Lackland DT, Lichtman JH, Mohl S, Sacco RL, Saver JL. Forecasting the future of stroke in the united states. Stroke. 2013;44(8):2361–75. https://doi.org/10.1161/STR.0b013e31829734f2.

Özbal S, Erbil G, Koçdor H, Tuğyan K, Pekçetin Ç, Özoğul C. The effects of selenium against cerebral ischemia-reperfusion injury in rats. Neurosci Lett. 2008;438(3):265–9. https://doi.org/10.1016/j.neulet.2008.03.091.

Parnham M, Sies H. Ebselen: prospective therapy for cerebral ischaemia. Expert Opin Investig Drugs. 2000;9(3):607–19. https://doi.org/10.1517/13543784.9.3.607.

Parnham MJ, Sies H. The early research and development of ebselen. Biochem Pharmacol. 2013;86(9):1248–53. https://doi.org/10.1016/j.bcp.2013.08.028.

Pillai R, Uyehara-Lock JH, Bellinger FP. Selenium and selenoprotein function in brain disorders. IUBMB Life. 2014;66(4):229–39. https://doi.org/10.1002/iub.1262.

Polonikov AV, Vialykh EK, Churnosov MI, Illig T, Freidin MB, Vasil'eva OV, Bushueva OY, Ryzhaeva VN, Bulgakova IV, Solodilova MA. The C718T polymorphism in the 3′-untranslated region of glutathione peroxidase-4 gene is a predictor of cerebral stroke in patients with essential hypertension. Hypertens Res. 2012;35(5):507–12. https://doi.org/10.1038/hr.2011.213.

Puisieux F, Deplanque D, Bulckaen H, Maboudou P, Gelé P, Lhermitte M, Lebuffe G, Bordet R. Brain ischemic preconditioning is abolished by antioxidant drugs but does not up-regulate superoxide dismutase and glutathion peroxidase. Brain Res. 2004;1027(1):30–7. https://doi.org/10.1016/j.brainres.2004.08.067.

Ramos P, Santos A, Pinto NR, Mendes R, Magalhães T, Almeida A. Anatomical regional differences in selenium levels in the human brain. Biol Trace Elem Res. 2015;163(1–2):89–96. https://doi.org/10.1007/s12011-014-0160-z.

Rodrigo R, Fernández-Gajardo R, Gutiérrez R, Manuel Matamala J, Carrasco R, Miranda-Merchak A, Feuerhake W. Oxidative stress and pathophysiology of ischemic stroke: novel therapeutic opportunities. CNS Neurol Disord-Dr. 2013;12(5):698–714.

Saenger AK, Christenson RH. Stroke biomarkers: progress and challenges for diagnosis, prognosis, differentiation, and treatment. Clin Chem. 2010;56(1):21–33.

Sakurai T, Kanayama M, Shibata T, Itoh K, Kobayashi A, Yamamoto M, Uchida K. Ebselen, a seleno-organic antioxidant, as an electrophile. Chem Res Toxicol. 2006;19(9):1196–204. https://doi.org/10.1021/tx0601105.

Salom JB, Pérez-Asensio FJ, Burguete MC, Marín N, Pitarch C, Torregrosa G, Romero FJ, Alborch E. Single-dose ebselen does not afford sustained neuroprotection to rats subjected to severe focal cerebral ischemia. Eur J Pharmacol. 2004;495(1):55–62. https://doi.org/10.1016/j.ejphar.2004.05.024.

Sampath D, Jackson GR, Werrbach-Perez K, Perez-Polo JR. Effects of nerve growth factor on glutathione peroxidase and catalase in PC 12 cells. J Neurochem. 1994;62(6):2476–9. https://doi.org/10.1046/j.1471-4159.1994.62062476.x.

Sarada SK, Himadri P, Ruma D, Sharma SK, Pauline T. Selenium protects the hypoxia induced apoptosis in neuroblastoma cells through upregulation of Bcl-2. Brain Res. 2008;1209:29–39. https://doi.org/10.1016/j.brainres.2008.02.041.

Savaskan NE, Bräuer AU, Kühbacher M, Eyüpoglu IY, Kyriakopoulos A, Ninnemann O, Behne D, Nitsch R. Selenium deficiency increases susceptibility to glutamate-induced excitotoxicity. FASEB J. 2003;17(1):112–4. https://doi.org/10.1096/fj.02-0067fje.

Savaskan NE, Hore N, Eyupoglu IY. Selenium and selenoproteins in neuroprotection and neuronal cell death. In: Metal ion in stroke. New York: Springer; 2012. p. 525–36. https://doi.org/10.1007/978-1-4419-9663-3_25.

Schweizer U, Seeher S. Selenoproteins in Brain. In: Selenium. 2015, pp. 479–496.

Schweizer U, Bräuer AU, Köhrle J, Nitsch R, Savaskan NE. Selenium and brain function: a poorly recognized liaison. Brain Res Rev. 2004a;45(3):164–78. https://doi.org/10.1016/j.brainresrev.2004.03.004.

Schweizer U, Schomburg L, Savaskan NE. The neurobiology of selenium: lessons from transgenic mice. J Nutr. 2004b;134(4):707–10.

Shi H, Liu S, Miyake M, Liu KJ. Ebselen induced C6 glioma cell death in oxygen and glucose deprivation. Chem Res Toxicol. 2006;19(5):655–60. https://doi.org/10.1021/tx0502544.

Skalny AV, Skalnaya MG, Nikonorov AA, Tinkov AA. Selenium antagonism with mercury and arsenic: from chemistry to population health and demography. In: Selenium. Basel: Springer International Publishing; 2016. p. 401–12. https://doi.org/10.1007/978-3-319-41283-2_34.

Skalny AV, Klimenko LL, Turna AA, Budanova MN, Baskakov IS, Savostina MS, Mazilina AN, Deyev AI, Skalnaya MG, Tinkov AA. Serum trace elements are interrelated with hormonal imbalance in men with acute ischemic stroke. J Trace Elem Med Biol. 2017a; https://doi.org/10.1016/j.jtemb.2016.12.018.

Skalny AV, Klimenko LL, Turna AA, Budanova MN, Baskakov IS, Savostina MS, Mazilina AN, Deyev AI, Skalnaya MG, Tinkov AA. Serum trace elements are associated with hemostasis, lipid spectrum and inflammatory markers in men suffering from acute ischemic stroke. Metab Brain Dis. 2017b;32(3):779–88. https://doi.org/10.1007/s11011-017-9967-6.

Smith S, Horgan F, Sexton E, Cowman S, Hickey A, Kelly P, McGee H, Murphy S, O'neill D, Royston M, Shelley E. The cost of stroke and transient ischaemic attack in Ireland: a prevalence-based estimate. Age Ageing. 2011;41(3):332–8. https://doi.org/10.1093/ageing/afr141.

Steinbrenner H, Sies H. Selenium homeostasis and antioxidant selenoproteins in brain: implications for disorders in the central nervous system. Arch Biochem Boiphys. 2013;536(2):152–7. https://doi.org/10.1016/j.abb.2013.02.021.

Stranges S, Marshall JR, Trevisan M, et al. Effects of selenium supplementation on cardiovascular disease incidence and mortality: secondary analyses in a randomized clinical trial. Am J Epidemiol. 2006;163:694–9. https://doi.org/10.1093/aje/kwj097.

Stranges S, Laclaustra M, Ji C, Cappuccio FP, Navas-Acien A, Ordovas JM, Rayman M, Guallar E. Higher selenium status is associated with adverse blood lipid profile in British adults. J Nutr. 2010;140(1):81–7. https://doi.org/10.3945/jn.109.111252.

Sui H, Wang W, Wang PH, Liu LS. Effect of glutathione peroxidase mimic ebselen (PZ51) on endothelium and vascular structure of stroke-prone spontaneously hypertensive rats. Blood Press. 2005;14(6):366–72. https://doi.org/10.1080/08037050500210781.

Sun JH, Tan L, Yu JT. Post-stroke cognitive impairment: epidemiology, mechanisms and management. Ann Transl Med. 2014;2(8) https://doi.org/10.3978/j.issn.2305-5839.2014.08.05.

Suwanwela NC, Poungvarin N. Stroke burden and stroke care system in Asia. Neurol India. 2016;64(7):46. https://doi.org/10.4103/0028-3886.178042.

Szydlowska K, Tymianski M. Calcium, ischemia and excitotoxicity. Cell Calcium. 2010;47(2):122–9. https://doi.org/10.1016/j.ceca.2010.01.003.

Takasago T, Peters EE, Graham DI, Masayasu H, Macrae IM. Neuroprotective efficacy of ebselen, an anti-oxidant with anti-inflammatory actions, in a rodent model of permanent middle cerebral artery occlusion. Br J Pharmacol. 1997;122(6):1251–6. https://doi.org/10.1038/sj.bjp.0701426.

Takizawa S, Matsushima K, Shinohara Y, Ogawa S, Komatsu N, Utsunomiya H, Watanabe K. Immunohistochemical localization of glutathione peroxidase in infarcted human brain. J Neurol Sci. 1994;122(1):66–73. https://doi.org/10.1016/0022-510X(94)90053-1.

Venardos KM, Kaye DM. Myocardial ischemia-reperfusion injury, antioxidant enzyme systems, and selenium: a review. Curr Med Chem. 2007;14(14):1539–49. https://doi.org/10.2174/092986707780831078.

Vinceti M, Mandrioli J, Borella P, Michalke B, Tsatsakis A, Finkelstein Y. Selenium neurotoxicity in humans: bridging laboratory and epidemiologic studies. Toxicol Lett. 2014;230(2):295–303. https://doi.org/10.1016/j.toxlet.2013.11.016.

Virtamo J, Valkeila E, Alfthan G, Punsar S, Huttunen JK, Karvonen MJ. Serum selenium and the risk of coronary heart disease and stroke. Am J Epidemiol. 1985;122(2):276–82. https://doi.org/10.1093/oxfordjournals.aje.a114099.

Voetsch B, Jin RC, Bierl C, Benke KS, Kenet G, Simioni P, Ottaviano F, Damasceno BP, Annichino-Bizacchi JM, Handy DE, Loscalzo J. Promoter polymorphisms in the plasma glutathione peroxidase (GPx-3) gene. Stroke. 2007;38(1):41–9. https://doi.org/10.1161/01.STR.0000252027.53766.2b.

Wang GS, Geng DQ, Wang YW, Chen XD, Yang TH, Chang CH. Protective effect of Na₂SeO₃ against cerebral ischemia-reperfusion injury to the hippocampal neurons in rats. J Southern Med Univ. 2010;30(10):2336–9.

Wei WQ, Abnet CC, Qiao YL, Dawsey SM, Dong ZW, Sun XD, Fan JH, Gunter EW, Taylor PR, Mark SD. Prospective study of serum selenium concentrations and esophageal and gastric cardia cancer, heart disease, stroke, and total death. Am J Clin Nutr. 2004;79(1):80–5.

Weisbrot-Lefkowitz M, Reuhl K, Perry B, Chan PH, Inouye M, Mirochnitchenko O. Overexpression of human glutathione peroxidase protects transgenic mice against focal cerebral ischemia/reperfusion damage. Mol Brain Res. 1998;53(1):333–8. https://doi.org/10.1016/S0169-328X(97)00313-6.

Weissman JD, Khunteev GA, Heath R, Dambinova SA. NR2 antibodies: risk assessment of transient ischemic attack (TIA)/stroke in patients with history of isolated and multiple cerebrovascular events. J Neurol Sci. 2011;300(1–2):97–102.

WHO. Media Centre. The top 10 causes of death. 2017. http://www.who.int/mediacentre/factsheets/fs310/en

Wirth EK, Conrad M, Winterer J, Wozny C, Carlson BA, Roth S, Schmitz D, Bornkamm GW, Coppola V, Tessarollo L, Schomburg L. Neuronal selenoprotein expression is required for interneuron development and prevents seizures and neurodegeneration. FASEB J. 2010;24(3):844–52. https://doi.org/10.1096/fj.09-143974.

Woodruff TM, Thundyil J, Tang SC, Sobey CG, Taylor SM, Arumugam TV. Pathophysiology, treatment, and animal and cellular models of human ischemic stroke. Mol Neurodegener. 2011;6(1):11. https://doi.org/10.1186/1750-1326-6-11.

Yamagata K, Ichinose S, Miyashita A, Tagami M. Protective effects of ebselen, a seleno-organic antioxidant on neurodegeneration induced by hypoxia and reperfusion in stroke-prone spontaneously hypertensive rat. Neuroscience. 2008;153(2):428–35. https://doi.org/10.1016/j.neuroscience.2008.02.028.

Yamaguchi T, Sano K, Takakura K, Saito I, Shinohara Y, Asano T, Yasuhara H. Ebselen in acute ischemic stroke. Stroke. 1998;29(1):12–7. https://doi.org/10.1161/01.STR.29.1.12.

Yoshizumi M, Kogame T, Suzaki Y, Fujita Y, Kyaw M, Kirima K, Ishizawa K, Tsuchiya K, Kagami S, Tamaki T. Ebselen attenuates oxidative stress-induced apoptosis via the inhibition of the c-Jun N-terminal kinase and activator protein-1 signalling pathway in PC12 cells. Br J Pharmacol. 2002;136(7):1023–32. https://doi.org/10.1038/sj.bjp.0704808.

Yousuf S, Atif F, Ahmad M, Hoda MN, Khan MB, Ishrat T, Islam F. Selenium plays a modulatory role against cerebral ischemia-induced neuronal damage in rat hippocampus. Brain Res. 2007;1147:218–25. https://doi.org/10.1016/j.brainres.2007.01.143.

Zhang F, Yu W, Hargrove JL, Greenspan P, Dean RG, Taylor EW, Hartle DK. Inhibition of TNF-α induced ICAM-1, VCAM-1 and E-selectin expression by selenium. Atherosclerosis. 2002;161(2):381–6. https://doi.org/10.1016/S0021-9150(01)00672-4.

Zhang X, Liu C, Guo J, Song Y. Selenium status and cardiovascular diseases: meta-analysis of prospective observational studies and randomized controlled trials. Eur J Clin Nutr. 2016;70(2):162–9. https://doi.org/10.1038/ejcn.2015.78.

Zhao R, Holmgren A. A novel antioxidant mechanism of ebselen involving ebselen diselenide, a substrate of mammalian thioredoxin and thioredoxin reductase. J Biol Chem. 2002;277(42):39456–62. https://doi.org/10.1074/jbc.M206452200.

Zhao R, Holmgren A. Ebselen is a dehydroascorbate reductase mimic, facilitating the recycling of ascorbate via mammalian thioredoxin systems. Antioxid Redox Signal. 2004;6(1):99–104. https://doi.org/10.1089/152308604771978390.

Zimmermann C, Winnefeld K, Streck S, Roskos M, Haberl RL. Antioxidant status in acute stroke patients and patients at stroke risk. Eur Neurol. 2004;51(3):157–61. https://doi.org/10.1159/000077662.

Chapter 12
Selenium Neurotoxicity and Amyotrophic Lateral Sclerosis: An Epidemiologic Perspective

Tommaso Filippini, Bernhard Michalke, Jessica Mandrioli,
Aristidis M. Tsatsakis, Jennifer Weuve, and Marco Vinceti

Abstract Selenium exposure has been proposed as possible risk factor for amyotrophic lateral sclerosis (ALS), due to the selective toxicity of the trace element, especially in its inorganic forms, toward motor neurons. The epidemiological evidence, in association with laboratory and veterinary findings, linking selenium exposure and ALS risk was originally suggested by the increased ALS mortality in an area characterized by high selenium content in soil, and subsequently confirmed in an Italian community. The latter was unintentionally exposed to high levels of inorganic hexavalent selenium through drinking water, and subsequently showed an increased incidence for neurodegenerative diseases, including ALS and Parkinson's disease. Review of the epidemiological studies addressing the association between

T. Filippini
CREAGEN, Environmental, Genetic and Nutritional Epidemiology Research Center;
Section of Public Health, Department of Biomedical, Metabolic and Neural Sciences,
University of Modena and Reggio Emilia, Modena, Italy

B. Michalke
Research Unit: Analytical BioGeoChemistry, Helmholtz Zentrum München – German
Research Center for Environmental Health GmbH, Neuherberg, Germany

J. Mandrioli
Department of Neurosciences, Azienda Ospedaliero-Universitaria di Modena, Sant Agostino
Estense Hospital, Modena, Italy

A. M. Tsatsakis
Department of Forensic Sciences and Toxicology, University of Crete, Heraklion, Greece

J. Weuve
Department of Epidemiology, Boston University School of Public Health, Boston, MA, USA

M. Vinceti (✉)
CREAGEN, Environmental, Genetic and Nutritional Epidemiology Research Center; Section
of Public Health, Department of Biomedical, Metabolic and Neural Sciences, University of
Modena and Reggio Emilia, Modena, Italy

Department of Epidemiology, Boston University School of Public Health, Boston, MA, USA
e-mail: marco.vinceti@unimore.it

© Springer International Publishing AG, part of Springer Nature 2018
B. Michalke (ed.), *Selenium*, Molecular and Integrative Toxicology,
https://doi.org/10.1007/978-3-319-95390-8_12

selenium exposure and ALS risk points out important lessons that should be considered in future research, in order to avoid misleading and biased evaluations of selenium's effects. These include the use of central nervous system indicator of exposure such as cerebrospinal fluid, and the implementation of speciation analysis, due to the different toxic and nutritional properties of the various selenium compounds.

Keywords Amyotrophic lateral sclerosis · Epidemiologic studies · Neurotoxicity · Speciation analysis · Selenium

Selenium and Neurological Disease

Selenium is a metalloid with both nutritional and toxicological interest showing an intriguing relation with human health, especially with cancer and other chronic diseases (Vinceti et al. 2016b, 2018a, b). In particular, adverse neurological effects of both selenium deficiency and selenium overexposure have been proposed in the recent years (Cicero et al. 2017; Pillai et al. 2014; Schweizer et al. 2011; Solovyev 2015; Trojsi et al. 2013; Vinceti et al. 2012b, 2014).

The neurotoxicity of excess selenium exposure has been originally suggested by observations in livestock from the seleniferous areas of the United States, where affected animals displayed a wide spectrum of neurological symptoms that encompassed wandering, stumbling, blindness, ataxia, disorientation, and generalized paralysis (Fan and Kizer 1990). In humans, early observations came from studies carried out in occupationally exposed subjects, subjects consuming misformulated Se supplements, and populations from seleniferous areas of China (Clark et al. 1996; Fordyce 1996; Helzlsouer et al. 1985; Nuttall 2006; Yang et al. 1983). The acute neurologic effects due to selenium intoxication may include tremor, tingling, ataxia, fatigue, confusion, irritability, delirium, coma, and eventually *postmortem* examinations showed in cases of presence of cerebral edema (Fan and Vinceti 2015; Nuttall 2006). Chronic selenium intoxication has been linked to neurological signs and symptoms encompassing peripheral anesthesia, acroparesthesia, pain to the extremities, numbness, hyperreflexia, convulsion, motor disturbances, and eventually hemiplegia (MacFarquhar et al. 2010; Nuttall 2006; Yang et al. 1983), with persistence for 90 days or more after cessation of impairment including tingling, muscle pain/aches, and even memory loss and mood changes (Fan and Vinceti 2015; MacFarquhar et al. 2010). A group of subjects after ingestion of high dose of selenium from misformulated dietary supplements showed persistence of neurological long-term side effects after 2.5-year follow-up, including dizziness, loss of balance, confusion or inability to concentrate, memory loss, numbness, and tingling in extremities (Morris and Crane 2013).

Finally, abnormal selenium exposure has been implicated also in the pathogenesis of three neurodegenerative diseases, amyotrophic lateral sclerosis (ALS), Parkinson's disease, and Alzheimer's disease (Vinceti et al. 2016b). For the two latter diseases, however, both increased and decreased selenium levels have been suggested to play a role in the etiology, thus yielding an extremely inconsistent and uncertain pattern and several uncertainties (Ellwanger et al. 2016; Raber et al. 2010; Vinceti et al. 2017a). Concerning ALS, a progressive and fatal neurodegenerative disease affecting lower and upper motor neurons, there is currently a rather wide spectrum of both human (epidemiologic) and animal laboratory studies addressing the relation between the etiology of this disease and selenium exposure. Though selenium deficiency has also been suggested to be involved in disease onset and progression (Orrell et al. 2008), by far the most common hypothesis underpinning the selenium and ALS relation is an etiologic role of selenium overexposure, possibly linked only to some chemical forms of the element (Vinceti et al. 2010a).

Selenium Exposure and ALS: Biological Plausibility

Evidence supporting biological plausibility of a relation between Se species, and selenite in particular, and ALS has been provided by several laboratory and animal studies. The higher toxicity of inorganic Se compounds, i.e., selenite (Se(IV)) followed by selenate (Se(VI)), in relation to other forms of selenium was observed by the earlier investigators of instances of selenium toxicity (Du et al. 2017; Rocha et al. 2017). The neurotoxic effects of selenium could be mediated by the electrophilic feature of these inorganic forms which can promote production of reactive oxygen species and catalyze the oxidation of thiol groups of biomolecules and proteins (Oliveira et al. 2017). It should be noted that also organic selenium species such as selenomethionine-bound Se (Se-Met) can induce oxidation of thiol-containing proteins (Dolgova et al. 2016), but inorganic selenium species and particularly Se(IV) and Se(VI) have shown stronger prooxidant effects, in sharp contrast with the antioxidant activity of selenoproteins (Mandrioli et al. 2017; Nogueira and Rocha 2011). The possible mechanisms underlying selenium neurotoxicity, particularly for Se(IV), Se(VI), and Se-Met, might involve the prooxidant properties and mitochondrial damage (D'Amico et al. 2013; Jablonska and Vinceti 2015; Rezacova et al. 2016). Recent *in vitro* observations showed that selenium, even at low concentrations, is able to trigger apoptotic process and decrease viability in a human neuron cell line, through for example copper/zinc superoxide dismutase translocation into mitochondria, and increase of inducible nitric oxide synthase (Maraldi et al. 2011).

Laboratory investigations on animal models have also provided evidence of possible mechanism for the specific motor neuron toxicity. In particular, high levels of sodium selenite in the environment of the nematode *Caenorhabditis elegans* can induce neurodegeneration and cell loss yielding motor function impairment and death through a decreased cholinergic signaling and increasing cytosolic muscle protein catabolism (Estevez et al. 2012, 2014). Similarly, selenium may alter neuromuscular functions in other animal models by depolarizing the nerve membrane (Lin-Shiau et al. 1990; Liu et al. 1989). In a toxicology study carried out on rat sciatic nerve fibers a selenite toxicity was found starting from 0.01 µM concentration, corresponding to a total selenium level of 0.8 µg/L (Ayaz et al. 2008); such a level is generally considered safe for humans (Vinceti et al. 2014, 2017c) and considerably lower levels may be commonly found in human blood (Christensen et al. 2015; Vinceti et al. 2015). In a fish model exposed to increasing waterborne selenium concentrations showed marked elevation of superoxide dismutase and glutathione S-transferase activity as well as inhibition of acetylcholinesterase activity in brain and muscle tissues (Kim and Kang 2015). In addition, recent findings in zebrafish treated with high selenium doses have showed an impairment of performances related to latent learning task (Naderi et al. 2017). In the fish brain, altered learning tasks were associated with the induction of oxidative stress and altered mRNA expression of dopamine receptors, tyrosine hydroxylase, and dopamine transporter genes.

Several veterinary observations have also provided biological evidence linking selenium exposure and ALS. In swine and cattle a specific toxicity to motor neurons with walking disturbances, paralysis, and death from respiratory failure, was pointed out after accidental intoxication with high dose of selenite (Casteignau et al. 2006; Davidson-York et al. 1999; Maag et al. 1960; Penrith 1995; Raber et al. 2010; SAC Consulting Veterinary Services 2010). The main and consistent anatomopathological findings demonstrated a bilaterally symmetrical focal poliomyelomalacia of spinal cord ventral horns in pigs (Casteignau et al. 2006; Harrison et al. 1983; Penrith and Robinson 1996; Raber et al. 2010; SAC Consulting Veterinary Services 2010) and polioencephalomalacia in selenium-exposed steers (Maag et al. 1960). Interestingly, these motor abnormalities have been experimentally reproduced in selenium-exposed swine (Panter et al. 1996), mainly due to the superior toxicity of inorganic selenium species although the higher body levels of selenium were achieved after supplementation with the organic forms. These lesions appear to mirror the pathological findings observed in the human affected by ALS.

Selenium Exposure and ALS: The Epidemiologic Evidence

The first association between selenium exposure and ALS was described in a report of four sporadic cases of the disease occurring in a sparse population from South Dakota (Kilness and Hochberg 1977). This cluster was composed of unrelated farmers living with a 15 km radius of each other in a region characterized by a natural occurrence of high selenium content in soil and within the local food chain, through contamination of grain and forage and livestock intoxication (Kilness and Hochberg 1977). Nevertheless, the etiological significance of these "sparse" observations was strongly challenged and was given limited attention, though on the basis of very limited epidemiologic evidence (Kurland 1977; Norris and Sang 1978). Interest in the potential relation was however renewed by the results of a study carried out in an Italian community (Vinceti et al. 2010a). In that study, conducted in the city of Reggio Emilia (Fig. 12.1) where a part of the municipal residents had been exposed to high level of environmental selenium of geologic origin through drinking water, an increased incidence of ALS was detected (Vinceti et al. 1996). In that community, from 1972 to 1988, a neighborhood ("Rivalta") was provided with municipal tap water characterized by unusually high levels of inorganic Se(VI) very close to the upper standard of 10 µg/L (Vinceti et al. 2013a) (Fig. 12.2). This high-Se-exposed cohort was unaware of the selenium content in tap water and had very similar sociodemographic characteristics compared to the remaining low-Se-exposed cohort from the rest of the municipal population; thus the high selenate content was the only distinctive feature detected comparing with drinking water distributed in the remaining municipal territory (Fig. 12.3) (Vinceti et al. 1996). These study settings made it possible to define what occurred in that community as a "natural experiment," usually of strong interest in environmental epidemiology (Rothman et al. 2008). A natural experiment mimics random allocation of subjects to conditions, including toxic exposure, which would be impossible to study with the paradigm of experimental studies, i.e., randomized control trials. After discontinuing the supply of this high-selenium well water, Se levels in municipal tap water distributed in Rivalta decreased to less than 1 µg/L; however, in the subsequent period (1986–1997) that community showed a slight increase in mortality from some malignant neoplasms, mainly due to an excess of melanoma and colorectal cancer in both sexes, kidney cancer in men, and lymphoid malignancies in women (Vinceti et al. 2016a), along with an increased mortality from cerebrovascular and neurodegenerative diseases, i.e., ALS and Parkinson's disease (Vinceti et al. 2000). The excess in mortality waned starting 10 years after the high-selenium exposure ended, especially for cancer malignancies; however increased rate ratios for neurodegenerative disease were still present after a long-term (1986–2012) follow-up (Vinceti et al. 2016a).

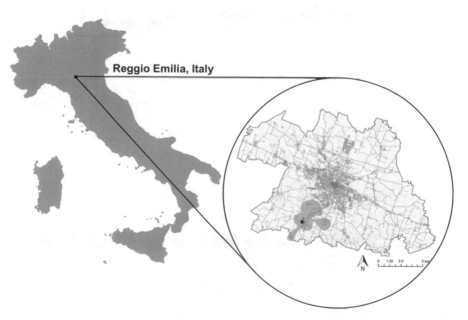

Fig. 12.1 Map of Reggio Emilia municipality showing Rivalta neighborhood (shaded area) and wells (black star) with high selenate content

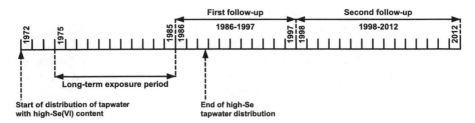

Fig. 12.2 Design of the retrospective cohort study, which involved residents of Reggio Emilia exposed to selenate (Se(VI)) through drinking water

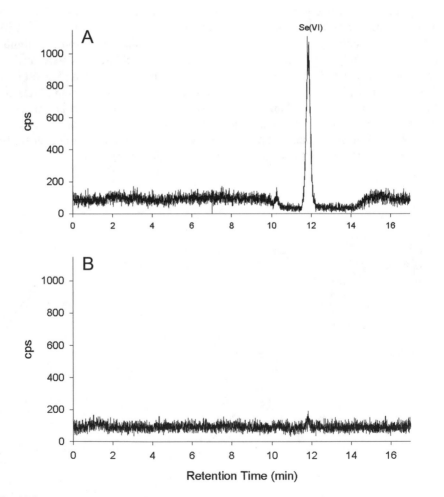

Fig. 12.3 Chromatograms showing the results of selenium speciation analysis for water samples distributed in the exposed (**A**) and unexposed (**B**) areas of Reggio Emilia municipality. *Cps* cycles per second, *Se(VI)* selenate

A number of case-control studies have also compared selenium levels in ALS cases and referent subjects, based on various indicators of exposure. The results of these studies are summarized in Table 12.1. Most of these studies investigated the overall Se content of body tissues without assessing the different chemical species of the metalloid. However, as noted previously, the biological function and toxicology of different Se compounds could be very different (Schweizer 2016; Solovyev 2015), thus increasing the value of speciation analysis to uncover the exact mechanism involved in brain damage (Michalke et al. 2018). Unfortunately, very few studies measured single-Se species (Mandrioli et al. 2017; Vinceti et al. 2013c). Instead, most measured overall Se content, probably due to high technology requirements of standardization and quality controls necessary in speciation analysis, and lack of standards for such selenoproteins, e.g., selenoprotein P (SELENOP) (Michalke et al. 2018). When the individual Se species were evaluated, the inorganic species (i.e., selenite and selenate) generally showed higher concentrations in ALS patients and an increased risk of ALS was specifically found for inorganic species, contrary to other Se forms (Vinceti et al. 2013c). Interestingly, these studies have shown that overall selenium content may not be associated with disease risk even when some specific inorganic and organic forms of the element correlate with the risk itself (Mandrioli et al. 2017; Vinceti et al. 2013c), thus suggesting the potential for bias of studies based on the simple determination of total selenium exposure.

Moreover, the levels of total Se and of specific Se compounds in the different body tissues may considerably vary, as may the correlation of concentrations of a given species between body compartments (Michalke et al. 2017; Solovyev et al. 2013). This hampers or even precludes the assessment of their concentrations in the target organs relevant for the disease on the basis of peripheral indicators of exposure (such as blood or toenail Se) or dietary intake of the metalloid (Behne et al. 2010; Vinceti et al. 2012a). This is particularly true within the brain due to the strict regulation of the blood–brain barrier, as showed by the independence of overall Se content in paired cerebrospinal fluid (CSF) and serum samples (Michalke et al. 2009), or by the lack of influence of plasma SELENOP deficiency on the brain content of this protein (Scharpf et al. 2007). These results were confirmed by recent speciation studies, showing that peripheral blood levels of some organic Se species (i.e., glutathione peroxidase-bound Se and thioredoxin reductase-bound Se) tend to reflect central nervous system (CNS) levels, yet other organic species, such as SELENOP, overall Se content, and particularly the inorganic forms of the element, selenate and selenite, did not show such correlation, thus suggesting that peripheral indicators of selenium exposure are not suitable for its CNS content (Michalke et al. 2017; Solovyev et al. 2013). Unfortunately, by far the majority of the human case-control studies based their exposure assessment on peripheral indicators, as serum or whole blood Se content, and they generally showed similar or lower level of selenium in ALS patients compared with controls. Conversely, studies using samples from central nervous system generally demonstrated higher Se content in ALS cases than in controls, measuring either Se level in spinal cord or CSF (see Table 12.1 for details).

Table 12.1 Characteristics and results of case-control studies comparing selenium levels in ALS

References	Country	Specimen	Cases/controls	Selenium levels[a] Cases	Controls	Notes
Kurlander and Patten (1979)	Houston, Texas (USA)	Spinal cord (µg/g)	7/12	Se levels not detectable in most subjects		Cases of MND, 5 ALS and 2 PMA. Non-healthy controls, 1 with PD and 1 with MS
Katsui et al. (1987), Nagata et al. (1985)	Kyoto, Japan	Dried blood cells (ng/mg)	40/25	1.16 (0.24)	0.84 (0.17)	↑ Higher levels in stage I/II (1.32) cases than stage III (1.14) or IV (1.18)
Gresham et al. (1986)	San Diego, California (USA)	Occupational exposure to Se	66/66	1 Case exposed and 2 controls exposed		↔
Mitchell et al. (1984, 1986a, b)	Edinburgh, UK	CSF	20/14	Reported only no difference		↔
		Spinal cord	5/5	Se level higher in spinal cord of cases ($P = 0.0094$)		↑
		Liver	5/5	Se level higher in liver of cases ($P = 0.014$)		↑
		Bone (thoracic spinous process)	5/5	Reported only no difference		↔
Khare et al. (1990)	Lexington, Kentucky (USA)	Spinal cord (ng/g)	21/20	110 (32.1)	128 (31.3)	↓/↔
		Bulk brain (ng/g)	29/98	166 (5.7)	175 (10.2)	↓/↔
		Motor neuron region (ng/g)	12/20	174 (3.7)	165 (4.7)	↑/↔
		Serum (ng/g)	40/29	95.4 (27.2)	116.0 (23.2)	↓
		Blood cells (ng/g)	28/12 M 9/7 F	140 (5.5) M 152 (3.3) F	148 (3.6) M 183 (2.8) F	↓/↔
		Nails (ng/g)	30/40	801 (5.8)	839 (6.6)	↓/↔

Study	Location	Tissue	Cases/controls	Cases	Controls	Comment	Direction
Oishi et al. (1990)	Japan	Hair (ppm)	11/1489			Reported only in figure, Se levels considerably high in two cases	↑/↔
Mitchell et al. (1991)	Edinburgh, UK	Spinal cord	15/7			Se level higher at the cervical (P = 0.044) and lumbar enlargements, but lower in the thoracic enlargement	↑/↔
		Liver				Se level higher in ALS cases (P = 0.0014)	↑
		Bone				Se level higher in ALS cases (P = 0.0066)	↑
Moriwaka et al. (1993)	Hokkaido, Japan	Plasma (ng/g)	21/35 13 Non-heathy controls with PD	81.20 (46.42)	120.61 (20.55)		↓ Higher levels in stage I–III cases (102.75) than stage IV (50.50)
		Blood cell (ng/g)	20/35	134.63 (73.36)	191.55 (35.88)		↓ Higher levels in stage I–III cases (176.03) than stage IV (84.02)
		Hair (ng/g)	2/0	Not reported			–
Ince et al. (1994)	Kentucky (US)	Lumbar spinal cord (ng/g)	38/22	142 (43)	100 (33)		↑ 16 Controls were neurological disease comparison cases
Lee (1994)	Massachusetts (USA)	Motor cortex (µg/g)	19/16	0.93 (0.35)	0.75 (0.24)		↑
		Cerebellum (µg/g)	13/8	0.74 (0.23)	1.09 (1.03)		↓
		Spinal cord (µg/g)	10/3	0.58 (0.23)	0.88 (0.22)		↓
Vinceti et al. (1997)	Reggio Emilia, Italy	Serum (µg/L)	16/39	68.6 (16.9)	76.8 (11.8)		↔/↓
				78.7 (12.0)	76.1 (14.5)		Subjects with limited degree of disability

(continued)

Table 12.1 (continued)

References	Country	Specimen	Cases/controls	Selenium levels[a] Cases	Controls	Notes
Pamphlett et al. (2001)	Sydney, Australia	Whole blood Plasma Blood cells	20/20	Not reported, only in figures showing comparable levels		↔
Bergomi et al. (2002)	Emilia-Romagna Region, Italy	Toenails (µg/g)	22/40	0.62 (0.54–0.70)	0.59 (0.53–0.70)	↔
Vinceti et al. (2010b)	Reggio Emilia, Italy	Se intake (drinking water and food)	41/82	High Se 8 Low Se 33	High Se 6 Low Se 76	High Se means ≥1 µg/L RR 3.3 (95% CI 1.0–11.0)
Roos et al. (2013)	Oslo, Norway	CSF (µg/L)	17/10	1.54 (0.25–2.86)[b]	1.74 (0.93–2.09)[b]	↔/↓
		Plasma (µg/L)	15/9	87.81 (57.05–166.02)[b]	89.28 (72.27–118.79)[b]	↔
Vinceti et al. (2013c)	Emilia-Romagna Region, Italy	CSF (µg/L)	38/38	0.765 (0.320–2.660)[c]	1.100 (0.140–8.380)[c]	↓ Total Se RR 0.3 (95% CI 0.1–0.9)
				0.765 (0.287–2.508)[c]	1.084 (0.053–8.284)[c]	↓ Organic Se RR 0.3 (95% CI 0.1–1.0)
				0.051 (0–0.169)[c]	0.026 (0–0.180)[c]	↑ Selenite (inorganic Se) RR 3.9 (95% CI 1.2–11.0)
De Benedetti et al. (2015)	Milan, Italy	Serum (µg/L)	7/5	97.71 (10.20)	89.54 (6.32)	↑/↔
Peters et al. (2016)	National Registry of Veterans with ALS, USA	Whole blood	163/229	Means not reported, overall range 11.9–73.5		Adjusted OR of doubling Se levels 0.5 (95% CI 0.2–1.0)

De Benedetti et al. (2017)	La Spezia, Italy	Serum (µg/L)	6/5	100 (12)	90 (8)	↑ Se higher in patients with the earliest onset
		Whole blood (µg/L)		110 (18)	121 (17)	↓
Forte et al. (2017)	Sardinia, Italy	Whole blood (µg/L)	34/30	137 (73.6–215)[d]	153 (106–182)[d]	↓/↔
		Hair (µg/g)		529 (230–1011)[d]	353 (166–844)[d]	↑
		Urine (µg/L)		16.2 (8.42–55.5)[d]	35.6 (6.10–70.3)[d]	↓
Mandrioli et al. (2017)	Milan, Modena, and Rome, Italy	CSF (µg/L)	9/42 One case TUBA4A carrier and 8 non-carriers	6.107 (12.042)	2.310 (1.204)	↑ Total Se
				5.576 (11.116)	1.923 (0.989)	↑ Organic Se
				0.449 (0.843)	0.246 (0.279)	↑ Inorganic Se
				0.313 (0.555)	0.141 (0.184)	↑ Selenite

ALS amyotrophic lateral sclerosis, *CI* confidence intervals, *CSF* cerebrospinal fluid, *F* females, *M* males, *MND* motor neuron disease, *MS* multiple sclerosis, *OR* odds ratio, *PD* Parkinson's disease, *PMA* progressive muscular atrophy, *RR* relative risk, *SD* standard deviation

[a]Mean (standard deviation), where not differently reported
[b]Mean (range)
[c]Median (interquartile range)
[d]Median (5th–95th)

Finally, the stage of the disease could have also influenced the apparent level of exposure, as during disease progression and with increasing muscle wasting, habits of patients, including diet, may considerably vary and thus influence their selenium status. This is particularly true for peripheral specimens, where selenium levels may have a shortened half-time, much more influenced by the selenium intake through diet and/or by the release of selenium from other body compartments (Behne et al. 2010), as well as by the intake of other dietary factors such as methionine (Vinceti et al. 2013b). Studies that measured selenium in ALS patients also showed that selenium was higher in those in the earliest clinical stages of the disease (De Benedetti et al. 2017; Moriwaka et al. 1993; Nagata et al. 1985; Vinceti et al. 1997; Oggiano et al. 2018). This means that case-control studies, if of any utility due to the risk of reverse causation, should be carried out only on newly diagnosed patients, use prospectively stored specimens (i.e., samples collected prior to the onset of symptoms), rely on CNS indicators of exposure, and perform Se speciation analyses. Finally, the control population should be carefully selected, in order to avoid misleading interpretations due to possible influence of selenium in the etiology of other neurological and non-neurological diseases (Vinceti et al. 2017a, c).

Selenium and ALS: Concluding Remarks

Overall, the epidemiological evidence indicates that exposure to some selenium species may represent a risk factor for ALS. In particular, the selenium inorganic species appear to be able to trigger the neurodegenerative process leading to ALS, through their powerful and highly specific toxicity toward motor neurons, as shown by the converging findings of laboratory and animal studies. Important lessons that should be learnt from conflicting results of previous epidemiological studies include the implementation of a comprehensive selenium speciation analysis, avoidance of use of misleading peripheral indicators, and eventually recruitment only of newly diagnosed participants, excluding the ALS cases with advanced disease.

Finally, the unique evidence generated by the South Dakota ALS cluster and by the "natural experiment" in the Italian community, consuming high levels of inorganic selenium through drinking water, suggests the need to investigate disease incidence in similar settings, e.g., working environments and/or seleniferous areas, characterized by unintentional though unusually high exposure to inorganic selenium compounds (Carsella et al. 2017; Chawla et al. 2015; Hurtado-Jimenez and Gardea-Torresdey 2007; Vinceti et al. 2017b), and eventually the reassessment of selenium standards in drinking water along with implementation of the management of selenium-laden wastewaters (Tan et al. 2016; Vinceti et al. 2013a).

References

Ayaz M, Dalkilic N, Tuncer S, Bariskaner H. Selenium-induced changes on rat sciatic nerve fibers: compound action potentials. Methods Find Exp Clin Pharmacol. 2008;30(4):271–5. https://doi.org/10.1358/mf.2008.30.4.1166220.

Behne D, Alber D, Kyriakopoulos A. Long-term selenium supplementation of humans: selenium status and relationships between selenium concentrations in skeletal muscle and indicator materials. J Trace Elem Med Biol. 2010;24(2):99–105. https://doi.org/10.1016/j.jtemb.2009.12.001.

Bergomi M, Vinceti M, Nacci G, Pietrini V, Bratter P, Alber D, Ferrari A, Vescovi L, Guidetti D, Sola P, Malagu S, Aramini C, Vivoli G. Environmental exposure to trace elements and risk of amyotrophic lateral sclerosis: a population-based case-control study. Environ Res. 2002;89(2):116–23.

Carsella JS, Sanchez-Lombardo I, Bonetti SJ, Crans DC. Selenium speciation in the fountain creek watershed (Colorado, USA) correlates with water hardness, Ca and Mg levels. Molecules. 2017;22(5):E708. https://doi.org/10.3390/molecules22050708.

Casteignau A, Fontan A, Morillo A, Oliveros JA, Segales J. Clinical, pathological and toxicological findings of a iatrogenic selenium toxicosis case in feeder pigs. J Vet Med A Physiol Pathol Clin Med. 2006;53(6):323–6. https://doi.org/10.1111/j.1439-0442.2006.00830.x.

Chawla R, Loomba R, Chaudhary RJ, Singh S, Dhillon KS. Impact of high selenium exposure on organ function and biochemical profile of the rural population living in seleniferous soils in Punjab, India. In: Banuelos GS, Lin Z-Q, Moraes MF, Guilherme LRG, dos Reis AR, editors. Global advance in selenium research from theory to application: Proceedings of the 4th International Conference on Selenium in the Environment and Human Health 2015. Sao Paulo: CRC Press; 2015. p. 93–4.

Christensen K, Werner M, Malecki K. Serum selenium and lipid levels: Associations observed in the National Health and Nutrition Examination Survey (NHANES) 2011-2012. Environ Res. 2015;140:76–84. https://doi.org/10.1016/j.envres.2015.03.020.

Cicero CE, Mostile G, Vasta R, Rapisarda V, Signorelli SS, Ferrante M, Zappia M, Nicoletti A. Metals and neurodegenerative diseases. A systematic review. Environ Res. 2017;159:82–94. https://doi.org/10.1016/j.envres.2017.07.048.

Clark RF, Strukle E, Williams SR, Manoguerra AS. Selenium poisoning from a nutritional supplement. JAMA. 1996;275(14):1087–8.

D'Amico E, Factor-Litvak P, Santella RM, Mitsumoto H. Clinical perspective on oxidative stress in sporadic amyotrophic lateral sclerosis. Free Radic Biol Med. 2013;65:509–27. https://doi.org/10.1016/j.freeradbiomed.2013.06.029.

Davidson-York D, Galey FD, Blanchard P, Gardner IA. Selenium elimination in pigs after an outbreak of selenium toxicosis. J Vet Diagn Investig. 1999;11(4):352–7. https://doi.org/10.1177/104063879901100410.

De Benedetti S, Lucchini G, Marocchi A, Penco S, Lunetta C, Iametti S, Gianazza E, Bonomi F. Serum metal evaluation in a small cohort of amyotrophic lateral sclerosis patients reveals high levels of thiophylic species. Peptidomics. 2015;2:29–34. https://doi.org/10.1515/ped-2015-0004.

De Benedetti S, Lucchini G, Del Bo C, Deon V, Marocchi A, Penco S, Lunetta C, Gianazza E, Bonomi F, Iametti S. Blood trace metals in a sporadic amyotrophic lateral sclerosis geographical cluster. Biometals. 2017;30(3):355–65. https://doi.org/10.1007/s10534-017-0011-4.

Dolgova NV, Hackett MJ, MacDonald TC, Nehzati S, James AK, Krone PH, George GN, Pickering IJ. Distribution of selenium in zebrafish larvae after exposure to organic and inorganic selenium forms. Metallomics. 2016;8(3):305–12. https://doi.org/10.1039/c5mt00279f.

Du Y, Yi X, Zheng W. Roles of selenium (Se) exposure in ALS development. J Trace Elem Med Biol. 2017;41S:4. https://doi.org/10.1016/j.jtemb.2017.03.024.

Ellwanger JH, Franke SI, Bordin DL, Pra D, Henriques JA. Biological functions of selenium and its potential influence on Parkinson's disease. An Acad Bras Cienc. 2016;88(3 Suppl):1655–74. https://doi.org/10.1590/0001-3765201620150595.

Estevez AO, Mueller CL, Morgan KL, Szewczyk NJ, Teece L, Miranda-Vizuete A, Estevez
    M. Selenium induces cholinergic motor neuron degeneration in *Caenorhabditis elegans*.
    Neurotoxicology. 2012;33(5):1021–32. https://doi.org/10.1016/j.neuro.2012.04.019.
Estevez AO, Morgan KL, Szewczyk NJ, Gems D, Estevez M. The neurodegenerative effects of
    selenium are inhibited by FOXO and PINK1/PTEN regulation of insulin/insulin-like growth
    factor signaling in *Caenorhabditis elegans*. Neurotoxicology. 2014;41C:28–43. https://doi.
    org/10.1016/j.neuro.2013.12.012.
Fan AM, Kizer KW. Selenium. Nutritional, toxicologic, and clinical aspects. West J Med.
    1990;153(2):160–7.
Fan AM, Vinceti M. Selenium and its compounds. In: Harbison RD, Bourgeois MM, Johnson GT,
    editors. Hamilton & Hardy's Industrial Toxicology. Hoboken, NJ: Wiley; 2015. p. 205–28.
    https://doi.org/10.1002/9781118834015.ch30.
Fordyce FM. Technical report WC/96/7R. Report of field visit and initial data from investigations
    into the prediction and remediation of human selenium imbalances in Enshi District, Hubei
    Province, China 8–16 November 1995. Nottingham: British Geological Survey; 1996.
Forte G, Bocca B, Oggiano R, Clemente S, Asara Y, Sotgiu MA, Farace C, Montella A, Fois AG,
    Malaguarnera M, Pirina P, Madeddu R. Essential trace elements in amyotrophic lateral scle-
    rosis (ALS): results in a population of a risk area of Italy. Neurol Sci. 2017;38(9):1609–15.
    https://doi.org/10.1007/s10072-017-3018-2.
Gresham LS, Molgaard CA, Golbeck AL, Smith R. Amyotrophic lateral sclerosis and occupational
    heavy metal exposure: a case-control study. Neuroepidemiology. 1986;5(1):29–38.
Harrison LH, Colvin BM, Stuart BP, Sangster LT, Gorgacz EJ, Gosser HS. Paralysis in swine due to
    focal symmetrical poliomalacia—possible selenium toxicosis. Vet Pathol. 1983;20(3):265–73.
Helzlsouer K, Jacobs R, Morris S. Acute selenium intoxication in the United States. Fed Proc.
    1985;44:1670.
Hurtado-Jimenez R, Gardea-Torresdey J. Evaluation of the exposure to selenium in Los Altos de
    Jalisco, Mexico. Salud Publica Mex. 2007;49(4):312–5.
Ince PG, Shaw PJ, Candy JM, Mantle D, Tandon L, Ehmann WD, Markesbery WR. Iron, selenium
    and glutathione peroxidase activity are elevated in sporadic motor neuron disease. Neurosci
    Lett. 1994;182(1):87–90.
Jablonska E, Vinceti M. Selenium and human health: Witnessing a Copernican Revolution?
    J Environ Sci Health C Environ Carcinog Ecotoxicol Rev. 2015;33(3):328–68. https://doi.org/
    10.1080/10590501.2015.1055163.
Katsui Y, Nagata H, Miyata S, Nakamura S, Kameyama M. Heavy metal concentrations in
    blood cells of patients with amyotrophic lateral sclerosis—study of five cases in Mie. Rinsho
    Shinkeigaku. 1987;27(1):19–22.
Khare SS, Ehmann WD, Kasarskis EJ, Markesbery WR. Trace element imbalances in amyotrophic
    lateral sclerosis. Neurotoxicology. 1990;11(3):521–32.
Kilness AW, Hochberg FH. Amyotrophic lateral sclerosis in a high selenium environment. JAMA.
    1977;237(26):2843–4.
Kim JH, Kang JC. Oxidative stress, neurotoxicity, and non-specific immune responses in juve-
    nile red sea bream, Pagrus major, exposed to different waterborne selenium concentrations.
    Chemosphere. 2015;135:46–52. https://doi.org/10.1016/j.chemosphere.2015.03.062.
Kurland LT. Amyotrophic Lateral Sclerosis and Selenium. JAMA. 1977;238(22):2365–6. https://
    doi.org/10.1001/jama.1977.03280230029005.
Kurlander HM, Patten BM. Metals in spinal cord tissue of patients dying of motor neuron disease.
    Ann Neurol. 1979;6(1):21–4. https://doi.org/10.1002/ana.410060105.
Lee RJ. Study of trace and minor elements in ALS (amyotrophic lateral sclerosis) patients.
    Research, Massachusetts Institute of Technology. 1994.
Lin-Shiau SY, Liu SH, Fu WM. Neuromuscular actions of sodium selenite on chick biventer cer-
    vicis nerve-muscle preparation. Neuropharmacology. 1990;29(5):493–501.
Liu SH, Fu WM, Lin-Shiau SY. Effects of sodium selenite on neuromuscular junction of the mouse
    phrenic nerve-diaphragm preparation. Neuropharmacology. 1989;28(7):733–9.

Maag DD, Orsborn JS, Clopton JR. The effect of sodium selenite on cattle. Am J Vet Res. 1960;21:1049–53.

MacFarquhar JK, Broussard DL, Melstrom P, Hutchinson R, Wolkin A, Martin C, Burk RF, Dunn JR, Green AL, Hammond R, Schaffner W, Jones TF. Acute selenium toxicity associated with a dietary supplement. Arch Intern Med. 2010;170(3):256–61. https://doi.org/10.1001/archinternmed.2009.495.

Mandrioli J, Michalke B, Solovyev N, Grill P, Violi F, Lunetta C, Conte A, Sansone VA, Sabatelli M, Vinceti M. Elevated levels of selenium species in cerebrospinal fluid of amyotrophic lateral sclerosis patients with disease-associated gene mutations. Neurodegener Dis. 2017;17(4–5):171–80. https://doi.org/10.1159/000460253.

Maraldi T, Riccio M, Zambonin L, Vinceti M, De Pol A, Hakim G. Low levels of selenium compounds are selectively toxic for a human neuron cell line through ROS/RNS increase and apoptotic process activation. Neurotoxicology. 2011;32:180–7. https://doi.org/10.1016/j.neuro.2010.10.008.

Michalke B, Grill P, Berthele A. A method for low volume and low Se concentration samples and application to paired cerebrospinal fluid and serum samples. J Trace Elem Med Biol. 2009;23(4):243–50. https://doi.org/10.1016/j.jtemb.2009.06.001.

Michalke B, Solovyev N, Vinceti M. Se-speciation investigations at neural barrier (NB). Se2017—200 Years of Selenium Research 1817–2017. 2017.

Michalke B, Willkommen D, Drobyshev E, Solovyev N. The importance of speciation analysis in neurodegeneration research. TrAC Trends Anal Chem. 2018;104:160–70. https://doi.org/10.1016/j.trac.2017.08.008.

Mitchell JD, Harris IA, East BW, Pentland B. Trace elements in cerebrospinal fluid in motor neurone disease. Br Med J (Clin Res Ed). 1984;288(6433):1791–2.

Mitchell JD, East BW, Harris IA, Pentland B. Trace element studies in amyotrophic lateral sclerosis (ALS). Acta Pharmacol Toxicol. 1986a;59:454–7. https://doi.org/10.1111/j.1600-0773.1986.tb02801.x.

Mitchell JD, East BW, Harris IA, Prescott RJ, Pentland B. Trace elements in the spinal cord and other tissues in motor neuron disease. J Neurol Neurosurg Psychiatry. 1986b;49(2):211–5.

Mitchell JD, East BW, Harris IA, Pentland B. Manganese, selenium and other trace elements in spinal cord, liver and bone in motor neurone disease. Eur Neurol. 1991;31(1):7–11.

Moriwaka F, Satoh H, Ejima A, Watanabe C, Tashiro K, Hamada T, Matsumoto A, Shima K, Yanagihara T, Fukazawa T, et al. Mercury and selenium contents in amyotrophic lateral sclerosis in Hokkaido, the northernmost island of Japan. J Neurol Sci. 1993;118(1):38–42.

Morris JS, Crane SB. Selenium toxicity from a misformulated dietary supplement, adverse health effects, and the temporal response in the nail biologic monitor. Nutrients. 2013;5(4):1024–57. https://doi.org/10.3390/nu5041024.

Naderi M, Salahinejad A, Jamwal A, Chivers DP, Niyogi S. Chronic dietary selenomethionine exposure induces oxidative stress, dopaminergic dysfunction, and cognitive impairment in adult zebrafish (Danio rerio). Environ Sci Technol. 2017;51(21):12879–88. https://doi.org/10.1021/acs.est.7b03937.

Nagata H, Miyata S, Nakamura S, Kameyama M, Katsui Y. Heavy metal concentrations in blood cells in patients with amyotrophic lateral sclerosis. J Neurol Sci. 1985;67(2):173–8.

Nogueira CW, Rocha JB. Toxicology and pharmacology of selenium: emphasis on synthetic organoselenium compounds. Arch Toxicol. 2011;85(11):1313–59. https://doi.org/10.1007/s00204-011-0720-3.

Norris FH Jr, Sang UK. Amyotrophic lateral sclerosis and low urinary selenium levels. JAMA. 1978;239(5):404.

Nuttall KL. Evaluating selenium poisoning. Ann Clin Lab Sci. 2006;36(4):409–20.

Oggiano R, Solinas G, Forte G, Bocca B, Farace C, Pisano A, Sotgiu MA, Clemente S, Malaguarnera M, Fois AG, Pirina P, Montella A, Madeddu R. Trace elements in ALS patients and their relationships with clinical severity. Chemosphere. 2018;197:457–66.

Oishi M, Takasu T, Tateno M. Hair trace elements in amyotrophtc lateral sclerosis. Trace Elements Med. 1990;7:182–5.

Oliveira CS, Piccoli BC, Aschner M, Rocha JBT. Chemical speciation of selenium and mercury as determinant of their neurotoxicity. Adv Neurobiol. 2017;18:53–83. https://doi.org/10.1007/978-3-319-60189-2_4.

Orrell RW, Lane RJ, Ross M. A systematic review of antioxidant treatment for amyotrophic lateral sclerosis/motor neuron disease. Amyotroph Lateral Scler. 2008;9(4):195–211. https://doi.org/10.1080/17482960801900032.

Pamphlett R, McQuilty R, Zarkos K. Blood levels of toxic and essential metals in motor neuron disease. Neurotoxicology. 2001;22(3):401–10.

Panter KE, Hartley WJ, James LF, Mayland HF, Stegelmeier BL, Kechele PO. Comparative toxicity of selenium from seleno-DL-methionine, sodium selenate, and Astragalus bisulcatus in pigs. Fundam Appl Toxicol. 1996;32(2):217–23.

Penrith ML. Acute selenium toxicosis as a cause of paralysis in pigs. J S Afr Vet Assoc. 1995;66(2):47–8.

Penrith ML, Robinson JT. Selenium toxicosis with focal symmetrical poliomyelomalacia in post-weaning pigs in South Africa. Onderstepoort J Vet Res. 1996;63(2):171–9.

Peters TL, Beard JD, Umbach DM, Allen K, Keller J, Mariosa D, Sandler DP, Schmidt S, Fang F, Ye W, Kamel F. Blood levels of trace metals and amyotrophic lateral sclerosis. Neurotoxicology. 2016;54:119–26. https://doi.org/10.1016/j.neuro.2016.03.022.

Pillai R, Uyehara-Lock JH, Bellinger FP. Selenium and selenoprotein function in brain disorders. IUBMB Life. 2014;66(4):229–39. https://doi.org/10.1002/iub.1262.

Raber M, Sydler T, Wolfisberg U, Geyer H, Burgi E. Feed-related selenium poisoning in swine. Schweiz Arch Tierheilkd. 2010;152(5):245–52. https://doi.org/10.1024/0036-7281/a000056.

Rezacova K, Canova K, Bezrouk A, Rudolf E. Selenite induces DNA damage and specific mitochondrial degeneration in human bladder cancer cells. Toxicol in Vitro. 2016;32:105–14. https://doi.org/10.1016/j.tiv.2015.12.011.

Rocha JBT, Piccoli BC, Oliveira CS. Biological and chemical interest in selenium: a brief historical account. ARKIVOC. 2017;2017:457–91. https://doi.org/10.3998/ark.5550190.p009.784.

Roos PM, Vesterberg O, Syversen T, Flaten TP, Nordberg M. Metal concentrations in cerebrospinal fluid and blood plasma from patients with amyotrophic lateral sclerosis. Biol Trace Elem Res. 2013;151(2):159–70. https://doi.org/10.1007/s12011-012-9547-x.

Rothman KJ, Greenland S, Lash TL. Modern epidemiology. Philadelphia, PA: Lippincott Williams & Wilkins; 2008.

SAC Consulting Veterinary Services. Selenium toxicity causes paralysis in Scottish pigs. Vet Rec. 2010;166(9):255–8. https://doi.org/10.1136/vr.c883.

Scharpf M, Schweizer U, Arzberger T, Roggendorf W, Schomburg L, Kohrle J. Neuronal and ependymal expression of selenoprotein P in the human brain. J Neural Transm (Vienna). 2007;114(7):877–84. https://doi.org/10.1007/s00702-006-0617-0.

Schweizer U. Selenoproteins in nervous system development, function and degeneration. In: Hatfield DL, Schweizer U, Tsuji PA, Gladyshev VN, editors. Selenium: its molecular biology and role in human health. Cham: Springer International Publishing; 2016. p. 427–39. https://doi.org/10.1007/978-3-319-41283-2_36.

Schweizer U, Dehina N, Schomburg L. Disorders of selenium metabolism and selenoprotein function. Curr Opin Pediatr. 2011;23(4):429–35. https://doi.org/10.1097/MOP.0b013e32834877da.

Solovyev ND. Importance of selenium and selenoprotein for brain function: from antioxidant protection to neuronal signalling. J Inorg Biochem. 2015;153:1–12. https://doi.org/10.1016/j.jinorgbio.2015.09.003.

Solovyev N, Berthele A, Michalke B. Selenium speciation in paired serum and cerebrospinal fluid samples. Anal Bioanal Chem. 2013;405(6):1875–84. https://doi.org/10.1007/s00216-012-6294-y.

Tan LC, Nancharaiah YV, van Hullebusch ED, Lens PNL. Selenium: environmental significance, pollution, and biological treatment technologies. Biotechnol Adv. 2016;34(5):886–907. https://doi.org/10.1016/j.biotechadv.2016.05.005.

Trojsi F, Monsurro MR, Tedeschi G. Exposure to environmental toxicants and pathogenesis of amyotrophic lateral sclerosis: state of the art and research perspectives. Int J Mol Sci. 2013;14(8):15286–311. https://doi.org/10.3390/ijms140815286.

Vinceti M, Guidetti D, Pinotti M, Rovesti S, Merlin M, Vescovi L, Bergomi M, Vivoli G. Amyotrophic lateral sclerosis after long-term exposure to drinking water with high selenium content. Epidemiology. 1996;7(5):529–32.

Vinceti M, Guidetti D, Bergomi M, Caselgrandi E, Vivoli R, Olmi M, Rinaldi L, Rovesti S, Solime F. Lead, cadmium, and selenium in the blood of patients with sporadic amyotrophic lateral sclerosis. Ital J Neurol Sci. 1997;18(2):87–92.

Vinceti M, Nacci G, Rocchi E, Cassinadri T, Vivoli R, Marchesi C, Bergomi M. Mortality in a population with long-term exposure to inorganic selenium via drinking water. J Clin Epidemiol. 2000;53(10):1062–8.

Vinceti M, Bonvicini F, Bergomi M, Malagoli C. Possible involvement of overexposure to environmental selenium in the etiology of amyotrophic lateral sclerosis: a short review. Ann Ist Super Sanita. 2010a;46(3):279–83. https://doi.org/10.4415/ANN_10_03_09.

Vinceti M, Bonvicini F, Rothman KJ, Vescovi L, Wang F. The relation between amyotrophic lateral sclerosis and inorganic selenium in drinking water: a population-based case-control study. Environ Health. 2010b;9:77. https://doi.org/10.1186/1476-069X-9-77.

Vinceti M, Crespi CM, Malagoli C, Bottecchi I, Ferrari A, Sieri S, Krogh V, Alber D, Bergomi M, Seidenari S, Pellacani G. A case-control study of the risk of cutaneous melanoma associated with three selenium exposure indicators. Tumori. 2012a;98(3):287–95. https://doi.org/10.1700/1125.12394.

Vinceti M, Fiore M, Signorelli C, Odone A, Tesauro M, Consonni M, Arcolin E, Malagoli C, Mandrioli J, Marmiroli S, Sciacca S, Ferrante M. Environmental risk factors for amyotrophic lateral sclerosis: methodological issues in epidemiologic studies. Ann Ig. 2012b;24(5):407–15.

Vinceti M, Crespi CM, Bonvicini F, Malagoli C, Ferrante M, Marmiroli S, Stranges S. The need for a reassessment of the safe upper limit of selenium in drinking water. Sci Total Environ. 2013a;443:633–42. https://doi.org/10.1016/j.scitotenv.2012.11.025.

Vinceti M, Crespi CM, Malagoli C, Del Giovane C, Krogh V. Friend or foe? The current epidemiologic evidence on selenium and human cancer risk. J Environ Sci Health C Environ Carcinog Ecotoxicol Rev. 2013b;31(4):305–41. https://doi.org/10.1080/10590501.2013.844757.

Vinceti M, Solovyev N, Mandrioli J, Crespi CM, Bonvicini F, Arcolin E, Georgoulopoulou E, Michalke B. Cerebrospinal fluid of newly diagnosed amyotrophic lateral sclerosis patients exhibits abnormal levels of selenium species including elevated selenite. Neurotoxicology. 2013c;38:25–32. https://doi.org/10.1016/j.neuro.2013.05.016.

Vinceti M, Mandrioli J, Borella P, Michalke B, Tsatsakis A, Finkelstein Y. Selenium neurotoxicity in humans: Bridging laboratory and epidemiologic studies. Toxicol Lett. 2014;230(2):295–303. https://doi.org/10.1016/j.toxlet.2013.11.016.

Vinceti M, Grill P, Malagoli C, Filippini T, Storani S, Malavolti M, Michalke B. Selenium speciation in human serum and its implications for epidemiologic research: a cross-sectional study. J Trace Elem Med Biol. 2015;31:1–10. https://doi.org/10.1016/j.jtemb.2015.02.001.

Vinceti M, Ballotari P, Steinmaus C, Malagoli C, Luberto F, Malavolti M, Rossi PG. Long-term mortality patterns in a residential cohort exposed to inorganic selenium in drinking water. Environ Res. 2016a;150:348–56. https://doi.org/10.1016/j.envres.2016.06.009.

Vinceti M, Burlingame B, Filippini T, Naska A, Bargellini A, Borella P. The epidemiology of selenium and human health. In: Hatfield DL, Schweizer U, Tsuji PA, Gladyshev VN, editors. Selenium: Its molecular biology and role in human health. Cham: Springer International Publishing; 2016b. p. 365–76. https://doi.org/10.1007/978-3-319-41283-2_31.

Vinceti M, Chiari A, Eichmuller M, Rothman KJ, Filippini T, Malagoli C, Weuve J, Tondelli M, Zamboni G, Nichelli PF, Michalke B. A selenium species in cerebrospinal fluid predicts conversion to Alzheimer's dementia in persons with mild cognitive impairment. Alzheimers Res Ther. 2017a;9(1):100. https://doi.org/10.1186/s13195-017-0323-1.

Vinceti M, Filippini T, Cilloni S, Bargellini A, Vergoni AV, Tsatsakis A, Ferrante M. Health risk assessment of environmental selenium: emerging evidence and challenges (Review). Mol Med Rep. 2017b;15(5):3323–35. https://doi.org/10.3892/mmr.2017.6377.

Vinceti M, Filippini T, Cilloni S, Crespi CM. The epidemiology of selenium and human cancer. Adv Cancer Res. 2017c;136:1–48. https://doi.org/10.1016/bs.acr.2017.07.001.

Vinceti M, Filippini T, Del Giovane C, Dennert G, Zwahlen M, Brinkman M, Zeegers MP, Horneber M, D'Amico R, Crespi CM. Selenium for preventing cancer. Cochrane Database Syst Rev. 2018a;1:CD005195.

Vinceti M, Filippini T, Rothman KJ. Selenium exposure and the risk of type 2 diabetes: a systematic review and meta-analysis. Eur J Epidemiol. 2018b;

Yang GQ, Wang SZ, Zhou RH, Sun SZ. Endemic selenium intoxication of humans in China. Am J Clin Nutr. 1983;37(5):872–81.

Part VI
The Role of Selenium in Cancer

Chapter 13
Therapeutic Potential of Selenium Compounds in the Treatment of Cancer

Arun Kumar Selvam, Mikael Björnstedt, and Sougat Misra

Abstract The potential applications of different selenium compounds as cancer chemotherapeutic agents is an active area of research within the field of cancer drug discovery. The antineoplastic efficacies of many of these small molecules have been extensively investigated, mainly in multiple preclinical models of cancer. Sodium selenite and Se-methylselenocysteine represent two of such selenium compounds, the cytotoxic and antiproliferative efficacies of which are discussed herein. These compounds differ in their mechanisms of action. Sodium selenite exerts its cytotoxic effects by directly oxidizing cellular free thiol pools. In contrast, Se-methylselenocysteine undergoes enzymatic transformation into methylselenol which is cytotoxic due to its ability to redox cycle with cellular thiols. Despite the inherent differences in their metabolic transformations, the disruption of the cellular redox balance and the activation of pro-death intracellular signaling pathways have been implicated as the most prevalent mechanisms of their cytotoxic effects. Both of these selenium compounds exert synergistic toxic effects with certain cancer chemotherapeutics. Together, the well-documented tumor-specific cytotoxic and antiproliferative effects of these compounds have paved the path for their clinical translation. In a phase I clinical trial, it has been shown that sodium selenite is well tolerated in human up to a dose of 10.2 mg/m^2 when administered daily for 5 days a week for 2 weeks. Similarly, Se-methylselenocysteine exhibits a favorable pharmacokinetic and safety profile during prolonged oral administration in healthy subjects. Further studies are warranted to investigate their cancer chemotherapeutic efficacies in clinical settings.

Keywords Cancer · Sodium selenite · Se-methylselenocysteine · Selenium metabolism · Phase I clinical trial · Chemotherapeutic agents

A. K. Selvam · M. Björnstedt · S. Misra (✉)
Division of Pathology F42, Department of Laboratory Medicine, Karolinska Institutet, Karolinska University Hospital Huddinge, Stockholm, Sweden
e-mail: Mikael.Bjornstedt@ki.se; Sougat.Misra@ki.se

© Springer International Publishing AG, part of Springer Nature 2018
B. Michalke (ed.), *Selenium*, Molecular and Integrative Toxicology,
https://doi.org/10.1007/978-3-319-95390-8_13

251

Introduction

Selenium is an essential trace element, the plasma levels of which has been shown to be inversely associated with cancer risk in several epidemiological studies (Kellen et al. 2006; Brinkman et al. 2006; Whanger 2004; Misra et al. 2015a; Finley 2006). The biological effects of selenium compounds are strictly concentration dependent and at low concentrations these molecules act as antioxidants. However, at supra-nutritional levels, selenium compounds exert prominent prooxidant properties with a quite narrow margin between antioxidant effects and toxicity (Tarze et al. 2007; Clark et al. 1996; Zeng 2009). Both organic and inorganic forms of selenium compounds have this dual activity, but their modes and mechanisms of actions in biological systems depend on the chemical species. A study in 1960 demonstrated inverse correlation between cancer mortality in a US population in relation to the selenium content in crop and/or soil, suggesting potential antitumor properties of plant-based selenium compounds (Shamberger and Frost 1969).

The biological effects of selenium compounds can be explained by the unique chemical properties of selenium. These are (a) specific incorporation of selenocysteine in selenoproteins and thus direct involvement in physiologically important redox processes; (b) redox cycling with thiols and oxygen; and (c) chelation of heavy metals (Mangiapane et al. 2014). Depending on the chemical properties of selenium compounds and their concentrations, the biological effects span a broad spectrum. At low doses, selenium compounds protect cells from oxidative damage, stimulate the immune response, and detoxify the intermediate metabolites of chemical carcinogens. While at higher doses, these molecules induce oxidative stress, apoptosis, and cell cycle arrest and reduce angiogenesis (Whanger 2004). Selenoproteins play key roles in rendering important physiological and cytoprotective effects. However, the expression of selenoproteins is saturated at higher intake levels and nonspecific effects arise beyond tolerance dose levels, either directly or indirectly (as metabolites). When in excess, cytotoxic effects are manifested which have consistently been exploited in preclinical studies aiming at their potential applications in cancer chemotherapy.

For clinical application as anticancer drugs, doses of selenium higher than dietary requirement are required. Hydrogen selenide (HSe-) and methylselenol are two intermediate key metabolites that are implicated with the antitumor effects of different selenium compounds. Both of these intermediates can effectively redox cycle with oxygen in the presence of NADPH and thiols, and thus exacerbate oxidative stress (Jackson and Combs 2008; Bjornstedt et al. 1992, 1995; Kumar et al. 1992). Selenium compounds can induce both caspase-dependent and caspase-independent apoptotic cell death pathways, depending on its chemical forms (Zeng 2009; Jackson and Combs 2008).

In addition, certain redox-active selenium compounds alter phase I and phase II enzyme activities (Ravn-Haren et al. 2008) induce antiproliferation activity *via* kinase signaling pathways (Park et al. 2012a; Pan et al. 2011) and caspase activation (Park et al. 2012a; Zuo et al. 2004), induce apoptosis (Park et al. 2012a; Zuo et al.

2004; Hussain et al. 2004; Nilsonne et al. 2006), and inhibit angiogenesis (Jiang et al. 1999; Bhattacharya 2011).

There is an ever-increasing interest in targeting cellular redox regulatory mechanisms in cancer. Metabolic oxidation/reduction (redox) reactions generate reactive oxygen species (ROS) (Hussain et al. 2003). ROS are known to be involved in both direct DNA damage and modulation of redox-regulated signaling pathways (Ray et al. 2012), which may be either beneficial or detrimental. Recent reports suggest that malignant cells in general harbor redox imbalance compared to benign and primary cells and the degree of oxidation or reduction varies with cancer types (Jorgenson et al. 2013). Normally, cancer cells exhibit higher basal levels of ROS compared to normal cells (reviewed in (Gorrini et al. 2013)), but cancer cells escape from ROS-induced cytotoxicity by activating a number of cellular pathways involved in antioxidant defense mechanisms. Such antioxidant-mediated defense mechanisms of tumor adaptation constitute amenable targets for anticancer therapy. One of such strategies involves the use of therapeutic agents that can increase cellular ROS levels beyond tolerance limits of cancer cells. An alternative approach would be inhibition of pathway/s involved in detoxification of ROS, the levels of which are usually higher in different cancer cells, as shown in several studies. Both the strategies ensure disproportionate ROS generation and induction of cell death *via* either apoptosis, necrosis, or any other modes of cell death pathways depending on the extent and duration of stimuli (Klaunig and Kamendulis 2004). To this end, redox-active selenium compounds fit uniquely. Not only many of these are implicated in ROS generation, but also these compounds target a multitude of pathways that are important for the survival of cancer cells (Misra et al. 2015b). Extensive bodies of preclinical studies clearly indicate the effectiveness of different selenium compounds in inducing cytotoxicity in prostate cancer (Zhong and Oberley 2001), breast cancer (Chen and Wong 2008), leukemia (Zuo et al. 2004), lung cancer (Bjorkhem-Bergman et al. 2002, 2005), and mesothelioma (Nilsonne et al. 2009).

In this chapter, we have briefly described the therapeutic potential of two important selenium compounds, sodium selenite and Se-methylselenocysteine (MSC).

Preclinical and Clinical Studies on Sodium Selenite as a Cancer Chemotherapeutic Agent

Rationale Behind Using Selenite as a Chemotherapeutic Agent

Sodium selenite (Na_2SeO_3) is a highly oxidizing agent and is spontaneously reduced to selenide upon reaction with low molecular weight and/or protein thiols (-SH group) (Fig. 13.1) (Painter 1941). This reaction produces superoxide upon further reduction of selenide into elemental selenium (Seko and Imura 1997). The superoxide radical is highly cytotoxic, unless superoxide dismutase catalytically converts it into hydrogen peroxide, which itself is an oxidizing agent. These cascades of

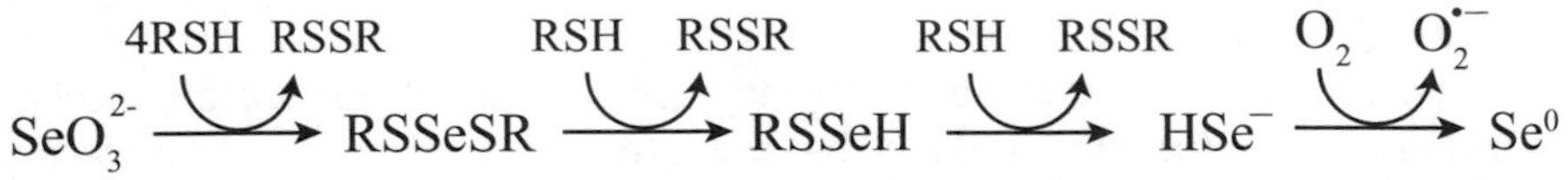

$$\text{SeO}_3^{2-} \xrightarrow[\text{4RSH}]{\text{RSSR}} \text{RSSeSR} \xrightarrow[\text{RSH}]{\text{RSSR}} \text{RSSeH} \xrightarrow[\text{RSH}]{\text{RSSR}} \text{HSe}^- \xrightarrow[\text{O}_2]{\text{O}_2^{\cdot-}} \text{Se}^0$$

Fig. 13.1 The reaction of selenite with thiols and subsequent formation of hydrogen selenide and the superoxide anion

reactions have certain important physiological implications, all of which antagonize cell survival. These are as follows: (a) loss of cellular thiols and other antioxidants including ascorbic acid; (b) potential oxidation of active functional -SH groups of certain enzymes, receptors, and transcription factors (Spyrou et al. 1995), thus potentially making these inactive; and (c) concomitant generation of reactive oxygen species and other secondary radicals. Together, selenite can blunt the functionalities of several cellular pathways that only function under a reductive milieu, along with induction of oxidative stress. Succession of these events eventually leads to cell death when the cellular damages are beyond repair.

The very nature of chemical metabolism of selenite indicates that these unfavorable reactions can manifest cytotoxicity in normal cells. However, several studies have shown that normal cells in culture are not as sensitive to selenite, as most of the cancer cells are (Nilsonne et al. 2006, 2009; Kim et al. 2007; Husbeck et al. 2005, 2006; Menter et al. 2000; Jonsson-Videsater et al. 2004). Indeed, there are some basic differences in the redox homeostasis between normal and cancer cells. One general observation is the elevated basal levels of ROS in cancer cells as outlined above. Under the assumption of equivalent amount of ROS generation upon selenite uptake, it is anticipated that cancer cells would incur much higher intracellular steady-state levels of ROS due to high basal levels of ROS. However, the initial assumption on similar uptake of selenite is not always the case, as there exist some major differences between the cellular transport of selenium from selenite in normal and cancer cells.

The transporter involved in selenite uptake is not very well characterized. In general, cellular transport of selenium from selenite is rather very poor in the absence of thiols in the transport medium in normal cells (Würmli et al. 1989; Scharrer et al. 1992). Earlier it has been shown that selenite transport process is pH dependent and anionic transporter inhibitor sensitive (Ganyc and Self 2008; Misra et al. 2012), suggesting the possible involvement of anionic transport systems in selenite uptake. However, small-molecule thiols are abundant both in the blood and interstitial fluid. The cystine/cysteine redox potential of a local cellular milieu depends largely on the expression of cystine/glutamate exchanger, also known as xCT (Bannai 1986). This antiporter transports cystine in the exchange of glutamate. Cystine is reduced to cysteine intracellularly and the latter is effluxed out of the cells. As a result, cysteine levels in the extracellular milieu is high enough (micromolar range) to facilitate selenium transport from selenite upon reduction into selenide or as a selenosulfide intermediate. A large number of cancer cells overexpress xCT under cell culture condition, while several malignant tumors inherently overexpress this antiporter compared to their normal counterparts. It is expected therefore that cellular uptake of selenium from selenite will be much higher in cells overexpressing xCT. In line with this, a correlation between extracellular thiols (mainly cysteine), cytotoxicity of selenite, and uptake of selenium was shown in several cell lines (Olm et al. 2009a). A relatively lower cytotoxicity of selenite in nonmalignant cells purportedly supports the role of xCT in selenite cytotoxicity.

In fact, the overexpression of xCT is associated with multidrug resistance and poor prognosis in cancer patients (Conrad and Sato 2012). We and others have shown that selenite exerts its superior cytotoxicity to drug-resistant cancer cells compared to their non-resistant counterparts (Jonsson-Videsater et al. 2004; Olm et al. 2009a; Caffrey and Frenkel 1992). We have also shown that selenite is a superior cytotoxic agent than conventional cytostatic drugs in isolated primary leukemic cells (Olm et al. 2009b).

In summary, certain intrinsic differences in xCT expression and steady-state ROS levels between normal and cancer cells partly explain as to why selenite is a superior cytotoxic agent to cancer cells. It is often being argued that a very high dose of selenite is required to kill cancer cells and thus it could be very toxic in humans. Our clinical study in fact suggests otherwise that selenite is very well tolerated in humans when administered intravenously in terminally ill cancer patients (Brodin et al. 2015). A mean plasma selenium concentration of about 23.0 µM was reached in patients receiving a dose of 10.2 mg/m^2, which was defined as maximum tolerated dose (MTD) of i.v.-administered selenite. There is outstanding evidence to suggest that many cancer cells in vitro can be sensitized at this dose level, as discussed below.

Mechanistic Insights into Selenite-Induced Cell Death

Dissecting the molecular pathways involved in drug-induced cell death is an important aspect of drug designing. Unregulated cell death augments inflammation and thus can blunt the efficacy of cytostatic drugs. For example, there exists a direct association between drug-induced augmentation of inflammatory pathways and the failure of chemotherapy, with subsequent onsets of metastasis (Vyas et al. 2014).

The nature of cell death, whether programmed (e.g., apoptosis) or unregulated (e.g., necrosis), depends on the cellular accumulation of a cytotoxic drug. While such cell death processes are often described independently, these could essentially be interconnected given that cellular drug accumulation is part of a continuum comprising influx, metabolism, and efflux. Therefore, the nature of toxic insults on cells is a function of cellular accumulation of drugs and bioactive metabolites at a given time point. Key pharmacological aspects along with understanding the modes and mechanisms of cell death induced by different selenium compounds are important to predict their systemic effects when applied in humans as a therapeutic agent.

Several in vitro studies have interrogated the pathway of selenite-induced cell death. Shen et al. reported that treatment with 10 μM of selenite resulted in superoxide formation followed by apoptotic cell death in HepG2 cells (Shen et al. 1999). Similarly, selenite was found to induce apoptotic cell death in prostate cancer cells (Menter et al. 2000; Vadgama et al. 2000). In ovarian cancer cell lines (A2780, HeyA8, and SKOV3iP1), it was shown that selenite treatment above 5.0 μM dose resulted in growth inhibitory effects and induced apoptosis (Park et al. 2012b). However, involvement of both apoptosis (both intrinsic and extrinsic) and autophagic cell death was found in human lung adenocarcinoma A549 cells (Park et al. 2012a). Treatment of these cells with 6.0 μM selenite resulted in increased expression of the pro-apoptotic protein BAX and death receptors such as FAS and DR4 and suppressed the expression of anti-apoptotic proteins such as BCL2 and BCL2L1 along with cleavage of PARP. The formation of LC3 puncta and increased incidence of apoptosis following Bafilomycin A treatment suggested autophagy-like cell death (Park et al. 2012a). In our laboratory, we interrogated the mode of cell death in HeLa cells, another cervical cancer cell line. A necroptosis-like cell death was found following treatment with 5.0 μM selenite for 24 h (Wallenberg et al. 2014). The above studies along with the others indicate that pharmacological concentrations of sodium selenite can induce a variety of pathways leading to cell death.

The tumor-suppressor protein TP53 can activate apoptosis pathway. Any DNA-damaging agent, including high dose of selenite, may potentially activate TP53 pathway. It was shown that prostate cancer cells with wild-type TP53 (LNCaP) were more sensitive to selenite than a TP53-null (PC3) and TP53-mutant (DU145) cells (Zhao et al. 2006). Although it is an interesting finding, no causal relationship between TP53 status and selenite cytotoxicity can be drawn, since a number of pathways other than TP53 are key determinants of selenite cytotoxicity.

Selenite in Acute Promyelocytic Leukemia (APL)

APL is a subtype of acute myeloid leukemia, associated with the t(15,17) (q22;q21) chromosomal translocation in the majority of patients. This translocation predominantly leads to fusion of the genes for promyelocytic leukemia (PML) and retinoic acid receptor alpha (RARα), resulting in the translation of fusion proteins PML/RARα and RARα/PML (Rowley et al. 1977; Mistry et al. 2003). PML is a zinc-finger protein and the zinc-finger domain confers its structural stability. Arsenic trioxide reacts with critical cystine residues of zinc-finger domain of PML and degrades this oncoprotein. Such a strategy has been successfully used to treat APL patients in combination with all-*trans*-retinoic acid (ATRA).

Based on the earlier findings on selenite-induced destabilization of zinc-thiolate coordination sites in zinc-finger protein SP1, we posited whether a similar interaction between selenite and PML/RARα could destabilize the oncoprotein and thus differentiate APL-originated NB4 cells when treated in combination with all-*trans*-retinoic acid (Misra et al. 2016). We showed that selenite degraded PML/RARα in a dose-dependent manner and induced multi-lineage maturation of NB4 cells when treated in combination with ATRA. However, selenite alone did not induce any differentiation in NB4 cells which was in disagreement with a previous study (Wang et al. 2015). Both of these in vitro studies indicate that selenite could potentially be considered as an investigational candidate drugs in the treatment of APL.

Sodium Selenite as an Experimental Therapeutic Agent in Terminally Ill Cancer Patients

Our research group was the first to perform a first-in-humans phase I clinical study to investigate the pharmacokinetics and preliminary efficacy of sodium selenite in 34 terminal cancer patients who didn't respond to standard chemotherapy (Brodin et al. 2015). The median half-life of plasma total selenium was 18.25 h. Fatigue, nausea, and vomiting (grades 1–2) were the main treatment-emergent adverse events at doses below or at MTD. The median survival of these patients was 6.5 months, which was a substantially long time given that all the patients had advanced disease (stage III or IV). Albeit the sample size was too small to draw any conclusions on drug effects from such a phase I study. This study provided substantial information on the pharmacokinetics of very high doses of sodium selenite in humans.

Selenite as an Ameliorating Agent Against Chemotherapeutic Drug-Induced Side Effects

Drug-induced side effects are often the key health concerns for a majority of the clinically used cytostatic drugs. To minimize the side effects without reducing the antitumor activity of a drug, various supplements in combination with the chemotherapeutic agents have been studied in several animal models. Since selenium compounds possess antineoplastic properties towards several tumors, these have been the key choices of supplements used in several studies with the aim to increase the therapeutic efficacies without reducing the anticancer properties of the administered cytostatic drugs. In line with this, it was shown that selenite pretreatment reduced the cisplatin-induced nephrotoxicity in BALB/c mice and Wistar rats (Baldew et al. 1989). When a single dose of selenite (i.p., 2 mg/kg) was administered in these animals prior to cisplatin treatment at different doses, a protective effect of selenite was observed as assessed by comparing the markers of kidney damage (blood, urea, nitrogen, and creatinine) between the control (only cisplatin-treated) and selenite-pretreated animals. At very high doses of cisplatin, the protective effects of selenite were partial.

The effects of daily selenium supplement (200 μg, as seleno-yeast) were evaluated in ovarian cancer patients who underwent post-surgical standard chemotherapy comprising cisplatin and cyclophosphamide (Sieja and Talerczyk 2004). Selenium was administered orally in the form of a capsule containing 15 mg β-carotene, 200 mg vitamin C, 4.5 mg riboflavin, and 45 mg niacin apart from 50 μg selenium. The control group received all the supplements, except for selenium in an identical manner. A significant decrease in side effects (abdominal pain, flatulence, hair loss, loss of appetite, malaise, and weakness) was observed in the treatment arm receiving the selenium-containing capsules for at least 2 months in comparison to the control group.

The above studies suggest that selenium in different chemical forms can alleviate the side effects exerted by certain forms of chemotherapeutics.

Methyl-Selenocysteine as an Anticancer Agent

The anticancer effects of different organic selenium compounds have been tested in several in vitro and in vivo models of different malignancies. Among these selenium compounds, the anticancer effects of selenocystine (please refer Chapter 14), selenomethionine (SeMet), and methyl-selenocysteine (MSC) have been widely studied. In the following section, a brief overview of the anticancer efficacy of MSC is discussed, with a specific focus on its metabolism.

MSC is essentially an inert compound, unless metabolized. It requires enzymatic transformation to generate active metabolites which are implicated in its antitumor and chemopreventive effects. MSC is actively metabolized by different enzymatic systems into methylated selenium compounds such as methylselenol (MS), dimethylselenide (DMSe), trimethylselenonium (TMSe+), and β-methylselenopyruvate (MSP). Among different metabolites, methylselenol is of a particular interest in pharmacology because of its prominent anticancer properties in controlling different cell signaling pathways, many of which antagonize the growth and survival of cancer cells (Gabel-Jensen et al. 2010). Methylselenol is extremely hydrophobic and it has a high vapor pressure and possesses higher nucleophilic properties than any corresponding thiols, which play a crucial role in antitumor effects, while MSP inhibits a number of histone-deacetylating enzymes (Andreadou et al. 1996; Cooper and Pinto 2005; Pinto et al. 2011).

Metabolism of MSC

MSC could be considered as a prodrug. It is metabolized by several enzymes to generate active compounds, which are efficient antitumor agents as indicated above (Vadhanavikit et al. 1993). Of these, the roles of kynurenine aminotransferases (KYATs; also known as KATs) are widely studied. There are four different KAT (KYAT I to KYAT IV) enzymes identified; of those KAT I (CCBL1) and KAT III (CCBL2) play a crucial role in metabolizing MSC (Andreadou et al. 1996;

Cooper et al. 2008; Akladios et al. 2012). KATs are multifunctional PLP-dependent enzymes involved in cleaving carbon-sulfur bonds, resulting in the conversion of the amino acid substrates into corresponding alpha-keto acids. The structural requirements of substrates suggest that these enzymes can metabolize selenium analogs of the respective sulfur-containing compounds as substrates. Earlier, it has been shown that MSC is a substrate for both CCBL1 and CCBL2, resulting in the formation of either β-methylselenopyruvate (transamination) or methylselenol (beta-elimination) as shown in Fig. 13.2. As there are very few published studies on

A. Transamination reaction of CCBL1

B. β-elimination reaction of CCBL1

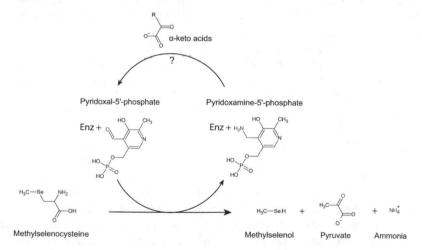

Fig. 13.2 The metabolism of methylselenocysteine by cysteine-*S*-conjugate beta-lyase enzymes. (**a**) The proposed catalytic mechanism of CCBL1 enzyme in metabolizing MSC into β-methylselenopyruvate and L-methionine in the presence of 2-ketomethiobutyrate as a co-substrate. (**b**) The beta-elimination reaction of CCBL1 converting MSC into methylselenol, pyruvate, and ammonium. Both the transamination and beta-elimination reactions involve the conversion of PLP to PMP. An excess of certain α-keto acids favors the beta-elimination reaction over the transamination reaction

CCBL2, and the mechanism of action is not yet completely delineated, we have chosen to focus on the metabolic transformation of MSC by CCBL1.

One of the key specialties of these enzymes is their involvement in both the transamination and beta-elimination activities. The nature of substrates and the concentrations of alpha-keto acids determine the fate of the reaction whether these will undergo transamination or beta-elimination. Besides the presence of pyridoxamine-5′-phosphate (PMP) and pyridoxal 5′-phosphate (PLP) plays a crucial role in determining the reaction path (Rossi et al. 2004; Han et al. 2010; Eliot and Kirsch 2004).

In general, KAT enzymes favor the transamination reactions over the beta-elimination reactions. During transamination reaction PLP is converted into PMP. For a beta-elimination reaction to happen, the enzyme needs PLP as a cofactor. So the addition of α-keto acids as co-substrates ensures to maintain the PLP form of an enzyme for an effective and continuous beta-elimination reaction (Stevens et al. 1986). The cysteine-Se-conjugate compounds are better substrates for beta-elimination activity of CCBL1 over corresponding cysteine-S-conjugate compounds. This may be due to a weaker C-Se bond compared to the C-S bond (Commandeur et al. 2000; Rooseboom et al. 2000).

CCBL1 is a homodimer containing one PLP per monomer. This enzyme possesses strong aminotransferase activity towards a wide variety of amino acids such as glutamine, phenylalanine, leucine, kynurenine, tryptophan, methionine, tyrosine, cysteine, asparagine, and histidine (Cooper et al. 2008). It is only catalytically active towards the L-form of amino acids. In terms of cysteine-S-conjugate substrates, the transamination competes with the beta-elimination reaction, with an estimated ratio of the transamination to beta-elimination of about 4:1 (Cooper et al. 2008). If a substrate has a strong nucleophilic group, then beta-elimination dominates over the transamination reaction. The addition of strong nucleophilic compounds as co-substrates such as phenyl pyruvate increases the beta-elimination reaction over the transamination (Cooper et al. 2008). The active pocket of this enzyme is large, so that it could accommodate two substrates, including large L-amino acids at a time. The active site of the enzyme remains always open even in the absence of substrates, but changes to tightly closed conformation by covalent attachment with substrate when bound to PLP. Beta-elimination is favored by the enzyme over the transamination when MSC is used as a substrate (Cooper et al. 2008; Han et al. 2010; Stevens et al. 1986). MSC is also a 100-fold more effective transamination substrate for CCBL1 than SeMet (Cooper et al. 2008). These findings together suggest that CCBL1 plays a key role in the anticancer efficacy of MSC upon metabolizing it into active metabolites, namely, methylselenol and methylselenopyruvate.

CCBL1 is mainly located in the cytosol, while CCBL2 is found in the mitochondria (Cooper and Pinto 2005). Such cellular compartmentalization together with higher beta-elimination activity of CCBL1 towards MSC indicates that cytosolic metabolism of MSC may serve as the key trigger in inducing cytotoxic effects. Also different tissues differ in their endogenous beta-elimination activities depending on the types and levels of expression of different beta-lyases. To this end, a better understanding of tissue-specific total beta-elimination activity is of particular importance to predict organ-specific toxicity following MSC administration in vivo. In line with this, it has been shown that whole-tissue lysates of kidney, liver, and brain of Wistar rats possess higher beta-elimination activity towards Se-conjugated compounds, followed by spleen, heart, large intestine, thyroid, lung, and small intestine, respectively (Rooseboom et al. 2002).

We have earlier shown that methylselenol is a better substrate for the thioredoxin and glutaredoxin systems compared to selenite and selenide (Fernandes et al. 2012). Such an observation has important implications on the cytotoxic effects of MSC given that it has been proposed that redox cycling of methylselenol generates ROS.

Cytotoxic Effects of MSC and the Associated Signaling Pathways

MSC is relatively nontoxic to cultured cancer cells when compared to other selenium compounds. As stated above, enzymatic transformation of MSC is a critical step in exerting its cytotoxicity. Thus, the involvement of both the transamination and beta-elimination reactions is critically important. These are not mutually exclusive reactions in the context of cellular metabolism of MSC. In fact, the products of these reactions, methylselenol and MSP, exert their cytotoxic and cell signaling modulatory effects independently, as outlined below.

Methylselenol has been shown to be involved in redox signaling, alters the cell signaling pathways and it exerts antiproliferative and pro-apoptotic properties to several malignant cells (Zeng 2009; Rooseboom et al. 2000; Zeng et al. 2009; Cooper et al. 2011). Using a methylselenol-generating system, it has been shown that methylselenol is implicated in reducing the invasiveness of tumor by inhibiting MMP-2 and induces cell cycle arrest and apoptosis via multiple cell signaling pathways (Zeng et al. 2009). It also upregulates tumor-suppressor genes such as *CDKN1C/p57^{KIP2}*, *HMOX1*, cell adhesion and signaling molecule genes *PECAM1* (which induces Bax-mediated apoptosis) and *PPARG* (increases growth inhibition apoptosis and differentiation of tumor cell populations). Methylselenol is also shown to downregulate *BCL2A1* (increased expression reduces the release of pro-apoptotic cytochrome C from mitochondria, thereby reducing the incidence of apoptosis), *HHIP*, a gene involved in the hedgehog signaling pathway, and *WIG1* which is a TP53 target gene. It also inhibits ERK1/2 phosphorylation and c-MYC oncoprotein expression in HT1080 cells, a fibrosarcoma cell line (Bhattacharya 2011; Zeng et al. 2006, 2009).

The transamination product, MSP, structurally resembles butyrate which is a known HDAC inhibitor. Nian and colleagues reported that the transamination metabolites of MSC and SeMet, MSP and KMSB, respectively, induced HDAC8 inhibition in a competitive manner (Nian et al. 2009). This inhibition triggered apoptosis and/or cell cycle arrest in cancer cells through chromatin remodeling.

In this study, they showed the increased incidence of apoptosis in HCT116 and HT29 colon cancer cell lines at 50 μM of MSP and KMSB, accompanied by cleavage of caspases -3, -6, -7, and -9 and PARP in a dose-dependent manner. Using prostate cancer cell lines, it was shown that treatment with 2.5 mM MSC did not affect HDAC activity, while 2.5 mM of MSP resulted in about 50% HDAC inhibition in LNCaP, C4-2, PC3, and DU145 cell lines (Lee et al. 2009a). This study also reported that MSC treatment resulted in increased accumulation of acetylated histone-H3. MSP was also reported to be involved in the regulation of several genes such as *HIF-1α, VEGF,* and *GLUT1* and abrogate transcription of androgen receptor (Cooper et al. 2011; Sinha et al. 2008).

In a human colorectal cancer cell line, COLO 205, the involvement of both death receptor (FASL) and ER-stress-mediated cell death pathways has been implicated, when a very high dose of MSC (200 μM, corresponding to about 30% cell survival at 24 h) was used (Tung et al. 2015). At this dose, there was increased expression of FAS, FASL, GADD 45, GADD 153, cleavage of PARP, procaspase 9, procaspase 3, and BAX, along with increased phosphorylation of P38 and JNK. It was suggested that MSC induced apoptosis via other pathways rather than ROS-induced apoptosis upon activating multiple kinase signaling pathways.

MSC was also shown to sensitize a TRAIL (tumor necrosis factor-related apoptosis-inducing ligand)-resistant human renal cancer cells (Caki cells) when used in combination with the ligand (Lee et al. 2009b). Increased apoptosis was associated with downregulation of *BCL-2*, both at mRNA and protein levels. These findings suggested direct transcriptional regulation of *BCL-2* by MSC or its metabolites. Similar findings on the inhibition of *BCL-2* by MSC have been reported in osteosarcoma cells, MG63 (Huang et al. 2015).

Coyne and colleagues investigated the combinatorial effect of MSC with gemcitabine and covalent bound immune-chemotherapeutic gemcitabine in combination with 15 μM of MSC against chemotherapy-resistant mammary adenocarcinoma (SKBr-3) (Coyne et al. 2015). In combination with MSC a dose of 10^{-10} M of gemcitabine has the same effect on 10^{-6} M of gemcitabine alone. This study demonstrated that MSC can increase the efficacy of certain cytostatic drugs and thereby increase the tumor cell killing efficiency at a reduced dose.

Experimental evidence suggests that MSC also functions as an anti-inflammatory agent. When RAW 264.7 murine macrophages were challenged with lipopolysaccharide (LPS) in the presence of MSC, there was a significant reduction of nitric oxide (NO) production (Pan et al. 2011). A concomitant downregulation of inducible nitric oxide synthase (iNOS) was found. Using a luciferase reporter assay, it was shown that this selenium compound inhibited the binding of NF-κB to the promoter region of the iNOS gene, thereby suggesting transcriptional inhibition. Such anti-inflammatory activity of MSC could potentially be exploited in cancer chemo- and immunotherapy when used in combination.

Taken together, it can be concluded that MSC alters a multitude of cell survival signaling pathways in a time- and dose-dependent manner. The majority of studies indicate apoptosis as the major pathway of cell death. In considering the chemopreventive effects of selenium, we posit that MSC requires a special attention since one of its key metabolites, β-methylselenopyruvate, modulates HDAC activity and methylselenol in fact is a good antioxidant at low concentrations.

Efficacy of MSC as an Anticancer Drug in Animal Models of Cancer

Some of the earlier studies on selenium and cancer were focused on the ability of selenium to inhibit chemically induced carcinogenesis in animal models. Ip and colleagues studied the anticancer potential of various selenium compounds in a rat model of DMBA-induced mammary carcinogenesis (Ip et al. 1991). Supplementation of 2.0 ppm selenium as MSC resulted in marked decrease in the incidence of tumor per animal. The findings from this study indicated that monomethylselenol-producing selenocompounds, including MSC, resulted in superior antitumor activity.

Further studies on mouse xenografts bearing human FaDu and A253 (head and neck squamous cell carcinoma) and HCT-8 and HT-29 (colon carcinoma) showed some remarkable anticancer efficacy of MSC in combination with cytostatic drugs (Cao et al. 2004). In this study, several cytostatic drugs such as irinotecan, FU, oxaliplatin, taxol, cisplatin, and doxorubicin were tested in combination with MSC and SeMet. The cure rate in the combination treatment with MSC was 100% in animals bearing xenografts of drug-sensitive tumor, i.e., FaDu and HCT-8, whereas only with cytostatic it was 30% and 20%, respectively. In animal xenografts with drug-resistant tumor cells A253 and HT-29, the cure rate was 60% and 20%, whereas the corresponding cytostatic drug administration alone incurred 10% and 0% cure in this model. It was also shown that in drug-sensitive tumors, only 50% of maximum tolerated dose (MTD) of the respective cytostatic drug is required in combination with MSC to obtain a complete cure. Together, this study provided substantial evidence that MSC is a potential and a selective modulator of drug-resistant tumors and provide protection against cytostatic drug-induced side effects. In a later study, the effect of MSC (0.2 mg/mouse/day) co-treatment with irinotecan in head and neck tumor (FaDu) bearing xenograft mice model was evaluated (Chintala et al. 2010). This study unveiled the inhibitory potential of MSC towards HIF-1α and its transcriptional targets VEGF and CAIX, thereby asserting antiangiogenic activity.

The effect of MSC in combination with anticancer drugs such as cyclophosphamide (CTX), cisplatin, oxaliplatin, and irinotecan was evaluated in xenografted athymic nude mice and Fischer rat models (Cao et al. 2014). MSC provided selective protection against toxicity induced by cytostatic drugs and it improved the therapeutic index in synergy. Furthermore, MSC protected against cisplatin-induced kidney and bladder toxicity and promoted hair growth after CTX treatment. It also provided protection against oxaliplatin-induced myelotoxicity, and showed higher complete remission in rats bearing advanced Ward colorectal carcinoma. Notably, MSC in combination with a lethal dose of cisplatin protected the normal tissues from toxicity.

Pharmacokinetic and Pharmacodynamics of MSC

The above-presented preclinical and clinical studies provide substantial evidence that MSC is a potent anticancer agent either alone or in combination with cytostatic drugs. However, clinical application of MSC as a chemotherapeutic agent requires a priori knowledge of its pharmacology. It is water soluble and easily absorbed in the gastrointestinal tract, which has additional advantages in its clinical application.

A study by Jonson and colleagues estimated the no observed adverse effect level (NOAEL) for MSC in rats and dogs following daily gavage for 28 days. Based on their data, the calculated NOAEL was <0.5 mg/kg/day for rats and <0.15 mg/kg/day for dogs (Johnson et al. 2008). In a subsequent study, acute and chronic toxicity of orally administered MSC was evaluated in BALB/c mice and Sprague-Dawley rats, respectively (Yang and Jia 2014). Following a single oral dose of MSC, the estimated LD_{50} was reported to be 12.6 mg (female) and 9.26 mg (male) per kg body weight. In rats, chronic daily intake of MSC to a maximum dose level of 0.9 mg/kg body weight/day for 90 days resulted in minor toxicity including hepatomegaly, albeit only at the higher dose levels. The calculated (NOAEL) oral dose was found to be 0.5 mg MSC/kg body weight/day for 90 days, corresponding to 0.22 mg Se/kg body weight/day, and was in excellent compliance with the previous study. This value was 0.14 mg Se/kg body weight/day for selenite when orally administered for a similar duration (Jia et al. 2005). When Benchmark Dose (BMD) approach was used, the BMD level was determined to be 0.34 mg MSC/kg body weight/day. Considering a default uncertainty factor of 100, the acceptable daily BMD intake level of MSC in human was found to be 3.4 μg MSC/kg body weight/day, equivalent to about 100 μg of Se per day. Notably, this study reported no genotoxic effects of MSC at pharmacological doses.

Recent studies provide some valuable information on the pharmacokinetic properties of MSC. The first-in-human randomized, double-blind study investigated the pharmacokinetics of orally administered single dose of MSC in healthy men. The study subjects received a single oral dose of 400, 800, or 1200 μg Se as MSC. No association between MSC administration and the occurrence of adverse events was found at any of the tested concentrations. The maximum plasma concentration of Se was found within 3–5 h of MSC administration. The base line-adjusted maximum plasma concentration (C_{max}) values (as Se; not MSC) were 22.8, 30.75, and 63.2 ng/mL for the study cohorts receiving 400, 800, and 1200 μg dose, respectively. This possibly indicates a nonlinear increase in plasma total selenium concentration at the highest dose level. An estimated half-life was calculated to be 29 h from the AUC values obtained from the cohort that received a dose of 1200 μg.

In a follow-up study, multiple-dose pharmacokinetics of MSC and SeMet were studied in a randomized, double-blind phase I trial (Marshall et al. 2017). A total of

29 healthy male subjects participated in the trial. The treatment arm consisted of 4 cohorts (5–7 volunteers) who received 400 and 800 µg of Se orally either as MSC or SeMet daily for 84 days. Incidence of two severe adverse events was recorded in the treatment arms and was judged to be unrelated to the test substances. The mean baseline plasma concentration in these groups of healthy subjects was 108 µg/L. Following long-term supplementation of MSC, only marginal increase in plasma total selenium was found. However, more than twofold increase (209–244 µg/L) in plasma selenium levels was found in the SeMet-supplemented cohorts. Plasma selenium C_{max} values on days 1 and 84 did not differ much (range 122–143 µg/L) in the subjects who received MSC treatment. However, it was much higher (mean range 252–319 µg/L) in the cohorts who received SeMet treatment. The AUC values (µg h/L) also reflected a similar trend. Apparently, any of these values were not baseline corrected as could be seen from the predose plasma total Se levels and the values from the earlier study. One of the key findings from this study is that long-term administration of MSC did not result in increased plasma level of selenium unlike SeMet, while plasma selenoprotein P and glutathione peroxidase levels remained similar at comparable administered doses. Thus, this study highlights as to why MSC can be a better source of selenium supplementation compared to SeMet.

Concluding Remarks

The use of selenium compounds for the treatment of cancer is not a new entity. The first report on the use of selenium for cancer treatment was published about 100 years ago (Watson-Williams 1919). There is substantial preclinical evidence to suggest that redox-active selenium compounds have potent anticancer efficacy by targeting multiple pathways that are critical for the survival and proliferation of malignant cells. Such multi-target nature of these experimental drugs makes it a compelling case for their clinical application. To this end, there has been very little development to bring these compounds into clinical practice. In pursuit of such goals, the utmost need is systematic investigations aimed at understanding the pharmacology and clinical applicability of these compounds.

Acknowledgments The authors would like to thank financial support from Barncancerfonden, Cancerfonden, Cancer- och Allergifonden, KI Fonder, Jochnick Foundation, Radiumhemmetsforsknings fonder, and the County Council of Stockholm.

References

Akladios FN, et al. Design and synthesis of novel inhibitors of human kynurenine aminotransferase-I. Bioorg Med Chem Lett. 2012;22(4):1579–81.
Andreadou I, et al. Synthesis of novel Se-substituted selenocysteine derivatives as potential kidney selective prodrugs of biologically active selenol compounds: evaluation of kinetics of beta-elimination reactions in rat renal cytosol. J Med Chem. 1996;39(10):2040–6.

Baldew GS, et al. Selenium-induced protection against cis-diamminedichloroplatinum(II) nephrotoxicity in mice and rats. Cancer Res. 1989;49(11):3020–3.

Bannai S. Exchange of cystine and glutamate across plasma membrane of human fibroblasts. J Biol Chem. 1986;261(5):2256–63.

Bhattacharya A. Methylselenocysteine: a promising antiangiogenic agent for overcoming drug delivery barriers in solid malignancies for therapeutic synergy with anticancer drugs. Expert Opin Drug Deliv. 2011;8(6):749–63.

Bjorkhem-Bergman L, et al. Drug-resistant human lung cancer cells are more sensitive to selenium cytotoxicity. Effects on thioredoxin reductase and glutathione reductase. Biochem Pharmacol. 2002;63(10):1875–84.

Bjorkhem-Bergman L, et al. Selenium prevents tumor development in a rat model for chemical carcinogenesis. Carcinogenesis. 2005;26(1):125–31.

Bjornstedt M, Kumar S, Holmgren A. Selenodiglutathione is a highly efficient oxidant of reduced thioredoxin and a substrate for mammalian thioredoxin reductase. J Biol Chem. 1992;267(12):8030–4.

Bjornstedt M, Kumar S, Holmgren A. Selenite and selenodiglutathione: reactions with thioredoxin systems. Methods Enzymol. 1995;252:209–19.

Brinkman M, et al. Use of selenium in chemoprevention of bladder cancer. Lancet Oncol. 2006;7(9):766–74.

Brodin O, et al. Pharmacokinetics and toxicity of sodium selenite in the treatment of patients with carcinoma in a phase I clinical trial: the SECAR study. Nutrients. 2015;7(6):4978–94.

Caffrey PB, Frenkel GD. Selenite cytotoxicity in drug resistant and nonresistant human ovarian tumor cells. Cancer Res. 1992;52(17):4812–6.

Cao S, Durrani FA, Rustum YM. Selective modulation of the therapeutic efficacy of anticancer drugs by selenium containing compounds against human tumor xenografts. Clin Cancer Res. 2004;10(7):2561–9.

Cao S, et al. Se-methylselenocysteine offers selective protection against toxicity and potentiates the antitumour activity of anticancer drugs in preclinical animal models. Br J Cancer. 2014;110(7):1733–43.

Chen T, Wong YS. Selenocystine induces S-phase arrest and apoptosis in human breast adenocarcinoma MCF-7 cells by modulating ERK and Akt phosphorylation. J Agric Food Chem. 2008;56(22):10574–81.

Chintala S, et al. Se-methylselenocysteine sensitizes hypoxic tumor cells to irinotecan by targeting hypoxia-inducible factor 1alpha. Cancer Chemother Pharmacol. 2010;66(5):899–911.

Clark LC, et al. Effects of selenium supplementation for cancer prevention in patients with carcinoma of the skin. A randomized controlled trial. Nutritional Prevention of Cancer Study Group. JAMA. 1996;276(24):1957–63.

Commandeur JN, et al. Bioactivation of selenocysteine Se-conjugates by a highly purified rat renal cysteine conjugate beta-lyase/glutamine transaminase K. J Pharmacol Exp Ther. 2000;294(2):753–61.

Conrad M, Sato H. The oxidative stress-inducible cystine/glutamate antiporter, system x (c) (-): cystine supplier and beyond. Amino Acids. 2012;42(1):231–46.

Cooper AJ, Pinto JT. Aminotransferase, L-amino acid oxidase and beta-lyase reactions involving L-cysteine S-conjugates found in allium extracts. Relevance to biological activity? Biochem Pharmacol. 2005;69(2):209–20.

Cooper AJL, et al. Substrate specificity of human glutamine transaminase K as an aminotransferase and as a cysteine S-conjugate beta-lyase. Arch Biochem Biophys. 2008;474(1):72–81.

Cooper AJ, et al. Cysteine S-conjugate beta-lyases: important roles in the metabolism of naturally occurring sulfur and selenium-containing compounds, xenobiotics and anticancer agents. Amino Acids. 2011;41(1):7–27.

Coyne CP, Jones T, Bear R. Simultaneous dual selective targeted delivery of two covalent gemcitabine immunochemotherapeutics and complementary anti-neoplastic potency of [Se]-methylselenocysteine. J Cancer Ther. 2015;6(1):62–89.

Eliot AC, Kirsch JF. Pyridoxal phosphate enzymes: mechanistic, structural, and evolutionary considerations. Annu Rev Biochem. 2004;73:383–415.

Fernandes AP, et al. Methylselenol formed by spontaneous methylation of selenide is a superior selenium substrate to the thioredoxin and glutaredoxin systems. PLoS One. 2012;7(11):e50727.

Finley JW. Bioavailability of selenium from foods. Nutr Rev. 2006;64(3):146–51.

Gabel-Jensen C, Lunoe K, Gammelgaard B. Formation of methylselenol, dimethylselenide and dimethyldiselenide in in vitro metabolism models determined by headspace GC-MS. Metallomics. 2010;2(2):167–73.

Ganyc D, Self WT. High affinity selenium uptake in a keratinocyte model. FEBS Lett. 2008;582(2):299–304.

Gorrini C, Harris IS, Mak TW. Modulation of oxidative stress as an anticancer strategy. Nat Rev Drug Discov. 2013;12(12):931–47.

Han Q, et al. Structure, expression, and function of kynurenine aminotransferases in human and rodent brains. Cell Mol Life Sci. 2010;67(3):353–68.

Huang G, et al. Analysis of selenium levels in osteosarcoma patients and the effects of Se-methylselenocysteine on osteosarcoma cells in vitro. Nutr Cancer. 2015;67(5):847–56.

Husbeck B, Peehl DM, Knox SJ. Redox modulation of human prostate carcinoma cells by selenite increases radiation-induced cell killing. Free Radic Biol Med. 2005;38(1):50–7.

Husbeck B, et al. Tumor-selective killing by selenite in patient-matched pairs of normal and malignant prostate cells. Prostate. 2006;66(2):218–25.

Hussain SP, Hofseth LJ, Harris CC. Radical causes of cancer. Nat Rev Cancer. 2003;3(4):276–85.

Hussain SP, et al. p53-induced up-regulation of MnSOD and GPx but not catalase increases oxidative stress and apoptosis. Cancer Res. 2004;64(7):2350–6.

Ip C, et al. Chemical form of selenium, critical metabolites, and cancer prevention. Cancer Res. 1991;51(2):595–600.

Jackson MI, Combs GF Jr. Selenium and anticarcinogenesis: underlying mechanisms. Curr Opin Clin Nutr Metab Care. 2008;11(6):718–26.

Jia X, Li N, Chen J. A subchronic toxicity study of elemental Nano-Se in Sprague-Dawley rats. Life Sci. 2005;76(17):1989–2003.

Jiang C, et al. Selenium-induced inhibition of angiogenesis in mammary cancer at chemopreventive levels of intake. Mol Carcinog. 1999;26(4):213–25.

Johnson WD, et al. Subchronic oral toxicity studies of Se-methylselenocysteine, an organoselenium compound for breast cancer prevention. Food Chem Toxicol. 2008;46(3):1068–78.

Jonsson-Videsater K, et al. Selenite-induced apoptosis in doxorubicin-resistant cells and effects on the thioredoxin system. Biochem Pharmacol. 2004;67(3):513–22.

Jorgenson TC, Zhong W, Oberley TD. Redox imbalance and biochemical changes in cancer. Cancer Res. 2013;73(20):6118–23.

Kellen E, Zeegers M, Buntinx F. Selenium is inversely associated with bladder cancer risk: a report from the Belgian case-control study on bladder cancer. Int J Urol. 2006;13(9):1180–4.

Kim EH, et al. Sodium selenite induces superoxide-mediated mitochondrial damage and subsequent autophagic cell death in malignant glioma cells. Cancer Res. 2007;67(13):6314–24.

Klaunig JE, Kamendulis LM. The role of oxidative stress in carcinogenesis. Annu Rev Pharmacol Toxicol. 2004;44:239–67.

Kumar S, Bjornstedt M, Holmgren A. Selenite is a substrate for calf thymus thioredoxin reductase and thioredoxin and elicits a large non-stoichiometric oxidation of NADPH in the presence of oxygen. Eur J Biochem. 1992;207(2):435–9.

Lee JI, et al. Alpha-keto acid metabolites of naturally occurring organoselenium compounds as inhibitors of histone deacetylase in human prostate cancer cells. Cancer Prev Res (Phila). 2009a;2(7):683–93.

Lee JT, et al. Se-methylselenocysteine sensitized TRAIL-mediated apoptosis via down-regulation of Bcl-2 expression. Int J Oncol. 2009b;34(5):1455–60.

Mangiapane E, Pessione A, Pessione E. Selenium and selenoproteins: an overview on different biological systems. Curr Protein Pept Sci. 2014;15(6):598–607.

Marshall JR, et al. Selenomethionine and methyl selenocysteine: multiple-dose pharmacokinetics in selenium-replete men. Oncotarget. 2017;8(16):26312–22.

Menter DG, Sabichi AL, Lippman SM. Selenium effects on prostate cell growth. Cancer Epidemiol Biomark Prev. 2000;9(11):1171–82.

Misra S, Kwong RWM, Niyogi S. Transport of selenium across the plasma membrane of primary hepatocytes and enterocytes of rainbow trout. J Exp Biol. 2012;215(9):1491–501.

Misra S, et al. Redox-active selenium compounds-from toxicity and cell death to cancer treatment. Nutrients. 2015a;7(5):3536–56.

Misra S, Wallenberg M, Brodin O, Bjornstedt M. Selenite in cancer therapy. In: Brigelius-Flohe R, Sies H, editors. Diversity of selenium functions in health and disease, vol. 38. Boca Raton: CRC Press; 2015b. p. 400.

Misra S, et al. Selenite promotes all-trans retinoic acid-induced maturation of acute promyelocytic leukemia cells. Oncotarget. 2016;7(46):74686–700.

Mistry AR, et al. The molecular pathogenesis of acute promyelocytic leukaemia: implications for the clinical management of the disease. Blood Rev. 2003;17(2):71–97.

Nian H, et al. Alpha-keto acid metabolites of organoselenium compounds inhibit histone deacetylase activity in human colon cancer cells. Carcinogenesis. 2009;30(8):1416–23.

Nilsonne G, et al. Selenite induces apoptosis in sarcomatoid malignant mesothelioma cells through oxidative stress. Free Radic Biol Med. 2006;41(6):874–85.

Nilsonne G, et al. Phenotype-dependent apoptosis signalling in mesothelioma cells after selenite exposure. J Exp Clin Cancer Res. 2009;28:92.

Olm E, et al. Extracellular thiol-assisted selenium uptake dependent on the x(c)- cystine transporter explains the cancer-specific cytotoxicity of selenite. Proc Natl Acad Sci U S A. 2009a;106(27):11400–5.

Olm E, et al. Selenite is a potent cytotoxic agent for human primary AML cells. Cancer Lett. 2009b;282(1):116–23.

Painter EP. The chemistry and toxicity of selenium compounds, with special reference to the selenium problem. Chem Rev. 1941;28(2):179–213.

Pan MH, et al. Se-methylselenocysteine inhibits lipopolysaccharide-induced NF-kappaB activation and iNOS induction in RAW 264.7 murine macrophages. Mol Nutr Food Res. 2011;55(5):723–32.

Park SH, et al. Induction of apoptosis and autophagy by sodium selenite in A549 human lung carcinoma cells through generation of reactive oxygen species. Toxicol Lett. 2012a;212(3):252–61.

Park JS, et al. The effects of selenium on tumor growth in epithelial ovarian carcinoma. J Gynecol Oncol. 2012b;23(3):190–6.

Pinto JT, et al. Chemopreventive mechanisms of alpha-keto acid metabolites of naturally occurring organoselenium compounds. Amino Acids. 2011;41(1):29–41.

Ravn-Haren G, et al. Effect of long-term selenium yeast intervention on activity and gene expression of antioxidant and xenobiotic metabolising enzymes in healthy elderly volunteers from the Danish Prevention of Cancer by Intervention by Selenium (PRECISE) pilot study. Br J Nutr. 2008;99(6):1190–8.

Ray PD, Huang B-W, Tsuji Y. Reactive oxygen species (ROS) homeostasis and redox regulation in cellular signaling. Cell Signal. 2012;24(5):981–90.

Rooseboom M, et al. Evaluation of the kinetics of beta-elimination reactions of selenocysteine Se-conjugates in human renal cytosol: possible implications for the use as kidney selective prodrugs. J Pharmacol Exp Ther. 2000;294(2):762–9.

Rooseboom M, et al. Tissue distribution of cytosolic beta-elimination reactions of selenocysteine Se-conjugates in rat and human. Chem Biol Interact. 2002;140(3):243–64.

Rossi F, et al. Crystal structure of human kynurenine aminotransferase I. J Biol Chem. 2004;279(48):50214–20.

Rowley JD, Golomb HM, Dougherty C. 15/17 translocation, a consistent chromosomal change in acute promyelocytic leukaemia. Lancet. 1977;1(8010):549–50.

Scharrer E, Senn E, Wollfram S. Stimulation of mucosal uptake of selenium from selenite by some thiols at various sites of rat intestine. Biol Trace Elem Res. 1992;33(1):109–20.

Seko Y, Imura N. Active oxygen generation as a possible mechanism of selenium toxicity. Biomed Environ Sci. 1997;10(2–3):333–9.

Shamberger RJ, Frost DV. Possible protective effect of selenium against human cancer. Can Med Assoc J. 1969;100(14):682.

Shen HM, Yang CF, Ong CN. Sodium selenite-induced oxidative stress and apoptosis in human hepatoma HepG2 cells. Int J Cancer. 1999;81(5):820–8.

Sieja K, Talerczyk M. Selenium as an element in the treatment of ovarian cancer in women receiving chemotherapy. Gynecol Oncol. 2004;93(2):320–7.

Sinha R, et al. Effects of naturally occurring and synthetic organoselenium compounds on protein profiling in androgen responsive and androgen independent human prostate cancer cells. Nutr Cancer. 2008;60(2):267–75.

Spyrou G, et al. AP-1 DNA-binding activity is inhibited by selenite and selenodiglutathione. FEBS Lett. 1995;368(1):59–63.

Stevens JL, Robbins JD, Byrd RA. A purified cysteine conjugate beta-lyase from rat kidney cytosol. Requirement for an alpha-keto acid or an amino acid oxidase for activity and identity with soluble glutamine transaminase K. J Biol Chem. 1986;261(33):15529–37.

Tarze A, et al. Extracellular production of hydrogen selenide accounts for thiol-assisted toxicity of selenite against Saccharomyces cerevisiae. J Biol Chem. 2007;282(12):8759–67.

Tung YC, et al. Se-Methyl-L-selenocysteine Induces Apoptosis via Endoplasmic Reticulum Stress and the Death Receptor Pathway in Human Colon Adenocarcinoma COLO 205 Cells. J Agric Food Chem. 2015;63(20):5008–16.

Vadgama J, et al. Effect of selenium in combination with adriamycin or taxol on. Anticancer Res. 2000;20:1391–414.

Vadhanavikit S, Ip C, Ganther HE. Metabolites of sodium selenite and methylated selenium compounds administered at cancer chemoprevention levels in the rat. Xenobiotica. 1993;23(7):731–45.

Vyas D, Laput G, Vyas AK. Chemotherapy-enhanced inflammation may lead to the failure of therapy and metastasis. Onco Targets Ther. 2014;7:1015.

Wallenberg M, et al. Selenium induces a multi-targeted cell death process in addition to ROS formation. J Cell Mol Med. 2014;18(4):671–84.

Wang S, et al. Dose-dependent effects of selenite (Se4+) on arsenite (As3+)-induced apoptosis and differentiation in acute promyelocytic leukemia cells. Cell Death Dis. 2015;6(1):e1596.

Watson-Williams E. A preliminary note on the treatment of inoperable carcinoma with selenium. Br Med J. 1919;2(3067):463–4.

Whanger PD. Selenium and its relationship to cancer: an update. Br J Nutr. 2004;91(1):11–28.

Würmli R, et al. Stimulation of mucosal uptake of selenium from selenite by L-cysteine in sheep small intestine. Biol Trace Elem Res. 1989;20(1):75–85.

Yang H, Jia X. Safety evaluation of Se-methylselenocysteine as nutritional selenium supplement: acute toxicity, genotoxicity and subchronic toxicity. Regul Toxicol Pharmacol. 2014;70(3):720–7.

Zeng H. Selenium as an essential micronutrient: roles in cell cycle and apoptosis. Molecules. 2009;14(3):1263–78.

Zeng H, et al. The selenium metabolite methylselenol inhibits the migration and invasion potential of HT1080 tumor cells. J Nutr. 2006;136(6):1528–32.

Zeng H, Wu M, Botnen JH. Methylselenol, a selenium metabolite, induces cell cycle arrest in G1 phase and apoptosis via the extracellular-regulated kinase 1/2 pathway and other cancer signaling genes. J Nutr. 2009;139(9):1613–8.

Zhao R, et al. Expression of p53 enhances selenite-induced superoxide production and apoptosis in human prostate cancer cells. Cancer Res. 2006;66(4):2296–304.

Zhong W, Oberley TD. Redox-mediated effects of selenium on apoptosis and cell cycle in the LNCaP human prostate cancer cell line. Cancer Res. 2001;61(19):7071–8.

Zuo L, et al. Sodium selenite induces apoptosis in acute promyelocytic leukemia-derived NB4 cells by a caspase-3-dependent mechanism and a redox pathway different from that of arsenic trioxide. Ann Hematol. 2004;83(12):751–8.

Chapter 14
Selenocystine and Cancer

Sougat Misra and Mikael Björnstedt

Abstract The diselenide compound selenocystine is a selenium analog of cystine. It is more reactive compared to cystine due to intrinsic differences in chemical properties between sulfur and selenium. Thioredoxin reductase or excess cysteine and glutathione reduces selenocystine to highly reactive selenolate. When selenocystine is present at high concentration, selenolate-mediated biochemical reactions perturb cellular redox homeostasis and induce oxidative stress. Limited pharmacokinetic studies indicate rather long half-life and biphasic elimination kinetics of selenocystine. It is well tolerated in mice and rats with a narrow window between no observed effects and toxicity. Several preclinical studies have interrogated its redox modulatory effects as an anticancer modality. Reported cytotoxic effects include DNA damage, S-phase arrest, activation of P53, alteration of MAPK and PI3K-AKT signaling pathways, loss of mitochondrial membrane potential, and release of cytochrome C. So far, findings from published studies suggest limited antineoplastic effects of selenocystine in various animal models of cancer.

Keywords Selenocystine · Redox reactions · Pharmacokinetics · Toxicity · Anticancer effects

Introduction

Selenocystine (also known as 3,3′-diselenodialanine) is the selenium analog of cystine. It contains two selenium molecules tethered by a diselenide bond. In 1936, the chemical synthesis of selenocystine was first reported (Fredga 1936). The synthesis involved the reaction between methyl ester of α-amino-β-chloropropionic acid hydrochloride and potassium diselenide in an aqueous solution with a yield of 30%. It was almost at the same time when reports on selenium toxicity in live stocks started to emerge, especially in animals grazing in the seleniferous soil of northern

S. Misra (✉) · M. Björnstedt
Division of Pathology F42, Department of Laboratory Medicine, Karolinska Institutet,
Karolinska University Hospital Huddinge, Stockholm, Sweden
e-mail: Sougat.Misra@ki.se

© Springer International Publishing AG, part of Springer Nature 2018
B. Michalke (ed.), *Selenium*, Molecular and Integrative Toxicology,
https://doi.org/10.1007/978-3-319-95390-8_14

part of the United States (reviewed in Trelease and Martin 1936). By then, it was known that plants can assimilate selenium when added to the soils as sodium selenite (Nelson et al. 1933). When grains and straw from these plants were fed to the animals, toxicosis manifested in the form of growth retardation and the animals died within few weeks. The authors indicated the presence of selenium "in intimate association with protein" which was experimentally shown by Franke (Franke 1934). It was then prominent that the organic forms of selenium were responsible for imparting toxicity in the experimental animals. Replacement of selenium in the place of sulfur in cystine and methionine in biological systems was proposed by Painter and Franke at the same time and thus brought selenocystine as a new entrant in the field of selenium toxicology. Further studies on this compound have revealed its chemical properties and biological functions including its potential applications in cancer chemotherapy. In this chapter, several aspects of selenocystine in biology with a specific focus on its therapeutic potential in the treatment of cancer are discussed.

Chemistry of Selenocystine

In describing the biological functions of selenium, Thressa C. Stadtman once wrote that "it is logical to assume that some unique chemical properties of an element are exploited when the element is used in biochemical systems as a catalyst" (Stadtman 1980). The diverse physiological functions of human selenoenzymes provide a direct evidence for the nature's choice of selenium as selenocysteine in the catalytic sites of these enzymes. T.C. Stadtman suggested that certain chemical properties of selenols (RSeH) make it a better choice as catalytic site of enzymes than the corresponding thiols (RSH). These are as follows: (a) organic selenium compounds are generally more reactive than the corresponding sulfur compounds; (b) in contrast to thiols, selenols are ionized at neutral pH, and thus remain in anionic form in the catalytic site; (c) selenols serve as good leaving groups being superior nucleophiles; and (d) the lower redox potential of selenols as compared with the corresponding thiols makes these better suited for redox catalysis. Since selenocystine can be reduced to corresponding selenol in the biological system, understanding the chemical and biochemical properties of selenocystine is important when the key interests are focused on the use of this compound in human health and diseases.

Physicochemical Properties of Selenium Atom

In the periodic table, selenium is the element number 34 with atomic weight 76.983 Da. It is located in period 4, group 16 which contains other chalcogens including oxygen, sulfur, and tellurium. The electron configuration of selenium is $[Ar]3d^{10}4s^24p^4$, which is equivalent to that of sulfur $[Ne]3s^23p^4$. This explains their similar atomic and physicochemical properties such as atomic sizes (both in ionic and covalent states), bond energies, ionization potentials, and electronegativities (Perrone et al. 2015). As selenium is heavier than sulfur, it is softer (polarizable) than sulfur, with a polarizability volume of 3.77 Å (Se) compared to 2.90 Å (S) (Lide 2006). The polarizability electronegativity of selenium is lower (2.31) than sulfur (2.49) (Nagle 1990). Based on the definition of electronegativity as the power in an atom to attract electron to itself, such differences of polarizability electronegativity between sulfur and selenium explain partly as to why these elements exhibit different properties in certain redox reactions involving transfer of electrons.

Some Key Chemical Properties of Selenocystine in Relation to Its Biological Activities

Selenocystine is not very soluble in water. However, it can be solubilized in acidic conditions. Optically active selenocystine is soluble in water to the extent of 6.3×10^{-4} mole/L, while the solubility of D,L-selenocystine in water (pH 7.0) is reported to be 2.35×10^{-3} mole/L (Odom (1983) and the references therein).

The antioxidant effects of selenocystine were first reported based on its ability to reduce lipid hydroperoxides in acidic condition (Caldwell and Tappel 1964). However, direct cleavage of hydroperoxides may have little biological effects since selenium-containing peroxidases are highly efficient in catalyzing such reactions.

Another key chemical property of selenocystine is its ability to oxidize thiols (cysteine, glutathione, and homocysteine) in the presence of hydroperoxides (Caldwell and Tappel 1965). Oxidation of cysteine is the highest among the tested thiols. It is a pH-dependent process in which the maximum oxidation of cysteine occurs at neutral pH. When tert-butyl hydroperoxide or cumene hydroperoxides were used as oxidants, the rate of cysteine oxidation was lower in comparison to hydrogen peroxide as an oxidant. Notably, selenocystine is much more efficient than cystine in protecting hydrogen peroxide-induced oxidative damage of yeast alcohol dehydrogenase and creatine kinase as shown in the activity assays. The proposed reaction mechanism involved hydroperoxide-mediated oxidation selenocystine to an intermediary monoselenide which reacted further with thiols to produce a sulfoselenide (Se-S bond). Such types of reactions indicate that in the presence of excess of thiols, selenocystine can catalyze a steady-state disproportionation of hydrogen peroxide to water and oxygen.

The reactions between selenocystine and thiols bring another complexity in connection with the physiological relevance of direct catalytic cleavage of hydrogen peroxide by selenocystine. Both cysteine and glutathione can completely reduce selenocystine to selenolate (Sec-Se⁻) when present in 1000-fold excess. It is very likely that such reactions can proceed at physiological concentration of thiols which is in millimolar range (Dickson and Tappel 1969). The catalytic mechanism involving hydroperoxides reduction by glutathione peroxidase (GPX4) explains the reaction between selenolate and hydroperoxides. Selenolate is rapidly oxidized by hydroperoxides to form a selenenic acid intermediate, which subsequently reacts with thiols to form an intermediate sulfoselenide (RSSeCys). Such sulfoselenide intermediate/s are subsequently reduced by a second thiol to produce an oxidized thiol and selenolate. Such redox reactions persist as long as reduced thiols are abundant. Therefore, it is plausible that in the presence of disulfide reductases (thioredoxin and glutaredoxin systems), selenocystine can catalyze an efficient reduction of hydroperoxides. This was shown in two independent studies using purified mammalian thioredoxin reductase (Björnstedt et al. 1995) and glutathione reductase/glutaredoxin/GSH systems (Björnstedt et al. 1997). First of all, like selenium-containing glutathione peroxidases, thioredoxin reductase possesses selenium-dependent peroxidase activity, but with a broad substrate specificity in reducing hydrogen peroxides, lipid hydroperoxides, and organic hydroperoxides (Björnstedt et al. 1995). Secondly, selenocystine is efficiently reduced by mammalian thioredoxin reductase with a K_m value of 6 μM and a high turnover rate (K_{cat}) of 3200 min^{-1}. These kinetic parameters show that selenocystine is an almost equally efficient substrate to mammalian thioredoxin reductase as the natural substrate oxidized thioredoxin and indicate a potential importance of this selenoenzyme in the reduction of selenocystine to selenocysteine. The presence of excess selenocysteine increases the efficacy even further as shown for the reduction of (15S)-hydroperoxy-(5Z), (8Z), 11(Z), 13E-eicosatetraenoic acid ((15S)-HPETE) to the corresponding alcohol, 15S-HETE, where selenocystine at a concentration of 2.5 μM increased the production of 15-HETE eightfold. Similar observation was made with glutathione reductase/glutaredoxin/GSH systems which regenerate GSH and thus facilitate reduction of selenocystine and oxidized glutathione and thereby result in increased reduction of hydroperoxides (Björnstedt et al. 1997). Together, these findings imply that enzyme-mediated reduction of disulfide bonds and selenocystine, together with inherent peroxidase activity of mammalian thioredoxin reductase, greatly accelerates the reduction of hydroperoxides.

Selenocystine is also an effective inhibitor of peroxynitrite-mediated oxidation and nitration with half-maximal inhibitory concentration of 2.5 and 30 μM, respectively (Briviba et al. 1996). Inhibition of peroxynitrite-induced DNA damage by selenocystine provides additional evidence for effective attenuation of such oxidative damage by peroxynitrite (Roussyn et al. 1996). Together, selenocystine at high dose can potentially alter the functionalities of certain cell types which are known to produce peroxynitrite as a mediator of cytotoxicity in inflammatory states.

Some of the above test tube-based studies were performed under certain reaction conditions including low pH and oxygen-free environment. Further in-depth studies are required to understand the potential biological effects of selenocystine in vivo. Both oxygen and thiols are abundant under physiological condition and majority of biochemical reactions take place at an alkaline condition. Earlier studies indicate that selenocystine undergoes autoxidation and decomposition at alkaline pH (Caldwell and Tappel 1965). However, the nature of the product upon autoxidation has not been elaborated. Besides, formation of a seleninic acid intermediate of selenocysteine is suggested at higher pH in an electrochemical study (Bai et al. 2009). Together, further spectroscopic studies are required to understand the stability and chemical equilibrium of selenocystine at physiological pH in the presence of oxygen.

Cellular Uptake, Biodistribution, and Elimination of Selenocystine

Transport: There are four known transporters (genes encoded by *SLC3A1, SLC7A9, SLC7A11,* and *SLC7A13*) for cystine uptake in human. The details of their transport properties have been described earlier (Misra and Björnstedt 2017). Based on the structural analogy, as is the case with methionine and selenomethionine, it has been suggested that selenocystine can be transported in a similar way as with their cognate substrate cystine.

Contradictory interpretations exist as to whether selenocystine is transported via the same transport systems as with cystine. Using everted gut sacs of hamsters, it has been shown that mucosal transport of D,L-selenocystine is not inhibited by the presence of tenfold excess of D,L-cystine dissolved in oxygen-saturated Krebs-Ringer bicarbonate medium (McConnell and Cho 1965). No net transmucosal movement against a chemical gradient was indicative of a passive transport process involving selenocystine uptake. In a later study using brush border membrane vesicles isolated from pig mid-jejunum, it has been shown that 100-fold excess of D,L-cystine inhibits the "initial" uptake (first 20 s) of D,L-selenocystine by 40% (Wolffram et al. 1989). These studies are not directly comparable due to fundamental differences in the conditions of uptake experiments and the relative ratios of selenocystine to cystine. Context-wise, different K_m values have been reported for L-cystine (0.11 ± 0.03 mM) and D,L-selenocystine (0.22 ± 0.05 mM) for b$^{0,+}$rBAT following the overexpression of the transporter in *Xenopus* oocytes (Nickel et al. 2009). Such differences in the K_m values indicate different affinity of the transporter for these two substrates.

The uptake of different chemical forms of selenium has been studied in Caco-2 cells. The apparent permeability coefficient (a unified measure of transport rate) of apical to basolateral transport of selenocystine was comparable to that of selenite transport (Leblondel et al. 2001). A recent study has reported similar findings in these cells (Takahashi et al. 2017). Interestingly, the cellular retention (both absorbed and adsorbed) of selenocystine was higher in comparison to selenite and selenomethionine while basolateral to apical transport was very low (Leblondel et al. 2001). Cysteine didn't inhibit the apical to basolateral transport of selenocystine. This indicates that that these compounds don't share a common transport pathway. Context-wise, it is important to address that Caco-2 cells lack the specificity and the presence of different amino acid transport systems.

Biodistribution and elimination: The biodistribution of selenocystine has been studied in different animal models. Intestinal absorption of selenocystine is comparable to that of selenomethionine in female Wistar rats following oral administration

(Thomson et al. 1975). The urinary and fecal excretions were 11.4% and 27.1% of the administered dose. The whole-body retention of selenocystine complied excellently with the urinary and fecal excretion values. Both the fecal and urinary excretions were much higher following the first 24 h post-administration of selenocystine when compared with selenomethionine. The accumulation of selenium from selenocystine was highest in the liver, followed by kidney. Serum selenium levels accounted for 1.1% of the administered dose after 10 weeks of dosing. This was comparable with the radiotracer level at the end of the first week, suggesting a high binding affinity of selenocystine with serum proteins with an apparent long half-life.

In a long-term feeding study spanning 9 weeks, male Sprague-Dawley rats were fed with torula yeast-based diet supplemented with 2.0 ppm Se in the form of selenocystine, selenomethionine, and selenite (Deagen et al. 1987). Plasma glutathione peroxidase (GPX) levels were comparable in animals receiving all forms of selenium. However, GPX activity in the liver and RBC was highest in the selenocystine-supplemented group. The total Se levels in these tissues were lower in the selenocystine-supplemented group in comparison to the rats that received selenomethionine. The total blood Se level was approximately the double in the latter group. Random incorporation of selenomethionine into protein partially explains such differences in the total selenium and GPX activity. One of the key findings from these two studies indicate that there exist remarkable similarities in the biodistribution pattern of Se- and tissue-specific glutathione peroxidase activities following long-term oral administration of selenite and selenocystine in rats.

The biological half-life of ^{75}Se-selenocystine has been reported to be 3 days following intravenous administration in mice (Anghileri and Marqués 1965). When high dosage of cystine or methionine (5 mg per animal) was co-injected intraperitoneally, greater than 59% of the total dose was retained in the body after 7 days (Anghileri 1966). However, methionine was more effective in delaying the whole-body clearance of Se from selenocystine. In a later study, it was shown that the whole-body elimination of L-selenocystine comprised of two phases in rats (Hasegawa 1972). The biological half-life of the first phase was about 6 days, while it was 17 days in the later phase. Interestingly, the elimination kinetics was described to be independent of the route of administration whether it was peroral or subcutaneous. The only notable difference was higher accumulation of selenium in the blood and liver following subcutaneous administration at the termination of experiment after 6 weeks. Time-course changes in plasma selenium level were reported in sheep following single intravenous administration of ^{75}Se-selenocystine in the jugular vein (Davidson and McMurray 1988). Following a fast disappearance, plasma ^{75}Se level increased slowly that was complete within 2 h. A steady-state level reached within 6–8 h, after which plasma radioactivity was slowly diminished. Interestingly, a substantial proportion of plasma radioactivity was labile following treatment with 2-mercaptoethanol, suggesting formation of an intermediate sulfoselenide bond with protein thiols. Furthermore, a comprehensive pharmacokinetic study on the D,L-selenocystine in mice has been reported following both oral and intravenous administrations. Following oral administration of 50 mg selenocystine/

kg, the plasma C_{max}, T_{max}, and 6 h AUC values were 3.27 µg/mL, 0.25 h, and 10.01 µg h/mL, respectively. When mice received an intravenous dose of 5 mg selenocystine/kg, the plasma C_{max}, T_{max}, and 6 h AUC values were 3.59 µg/mL, 0.08 h, and 3.58 µg h/mL, respectively. Apparently, it required tenfold higher oral dose (which is toxic) to attain a similar C_{max} value when compared with intravenous administration. The erythrocytes contained five times higher levels of selenium than the plasma concentration at 6 h, following high dose of oral administration of selenocystine. Liver total selenium was comparable after 1 h of selenium administration via both routes despite differences in the administered dosage. However, intravenous dosing resulted in fast elimination from liver in subsequent 5 h, followed by a slow elimination. In mice that received peroral treatment, about 30% of selenium was lost from the high-molecular-weight cytosolic fractions of liver following 24 h of dialysis in the presence of 2-mercaptoethanol. This again suggests the mercaptan-labile nature of protein-bound selenium when administered as selenocystine.

Selenocystine Toxicity in Animals

The first published experimental toxicity of selenocystine was studied in albino rats following intraperitoneal injection (Moxon 1940). Range of dosage used in this study varied from 3.0 to 30.0 mg Se/kg body weight. The minimum fatal dose (amount of Se to cause death in 75% of animals within 2 days) was determined to be 4.0 mg Se/kg body weight, equivalent to 17.4 mg selenocystine/kg body weight. In a later study, the effect of long-term dietary supplementation of different enantiomorphs of selenocystine in albino rats was reported (Moxon et al. 1941). The calculated average total selenocystine (optically inactive form) consumption per animal was between 20.3 and 24.4 mg over a period of 40 days, while it was 51.5 and 52.5 mg over a period of 80 days. Two out of six animals died in the treatment group during the course of the experimentation. Dietary selenocystine administration resulted in a considerably low food intake along with severe growth inhibition. The average weight of the surviving animals receiving selenocystine was about the half of the control animals at the termination of experiments. At necropsy, the histological examinations indicated necrosis and atrophy of livers with evidence of hemochromatosis. The same study also reported the effects of dietary supplementation (20 mg/kg diet) of optically active D- and L-selenocystine, although the study durations of this series of experiments were not mentioned in the original publication. The authors noted that L-selenocystine was more toxic than D-selenocystine based on the evaluation on the mortality rates, growth rates, pathological examinations of livers (higher prevalence of hypertrophy of the caudate and lateral lobes), and general condition of the experimental animals.

The acute and subacute toxicity of orally administered D,L-selenocystine has been studied in ICR mice (Sayato et al. 1993). Following a single oral dose, the calculated 10-day LD_{50} for selenocystine was reported to be 76.0 mg/kg (confidence interval ranged between 64.4 and 89.7 mg/kg). Peroral administration of a single dose of 50.0 mg/kg selenocystine resulted in elevated levels of alanine aminotransferase (ALT), aspartate aminotransferase (AST), urea-nitrogen, and phosphorus along with a significant reduction of plasma calcium. Alterations in the levels of these key biomarkers of liver and kidney functions were transient in nature and returned to the base levels within 3 days of treatment. In subacute toxicity study, the mice received different dosages of selenocystine (10, 20, 30, and 40 mg/kg/day) for 30 days. Mice that received 30 and 40 mg selenocystine/kg/day died within 25 and 10 days, respectively. No incidences of histopathological lesions of livers were observed in animals treated with either 10 or 20 mg selenocystine/kg/day. However, plasma ALT and AST values were higher in animals that received a dose of 20 mg selenocystine/kg/day. In a follow-up study, the effects of long-term administration of different dosage of selenocystine (5, 10, and 15 mg/kg/day) have been reported in the same mice strain (Hasegawa et al. 1994). Growth retardation and increased activities of plasma ALT and AST were observed in animals receiving 10 or 15 mg selenocystine/kg/day for 90 days. No histopathological changes were observed at any of the administered dosage of selenocystine at the end of the experiments. The cytosolic fraction of liver homogenate contained the maximum levels of selenium (ranging from 68 to 72% of total selenium) at the highest treatment dose.

With reference to an earlier study (Moxon 1940) as outlined above, orally administered selenocystine appears to be less toxic. It is important to note that different enantiomers of selenocystine were used in these studies. Also, the purity of the study compound used in the first two studies could be an important limiting factor. In summary, oral administration of 5 mg selenocystine/kg/day for 90 days appears to be a safe dose in mice with no notable signs of toxicity as could be assessed from the growth, histopathological assessment, and plasma levels of ALT and AST.

Selenocystine in Cancer

The early history of cancer treatment with selenium goes back to more than a century ago (documented in Misra and Björnstedt 2017). Despite remarkable antitumor effects of different selenium compounds in animal models of cancer, lack of clinical trials has limited the possibility to understand their safety and efficacy in the treatment of human cancers. In this section below, antitumor effects of selenocystine in different animal models are discussed.

In transplantable tumor: The effect of intraperitoneal administration of selenocystine was evaluated in ICR mice that received freshly isolated transplantable Ehrlich ascites tumor cells (EATC) originated from donor animals (Greeder and Milner 1980). The mice were inoculated with EATC and selenocystine (2.0 μg Se/g initial body weight) was administered by intraperitoneal injection at day 0. These mice also received nine additional treatments until day 21 when treatment was terminated and tumor incidence was recorded in half of the treated mice. No incidence of malignancy was reported in the selenocystine-treated mice neither at day 21 nor at day 42, while all control mice developed ascites tumors. In a parallel experiment, when tumor-bearing mice received 1.0 µg Se as selenocystine/g initial body weight under an identical experimental setup, none of the treated mice developed tumors. However, at lower dose of selenocystine (0.5 µg Se/g initial body weight), two out of five animals developed tumors. The volume of ascitic fluid in these animals was much lower in comparison to the control animals. When the same mice strain received four doses of about 0.25 µg Se as selenocystine/g initial body weight under similar experimental conditions, the incidence of EATC was recorded in nine out of ten mice after 5 weeks (Poirier and Milner 1983). In a later study, the effects of selenocystine treatment were studied in a transplanted lymphocytic leukemia model harboring L1210 cells (Milner and Hsu 1981). Following transplantation of 1.06×10^2 cells, the mice were treated daily with selenocystine (40 µg Se/day) for 10 days. The mean survival time was longer in the treated mice compared to the control mice. None of the selenocystine-treated animals survived until 60 days while 90% of the sodium selenite-treated animals survived during this period with further treatment.

It is important to note that the site of tumor cell inoculation and treatment overlapped in all the studies as outlined above. Also, the treatment was initiated on the same day as with transplantation. Although neither of these observations can overrule the efficacy or failure of selenium treatment, further in vivo studies are required to assess the efficacy of selenocystine in pertinent animal models of cancer.

In chemically-induced carcinogenesis model: The anticarcinogenic effects on different selenium compounds have been extensively studied in different animal models. However, there is a dearth of information concerning the anticarcinogenic effect of selenocystine. The effect of a tobacco-specific carcinogen, 4-(methylnitrosamino)-1-(3-pyridyl)-1-butanone (NNK), has been studied in female A/J mice (Li et al. 2006). Mice were fed with L-selenocystine-supplemented diet (15 ppm Se) for 1 week prior to NNK treatment and received the same diet for another 16 weeks posttreatment. A lower mean lung adenoma multiplicity (number of lung tumors/mouse) was found in the L-selenocystine-treated group (4.6) in comparison to the control group (7.2). The effect of treatment on the tumor size has not been reported in the same study. Although limited feed intake was associated with the lower adenoma multiplicity upon supplementation of L-selenocystine, feed consumption in these animals was not reported.

It shall be emphasized that the mechanisms of chemical carcinogenicity depend on the exposure dose, time, and structure-activity relationships. Hence, it may simply be an overestimation that selenium can prevent different modes of carcinogenesis within the realms of its limited biological activities in different chemical forms. The anticarcinogenic effect of selenocystine, as outlined above, perhaps does not deviate from such an assumption.

Selenocystine as a Single Agent in Targeting Cancer Cells: In Vitro and Molecular Studies

Several in vitro studies have documented the cytotoxic effects of selenocystine in different types of nonhuman and human cancer cells. Milner and colleagues studied the effects of selenocystine on the growth of relatively resistant canine mammary tumor cell lines CMT-11 and CMT-13, along with normal cells isolated from a canine normal mammary gland (Fico et al. 1986). Selenocystine at a concentration of 9.75 µM dose inhibited the growth of CMT-13 cells by 29% within 48 h, but the proliferation of CMT-11 and nonneoplastic normal cells remained unaffected under similar condition. In a human myeloid cell line, HL-60, 72 h IC_{50} was reported to be 10.5 µM (Batist et al. 1986). When 1.0 mM GSH was added in the extracellular medium, 72-h IC_{50} value for selenocystine was shifted to 20.0 µM in these cells. A similar observation has been made in murine melanoma B16 and pB16 cells (Siwek et al. 1994). When these cells were preincubated with 50 µM GSH for 24 h prior to treatment with selenocystine, viability was higher in GSH-pretreated cells compared to the control cells in both the cell lines. In an earlier study, we reported that the co-incubation with monosodium glutamate and 5,5'-dithiobis-2-nitrobenzoic acid (DTNB) abrogated the cytotoxicity of seleno-L-cystine in H157 cells (Olm et al. 2009). In Chinese hamster lung fibroblasts, 48 h IC_{50} value (MTS assay) for L-selenocystine was reported to be 34.0 µM, while for D-selenocystine, it was 39.0 µM (Short et al. 2003). Findings from this study suggest that D-selenocystine is toxic, but is not efficient in increasing the glutathione peroxidase activity when measured 48 h after exposure to an identical concentration of both isomers in these cells. Chen and Wong have studied the cytotoxicity of L-selenocystine in different human-originated cancer cell lines (Chen and Wong 2009). The reported 72 h IC_{50} values (MTT assay) ranged between 3.7 and 37.0 µM in these cell lines. However, the 72 h IC_{50} values for selenocystine in HL-60 and HepG2 cell lines in this study differed from the other studies (Batist et al. 1986; Hoefig et al. 2011), in which a higher cytotoxicity of selenocystine was observed. Interestingly, selenocystine was very ineffective in inducing cytotoxicity in human normal fibroblast cells (HS68), as shown by two different cell death assays. Apoptosis was found to be the major pathway of cell death mediated by selenocystine, as shown in A375 (melanoma), HepG2 (hepatocellular carcinoma), and MCF-7 (breast adenocarcinoma) cell lines. In line with the previous studies, pretreatment with high level of GSH (5.0 mM) prevented DNA strand break and the number of apoptotic cells was lower in MCF-7 cell line.

On the Mechanisms of Selenocystine Cytotoxicity

Involvement of multiple cellular pathways has been implicated in the cytotoxicity of selenocystine. Several studies have shown that reactive oxygen species (ROS), metabolic by-products of selenocystine metabolism, play key roles in the observed cytotoxicity. Autoxidation of selenolate (Sec-Se⁻) to selenocystine in the presence of oxygen leads to ROS generation (Wallenberg et al. 2010).

High levels of ROS generation and thiol oxidation are implicated in the opening of mitochondrial transition pore (MTP) and subsequent release of cytochrome C from mitochondria. Such cellular events are often associated with apoptotic cell death. In line with this, it was shown that treatment of HepG2 cells with 10 µM L-selenocystine resulted in loss of mitochondrial membrane potential and subsequent release of cytochrome C into cytosol (Kim et al. 2003). Similar observation was made in isolated rat liver mitochondria upon treatment with a high dose (100 µM) of selenocystine.

Chen and colleagues have extensively studied the mechanisms of selenocystine cytotoxicity in different cancer cell lines. It was shown that selenocystine induced S-phase arrest in a dose-dependent manner in human breast adenocarcinoma MCF-7 cells (Chen and Wong 2008a). This was associated with decreased expression of cyclin D1, cyclin D3, and cyclin-dependent kinases CDK 4 and CDK 6. An elevated expression of P53 was found only at higher dose (20 µM). When these cells were preincubated with different inhibitors of MAPK pathway 1 h prior to selenocystine treatment, only ERK inhibitor provided protection against selenocystine cytotoxicity. When the involvement of PI3K-AKT pathway in selenocystine-mediated cytotoxicity was interrogated, it was found that following an initial increase in phosphorylated-AKT, its level significantly reduced at 24 h. However, pretreatment with a PI3K inhibitor provided significant protection against selenocystine cytotoxicity. Such findings indicate possible signaling modulatory effects of selenocystine upstream of AKT. However, it remains to be understood whether these above-mentioned effects of selenocystine are mediated by itself or via generation of ROS, given that both MAPK and PI3K-AKT signaling pathways are regulated by ROS and thioredoxins, mainly via oxidation of protein thiols (Ray et al. 2012).

Selenocystine-induced DNA damage and activation of P53 pathway were investigated in A375 cells (Chen and Wong 2008b). High doses of selenocystine induced DNA damage as measured by olive tail movement in comet assay. A concomitant increase in the phosphorylation of serine 139 residue of histone H2A.X was found. Selenocystine treatment also increased the expression of P53 and phosphorylated serine 15 residue of P53, often implicated as a response to DNA damage. The inhibition of selenocystine cytotoxicity by P53 siRNA suggested that P53 may play a key role in selenocystine cytotoxicity in these cells. Further studies on human breast cancer cell lines showed that selenocystine treatment resulted in both necrotic and apoptotic cell death along with cell cycle arrest at S phase (Long et al. 2015).

Findings from the above studies indicate that exposure to high doses of selenocystine results in DNA damage, S-phase arrest, activation of P53, alteration of MAPK and PI3K-AKT signaling pathways, loss of mitochondrial membrane potential, and release of cytochrome C and eventually leads to cell death either by necrosis or apoptosis. However, different cell types differ in their sensitivity to this selenium compound. To this end, further studies are required to understand the transport mechanism/s of selenocystine in both normal and cancer cells under physiologically relevant conditions.

Selenocystine in Combination with Cytostatic Drugs: In Vitro Studies

A number of in vitro studies have investigated the possible synergistic or additive effects of selenocystine and cancer chemotherapeutic drugs using different cancer cell lines. In combination with 5-FU, selenocystine was found to be more cytotoxic than a single agent in A375 cells (Fan et al. 2013). In the combined treatment, there were significant loss of mitochondrial membrane potential, along with increased expression of proapoptotic proteins Bax and Bad, while it was opposite for anti-apoptotic proteins Bcl-2 and BCL-xL. A concomitant increase in apoptotic cell population was reported in the combined treatment. A significant inhibition of cell death was found following pretreatment with an ERK inhibitor, U0126, in the combined treatment. Thus, the involvement of the ERK pathway has been implicated in the observed cytotoxic effects of the combined treatment. A synergistic cytotoxic effect of selenocystine and auranofin was reported in MCF-7 cells (Liu et al. 2013). Unlike an earlier report describing S-phase arrest following selenocystine treatment in these cells (Chen and Wong 2008a), no such inhibitory effect was found in this study at identical exposure concentration (20.0 μM). Also, PI3K inhibitor, LY294002, was ineffective in protecting cell viability against the combined treatment, while it was effective against selenocystine in the same cell line. Hence, a complex interplay between LY294002 and auranofin on cell viability could be postulated.

In recent years, the inhibition of thioredoxin reductases has been investigated as a potential therapeutic strategy in cancer. A number of candidate molecules, including auranofin, are potent inhibitors of thioredoxin reductases. In line with this, single or combined cytotoxic effects of selenocystine and auranofin were investigated in A549 cells, a human lung adenocarcinoma cell line (Fan et al. 2014a). When these cells were pretreated with selenocystine for different time intervals and subsequently treated with auranofin for another 6 h, a time-dependent increase in cytotoxicity was observed in these cells. Combined treatment resulted in increased numbers of apoptotic cells as assessed by sub-G1 cell population. A concomitant downregulation of phosphorylated AKT and ERK was found in the combined treatment. Additionally, when cells were pretreated with chemical inhibitors of AKT and ERK, significant reduction of cell viability was found in the combined treatment in comparison to control cells treated with the combination of selenocystine and auranofin. As mentioned in earlier studies, pretreatment of cells with GSH (10 mM) protected against the combined treatment. Chen and colleagues reported similar synergistic cytotoxic effects of doxorubicin and selenocystine in a human hepatocellular carcinoma cell line, HepG2 (Fan et al. 2014b).

Selenocystine in the Treatment of Human Cancer

Weisberger and Shurland have described the treatment effect of high doses of sele-nocystine in a case series involving four leukemia patients (Weisberger and Suhrland 1956). Two of these patients had acute leukemia (one with stem cell and another with childhood leukemia) and two others had chronic myeloid leukemia. All of these patients received selenocystine orally, ranging between 50 and 200 mg/day for a period ranging between 10 and 57 days. One patient with acute leukemia received a total of 5.2 g of selenocystine over a period of 50 days.

In all patients, there was a rapid decrease in the total leukocyte count and spleen size following treatment with selenocystine. Immature granulocytes disappeared more rapidly than the mature ones. Interestingly, one patient regained sensitivity to an earlier chemotherapeutic agent following selenocystine treatment. Two out of four patients deceased during the course of treatment and the cause of death was found to be unrelated to selenocystine treatment at autopsy. The other two patients had partial remission and continued on other chemotherapeutics due to side effects of selenocystine treatment.

Selenocystine at the administered dose manifested severe side effects including nausea, vomiting, diarrhea, alopecia, and damage to the fingernails. The latter two side effects were reversible when treatment was withdrawn. However, no changes in hepatic or renal functions were found during the entire course of study in all these patients.

In summary, this study on human was the first to demonstrate substantial indica-tions of antitumor effects of selenocystine, specifically in different hematological malignancies.

Concluding Remarks

We have already gathered substantial knowledge on the chemistry, toxicity, biodis-tribution, and modes and mechanisms of action of selenocystine, specifically in multitude of cancer cells in vitro. There is outstanding evidence to suggest that selenocystine has a very good potential as an anticancer agent. There are indications from few in vivo studies that this compound can be used in combination with che-motherapeutic agents to achieve a better therapeutic effect. Further clinical trials are needed to explore such key potentials of selenocystine in the treatment of cancer.

Acknowledgments The authors would like to thank financial support from Barncancerfonden, Cancerfonden, Cancer- och Allergifonden, KI Fonder, Jochnick Foundation, Radiumhemmetsforsknings fonder, and the County Council of Stockholm.

References

Anghileri LJ. Effects of cystine and methionine on the 75 Se selenocystine metabolism in mice. Naturwissenschaften. 1966;53(10):256.

Anghileri LJ, Marqués R. Fate of injected Se75-methionine and Se75-cystine in mice. Arch Biochem Biophys. 1965;111(3):580–2.

Bai Y, Wang T, Liu Y, Zheng W. Electrochemical oxidation of selenocystine and selenomethionine. Colloids Surf B Biointerfaces. 2009;74(1):150–3.

Batist G, Katki AG, Klecker RW, Myers CE. Selenium-induced cytotoxicity of human leukemia cells: interaction with reduced glutathione. Cancer Res. 1986;46(11):5482–5.

Björnstedt M, Hamberg M, Kumar S, Xue J, Holmgren A. Human thioredoxin reductase directly reduces lipid hydroperoxides by NADPH and selenocystine strongly stimulates the reaction via catalytically generated selenols. J Biol Chem. 1995;270(20):11761–4.

Björnstedt M, Kumar S, Björkhem L, Spyrou G, Holmgren A. Selenium and the thioredoxin and glutaredoxin systems. Biomed Environ Sci.: BES. 1997;10(2–3):271–9.

Briviba K, Roussyn I, Sharov VS, Helmut S. Attenuation of oxidation and nitration reactions of peroxynitrite by selenomethionine, selenocystine and ebselen. Biochem J. 1996;319(1):13–5.

Caldwell KA, Tappel AL. Reactions of Seleno- and Sulfoamino acids with hydroperoxides. Biochemistry. 1964;3:1643–7.

Caldwell KA, Tappel AL. Acceleration of sulfhydryl oxidations by selenocystine. Arch Biochem Biophys. 1965;112(1):196–200.

Chen T, Wong Y-S. Selenocystine induces S-phase arrest and apoptosis in human breast adeno-carcinoma MCF-7 cells by modulating ERK and Akt phosphorylation. J Agric Food Chem. 2008a;56(22):10574–81.

Chen T, Wong Y-S. Selenocystine induces reactive oxygen species–mediated apoptosis in human cancer cells. Biomed Pharmacother. 2009;63(2):105–13.

Chen T, Wong Y. Selenocystine induces apoptosis of A375 human melanoma cells by activat-ing ROS-mediated mitochondrial pathway and p53 phosphorylation. Cell Mol Life Sci. 2008b;65(17):2763–75.

Davidson W, McMurray C. 75Selenium-labeled sheep plasma: The time course of changes in 75selenium distribution. J Inorg Biochem. 1988;34(1):1–9.

Deagen J, Butler J, Beilstein M, Whanger P. Effects of dietary selenite, selenocystine and sele-nomethionine on selenocysteine lyase and glutathione peroxidase activities and on selenium levels in rat tissues. J Nutr. 1987;117(1):91–8.

Dickson RC, Tappel AL. Reduction of selenocystine by cysteine or glutathione. Arch Biochem Biophys. 1969;130(1):547–50.

Fan C, Chen J, Wang Y, Wong Y-S, Zhang Y, Zheng W, et al. Selenocystine potentiates cancer cell apoptosis induced by 5-fluorouracil by triggering reactive oxygen species-mediated DNA dam-age and inactivation of the ERK pathway. Free Radic Biol Med. 2013;65:305–16.

Fan C, Zheng W, Fu X, Li X, Wong Y-S, Chen T. Strategy to enhance the therapeutic effect of doxorubicin in human hepatocellular carcinoma by selenocystine, a synergistic agent that regu-lates the ROS-mediated signaling. Oncotarget. 2014a;5(9):2853.

Fan C, Zheng W, Fu X, Li X, Wong Y, Chen T. Enhancement of auranofin-induced lung cancer cell apoptosis by selenocystine, a natural inhibitor of TrxR1 in vitro and in vivo. Cell Death Dis. 2014b;5(4):e1191.

Fico M, Poirier K, Watrach A, Watrach M, Milner J. Differential effects of selenium on normal and neoplastic canine mammary cells. Cancer Res. 1986;46(7):3384–8.

Franke KW. A new toxicant occurring naturally in certain samples of plant foodstuffs. J Nutr. 1934;8:609–12.

Fredga A. Selensubstituierte Aminosauren. I Synthese von aa'-Diamino Diselen-Dihydrakrylsaure(Selencystin). Sven Kem Tidskr. 1936;48:160.

Greeder G, Milner J. Factors influencing the inhibitory effect of selenium on mice inoculated with Ehrlich ascites tumor cells. Science. 1980;209(4458):825–7.

Hasegawa A. Study on the body retention and excretion of sodium selenite and L-selenocystine. J Hygien Chem. 1972;18(2):70–5.

Hasegawa T, Taniguchi S, Mihara M, Nakamuro K, Sayato Y. Toxicity and chemical form of selenium in the liver of mice orally administered selenocystine for 90 days. Arch Toxicol. 1994;68(2):91–5.

Hoefig CS, Renko K, Köhrle J, Birringer M, Schomburg L. Comparison of different selenocompounds with respect to nutritional value vs. toxicity using liver cells in culture. J Nutr Biochem. 2011;22(10):945–55.

Kim T-S, Yun BY, Kim IY. Induction of the mitochondrial permeability transition by selenium compounds mediated by oxidation of the protein thiol groups and generation of the superoxide. Biochem Pharmacol. 2003;66(12):2301–11.

Leblondel G, Mauras Y, Cailleux A, Allain P. Transport measurements across Caco-2 monolayers of different organic and inorganic selenium. Biol Trace Elem Res. 2001;83(3):191–206.

Li L, Xie Y, El-Sayed WM, Szakacs JG, Franklin MR, Roberts JC. Chemopreventive activity of selenocysteine prodrugs against tobacco-derived nitrosamine (NNK) induced lung tumors in the A/J mouse. J Biochem Mol Toxicol. 2006;19(6):396–405.

Lide DR, editor. CRC Handbook of Chemistry and Physics, vol. 87. Boca Raton: CRC Press; 2006.

Liu C, Liu Z, Li M, Li X, Wong Y-S, Ngai S-M, et al. Enhancement of auranofin-induced apoptosis in MCF-7 human breast cells by selenocystine, a synergistic inhibitor of thioredoxin reductase. PLoS One. 2013;8(1):e53945.

Long M, Wu J, Hao J, Liu W, Tang Y, Li X, et al. Selenocystine-induced cell apoptosis and S-phase arrest inhibit human triple-negative breast cancer cell proliferation. In Vitro Cell Dev Biol Anim. 2015;51(10):1077–84.

McConnell KP, Cho GJ. Transmucosal Movement of Selenium. Am J Phys. 1965;208:1191–5.

Milner J, Hsu C. Inhibitory effects of selenium on the growth of L1210 leukemic cells. Cancer Res. 1981;41(5):1652–6.

Misra S, Björnstedt M. Metabolism of Selenium/Selenocystine and their roles in the prevention and treatment of human cancer organoselenium compounds in biology and medicine; 2017. p. 377–400.

Moxon A, Du Bois K, Potter R. The toxicity of optically inactive, d-and l-selenium-cystine. J Pharmacol Exp Ther. 1941;72(2):184–95.

Moxon AL. Toxicity of selenium-cystine and some other organic selenium compounds. J Am Pharm Assoc (Scientific ed). 1940;29(6):249–51.

Nagle JK. Atomic polarizability and electronegativity. J Am Chem Soc. 1990;112(12):4741–7.

Nelson EM, Hurd-Karrer AM, Robinson WO. Selenium as an insecticide. Science. 1933;78(2015):124.

Nickel A, Kottra G, Schmidt G, Danier J, Hofmann T, Daniel H. Characteristics of transport of selenoamino acids by epithelial amino acid transporters. Chem Biol Interact. 2009;177(3):234–41.

Odom JD. Selenium biochemistry chemical and physical studies, Inorganic Elements in Biochemistry. Berlin: Springer; 1983. p. 1–26.

Olm E, Fernandes AP, Hebert C, Rundlof AK, Larsen EH, Danielsson O, et al. Extracellular thiol-assisted selenium uptake dependent on the x(c)- cystine transporter explains the cancer-specific cytotoxicity of selenite. [Research Support, Non-U.S. Gov't]. Proc Natl Acad Sci U S A. 2009;106(27):11400–5.

Perrone D, Monteiro M, Nunes JC. The chemistry of selenium. In: Preedy VR, editor. Selenium: chemistry, analysis, function and effects. London: The Royal Society of Chemistry; 2015. p. 642.

Poirier KA, Milner JA. Factors influencing the antitumorigenic properties of selenium in mice. J Nutr. 1983;113(11):2147–54.

Ray PD, Huang B-W, Tsuji Y. Reactive oxygen species (ROS) homeostasis and redox regulation in cellular signaling. Cell Signal. 2012;24(5):981–90.

Roussyn I, Briviba K, Masumoto H, Sies H. Selenium-Containing Compounds Protect DNA from Single-Strand Breaks Caused by Peroxynitrite. Arch Biochem Biophys. 1996;330(1):216–8.

Sayato Y, Hasegawa T, Taniguchi S, Maeda H, Ozaki K, Narama I, et al. Acute and subacute oral toxicity of selenocystine in mice. Jpn J Toxic Environ Health. 1993;39(4):289–96.

Short MD, Xie Y, Li L, Cassidy PB, Roberts JC. Characteristics of selenazolidine prodrugs of selenocysteine: toxicity and glutathione peroxidase induction in V79 cells. J Med Chem. 2003;46(15):3308–13.

Siwek B, Bahbouth E, Serra M-Á, Sabbioni E, de Pauw-Gillet M-C, Bassleer R. Effect of selenium compounds on murine B16 melanoma cells and pigmented cloned pB16 cells. Arch Toxicol. 1994;68(4):246–54.

Stadtman TC. Biological functions of selenium. Trends Biochem Sci. 1980;5(8):203–6.

Takahashi K, Suzuki N, Ogra Y. Bioavailability Comparison of Nine Bioselenocompounds In Vitro and In Vivo. Int J Mol Sci. 2017;18(3):506.

Thomson CD, Robinson BA, Stewart R, Robinson MF. Metabolic studies of [75Se] selenocystine and [75Se] selenomethionine in the rat. Br J Nutr. 1975;34(3):501–9.

Trelease SF, Martin AL. Plants made poisonous by selenium absorbed from the soil. Bot Rev. 1936;2(7):373–96.

Wallenberg M, Olm E, Hebert C, Björnstedt M, Fernandes AP. Selenium compounds are substrates for glutaredoxins: a novel pathway for selenium metabolism and a potential mechanism for selenium-mediated cytotoxicity. Biochem J. 2010;429(1):85–93.

Weisberger AS, Suhrland LG. Studies on analogues of l-cysteine and l-cystine III. The Effect of Selenium Cystine on Leukemia. Blood. 1956;11(1):19–30.

Wolffram S, Berger B, Grenacher B, Scharrer E. Transport of selenoamino acids and their sulfur analogues across the intestinal brush border membrane of pigs. J Nutr. 1989;119(5):706–12.

Chapter 15
Selenium in Radiation Oncology

Oliver Micke, Jens Buentzel, and Ralph Mücke

Abstract Selenium measurement and supplementation in radiation oncology is a controversial issue. Selenium has been shown to possess cancer-preventive and cytoprotective activities in both animal models and humans. Recent clinical trials showed the importance of selenium for clinical radiation oncology. This overview outlines the most important results from literature and our own experience. Additionally, we want to point out the future scientific topics. Moreover, we highlight strategies for identifying those tumor patients who might benefit most from selenium, and we discuss the potential benefits and risks of this selenium supplementation. In conclusion, selenium supplementation yielded promising results concerning radioprotection in tumor patients and should be considered as a meaningful adjuvant treatment option in subjects with a low selenium status.

Keywords Selenium · Selenoproteins · Radiotherapy · Radiation oncology · Free radicals · Side effects · Cytoprotection · Radioprotection · Antioxidants

Introduction

Selenium measurement and supplementation is a controversial issue in radiation oncology (Muecke et al. 2010c). The essential trace element selenium, which is a crucial cofactor in the most important endogenous antioxidative systems of the human body, attracts more and more attention of radiation oncology expert groups (Micke et al. 2010a, b).

O. Micke (✉)
Klinik für Strahlentherapie und Radioonkologie, Franziskus Hospital Bielefeld,
Bielefeld, Germany
e-mail: omicke@trace-elements.de

J. Buentzel
Klinik für Hals-Nasen-Ohren-Heilkunde, Südharz Klinikum, Nordhausen, Germany

R. Mücke
Strahlentherapie RheinMainNahe, Bad Kreuznach, Germany

© Springer International Publishing AG, part of Springer Nature 2018
B. Michalke (ed.), *Selenium*, Molecular and Integrative Toxicology,
https://doi.org/10.1007/978-3-319-95390-8_15

287

Selenium is a constituent of the small group of selenocysteine-containing seleno-proteins and elicits important structural and enzymatic functions. Selenium deficiency has been linked to increased infection risk and adverse mood states. It has been shown to possess cancer-preventive and cytoprotective activities in both animal models and humans. It is well established that selenium has a key role in redox regulation and antioxidant function, and hence in membrane integrity, energy metabolism, and protection against DNA damage. These and other functions are mediated through a small number of approximately 50 different selenoproteins encoded by 25 separate human genes, which require adequate selenium availability for their regular biosynthesis and expression. Selenoproteins include several forms of the enzymes glutathione peroxidase (GPX), thioredoxin reductase, and iodothyronine deiodinase (Papp et al. 2007; Rayman 2000; Schomburg et al. 2004).

Blood plasma concentration is the most commonly used indicator of selenium status in humans. Low selenium intakes, plasma selenium concentrations, and GPX activities have direct, linear associations up to a threshold plasma selenium concentration (70–100 µg/L), beyond which GPX activity plateaus. This maximum GPX concentration is thought to represent repletion, and commensurate selenium intake forms the basis of recommended dietary requirements. Concentrations of other selenoproteins are also influenced by selenium intake and may have a role as functional indicators of the selenium status. The mammalian organism has developed a hierarchical supply system ensuring that the most important selenoproteins in the essential tissues are preferentially supplied with selenium in times of deficiency. However, we do not clearly understand the health implications of submaximal expression levels of the selenoproteins, and the effects of different selenocompounds on the intermediary metabolism (Burk et al. 2001; Coombs 2001; Hoefig et al. 2011; Rayman 2000, 2012).

In last years, there has been growing evidence for the increasing popularity of selenium use in particular among cancer patients. They hope to improve their quality of life, alleviate symptoms, prolong life, cure their disease, and boost their immune system. Additionally, self-treatment is most often not reported by the patients or addressed by the treating oncologist (Micke et al. 2009; Muecke et al. 2014a).

For obvious reasons, the clinically working radiation oncologist should be mainly interested in the following medical aspects of selenium: radioprotection of normal tissues, radiosensitizing effects of selenium in malignant tumors, antiedematous effects, prognostic impact of selenium, and effects in primary and secondary cancer prevention.

Selenium Deficiency in Cancer Patients

Various epidemiological studies have shown an association between low selenium levels and an increased risk of cancer incidence. Some authors correlated the decreased levels of selenium in blood, serum, or plasma with reduced selenium-dependent enzymatic antioxidant capacities in patients with malignant diseases

(Brooks et al. 2001; Kellen et al. 2006; Knekt et al. 1990; Pawlowicz et al. 1991; Rayman 2000; Torun et al. 1995). The issue of whether this difference is secondary to the malignancy or represents a predisposing risk factor leading to higher cancer incidence is at present unresolved. Furthermore, the potential of selenium as a natural anticancer agent is well documented by clinical interventional trials (Clark et al. 1996; Shu-You et al. 1991), but has recently been called into question by the results of the large supplementation study SELECT (Lippman et al. 2009).

Our working group has conducted several studies in which selenium status was monitored. Hereby, we were able to confirm the notion that cancer patients display on average a reduced selenium status as compared to control probands; this finding might be of specific importance for regions with a general low regular supply, e.g., for most countries of the European Union (Kvicala et al. 2011), and it might moreover even be restricted to these countries, for a constant high selenium intake by the regular nutrition might overrun the developing deficit and thereby become undetectable. The majority of our tumor patients with different diagnoses (carcinomas of the uterus, head and neck cancer, lung cancer, rectal cancer, and prostate cancer) had a relative selenium deficiency in whole blood and serum in comparison to the published normal reference range. In patients with prostate cancer, tissue selenium levels are reduced in the compartment surrounding the carcinoma in comparison to patients with benign prostatic hyperplasia and circulating selenium and selenoprotein concentrations are lower compared to controls (Buentzel et al. 2010a, d; Muecke et al. 2000a, 2009a, b; Meyer et al. 2009). These results prompted to consider selenium supplementation in our tumor patients as an adjuvant treatment option and created the data basis and scientific rationale for our respective clinical studies.

Preclinical Studies on Radioprotection and Radiosensitization by Selenium

Preclinical experimental evidence indicated that selenium might function as an effective radioprotector with the ability to alleviate side effects of tumor-specific radiotherapy treatments (Breccia et al. 1969; Diamond et al. 1996; Doerr 2006; Gehrisch and Doerr 2007; Margulies et al. 2008; Mutlu-Tuerkoglu et al. 2000; Patchen et al. 1990; Puspitasari et al. 2017; Rodemann et al. 1999; Schleicher et al. 1999; Schueller et al. 2001; Weiss et al. 1987). Due to its antioxidant properties, selenium has traditionally been thought to possess protective capacities against the effects of radiation. Reactions of free radicals with sulfhydryl groups from solute cysteine or peptides and proteins containing cysteine are thought to promote radiation protection (Weiss and Landauer 2009). The most powerful cysteine-containing natural antioxidant is glutathione. Artificial cytoprotectants like amifostine have been developed during recent years that also make use of the binding of SH groups to free radicals. The radioprotective effect of these drugs including selenium is supported by experimental animal data (Patchen et al. 1990).

There are five known forms of glutathione peroxidases (GPX) containing selenium (Arthur 2000; Kryukov et al. 2003). GPX isoenzymes catalyze the elimination of hydrogen peroxide as well as organic peroxides by oxidation of GSH. They contain a covalently bound selenium in the form of selenocysteine residue in their active center (Epp et al. 1983). The substitution of selenocysteine with normal cysteine at the active site of Gpx has been shown to dramatically reduce the enzymatic activity. Gpx-1 and Gpx-2 are soluble enzymes found in the cytosol, while Gpx-3 is a secreted enzyme found in the plasma. Gpx-4 performs special functions in the metabolism of phospholipid hydroperoxides, while expression of Gpx6 has been described in embryos and olfactory epithelium only. Both overexpression and knockout models point to an important role of these enzymes in the protection against oxidative attacks, like ionizing radiation (Conrad and Schweizer 2010).

For glioma cells, a Chinese group showed that they possess antioxidant enzymes (superoxide dismutase, catalase) and that their sensitivity to glutathione-modifying drugs like BCNU is correlated to the catalase activity in these cells (Zhung et al. 1999).

A Turkish group demonstrated a protective effect of selenium and vitamin E on rat intestine that correlated with an increase of intestinal GPx activity (Mutlu-Tuerkoglu et al. 2000). These results suggest a radioprotective effect of selenium on normal tissue. A German group from Tuebingen showed a radioprotective effect of selenium in normal tissue (fibroblasts) but not in tumor cells (Hehr et al. 1999). Another German group found a stronger radioprotective effect in human endothelial cell lines than in cervix squamous carcinoma cells (Schleicher et al. 1999).

Gehrisch and Doerr investigated the effects of systemic or topical administration of sodium selenite on early radiation effects (oral mucositis) in the mouse oral mucosa model. They found that the administration of sodium selenite during clinically relevant fractionated irradiation protocols has a significant effect during the initial treatment phase. Therefore, in clinical radiotherapy, the latent time to manifestation of confluent mucositis may be significantly prolonged, and hence the burden for the patient can be reduced by selenium (Gehrisch and Doerr 2007). Margulies et al. showed that radiation therapy differentially decreased cell number; with osteoblasts being shown to be the least sensitive to irradiation, the tumor cells had an intermediate sensitivity and monocytes were the most sensitive. Sodium selenite protected chondrocytes and osteoblasts from the negative effects of irradiation while not protecting the tumor cells (Margulies et al. 2008).

All these experimental findings might be the basis for an improvement of the therapeutic ratio.

On the other hand, there are several experimental data that illustrate the radiosensitizing capacities of selenium (Davis and Spallholz 1996; Evans et al. 2017; Hehr et al. 1999; Spallholz 1994; Lanfear et al. 1994; Lu et al. 1994; Rodemann et al. 1999; Shin et al. 2007; Stewart et al. 1999). One group found that catalytically active selenium compounds can induce apoptosis and exert a cytotoxic effect by generating superoxide radicals (Stewart et al. 1999). The generation of superoxide is thought to be the main mechanism of selenium toxicity. It was shown to be dose related and limited to such compounds that react to form the selenite anion (Spallholz

1994). These results were independently confirmed by other authors who found selenite-induced DNA strand breaks and apoptosis and proposed various mechanisms for their coming about (oxidative stress by oxidation of glutathione, selenite-induced endonuclease activity) (Davis and Spallholz 1996; Lanfear et al. 1994; Lu et al. 1994). A Korean group showed that the combined treatment of the cancer cell lines with selenomethionine and ionizing radiation resulted in increased cell killing as assessed by clonogenic survival assay, and the increased radiosensitivity in the cancer cells was correlated with the attenuation of the key proteins involved in either cell survival signaling (Akt, EGFR (epidermal growth factor receptor), ErbB2 and Raf1), or DNA damage response (Mre11, Rad50, Nbs1, Ku80, 53BP1, and DNAPK). These data provide possible clinical applications, as selenium selectively enhanced the radiosensitivity of the tumor cells whereas that of the normal cells was nearly unaffected (Shin et al. 2007). Only one study group investigated the influence of low doses of selenite on human glioma cells and thus did not find any influence of selenite on radiosensitivity (Frisk et al. 1997).

An experimental study of our group showed a radiosensitizing effect of selenite in irradiated rat glioma cells at medium, nontoxic concentrations of 2 to 3 µM, particularly at radiation doses >2 Gy (Fig. 15.1). This study confirms similar data from other working groups. If there really is a radiosensitizing effect of selenite on tumor cells at medium concentrations—as our results indicate—and at the same time a radioprotective effect on normal tissue—as the other results suggest—then selenite might be able to increase the therapeutic ratio for clinical radiotherapy (Schueller et al. 2004, 2005). This hypothesis is also supported by the results from Hehr et al.

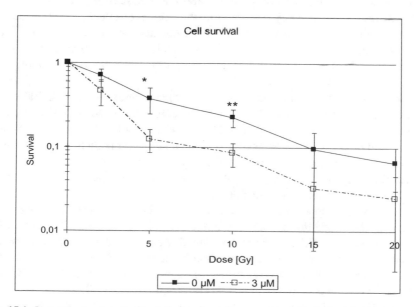

Fig. 15.1 Logarithmic plot of cell survival at doses between 0 and 20 Gy for selenite concentrations of 0 and 3 µM. Bars denote 95% confidence intervals. Asterisks denote significant values ($*p < 0.05$; $**p < 0.01$)

(1999), who showed a radioprotective effect of selenium in normal tissue (fibroblasts) but not in tumor cells (squamous cell carcinoma) (Hehr et al. 1999). Moreover, Rodemann et al. described a pro-apoptotic effect (Rodemann et al. 1999).

Moreover, the question of radiation sensitization or protection might also be a concentration issue: protection by its antioxidant properties at low concentrations versus sensitization by generation of superoxide at high, but nontoxic, concentrations. Besides the antioxidative capacity via increased biosynthesis of the different Gpx and thioredoxin reductase isoenzymes, a selective unusual activation of wild-type p53 in healthy cells by selenium-dependent reduction of two critical cysteine residues by Ref-1 might be responsible for consecutive activation of DNA repair that could be responsible for radioprotection of healthy cells (Gudkov 2002; Fischer et al. 2007). In addition, selenium may reduce translocation of the inflammatory transcription factor NFkB into the nucleus and thereby reduce cytokine production and release (Beck et al. 2001; Vunta et al. 2007).

Clinical Studies on Radioprotection by Selenium

Radio- and chemotherapy as well as suboptimal nutrition of cancer patients in the clinics might aggravate the situation in selenium-deficient patients even further and increase the likelihood of radiation-induced side effects during and after therapy (Buentzel et al. 2000, 2005; Schueller et al. 2001).

There is some clinical evidence indicating that selenium might function as an effective radio- and chemoprotector with the ability to alleviate side effects of tumor-specific chemotherapy or radiation treatments (Asfour et al. 2006, 2007, 2009; Buentzel et al. 2005, 2010c; Dennert and Horneber 2006; Funke 1999; Fraunholz et al. 2001; Hehr et al. 1997; Hu et al. 1997; Puspitasari et al. 2014; Sieja and Talerczyk 2004; Weijl et al. 2004).

A large retrospective study showed a positive correlation between initial serum selenium levels and dose delivery osf chemotherapy and outcome in patients with aggressive non-Hodgkin's lymphoma. In light of the results of a following experimental study the authors concluded that the selenium compounds methylseleninic acid and selenodiglutathione induce cell death in lymphoma cell lines and primary lymphoma cultures, which may be partly attributable to the generation of reactive oxygen species (Last et al. 2003, 2006).

Our working conducted a randomized phase III clinical studies to examine the radioprotective properties of sodium selenite in radiation oncology. The aim of the study was to assess whether an adjuvant supplementation with selenium improves the selenium status and reduces the radiation-induced side effects of patients treated by pelvic radiotherapy for cervical and uterine cancer (Muecke et al. 2010d, 2014b). A total of 81 patients were randomized. Thirty-nine were enrolled in the selenium group (SeG) and 42 in the control group (CG). Plasma and whole-blood selenium concentrations increased in the SeG and the actuarial incidence of at least CTC 2 diarrhea was significantly reduced compared to the CG (Fig. 15.2). The 10-year overall survival rate of patients in the SeG was calculated to be 55.3% compared to

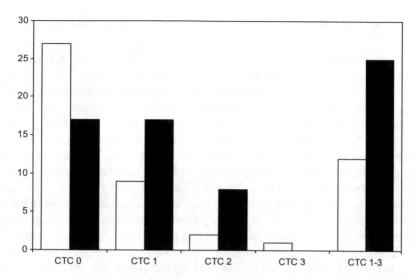

Fig. 15.2 Number of patients with radiation-induced diarrhea according to CTC criteria in RT week 4 depending on the supplementation of selenium (colorless bars: with selenium; black bars: without Se)

42.7% in the CG ($p = 0.09$), and the 10-year disease-free survival rate of patients in the SeG was calculated to be 80.1% compared to 83.2% in the CG ($p = 0.65$) (Muecke et al. 2010d, 2014b). In particular, the patients with higher plasma and whole-blood selenium levels tolerated the side effects of radiotherapy significantly better without any obvious impairment of survival data. We would like to stress the fact that the long-term survival rates do not differ between the groups, since it shows that a protection of tumor cells by selenium, as is often assumed and suspected by many oncologists, has not taken place (Muecke et al. 2010d, 2014b).

A second randomized trial of our group enrolled head and neck tumor patients undergoing radiation therapy. A total of 39 patients were randomized. Twenty-two were enrolled in the SeG and 17 in the CG. We observed the following serious toxicities (SeG vs. CG): dysphagia 22.7% versus 35.3%, loss of taste 22.7% versus 47.1%, dry mouth 22.7% versus 23.5%, and stomatitis 36.4% versus 23.5%. A statistical trend was seen in loss of taste ($p = 0.172$). The analysis per week showed a significant reduction of dysphagia in the SeG at the last week of irradiation ($p = 0.04$). The small randomized trial showed limited effects of selenium in the prevention of ageusia (loss of taste) and dysphagia due to radiotherapy because of head and neck cancer. Due to the small number of included patients a clinical relevant radioprotection was not observed (Buentzel et al. 2010a, b).

Overall, 16 clinical studies on the use of selenium in radiotherapy were worldwide performed between 1987 and 2012. Selenium supplementation improved the general conditions of the patients, improved their quality of life, and reduced the side effects of radiotherapy. Selenium supplementation did not reduce the effectiveness of radiotherapy, and no toxicities were reported (Puspitasari et al. 2014).

Selenium Supplementation in Patients with Lymphedemas

Selenium is a further interesting therapeutic option for patients suffering from lymphedema. However, the antiedematous effect of it is proven but not widely published or accepted. Early clinical studies have shown that oral selenium supplementation lowers oxygen radical production, causes a spontaneous reduction in lymphedema volume, increases the efficacy of physical therapy for lymphedema, and reduces the incidence of erysipelas infections in patients with chronic lymphedema at various sites. Unfortunately, these studies did not include large numbers of patients or use a standardized classification system for lymphedema, making objective evaluation of their outcomes difficult (Bruns et al. 2004; Pfister et al. 2016). Kasseroller reported promising results of a placebo-controlled, double-blinded study of selenium in 179 postmastectomy patients suffering from secondary lymphedema. He described a significant reduction in edema volume, as well as improvement in skinfold index in subjects with arm edemas. The incidence of erysipelas was also reduced in the selenium-treated group compared with the placebo group (Kasseroller 1998).

These results encouraged us to perform an own study using sodium selenite for the treatment of radiation-induced lymphedema. The results of this exploratory study involving 48 patients suggest that selenium has a positive effect on radiation-associated secondary lymphedema in patients with limb edemas as well as in the head and neck region, including endolaryngeal edema. The majority of patients showed a reduction in edema characteristics as classified by the Földi and Miller scoring systems. We also estimated that 65% of patients with interstitial grade III or IV endolaryngeal edema, who normally would require tracheotomy for treatment, could avoid surgical intervention. Although we could demonstrate a reduction in the circumferential difference between affected and unaffected sites in patients treated with selenium, as well as improvement in the skinfold index and patient quality of life (as measured by a visual analogue scale), only the improvement in quality of life reached statistical significance. This is likely due to the small sample size (Micke et al. 2003).

A few years later, Zimmermann et al. (Zimmermann et al. 2005) performed a small double-blind, randomized study ($n = 20$) to establish whether sodium selenite administered orally or intravenously reduces postoperative lymphedema after oral tumor surgery. They showed a significant reduction of lymphedema in the sodium selenite-treated group.

The exact pharmacologic mechanisms of selenium effects in lymphedema are unknown. In the affected tissues of patients with chronic lymphedema, the production of free reactive oxygen radicals is enhanced as a result of lymphostasis, mechanical tissue compression, and chronic inflammation processes triggered by an excess of interstitial proteins and cellular debris. This promotes a variety of degenerative processes, worsening lymphostasis, and inflammation by tissue fibrosis. A reduction of free radicals caused by selenium-induced activation of GPX probably plays an important role in this pathological process (Brenke et al. 1997;

Pfister et al. 2016; Schrauzer 1997). Other preclinical studies have shown that selenium can protect human endothelial cells from oxidative damage by inducing GPX and thioredoxin reductase (Miller et al. 2001).

Conclusions and Prospects

In tumor patients with different diagnoses we observed a selenium deficiency in whole blood or serum and in tissue surrounding the carcinoma. Supplementation of selenium yielded encouraging results concerning radioprotection and lymphedema treatment in tumor patients. Nevertheless, a much better understanding of selenium biology is needed in order to justify selenium supplementation as an adjuvant treatment option in radiation oncology. Unfortunately, the field of selenium research and adjuvant supplementation of cancer patients has suffered a serious drawback recently, when data were published indicating a somewhat increased risk of developing diabetes mellitus with constant high selenium intake (Lippman et al. 2009; Stranges et al. 2007). These studies indicated again the narrow therapeutic width of selenium intake in humans and the potential risk associated with selenium supplementation.

In a 2008 published representative sample of the US population with 13,887 adult participants a nonlinear association between serum selenium levels and all-cause and cancer mortality was found. Increasing serum selenium levels were associated with decreased mortality up to 130 ng/mL. These results, however, raise the concern that higher serum selenium levels may be associated with increased mortality (Bleys et al. 2008). Still, we strongly suggest measuring the selenium status in the patients prior to and during therapy to avoid side effects and optimize the odds for a positive selenium supplementation effect in the clinics (Micke et al. 2010a, b; Muecke et al. 2010a, b, c).

Nevertheless, given the relative selenium deficiency of most Europeans, the benefit-risk ratio of our cancer patients is clearly on the positive side, for they are insufficiently supplied with this essential trace element and the disease appears to cause a further decline in selenium status which seems to aggravate the disease and hampers fast and uncomplicated recovery.

Unfortunately, there is no general recommendation in favor of or against selenium supplementation in cancer patients (Dennert and Horneber 2006). Nevertheless, more than a few patients treated with curative or palliative radiotherapy are using adjuvant selenium supplementation (Buentzel et al. 2011; Micke et al. 2009). Still, we strongly advocate to take the selenium status of tumor patients under oncological therapy and aftercare situation more seriously into account and to consider a respective supplementation prior when the current selenium status appears insufficient (Micke et al. 2013).

A new and encouraging aspect of selenium is the use of selenium nanoparticles in oncology and particularly in radiotherapy (Wadhwani et al. 2016). Recent experimental studies described radioprotective (Du et al. 2017; El-Ghazaly et al. 2017) as well as radiosensitizing properties (Du et al. 2017; Chan et al. 2017; Yu et al. 2016). However, despite this promising data, selenium nanoparticles are still not used in clinical practice, but these results will open a new window in selenium research.

Overall, it can be concluded that selenium (and its compounds) is one of the most exciting natural elements for the radiation oncologist.

References

Arthur JR. The glutathione peroxidases. Cell Mol Life Sci. 2000;57:1825–35.

Asfour IA, Shazly SE, Fayek MH, Hegab HM, Raouf S, Moussa MA. Effect of high-dose sodium selenite therapy on polymorphonuclear leukocyte apoptosis in non-Hodgkin's lymphoma patients. Biol Trace Elem Res. 2006;110:19–32.

Asfour IA, Fayek MH, Raouf S, Soliman M, Hegab HM, El-Desoky H, Saleh R, Moussa MA. The impact of high-dose sodium selenite therapy on Bcl-2 expression in adult non-Hodgkin's lymphoma patients: correlation with response and survival. Biol Trace Elem Res. 2007;120:1–10.

Asfour IA, El-Tehewi MM, Ahmed MH, Abdel-Sattar MA, Moustafa NN, Hegab HM, Fathey OM. High-dose sodium selenite can induce apoptosis of lymphoma cells in adult patients with non-Hodgkin's lymphoma. Biol Trace Elem Res. 2009;127:200–10.

Beck MA, Nelson HK, Shi Q, Van Dael P, Schiffrin EJ, Blum S, Barclay D, Levander OA. Selenium deficiency increases the pathology of an influenza virus infection. FASEB J. 2001;15:1481–3.

Bleys J, Navas-Acien A, Guallar E. Serum selenium levels and all cause, cancer, and cardiovascular mortality among US adults. Arch Intern Med. 2008;168:404–10.

Breccia A, Badiello R, Trenta M, Mattii M. On the chemical radioprotection by organic selenium compounds in vivo. Radiat Res. 1969;38:483–92.

Brenke R, Siems W, Grune T. Measures for therapy optimization in chronic lymphedema. Z Lymphol. 1997;21:1–29.

Brooks JD, Metter EJ, Chan DW. Plasma selenium level before diagnosis and the risk of prostate cancer development. J Urol. 2001;166:2034–8.

Bruns F, Buentzel J, Muecke R, Schoenekaes K, Kisters K, Micke O. Selenium in the treatment of head and neck lymphedema. Med Princ Pract. 2004;13:185–90.

Buentzel J, Muecke R, Micke O. Mineral status and enzymatic antioxidative capacities during radiochemotherapy in patients with advanced head and neck cancer. Trace Elem Electrolytes. 2000;18:98.

Buentzel J, Micke O, Muecke R, Schoenekaes KG, Schaefer U, Kisters K, Bruns F. Amifostine and selenium during simultaneous radiochemotherapy in head and neck cancer—redox status data. Trace Elem Electrolytes. 2005;22:211–5.

Buentzel J, Micke O, Kisters K, Bruns F, Glatzel M, Schoenekaes KG, Schaefer U, Muecke R. Selenium substitution during radiotherapy of solid tumours—laboratory data from two observation studies in gynaecologic and head and neck cancer patients. Anticancer Res. 2010a;30:1783–6.

Buentzel J, Riesenbeck D, Glatzel M, Berndt-Skorka R, Riedel T, Muecke R, Kisters K, Schoenekaes KG, Schaefer U, Bruns F, Micke O. Limited effects of selenium substitution in the prevention of radiation-associated toxicities. Results of a randomized study in head neck cancer patients. Anticancer Res. 2010b;30:1829–32.

Buentzel J, Micke O, Glatzel M, Schaefer U, Riesenbeck D, Kisters K, Bruns F, Schoenekaes KG, Dawczynski H, Muecke R. Selenium substitution during radiotherapy in head and neck cancer. Trace Elem Electrolytes. 2010c;27:235–9.

Buentzel J, Knolle U, Garayev A, Muecke R, Schaefer U, Kisters K, Schoenekaes KG, Hunger R, Bruns F, Glatzel M, Micke O. Trace elements selenium and zinc as tumor markers in patients with advanced head and neck cancer. Trace Elem Electrolytes. 2010d;27:246–9.

Buentzel J, Büntzel H, Micke O, Kisters K, Bruns F, Glatzel M, Muecke R, Schoenekaes KG, Schaefer U. Complementary and alternative medicine (CAM) use in terminally ill patients. Trace Elem Electrolytes. 2011;28:49–51.

Burk RF, Hill KE, Motley AK. Plasma selenium in specific and non-specific forms. Biofactors. 2001;14:107–14.

Chan L, He L, Zhou B, Guan S, Bo M, Yang Y, Liu Y, Liu X, Zhang Y, Xie Q, Chen T. Cancer-targeted selenium nanoparticles sensitize cancer cells to continuous γ radiation to achieve synergetic chemo-radiotherapy. Chem Asian J. 2017;12:3053–60.

Clark LC, Combs GF, Turnbull BW, Slate EH, Chalker DK, Chow J, Davis LS, Glover RA, Graham GF, Gross EG, Krongrad A, Lesher JL, Park HK, Sanders BB, Smith CI, Taylor JR. Effects of selenium supplementation for cancer prevention in patients with carcinoma of the skin. JAMA. 1996;276:1957–63.

Conrad M, Schweizer U. Unveiling the molecular mechanisms behind selenium-related diseases through knockout mouse studies. Antioxid Redox Signal. 2010;12:851–65.

Coombs GF Jr. Selenium in global food systems. Br J Nutr. 2001;85:517–47.

Davis RL, Spallholz JE. Inhibition of selenite-catalyzed superoxide generation and formation of elemental selenium (Se0) by copper, zinc, and aurintricarboxylic acid (ATA). Biochem Pharmacol. 1996;51:1015–20.

Dennert G, Horneber M. Selenium for alleviating the side effects of chemotherapy, radiotherapy and surgery in cancer patients. Cochrane Database Syst Rev. 2006;3:CD005037.

Diamond AM, Dale P, Murray JL, Grdina DJ. The inhibition of radiation-induced Mutagenesis by the combined effects of selenium and the aminothiol WR-1065. Mutat Res. 1996;356:147–54.

Doerr W. Effects of selenium on radiation responses of tumor cells and tissue. Strahlenther Onkol. 2006;182:693–5.

Du J, Gu Z, Yan L, Yong Y, Yi X, Zhang X, Liu J, Wu R, Ge C, Chen C, Zhao Y. Poly(Vinylpyrrolidone)- and selenocysteine-Modified Bi_2Se_3 nanoparticles enhance radiotherapy efficacy in tumors and promote radioprotection in normal tissues. Adv Mater. 2017;29

El-Ghazaly MA, Fadel N, Rashed E, El-Batal A, Kenawy SA. Anti-inflammatory effect of selenium nanoparticles on the inflammation induced in irradiated rats. Can J Physiol Pharmacol. 2017;95:101–10.

Epp O, Ladenstein R, Wendel A. The refined structure of the selenoenzyme glutathione peroxidase at 0.2 nm resolution. Eur J Biochem. 1983;133:51–69.

Evans SO, Khairuddin PF, Jameson MB. Optimising selenium for modulation of cancer treatments. Anticancer Res. 2017;37:6497–509.

Fischer JL, Mihelc EM, Pollok KE, Smith ML. Chemotherapeutic selectivity conferred by selenium: a role for p53-dependent DNA repair. Mol Cancer Ther. 2007;6:355–61.

Fraunholz I, Jueling-Pohlit L, Boettcher H. Influence of selenium on acute mucositis in radiochemotherapy of head and neck tumors. Trace Elem Electrolytes. 2001;18:98–9.

Frisk P, Saetre A, Couce B, Stenerlow B, Carlsson J, Lindh U. Effects of Pb2+, Ni2+, Hg2+ and Se4+ on cultured cells. Analysis of uptake, toxicity and influence on radiosensitivity. Biometals. 1997;10:263–70.

Funke AM. Potential of selenium in gynecological oncology. Med Klin. 1999;94:42–4.

Gehrisch A, Doerr W. Effects of systemic or topical administration of sodium selenite on early radiation effects in mouse oral mucosa. Strahlenther Onkol. 2007;183:36–42.

Gudkov AV. Converting p53 from a killer to a healer. Nat Med. 2002;8:1196–8.

Hehr T, Hoffmann W, Bamberg M. Role of sodium selenite as an adjuvant in radiotherapy of rectal carcinoma. Med Klin. 1997;92(Suppl. 3):48–9.

Hehr T, Bamberg M, Rodemann HP. Präklinische und klinische relevanz der radiopro-tektiven Wirkung von Natriumselenit. InFoOnkologie. 1999;2(Suppl 2):25–9.

Hoefig CS, Renko K, Köhrle J, Birringer M, Schomburg L. Comparison of different selenocompounds with respect to nutritional value vs. toxicity using liver cells in culture. J Nutr Biochem. 2011;22:945–55.

Hu YJ, Chen Y, Zhang YQ, Zhou MZ, Song XM, Zhang BZ, Luo L, Xu PM, Zhao YN, Zhao YB, Cheng G. The protective role of selenium on the toxicity of cisplatinum-contained chemotherapy regimen in cancer patients. Biol Trace Elem Res. 1997;56:331–41.

Kasseroller R. Sodium selenite as prophylaxis against erysipelas in secondary lymphedema. Anticancer Res. 1998;18:2227–30.

Kellen E, Zeegers M, Buntinx F. Selenium is inversely associated with bladder cancer risk: a report from the Belgian case-control study on bladder cancer. Int J Urol. 2006;13:1180–4.

Knekt P, Aromaa A, Mantela J. Serum selenium and subsequent risk of cancer among Finnish men and woman. J Natl Cancer Inst. 1990;82:864–8.

Kryukov GV, Castellano S, Novoselov SV, Lobanov AV, Zehtab O, Guigo R, Gladyshev VN. Characterization of mammalian selenoproteomes. Science. 2003;300:1439–43.

Kvicala J, Zamrazil V, Nemecek J, Jiranek V. Influence of long-term supplementation by various quantities of yeast-bound selenium upon selenium-status of South Bohemia seniors. Trace Elem Electrolytes. 2011;28:11–7.

Lanfear J, Fleming J, Wu L, Webster G, Harrison PR. The selenium metabolite selenodiglutathione induces p53 and apoptosis: relevance to the chemoprotective effects of selenium? Carcinogenesis. 1994;15:1387–92.

Last KW, Cornelius V, Delves T, Sieniawska CH, Fitzgibbon J, Norton A, Amess J, Wilson A, Rohatiner A, Lister AT. Presentation serum selenium predicts for overall survival, dose delivery, and first treatment response in aggressive non-Hodgkin's lymphoma. J Clin Oncol. 2003;21:2335–41.

Last K, Maharaj L, Perry J, Strauss S, Fitzgibbon J, Lister TA, Joel S. The activity of methylated and non-methylated selenium species in lymphoma cell lines and primary tumours. Ann Oncol. 2006;17:773–9.

Lippman SM, Klein EA, Goodman PJ, Lucia MS, Thompson IM, Ford LG, Parnes HL, Minasian LM, Gaziano JM, Hartline JA, Parsons JK, Bearden JD, Crawford ED, Goodman GE, Claudio J, Winquist E, Cook ED, Karp DD, Walther P, Lieber MM, Kristal AR, Darke AK, Arnold KB, Ganz PA, Santella RM, Albanes D, Taylor PR, Probstfield JL, Jagpal TJ, Crowley JJ, Meyskens FL, Baker LH, Coltman CA. Effect of selenium and vitamin E on risk of prostate cancer and other cancers: The selenium and vitamin E cancer prevention trial (SELECT). JAMA. 2009;301:39–51.

Lu JX, Kaeck M, Jiang C, Wilson AC, Thompson HJ. Selenite induction of DNA strand breaks and apoptosis in mouse leukemic L1210 cells. Biochem Pharmacol. 1994;47:1531–5.

Margulies BS, Damron TA, Allen MJ. The differential effects of the radioprotectant drugs amifostine and sodium selenite treatment in combination with radiation therapy on constituent bone cells, Ewing's sarcoma of bone tumor cells, and rhabdomyosarcoma tumor cells in vitro. J Orthop Res. 2008;26:1512–9.

Meyer HA, Hollenbach B, Stephan C, Endermann T, Morgenthaler NG, Cammann H, Kohrle J, Jung K, Schomburg L. Reduced serum selenoprotein P concentrations in German prostate cancer patients. Cancer Epidemiol Biomark Prev. 2009;18:2386–90.

Micke O, Bruns F, Muecke R, Schaefer U, Glatzel M, DeVries AF, Schoenekaes K, Kisters K, Büntzel J. Selenium in the treatment of radiation-associated secondary lymphedema. Int J Radiat Oncol Biol Phys. 2003;56:40–9.

Micke O, Bruns F, Glatzel M, Schoenekaes KG, Micke P, Muecke R, Buentzel J. Predictive factors for the use of complementary and alternative medicine (CAM) in radiation oncology. Eur J Integr Med. 2009;1:22–30.

Micke O, Schomburg L, Buentzel J, Kisters K, Muecke R. Selenium in oncology—an update. Trace Elem Electrolytes. 2010a;27:250–7.

Micke O, Muecke R, Buentzel J, Kisters K, Schaefer U. Some more steps on the way to clinical elementology. Trace Elem Electrolytes. 2010b;27:29–34.

Micke O, Schomburg L, Kisters K, Buentzel J, Huebner J, Muecke R. Selenium and hypertension: do we need to reconsider selenium supplementation in cancer patients? J Hypertens. 2013;31:1049–50.

Miller S, Walker SW, Arthur JR, Nicol F, Pickard K, Lewin MH, Howie AF, Beckett GJ. Selenite protects human endothelial cells from oxidative damage and induces thioredoxin reductase. Clin Sci. 2001;100:543–50.

Muecke R, Micke O, Schoenekaes KG. Serum selenium levels, glutathione peroxidase activities and serum redox potential levels in patients with untreated non-small cell lung cancer and adenocarcinoma of the rectum. Trace Elem Electrolytes. 2000a;17:119–23.

Muecke R, Klotz T, Giedl J, Buentzel J, Kundt G, Kisters K, Prott FJ, Micke O. Whole blood selenium levels (WBSL) in patients with prostate cancer (PC), benign prostatic hyperplasia (BPH) and healthy male inhabitants (HMI) and prostatic tissue selenium levels (PTSL) in patients with PC and BPH. Acta Oncol. 2009a;48:239–46.

Muecke R, Buentzel J, Glatzel M, Bruns F, Kisters K, Prott FJ, Schmidberger H, Micke O. Postoperative serum and whole blood selenium levels in patients with squamous cell and adenocarcinomas of the uterus after curative surgical treatment. Trace Elem Electrolytes. 2009b;26:78–82.

Muecke R, Schomburg L, Buentzel J, Gröber U, Holzhauer P, Micke O. Komplementärer Seleneinsatz in der Onkologie. Onkologe. 2010a;16:181–6.

Muecke R, Schomburg L, Buentzel J, Kisters K, Micke O. Blood selenium status in tumor patients—Omnia sunt venena, nihil est sine veneno. Sola dosis facit venenum. Trace Elem Electrolytes. 2010b;27:181–4.

Muecke R, Schomburg L, Buentzel J, Kisters K, Micke O. Selenium or no selenium—that is the question in tumor patients: a new controversy. Integr Cancer Ther. 2010c;9:136–41.

Muecke R, Schomburg L, Glatzel M, Bernd-Skorka R, Baaske D, Reichl B, Buentzel J, Kundt G, Prott FJ, De Vries A, Stoll G, Kisters K, Bruns F, Schaefer U, Willich N, Micke O. Multicenter, phase III trial comparing selenium supplementation with observation in gynecologic radiation oncology. Int J Radiat Oncol Biol Phys. 2010d;70:828–35.

Muecke R, Micke O, Schomburg L, Kisters K, Buentzel J, Huebner J, Kriz J. Selenium supplementation in radiotherapy patients: do we need to measure selenium levels in serum or blood regularly prior radiotherapy? Radiat Oncol. 2014a;9:289.

Muecke R, Micke O, Schomburg L, Glatzel M, Reichl B, Kisters K, Schaefer U, Huebner J, Eich HT, Fakhrian K, Adamietz IA, Buentzel J. Multicenter, phase III trial comparing selenium supplementation with observation in gynecologic radiation oncology: follow-up analysis of the survival data 6 years after cessation of randomization. Integr Cancer Ther. 2014b;13:463–7.

Mutlu-Tuerkoglu UE, Erbil Y, Oztezcan S, Olgac V, Toker G, Uysal M. The effect of selenium and/or vitamin E treatments on radiation-induced intestinal injury in rats. Life Sci. 2000;66:1905–13.

Papp LV, Lu J, Holmgren A, Khanna KK. From selenium to selenoproteins: synthesis, identity, and their role in human health. Antioxid Redox Signal. 2007;9:775–806.

Patchen ML, MacVittie TJ, Weiss JF. Combined modality radioprotection: the use of glucan and selenium with WR-2721. Int J Radiat Oncol Biol Phys. 1990;18:1069–75.

Pawlowicz Z, Zachara BA, Trafikowska U, Maciag A, Marchaluk E, Nowicki A. Blood selenium concentrations and glutathione peroxidase activities in patients with breast cancer and with advanced gastrointestinal cancer. J Trace Elem Electrolytes Health Dis. 1991;5:272–7.

Pfister C, Dawczynski H, Schingale FJ. Sodium selenite and cancer related lymphedema: Biological and pharmacological effects. J Trace Elem Med Biol. 2016;37:111–6.

Puspitasari IM, Abdulah R, Yamazaki C, Kameo S, Nakano T, Koyama H. Updates on clinical studies of selenium supplementation in radiotherapy. Radiat Oncol. 2014;9:125.

Puspitasari IM, Yamazaki C, Abdulah R, Putri M, Kameo S, Nakano T, Koyama H. Protective effects of sodium selenite supplementation against irradiation-induced damage in non-cancerous human esophageal cells. Oncol Lett. 2017;13:449–54.

Rayman MP. The importance of selenium to human health. Lancet. 2000;356:233–41.

Rayman MP. Selenium and human health. Lancet. 2012;379:1256–68.

Rodemann HP, Hehr T, Bamberg M. Relevance of the radioprotective effect of sodium selenite. Med Klin (Munich). 1999;94(Suppl 3):39–41.

Schleicher UM, Lopez Cotarelo C, Andreopoulos D, Handt S, Ammon J. Radioprotection of human endothelial cells by sodium selenite. Med Klin (Munich). 1999;94(Suppl 3):35–8.

Schomburg L, Schweizer U, Koehrle J. Selenium and selenoproteins in mammals: extraordinary, essential, enigmatic. Cell Mol Life Sci. 2004;61:1988–95.

Schrauzer GN. Selenium in the therapy of chronic lymphedema—mechanistic perspectives and practical applications. Z Lymphol. 1997;21:16–9.

Schueller P, Puettmann S, Muecke R, Senner V, Schaefer U, Kisters K, Micke O. From the radiolysis of water to the role of trace elements in radiobiology and clinical radiation therapy: following a logical chain. Trace Elem Electrolytes. 2001;18:186–92. 34–36.

Schueller P, Puettmann S, Micke O, Senner V, Schaefer U, Willich N. Selenium influences the radiation sensitivity of C6 rat glioma cells. Anticancer Res. 2004;24:2913–7.

Schueller P, Puettmann S, Micke O, Senner V, Schaefer U, Willich N. Selenium—A novel radiosensitizer? Trace Elem Electrolytes. 2005;22:201–6.

Shin SH, Yoon MJ, Kim M, Kim JI, Lee SJ, Lee YS, Bae S. Enhanced lung cancer cell killing by the combination of selenium and ionizing radiation. Oncol Rep. 2007;17:209–16.

Shu-You Y, Ya-Jun Z, Li W-G, Qui-Sheng H, Zhi-Huang C, Qi-Nan Z, Chong H. A preliminary report on the intervention trials of primary liver cancer in high-risk populations with nutritional supplementation of selenium in china. Biol Trace Elem Res. 1991;29:289–94.

Sieja K, Talerczyk M. Selenium as an element in the treatment of ovarian cancer in women receiving chemotherapy. Gynecol Oncol. 2004;93:320–7.

Spallholz JE. On the nature of selenium toxicity and carcinostatic activity. Free Radic Biol Med. 1994;17:45–64.

Stewart MS, Spallholz JE, Neldner KH, Pence BC. Selenium compounds have disparate abilities to impose oxidative stress and include apoptosis. Free Radic Biol Med. 1999;26:42–8.

Stranges S, Marshall JR, Natarajan R, Donahue RP, Trevisan M, Combs GF, Cappuccio FP, Ceriello A, Reid ME. Effects of long-term selenium supplementation on the incidence of type 2 diabetes: a randomized trial. Ann Intern Med. 2007;147:217–23.

Torun M, Aldemir H, Yardim S. Serum selenium levels in various cancer types. Trace Elem Electrolytes. 1995;12:186–90.

Vunta H, Davis F, Palempalli UD, Bhat D, Arner RJ, Thompson JT, Peterson DG, Reddy CC, Prabhu KS. The anti-inflammatory effects of selenium are mediated through 15-deoxy-Delta12,14-prostaglandin J2 in macrophages. J Biol Chem. 2007;282:17964–73.

Wadhwani SA, Shedbalkar UU, Singh R, Chopade BA. Biogenic selenium nanoparticles: current status and future prospects. Appl Microbiol Biotechnol. 2016;100:2555–66.

Weijl NI, Elsendoorn TJ, Lentjes EG, Hopman GD, Wipkink-Bakker A, Zwinderman AH, Cleton FJ, Osanto S. Supplementation with antioxidant micronutrients and chemotherapy-induced toxicity in cancer patients treated with cisplatin-based chemotherapy: a randomised, double-blind, placebo-controlled study. Eur J Cancer. 2004;40:1713–23.

Weiss JF, Landauer MR. History and development of radiation-protective agents. Int J Radiat Biol. 2009;85:539–73.

Weiss JF, Hoover RL, Kumar KS. Selenium enhances the radioprotective effect and reduces the lethal toxicity of WR-2721. Free Radic Res Commun. 1987;3:33–8.

Yu B, Liu T, Du Y, Luo Z, Zheng W, Chen T. X-ray-responsive selenium nanoparticles for enhanced cancer chemo-radiotherapy. Colloids Surf B: Biointerfaces. 2016;139:180–9.

Zhung W, Yan T, Lim R, Oberley LW. Expression of superoxide dismutases, catalase, and glutathione peroxidase in glioma cells. Free Radic Biol Med. 1999;27:1334–45.

Zimmermann T, Leonhardt H, Kersting S, Albrecht S, Range U, Eckelt U. Reduction of post-operative lymphedema after oral tumor surgery with sodium selenite. Biol Trace Elem Res. 2005;106:193–203.

Part VII
The Role of Selenium in Various Diseases and Health Issues

Chapter 16
Selenium and Cardiovascular Disease: Epidemiological Evidence of a Possible U-Shaped Relationship

Xi Zhang, Xinli Li, Weili Zhang, and Yiqing Song

Abstract Selenium is an essential mineral that plays a crucial role in the regulation of cardiovascular system. The relation between selenium and cardiovascular disease (CVD) has been studied extensively over the last decades. In human prospective observational studies, there seems a U-shaped association between baseline selenium status and CVD risk, indicating possible adverse cardiometabolic effects of very low and high selenium levels. A few randomized controlled trials (RCTs) have evaluated the effects of selenium on CVD but showed no obvious benefits or risks. However, different population selenium status, selenium formulae, dosage, and intervention durations as well as trial quality may have contributed to between-trial heterogeneity, which largely prevents us from drawing causal conclusions. This chapter focuses on current evidence from prospective data, which helps to gain a more comprehensive insight into the selenium-CVD relationship and provide reasonable explanations of the discrepancies between results from human observational and interventional studies.

Xi Zhang and Xinli Li contributed equally to this work.

X. Zhang
Clinical Research Unit, Xin Hua Hospital Affiliated to Shanghai Jiao Tong University School of Medicine, Shanghai, China

X. Li
Department of Nutrition and Food Hygiene, School of Public Health, Medical College of Soochow University, Suzhou, Jiangsu, China

W. Zhang
State Key Laboratory of Cardiovascular Disease, FuWai Hospital, National Center for Cardiovascular Diseases, Peking Union Medical College and Chinese Academy of Medical Sciences, Beijing, China

Y. Song (✉)
Department of Epidemiology, Richard M. Fairbanks School of Public Health, Indiana University, Indianapolis, IN, USA
e-mail: yiqsong@iu.edu

© Springer International Publishing AG, part of Springer Nature 2018
B. Michalke (ed.), *Selenium*, Molecular and Integrative Toxicology,
https://doi.org/10.1007/978-3-319-95390-8_16

Keywords Selenium · Cardiovascular disease (CVD) · Supplementation ·
Selenoproteins · Glutathione peroxidase (GPX) · Observational studies ·
Randomized controlled trials (RCTs) · Meta-analysis · Systematic review

Introduction

Selenium is a trace element that plays essential roles in human health and disease.
Its nutritional function mainly involves selenoproteins, which were first identified in
the 1970s (Stadtman 1974; Cone et al. 1976). Selenium mediates its pleiotropic
effects on various aspects of cell function and physiological function mainly through
incorporation into different selenoproteins and selenium-dependent enzymes (Polo
et al. 2016). The amount of selenium in plants depends largely on geographical factors, including the chemical structure of selenium in soil, pH, amounts of organic
matter and compounds, amounts of sulfur, amount of rainfall, and soil microbes
(Haug et al. 2007; Jones et al. 2017). Therefore, dietary selenium intake varies
hugely worldwide depending on the soil on which crops and fodder are grown,
ranging from 7 to 4990 μg/day per person (Reilly 2006; Navarro-Alarcon and
Cabrera-Vique 2008). Selenium is both an essential element for human nutrition
and a toxicant, i.e., there is a very narrow margin between nutritionally optimal and
potentially toxic dietary exposures (Sun et al. 2013). The US-recommended dietary
allowance (RDA) of selenium is 55 μg/day for adults, 60 μg/day for pregnant
women, and 70 μg/day for lactating women, while the tolerable upper intake level
(TUIL) is 400 μg/day (Trumbo et al. 2001). Dietary selenium levels are closely correlated with circulating selenium: normal serum and plasma selenium levels are
70–150 ng/mL (or μg/L), and levels less than 70 ng/mL or 0.8 μmol/L suggest a
selenium deficiency across age groups (Muntau et al. 2002; Neve 1995).

There is long-standing interest in the cardiovascular disease (CVD) research
community regarding the potential yet unproven benefits or risks of selenium intake
on the development and progression of CVD. First, previous experimental evidence
indicates that selenium, as a constituent of selenoproteins, plays an important role
in the regulation of redox signaling, antioxidant defense, DNA synthesis and methylation, inflammation, immune response, thyroid hormone function, lipoprotein
metabolism, glucose and insulin metabolism, nitric oxide synthesis, and platelet
aggregation (Bleys et al. 2008; Steinbrenner and Sies 2009; Rayman et al. 2011;
Murr et al. 2007). Second, there is relevant evidence from human observational
studies. Earlier retrospective case-control studies showed that blood selenium concentrations of CVD patients were lower than those of healthy subjects, indicating an
inverse correlation between selenium levels and risk of CVD (Navarro-Alarcon and
MC 2000; Flores-Mateo et al. 2006). However, because these cross-sectional or
retrospective studies are potentially biased by reverse causation and many confounding factors, their results need to be interpreted cautiously. Nevertheless, these
data can help to postulate hypotheses, implicating a role of selenium in the etiology
of CVD. In observational studies, prospective cohort design is considered optimal
for the study of long-term nutrient intake in the primary prevention of chronic

diseases. Prospective observational studies of the relationship between blood selenium levels and CVD have yielded inconsistent results in different populations with different levels of selenium intake or blood selenium. Our previous meta-analysis of 16 prospective observational studies identified a significant inverse and U-shaped association between selenium status and CVD risk, indicating possible adverse cardiometabolic effects of high selenium levels (Flores-Mateo et al. 2006). Third, a few randomized controlled trials have evaluated the effects of selenium on cardiovascular outcomes (Eaton et al. 2010; Lubos et al. 2010; Xun et al. 2010; Rajpathak et al. 2005) but showed no obvious benefits. Of note, these individual trials used different selenium formulae and dosage. They also utilized small sample sizes and a variety of intervention periods, reducing their power to address optimal selenium dose and concentrations for cardiovascular health. Overall the persistent disagreement between observational studies and RCTs largely prevents us from drawing valid conclusions.

This chapter reviews current evidence regarding selenium status and CVD, focusing particularly on prospective data from human observational studies and randomized controlled trials, which helps to elucidate the causal association between selenium status and CVD development. We first summarize current thinking regarding the mechanisms whereby selenium status and CVD are interrelated. Then we offer an updated meta-analysis of prospective observational studies and a critique of trial data in a comprehensive assessment of available human evidence. Finally, we comment on unanswered research questions, future research directions, and implications for dietary recommendations.

Mechanisms Underlying a Possible U-Shaped Relation Between Selenium and CVD

Evidence suggests that oxidative stress may play a crucial role in the pathophysiology of cardiometabolic diseases (Mahjoub and Masrour-Roudsari 2012; Heyland et al. 2005); selenium is the key component of a number of selenoproteins that protect against oxidative stress initiated by excess reactive oxygen species (ROS) and reactive nitrogen species (NOS) (Forman and Torres 2002; Guo et al. 2012). Accumulating evidence from animal models supports an important role of selenoproteins, especially glutathione peroxidase (GPX), in protection against the oxidative stress that leads to atherosclerosis.

Numerous experimental studies have implied a pathophysiological link between selenium deficiency and oxidative stress linked to cardiometabolic disorders (Fig. 16.1). When selenium status is physiologically normal, proposed mechanisms for the cardiovascular benefits of selenium include preservation of the plasma antioxidant capacity of glutathione, decreased protein and lipid oxidation, inhibition of platelet aggregation, anti-inflammatory effects, improved endothelial function and lipid metabolism, reduced myocardial injury and damage, accelerated recovery of

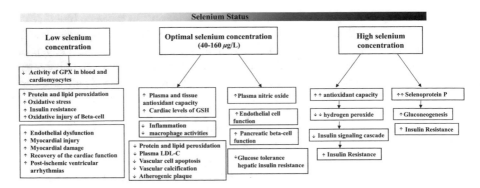

Fig. 16.1 Schematic figure showing the hypothetic mechanisms for a link between selenium status and CVD

ventricular remodeling after myocardial infarction, and decreasing postischemic ventricular arrhythmias (Maulik and Das 2008; Ago and Sadoshima 2006; Venardos et al. 2004; Cui et al. 2013; Tanguy et al. 1998, 2004, 2011). Selenium supplementation has also demonstrated antidiabetic and insulin-mimetic effects (Stapleton 2000). In 1990, Ezaki first discovered that selenate promotes the transport of glucose to adipocytes in *in vitro* mouse cell studies (Ezaki 1990). A similar role was also confirmed in rat muscle tissue (Furnsinn et al. 1996). The hypoglycemic effect of selenate was later confirmed in an *in vivo* rat experiment (McNeill et al. 1991). Further cellular mechanism studies have shown that, like insulin, selenium regulates glucose uptake and glucose metabolism mainly through the regulation of insulin-signaling pathways involving insulin receptors, glucose transporters, and key enzymes in glycolysis and gluconeogenesis (Ghosh et al. 1994; Berg et al. 1995; Shepherd et al. 1995; Magnuson et al. 1989).

Of note, the selenium dose required for the insulin-mimetic effect seems to be close to the toxic limit for human beings. The high selenium could increase the risk of type 2 diabetes, since high antioxidant activity of GPX1 would interfere with insulin signaling, for which hydrogen peroxide acts as a second messenger (Bleys et al. 2007a; Czernichow et al. 2006; Stranges et al. 2011; Laclaustra et al. 2009; Gao et al. 2007). There is some evidence that selenoprotein P (SELENOP), a major component of selenium in plasma, has the opposite effect and can induce insulin resistance and increase glucose intolerance by regulating gluconeogenic enzymes. The results from human studies have shown significantly higher SELENOP levels in patients with type 2 diabetes or prediabetes than in those with normal glucose tolerance, although longitudinal and prospective data for higher selenium exposure are lacking. Overall, the mechanisms underlying the relation between high selenium levels and increased CVD risk remain largely undefined due to lack of convincing evidence. Further investigation in well-designed metabolic studies is warranted to elucidate the genuine effects of selenoproteins on cardiometabolic outcomes across a broad range of their activities and levels.

Evidence from Human Observational Studies

The relationship between selenium and CVD has been studied extensively for nearly 40 years. The first evidence in the literature appears in 1979 (Keshan and Disease Research Group of the Chinese Academy of Medical Sciences 1979a), when an epidemiologic study in China reported a correlation between selenium deficiency and Keshan disease, a congestive cardiomyopathy. Supplementation of sodium selenite was reported to prevent Keshan disease in selenium-deficient areas of China (Keshan and Disease Research Group of the Chinese Academy of Medical Sciences 1979b). Subsequently, the majority of epidemiologic data relating selenium intake or status to the cardiovascular system has been provided by numerous cross-sectional studies. Results from most (but not all) cross-sectional studies suggest that low selenium levels are associated with CVD in diverse populations. For example, one clinical study from the mid-1980s reported that low selenium concentrations in blood (lower than 45 µg/L) and toenails were frequent among heart-failure patients (Virtamo et al. 1985). Another cross-sectional study of 1110 men aged 55–74 years in two rural areas of Finland evaluated the association between serum selenium levels and 5-year all-cause and cardiovascular mortality and found a significantly high risk of overall mortality and cardiovascular mortality among men with serum selenium lower than 45 µg/L (Virtamo et al. 1985). However, evidence from cross-sectional studies does not necessarily imply any causal relation because of the inherent limitations of that study design.

In observational studies, prospective cohort design is considered optimal for understanding the etiology of chronic diseases. Meta-analysis in epidemiological research is a useful tool, since combining evidence across studies reduces sampling error and increases statistical power despite the inconsistencies of study results. In a meta-analysis of 25 observational studies (14 cohorts and 11 case-control studies), Flores-Mateo et al. showed an inverse association between blood or toenail selenium levels and coronary heart disease; the pooled relative risk in a comparison of the highest versus the lowest selenium level categories was 0.85 (95% CI: 0.74–0.99) in cohort studies and 0.43 (0.29–0.66) in case-control studies (Flores-Mateo et al. 2006). Their findings were consistent with our previous meta-analysis results based on available prospective data published up to December 2013 (Zhang et al. 2016). In our meta-analysis of 16 prospective observational studies involving 35,607 participants and 4421 incident CVD cases, the pooled RR for the highest versus the lowest category of baseline blood (serum/plasma/erythrocyte) selenium levels was 0.87 (95% CI: 0.76–0.99), indicating a significant but modest association (Zhang et al. 2016). Our further dose-response meta-analysis also showed a nonlinear relation of CVD risk with blood selenium concentrations across a wide range of 30–165 µg/L, but a significantly inverse association was observed within a narrow range of 55–145 µg/L (Zhang et al. 2016).

To provide an up-to-date systematic review and meta-analysis, we searched MEDLINE and EMBASE databases for all relevant articles on the association between blood selenium and the risk of CVD published up to December 30, 2017.

Figure 16.2 is a forest plot summarizing the results from a total of 19 prospective studies involving 60,540 participants and 7770 incident CVD cases in the meta-analysis. Of the 19 studies, 12 were cohort studies and 7 were nested case-control studies. Compared with data prior to 2014 (Zhang et al. 2016), these updated numbers of total participants and incident CVD cases reflect an increase of 70–75%. When the data from these independent prospective cohorts were combined via meta-analysis, the pooled estimate of RRs comparing the highest category (median: 102.81 µg/L) of circulating selenium concentrations with the lowest category (median: 68.77 µg/L) were 0.84 (95% CI: 0.77–0.92), indicating a significant inverse association between baseline selenium concentrations and CVD risk (Fig. 16.2). There was weakly significant between-study heterogeneity. Assuming a linear relation between selenium levels and CVD, the pooled RR was estimated to be 0.94 (95% CI: 0.92, 0.97) for each 25 µg/L increment in circulating selenium levels.

To further explore the threshold effect for the relation between selenium levels and CVD events, we specifically assessed the overall dose-response relationship between a broad range of blood selenium levels (17–165 µg/L) and CVD risk. Our analysis, modeled by restricted cubic spline, suggested a reasonably nonlinear U-shaped relationship between selenium intake and CVD risk (Fig. 16.3). Based on seven independent prospective studies with available data, the curve showed that selenium concentrations in the range of 40–160 µg/L (with a nadir at 125 µg/L) were significantly associated with lower risk of CVD compared to low selenium concentrations (median: 52.8 µg/L in the lowest categories from all included studies). The association became the null when selenium concentrations exceeded 160 µg/L. Given such sparse data, current evidence is insufficient to make any

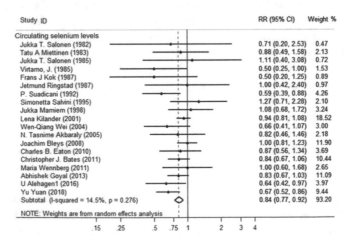

Fig. 16.2 A random-effect meta-analysis of 19 independent prospective studies involving 60,540 participants and 7770 incident CVD cases with adjusted relative risk (RR) and 95% confidence interval (CI) of CVDs in relation to blood selenium concentrations (the highest versus the lowest category). Black solid circles indicate RR in each study and horizontal line represents the 95% CI in each study. The pooled RR and 95% CI are indicated by the unshaded diamond

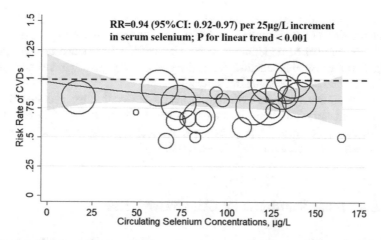

Fig. 16.3 Dose-response relation between baseline concentrations of selenium and the risk of CVDs in seven independent prospective studies. The relation is fitted by the quadratic regression model. Circles indicate RR in each study. The circle size is proportional to the precision of the RR (inverse of variance). The grey-shaded region shows the 95% CIs around the regression line. The selenium concentrations were across the range from 17.2 to 164.6 µg/L; the median concentrations in all the control groups were 52.8 µg/L

conclusions regarding the relationship between CVD risk and selenium concentrations above 160 µg/L.

Inconsistent findings from individual prospective observational studies may be due to differences in selenium intake and status among various populations, sample size, follow-up duration, and population characteristics. Our stratified analyses yielded a significant interaction by duration of follow-up (P for interaction <0.0001); the inverse associations were stronger among studies with <10 years of follow-up (RR, 0.70; 95% CI: 0.60, 0.82) than those with longer follow-up (≥10 years) (RR, 0.92; 95% CI: 0.84, 1.00). Though many factors may explain heterogeneity across studies, none of the following significantly modified the inverse association, although they were all potential effect modifiers: sex, sample size, baseline selenium levels, adjustment for BMI or smoking, and CVD endpoints. Also, though the source of biospecimen (blood/serum/plasma/tissue) for assessment may modify this association, our updated meta-analysis did not identify significant differences by serum or other specimen source.

Despite the considerable controversy regarding the association between toenail selenium levels and CVD, toenail selenium has been proposed as a reliable biomarker of long-term selenium exposure. Since 2011, there has been a lack of new prospective data on toenail selenium and CVD. As we previously reported (Zhang et al. 2016), we found no significant relation between toenail selenium concentrations and CVD based on two prospective studies.

Additionally, epidemiologic data provide further support for a pivotal role of selenium in other cardiometabolic diseases, including type 2 diabetes, hypertension, and dyslipidemia. A significant U-shaped relationship between serum selenium levels and type 2 diabetes was also identified (Wang et al. 2016). These findings raise concern that high selenium may lead to insulin resistance or type 2 diabetes, at least in well-nourished populations. Also, observational evidence on hypertension and lipid profile is also inconclusive, and the studies vary greatly in terms of population, design, and baseline selenium status.

Considering the available evidence, it seems reasonable to speculate that high selenium concentrations may be related to some intermediate CVD risk factors, including dyslipidemia and type 2 diabetes, and may thus diminish the inverse association, perhaps even leading to increased risk of CVD.

Evidence from Randomized Controlled Trials

Randomized controlled trials can provide direct evidence for causality. In human intervention studies, a randomized double-blinded, placebo-controlled trial is considered the best approach to examine a cause-effect relation. However, the available controlled trials are usually small with short follow-up and are carried out in the secondary prevention setting of chronic disease because of cost and logistical considerations. Numerous small clinical trials have assessed the therapeutic effect of selenium supplements in cardiovascular diseases but yielded inconsistent results. Many factors may have contributed to inconsistency across trials, including small sample size, incomplete randomization, lack of blinding in design, variable duration of follow-up, high rates of noncompliance, as well as differences in selenium treatment protocols, formulation and dose, and study populations. The findings from a few trials suggest that low-dose selenium (100 or 200 μg/day) combined with coenzyme Q10 supplementation can reduce the risk of CVD (Alehagen et al. 2013; Kuklinski et al. 1994). Most RCT studies with that dosage range found null associations.

In a meta-analysis of six randomized trials involving 17,766 participants published between 1989 and 2004, Flores-Mateo et al. showed a nonsignificant 11% reduction in CVD risk comparing those taking selenium supplements with the placebo groups (the pooled RR: 0.89; 95% CI: 0.68–1.17) (Flores-Mateo et al. 2006). In a Cochrane review and meta-analysis (Rees et al. 2013), Rees et al. included only 12 randomized controlled trials involving 19,715 participants and found that selenium supplementation had no significant effects on all-cause mortality (the pooled RR: 0.97; 95% CI: 0.88–1.08), CVD mortality (0.97; 95% CI: 0.79–1.20), nonfatal CVD events (0.96; 95% CI: 0.89–1.04), or all CVD events (fatal and nonfatal) (1.03; 95% CI: 0.95–1.11). In agreement, the results of our meta-analysis of nine randomized controlled trials published up to December 2013 indicate that oral selenium supplements (75–300 μg/day; median dose: 100 μg/day) for 6 to 114 months (median duration: 60 months) did not significantly decrease the incidence of CVD (the pooled RR: 0.91; 95% CI: 0.74–1.10) compared with placebo (Zhang et al. 2016). In addition, we also found some evidence of possible publication bias in previous randomized trial data, which might explain the significant results of some individual trials. In particular, most large trials with longer durations reported null findings, suggesting substantial publication bias due to selective publication of small trials with positive results.

Although previous meta-analyses of RCTs consistently found no significant effect of selenium supplementation on CVD (Zhang et al. 2016; Rees et al. 2013), that null effect could be modified by the significant between-study heterogeneity in selenium dosage, formula, duration, and combinations of supplements. Our subgroup analysis by selenium dose showed no differential effects; the pooled RR was 0.78 (95% CI: 0.49, 1.26) for six trials with dose of ≤100 µg/day (only one is 75 µg/day) and 0.91 (95% CI: 0.69, 1.21) for three trials with 200 µg/day selenium intake (Zhang et al. 2016). Recently, Rayman et al. conducted a double-blind, randomized, controlled trial of selenium supplementation and all-cause and cardiovascular mortality in 491 healthy and elderly residents of Denmark with moderately low selenium status (Rayman et al. 2018). The hazard ratios for all-cause mortality comparing 300 µg/day selenium supplementation via yeast to placebo were 1.62 (0.66 to 3.96) after 5 years of treatment and 1.59 (1.02 to 2.46) over the entire follow-up. For CVD mortality, the HR was 2.17 (0.40, 11.85) and 1.51 (0.69, 3.33), respectively. These results suggest a high-dose harmful effect of selenium supplementation on cardiovascular mortality and all-cause mortality.

Selenium dosage varied across RCTs; most published trials used 100 and 200 µg/L. These differences might have affected results and led to difficulties in identifying the optimal dose of selenium supplements. Our meta-analysis of ten RCTs showed that oral selenium supplementation (median dose: 200 µg/day) for 6.5 months (range: 2 weeks to 144 months) significantly raised blood selenium concentrations by 56.4 µg/L from a median of 98.5 µg/L (95% CI for weighted mean differences [WMD]: 40.9, 72.0 µg/L) and reached a maximum of 150 µg/L, which is at the high end of the range of 40–160 µg/L associated with significant CVD risk reduction but may not be optimal for CVD health. Nevertheless, evidence from doses ≥300 µg/day is both limited and inconclusive. Only one RCT reported a significant increment of selenium concentrations by 41.2 µg/L (29.9–51.3) after a high dose of 300 µg/day selenium supplementation for 12 weeks (Ghosh et al. 1994).

The mechanism underlying a high-dose side effect might be related to the activity of selenoproteins, including antioxidant enzyme. The findings from our meta-analysis of activity may explain the disparity in results between observational studies and RCTs for cardiovascular health by selenium. Our meta-analysis of activity showed that activity increased abruptly at 1–2 weeks after oral selenium supplementation and then reached maximal levels (12%) at 12 weeks. However, it is questionable whether increment in activity is sustained in more than 12 weeks and largely explains the long-term effects of selenium on CVD. Hurst et al. comprehensively evaluated the dose-response relations for different forms of selenium among 119 healthy men and women aged 50–64 years living in the UK (Hurst et al. 2010). Selenoproteins are probably saturated at a plasma selenium concentration of ~125 µg/L after 6-week supplementation with a dose as low as 50 µg/day. Although a higher dose further increased levels of plasma selenium, the selenoproteins changed only slightly (Hurst et al. 2010). Consistently, Deitrich et al. explored the dose- and duration-response relationship between selenium supplementation and plasma selenium and selenoprotein concentrations in a small number of participants and found an unparalleled change of plasma selenium and selenoproteins as selenium doses increased (Rayman et al. 2018). While serum selenium concentrations increased markedly from 6 months to 5 years, the concentrations of selenoproteins fell significantly at the two groups with high doses (Rayman et al. 2018).

Taken together, evidence suggests that long-term treatment with selenium does not yield beneficial effects on health but may lead instead to selenoprotein depletion and negative health consequences. The harmful effect of high-dose selenium supplementation on cardiovascular diseases may not be related to selenoprotein activity, but the exact mechanisms have not yet been fully elucidated. Overall, the evidence remains unconvincing due to the relatively limited data, and further investigation via prospective studies with sufficient numbers of cases of CVD is warranted.

Implications and Conclusions

As the evidence from observational studies and randomized clinical trials accumulates, a U-shaped relationship between selenium status or selenium supplementation and CVD has become clearer. Among those with low selenium status (<67.1 μg/L), the risks of cardiovascular diseases, cardiovascular mortality, and diabetes mellitus are moderately higher than among those with normal selenium status. Selenium supplementation <300 μg/day can improve selenium status and selenoprotein activity, enhancing metabolic profiles among those with selenium deficiencies. In contrast, prevalence of diabetes, hyperlipidemia, and hypertension is higher among participants with high selenium. Consistently, moderate-to-high selenium supplementation in populations with adequate selenium status only elevated blood selenium levels, but did not improve the activity of selenoproteins; that might even have an adverse cardiometabolic effect (Rayman et al. 2011; Bleys et al. 2007a, b; Laclaustra et al. 2009; Lockitch 1989). Therefore, we suggest that the selenium-CVD relationship is U-shaped. We also propose that the cardiometabolic benefits of selenium depend on three critical factors: population selenium status, selenium dosage, and duration of supplementation. In other words, selenium supplementation should be implemented among those in need, given certain restrictions on dosage and duration.

Current evidence from observational and randomized trials has provided clues to the range of selenium concentrations that indicate selenium deficiency. The upper limits of selenium deficiency ranged from 45 to 70 μg/L according to current evidence. Researcher used the nationwide data from the National Health and Nutrition Examination Survey for the period 2011–2012 to determine normal reference ranges and percentile distributions for selenium in blood. The limits of normal reference ranges for blood selenium (defined as the 2.5th and 97.5th percentiles for the overall US population) were 146.8 μg/L and 247.3 μg/L (Jain and Choi 2015). However, selenium levels in the serum of populations throughout the world vary wildly, from 41.7 μg/L in Finland to 158.2 μg/L in Canada (Lockitch 1989). To answer the question of whether selenium supplementation is necessary in a particular population, further well-designed studies on blood selenium limits are critical. While much uncertainty exists regarding the validity of epidemiologic studies, the best approach to confirm a cause-effect relation is obviously to perform a randomized, double-blinded, placebo-controlled trial. Our findings thus indicate the need for future long-term RCTs focused on identifying optimal selenium supplement dose and safety. At present, available evidence is insufficient to support the widespread use of selenium or selenium-containing supplements for CVD prevention.

The precise mechanisms underlying selenium metabolism are far from clear. Recent genetic studies of selenoprotein genes or other genetic variants significantly associated with selenium or selenoprotein levels have shed light on the underlying molecular basis of selenium metabolism and helped identify genetic variants that modify the metabolic effects of selenium intake. Recent studies have implicated the epigenetic effects by selenium supplementation and status. Alterations of the epigenome are also linked to the onset and progression of CVD. From a mechanistic perspective, there is a compelling need for comprehensive information of multi-omics signatures in response to selenium supplementation, which will help us gain important insights into the pathophysiological mechanisms underlying cardiometabolic abnormalities in response to selenium supplementation. Additionally, serum selenium is considered a marker for selenium status, but reliable and sensitive biomarkers of the biological activity or function of selenoproteins remain to be identified.

In summary, the relationship between selenium and CVD, based on human observational data, may be U-shaped, with possible harmful effects both below and above certain ranges of selenium levels. Although data for higher selenium status are sparse, our suggestive evidence from a meta-analysis of prospective studies published up to December 2017 raises a red flag about the potential adverse effects of high selenium status on the cardiovascular system. Available evidence from randomized controlled trials does not support any beneficial or harmful effects of selenium or selenium-containing supplements on CVD risk. Further investigation is warranted to elucidate the optimal duration of selenium supplementation and the mechanisms underlying the selenium-cardiometabolic association; optimize the amount of selenium required for health benefits; identify individuals who are at high risk and may benefit most from increasing selenium intake; and tailor intervention strategies for the prevention of cardiometabolic diseases. Nevertheless, until more definitive data are available, the collective evidence is not sufficient to recommend for or against selenium supplements for primary prevention of CVD.

References

Ago T, Sadoshima J. Thioredoxin and ventricular remodeling. J Mol Cell Cardiol. 2006;41:762–73.

Alehagen U, Johansson P, Bjornstedt M, Rosen A, Dahlstrom U. Cardiovascular mortality and N-terminal-proBNP reduced after combined selenium and coenzyme Q10 supplementation: a 5-year prospective randomized double-blind placebo-controlled trial among elderly Swedish citizens. Int J Cardiol. 2013;167:1860–6.

Berg EA, Wu JY, Campbell L, Kagey M, Stapleton SR. Insulin-like effects of vanadate and selenate on the expression of glucose-6-phosphate dehydrogenase and fatty acid synthase in diabetic rats. Biochimie. 1995;77:919–24.

Bleys J, Navas-Acien A, Guallar E. Serum selenium and diabetes in U.S. adults. Diabetes Care. 2007a;30:829–34.

Bleys J, Navas-Acien A, Guallar E. Selenium and diabetes: more bad news for supplements. Ann Intern Med. 2007b;147:271–2.

Bleys J, Navas-Acien A, Guallar E. Serum selenium levels and all-cause, cancer, and cardiovascular mortality among US adults. Arch Intern Med. 2008;168:404–10.

Cone JE, Del Rio RM, Davis JN, Stadtman TC. Chemical characterization of the selenoprotein component of clostridial glycine reductase: identification of selenocysteine as the organoselenium moiety. Proc Natl Acad Sci U S A. 1976;73:2659–63.

Cui J, Li Z, Qian LB, et al. Reducing the oxidative stress mediates the cardioprotection of bicyclol against ischemia-reperfusion injury in rats. J Zhejiang Univ Sci B. 2013;14:487–95.

Czernichow S, Couthouis A, Bertrais S, et al. Antioxidant supplementation does not affect fasting plasma glucose in the Supplementation with Antioxidant Vitamins and Minerals (SU.VI.MAX) study in France: association with dietary intake and plasma concentrations. Am J Clin Nutr. 2006;84:395–9.

Eaton CB, Abdul Baki AR, Waring ME, Roberts MB, Lu B. The association of low selenium and renal insufficiency with coronary heart disease and all-cause mortality: NHANES III follow-up study. Atherosclerosis. 2010;212:689–94.

Ezaki O. The insulin-like effects of selenate in rat adipocytes. J Biol Chem. 1990;265:1124–8.

Flores-Mateo G, Navas-Acien A, Pastor-Barriuso R, Guallar E. Selenium and coronary heart disease: a meta-analysis. Am J Clin Nutr. 2006;84:762–73.

Forman HJ, Torres M. Reactive oxygen species and cell signaling: respiratory burst in macrophage signaling. Am J Respir Crit Care Med. 2002;166:S4–8.

Furnsinn C, Englisch R, Ebner K, Nowotny P, Vogl C, Waldhausl W. Insulin-like vs. non-insulin-like stimulation of glucose metabolism by vanadium, tungsten, and selenium compounds in rat muscle. Life Sci. 1996;59:1989–2000.

Gao S, Jin Y, Hall KS, et al. Selenium level and cognitive function in rural elderly Chinese. Am J Epidemiol. 2007;165:955–65.

Ghosh R, Mukherjee B, Chatterjee M. A novel effect of selenium on streptozotocin-induced diabetic mice. Diabetes Res. 1994;25:165–71.

Guo F, Monsefi N, Moritz A, Beiras-Fernandez A. Selenium and cardiovascular surgery: an overview. Curr Drug Saf. 2012;7:321–7.

Haug A, Graham RD, Christophersen OA, Lyons GH. How to use the world's scarce selenium resources efficiently to increase the selenium concentration in food. Microb Ecol Health Dis. 2007;19:209–28.

Heyland DK, Dhaliwal R, Suchner U, Berger MM. Antioxidant nutrients: a systematic review of trace elements and vitamins in the critically ill patient. Intensive Care Med. 2005;31:327–37.

Hurst R, Armah CN, Dainty JR, et al. Establishing optimal selenium status: results of a randomized, double-blind, placebo-controlled trial. Am J Clin Nutr. 2010;91:923–31.

Jain RB, Choi YS. Normal reference ranges for and variability in the levels of blood manganese and selenium by gender, age, and race/ethnicity for general U.S. population. J Trace Elem Med Biol. 2015;30:142–52.

Jones GD, Droz B, Greve P, et al. Selenium deficiency risk predicted to increase under future climate change. Proc Natl Acad Sci U S A. 2017;114:2848–53.

Keshan and Disease Research Group of the Chinese Academy of Medical Sciences. Epidemiologic studies on the etiologic relationship of selenium and Keshan disease. Chin Med J. 1979a;92:477–82.

Keshan and Disease Research Group of the Chinese Academy of Medical Sciences. Observations on effect of sodium selenite in prevention of Keshan disease. Chin Med J. 1979b;92:471–6.

Kuklinski B, Weissenbacher E, Fahnrich A. Coenzyme Q10 and antioxidants in acute myocardial infarction. Mol Asp Med. 1994;(15 Suppl):s143–7.

Laclaustra M, Navas-Acien A, Stranges S, Ordovas JM, Guallar E. Serum selenium concentrations and diabetes in U.S. adults: National Health and Nutrition Examination Survey (NHANES) 2003–2004. Environ Health Perspect. 2009;117:1409–13.

Lockitch G. Selenium: clinical significance and analytical concepts. Crit Rev Clin Lab Sci. 1989;27:483–541.

Lubos E, Sinning CR, Schnabel RB, et al. Serum selenium and prognosis in cardiovascular disease: results from the AtheroGene study. Atherosclerosis. 2010;209:271–7.

Magnuson MA, Andreone TL, Printz RL, Koch S, Granner DK. Rat glucokinase gene: structure and regulation by insulin. Proc Natl Acad Sci U S A. 1989;86:4838–42.

Mahjoub S, Masrour-Roudsari J. Role of oxidative stress in pathogenesis of metabolic syndrome. Caspian J Int Med. 2012;3:386–96.

Maulik N, Das DK. Emerging potential of thioredoxin and thioredoxin interacting proteins in various disease conditions. Biochim Biophys Acta. 2008;1780:1368–82.

McNeill JH, Delgatty HL, Battell ML. Insulinlike effects of sodium selenate in streptozocin-induced diabetic rats. Diabetes. 1991;40:1675–8.

Muntau AC, Streiter M, Kappler M, et al. Age-related reference values for serum selenium concentrations in infants and children. Clin Chem. 2002;48:555–60.

Murr C, Talasz H, Artner-Dworzak E, et al. Inverse association between serum selenium concentrations and parameters of immune activation in patients with cardiac disorders. Clin Chem Lab Med. 2007;45:1224–8.

Navarro-Alarcon M, Cabrera-Vique C. Selenium in food and the human body: a review. Sci Total Environ. 2008;400:115–41.

Navarro-Alarcon M, MC L-M. Essentiality of selenium in the human body: relationship with different diseases. Sci Total Environ. 2000;249:347–71.

Neve J. Human selenium supplementation as assessed by changes in blood selenium concentration and glutathione peroxidase activity. J Trace Elem Med Biol. 1995;9:65–73.

Polo A, Colonna G, Guariniello S, Ciliberto G, Costantini S. Deducing the functional characteristics of the human selenoprotein SELK from the structural properties of its intrinsically disordered C-terminal domain. Mol BioSyst. 2016;12:758–72.

Rajpathak S, Rimm E, Morris JS, Hu F. Toenail selenium and cardiovascular disease in men with diabetes. J Am Coll Nutr. 2005;24:250–6.

Rayman MP, Stranges S, Griffin BA, Pastor-Barriuso R, Guallar E. Effect of supplementation with high-selenium yeast on plasma lipids: a randomized trial. Ann Intern Med. 2011;154:656–65.

Rayman MP, Winther KH, Pastor-Barriuso R, et al. Effect of long-term selenium supplementation on mortality: results from a multiple-dose, randomised controlled trial. Free Radic Biol Med. 2018.

Rees K, Hartley L, Day C, Flowers N, Clarke A, Stranges S. Selenium supplementation for the primary prevention of cardiovascular disease. Cochrane Database Syst Rev. 2013:CD009671.

Reilly C. Selenium in Food and Health. 2nd ed. New York: Springer; 2006.

Shepherd PR, Nave BT, Siddle K. Insulin stimulation of glycogen synthesis and glycogen synthase activity is blocked by wortmannin and rapamycin in 3T3-L1 adipocytes: evidence for the involvement of phosphoinositide 3-kinase and p70 ribosomal protein-S6 kinase. Biochem J. 1995;305(Pt 1):25–8.

Stadtman TC. Selenium biochemistry. Science. 1974;183:915–22.

Stapleton SR. Selenium: an insulin-mimetic. Cellular and molecular life sciences. CMLS. 2000;57:1874–9.

Steinbrenner H, Sies H. Protection against reactive oxygen species by selenoproteins. Biochim Biophys Acta. 2009;1790:1478–85.

Stranges S, Galletti F, Farinaro E, et al. Associations of selenium status with cardiometabolic risk factors: an 8-year follow-up analysis of the Olivetti Heart study. Atherosclerosis. 2011;217:274–8.

Sun M, Liu G, Wu Q. Speciation of organic and inorganic selenium in selenium-enriched rice by graphite furnace atomic absorption spectrometry after cloud point extraction. Food Chem. 2013;141:66–71.

Tanguy S, Boucher F, Besse S, Ducros V, Favier A, de Leiris J. Trace elements and cardioprotection: increasing endogenous glutathione peroxidase activity by oral selenium supplementation in rats limits reperfusion-induced arrhythmias. J Trace Elem Med Biol. 1998;12:28–38.

Tanguy S, Morel S, Berthonneche C, et al. Preischemic selenium status as a major determinant of myocardial infarct size in vivo in rats. Antioxid Redox Signal. 2004;6:792–6.

Tanguy S, Rakotovao A, Jouan MG, Ghezzi C, de Leiris J, Boucher F. Dietary selenium intake influences Cx43 dephosphorylation, TNF-alpha expression and cardiac remodeling after reperfused infarction. Mol Nutr Food Res. 2011;55:522–9.

Trumbo P, Yates AA, Schlicker S, Poos M. Dietary reference intakes: vitamin A, vitamin K, arsenic, boron, chromium, copper, iodine, iron, manganese, molybdenum, nickel, silicon, vanadium, and zinc. J Am Diet Assoc. 2001;101:294–301.

Venardos K, Harrison G, Headrick J, Perkins A. Effects of dietary selenium on glutathione peroxidase and thioredoxin reductase activity and recovery from cardiac ischemia-reperfusion. J Trace Elem Med Biol. 2004;18:81–8.

Virtamo J, Valkeila E, Alfthan G, Punsar S, Huttunen JK, Karvonen MJ. Serum selenium and the risk of coronary heart disease and stroke. Am J Epidemiol. 1985;122:276–82.

Wang XL, Yang TB, Wei J, Lei GH, Zeng C. Association between serum selenium level and type 2 diabetes mellitus: a non-linear dose-response meta-analysis of observational studies. Nutr J. 2016;15:48.

Xun P, Liu K, Morris JS, Daviglus ML, He K. Longitudinal association between toenail selenium levels and measures of subclinical atherosclerosis: the CARDIA trace element study. Atherosclerosis. 2010;210:662–7.

Zhang X, Liu C, Guo J, Song Y. Selenium status and cardiovascular diseases: meta-analysis of prospective observational studies and randomized controlled trials. Eur J Clin Nutr. 2016;70:162–9.

Chapter 17
Selenium and Diabetes

Ji-Chang Zhou, Jun Zhou, Liqin Su, Kaixun Huang, and Xin Gen Lei

Abstract The relationship between selenium (Se) and diabetes remains an evolving field. Early studies were focused on antioxidant benefits of Se in diabetic animals and patients. However, the discovery of type 2 diabetes-like phenotype in the glutathione peroxidase (GPX) 1 overexpression mice and the pro-diabetic potential of Se supplementation in cancer subjects have provoked both research and public interests on its role in diabetes. Limited human data indicate a Se baseline-dependent risk for diabetes associated with Se supplementations: potentiating the risk for diabetes only in subjects with high-Se status. Among the 25 selenoproteins, GPX1 exhibits dual roles in insulin synthesis, secretion, and signaling via regulation of redox homeostasis, and selenoprotein P has the counteraction effect on insulin signaling. Both GPX3 and selenoprotein S may play roles in diabetic etiology via mediating inflammation. Dysregulations of the two endoplasmic reticulum (ER)-resident selenoproteins, selenoproteins M and T, may disturb the redox homeostasis in ER, causing ER stress and increasing the diabetes risk. Iodothyronine deiodinases catalyze the metabolism of thyroid hormones and thus may affect the metabolism of glucose, lipids, and protein in the diabetic status. Polymorphism of selenoprotein genes in humans offers clues to the association of Se/selenoproteins and diabetes risk. In conclusion, effects of Se intake on the risk of diabetes are dose and baseline dependent. While underlying mechanisms for this paradox are partly

J.-C. Zhou
School of Public Health (Shenzhen), Sun Yat-sen University, Shenzhen, China

Molecular Biology Laboratory, Shenzhen Center for Chronic Disease Control, Shenzhen, China

J. Zhou · K. Huang
Hubei Key Laboratory of Bioinorganic Chemistry and Materia Medica, School of Chemistry and Chemical Engineering, Huazhong University of Science and Technology, Wuhan, China

L. Su
Department of Soil Quality and Health Monitoring, National Institute of Environmental Health, Chinese Center for Disease Control and Prevention, Beijing, China

X. G. Lei (✉)
Department of Animal Science, Cornell University, Ithaca, NY, USA
e-mail: XL20@cornell.edu

© Springer International Publishing AG, part of Springer Nature 2018
B. Michalke (ed.), *Selenium*, Molecular and Integrative Toxicology,
https://doi.org/10.1007/978-3-319-95390-8_17

317

understood through animal studies on the functions of several selenoproteins, appropriate Se intakes for the general public to prevent or treat diabetes warrant future research.

Keywords Animal · Diabetes · Endoplasmic reticulum · Glutathione peroxidase · Human · Insulin · Reactive oxygen species · Selenoprotein · Signaling

Abbreviations

AKT	Protein kinase B
AMPK	Adenosine monophosphate-activated protein kinase
BMI	Body mass index
BW	Body weight
CAT	Catalase
CI	Confidence interval
Cys	Cysteine
DIO	Iodothyronine deiodinase
DM	Diabetes mellitus
ER	Endoplasmic reticulum
FOXA2	Forkhead box A2
FOXO1a	Forkhead box O1a
FPG	Fasting plasma glucose
FPI	Fasting plasma insulin
G6P	Glucose-6-phosphatase
GDM	Gestational diabetes mellitus
GPX	Glutathione peroxidase
GSIS	Glucose-stimulated insulin secretion
HOMA-IR	Homeostasis model assessment of insulin resistance
INSR	Insulin receptor
IRS	Insulin receptor substrate
MS	Metabolic syndrome
MSRB1	Methionine-R-sulfoxide reductase B1
NCD	Noncommunicable disease
NF-κB (NFKB1 in GenBank)	Nuclear factor kappa B subunit 1
OR	Odds ratio
PACAP	Pituitary adenylate cyclase-activating polypeptide
PDX1	Pancreatic duodenal homeobox 1
PEPCK/PCK	Phosphoenolpyruvate carboxykinase

PGC1α (PPARGC1A in GenBank)	Peroxisome proliferator-activated receptor gamma coactivator 1 alpha
PI3K	Phosphatidylinositol 3-kinase
PPARγ (PPARG in GenBank)	Peroxisome proliferator-activated receptor gamma
PTP1B (PTPN1 in GenBank)	Protein-tyrosine phosphatase 1B (non-receptor type 1)
RCT	Randomized controlled trial
ROS	Reactive oxygen species
SAA	Serum amyloid A
Scly	Selenocysteine lyase
Se	Selenium
Sec	Selenocysteine
SELENOM	Selenoprotein M
SELENOP	Selenoprotein P
SELENOS	Selenoprotein S
SELENOT	Selenoprotein T
SeMet	Selenomethionine
SNP	Single-nucleotide polymorphism
SOD	Superoxide dismutase
T1D	Type 1 diabetes
T2D	Type 2 diabetes
T3	3,5,3′-Triiodothyronine
T4	3,5,3′,5′-Tetraiodothyronine
UCP	Uncoupling protein
UTR	Untranslated region

Introduction

Diabetes mellitus (DM) or diabetes is one of the top noncommunicable diseases (NCDs) worldwide today. Estimated by NCD Risk Factor Collaboration, 8.5% of the adults (422 million) lived with diabetes in 2014 (NCD-RisC 2016). More than 90% of DM are categorized as type 2 diabetes (T2D), and the rest are type 1 diabetes (T1D), gestational diabetes (GDM), and other very rare types. All types of DM have common apparent phenotypes of higher circulating glucose concentration than the normal range at overnight fasting, and/or after food, glucose, and/or insulin challenges, along with dysregulated lipid and protein metabolism. Moreover, T1D is characterized by insulin deficiency due to destructed pancreatic islets, while both T2D and GDM are characterized by insulin resistance and impaired glucose clearance from circulation. GDM might be temporal and recovers after giving birth. Though the etiology of DM has not fully been elucidated, a disturbed redox homeostasis might be an important mechanism.

Selenium (Se) is an essential nutrient for humans and animals, with diverse physiologic functions mainly in the form of 24–25 selenoproteins (Kryukov et al. 2003) (see Chapter 3.1). The well-known or -studied selenoproteins include oxidoreductases [glutathione peroxidases (GPXs) and thioredoxin reductases (TXNRDs)], metabolic enzymes of thyroid hormones [iodothyronine deiodinases (DIOs)], Se transporter [selenoprotein P (SELENOP)], and proteins involved in other various functions [methionine-R-sulfoxide reductase B1 (MSRB1), selenoprotein M (SELENOM), selenoprotein N (SELENON), selenoprotein S (SELENOS), selenoprotein T (SELENOT), etc.] (Papp et al. 2007; Brigelius-Flohe and Flohe 2017). Dietary Se is mainly selenomethionine (SeMet) in plant foods and selenocysteine (Sec) in meats (Rayman et al. 2008). Besides, Se can also be obtained as sodium selenite, sodium selenate, and Se-enriched yeast via nutritional supplements (Rayman 2012). Metabolism of various forms of Se converges at hydrogen selenide (Rayman et al. 2008) that supplies Se for the cellular biosynthesis of selenoproteins or is transformed to the forms for clearance. Se compounds were found to improve pancreatic β-cell function and to mimic the action of insulin on its major target cells. Dietary Se has a U-shaped dose-response curve with a rather narrow "safe window" (Rayman 2012; Fairweather-Tait et al. 2011) compared with other micronutrients. The nutrient requirement of Se by rodents is 0.15 mg Se/kg of feed (NRC 1995), and 5 mg Se/kg of feed slows growth and causes deterioration of biochemical and molecular markers (Sunde and Raines 2011). For humans, the dietary recommended intake of Se is 55–75 µg/day in Europe and USA (Fairweather-Tait et al. 2011), and 300–450 µg/day is the "tolerable upper intake level" (Division for Nutrition 2006).

Observed Relationships Between Se and DM

Se and Diabetic Phenotypes in Animal Studies

Earlier Work on Se as an Insulin Mimic

In earlier studies, inorganic Se was found to act as an insulin mimic (Stapleton 2000), stimulate glucose uptake (Furnsinn et al. 1996), activate serine/threonine kinases (Ezaki 1990; Hei et al. 1998; Pillay and Makgoba 1992; Stapleton et al. 1997), improve glucose homeostasis (McNeill et al. 1991; Berg et al. 1995; Becker et al. 1996; Battell et al. 1998; Mueller et al. 2003; Mueller and Pallauf 2006), and restore the vascular architecture and function (Aydemir-Koksoy and Turan 2008) in diabetic animals. This gave an antidiabetic label to sodium selenate, sodium selenite (Mukherjee et al. 1998; Ayaz et al. 2002; Sheng et al. 2005; Ozdemir et al. 2005; Can et al. 2005; Ulusu and Turan 2005; Hwang et al. 2007; Zeng et al. 2009; Campbell et al. 2008), SeMet (Douillet et al. 1998; Erbayraktar et al. 2007), and Se-rich yeast (Agbor et al. 2007). The molecular mechanisms for their effects were reviewed elsewhere (Mueller et al. 2009a). The beneficial effects of Se on glucose regulation and diabetes prevention are largely interpreted by similar insulin-mimetic effects of many other elements and merely represent a manifestation of the stress response (Steinbrenner et al. 2011). However, these insulin-like effects were observed only at very high Se doses (e.g., 10–15 μmol/kg body weight (BW)/day, by intraperitoneal injection), and the clinical application in humans is not practical. In comparison, Se deficiency impaired antioxidant defense and glucose or lipid metabolism in the pancreas, liver, muscle, fat tissue, and/or adipocytes (Thompson and Scott 1970; Huang et al. 2011; Bunk and Combs 1981; Souness et al. 1983; Asayama et al. 1986; Reddi and Bollineni 2001), and aggravated reactive oxygen species (ROS)-mediated injury implicated in the onset of diabetes (Lei and Vatamaniuk 2011). A rarely focused Se compound, Se-containing phycocyanin, inhibited the fibrillation of human islet amyloid polypeptide and suppressed the formation of ROS to prevent β-cell apoptosis (Li et al. 2014).

Current Findings on Pro-diabetic Potential of High Se Intakes

Several animal studies have provided compelling evidences that high Se intakes potentiate diabetic risk. After sodium selenite was administrated to rats by intraperitoneal injection at relatively high dose [1.6 mg or more Se/kg BW at once (Rasekh et al. 1991) or 5 μmol/kg BW/day for 5 weeks (Ozdemir et al. 2005)], hyperglycemia was produced in a time- and dose-dependent manner. While the injections did not change plasma insulin levels in either fasted or fed animals, the increase in corticosterone levels suggested the involvement of gluconeogenesis in this hyperglycemic response. In high-fat diet/streptozotocin-induced diabetic mice, oral gavage with 2 mg sodium selenite (i.e., 0.9 mg Se)/kg BW/day for 4 weeks further increased the fasting plasma insulin (FPI) concentration and homeostasis model assessment of insulin resistance (HOMA-IR) (Zhou et al. 2015a).

Meanwhile, a number of recent animal studies in different species have shown the link of supranutritional Se intakes, rather than toxic levels of Se, to diabetes (Table 17.1).

Se and DM in Human Studies

The insulin-mimic property and the antioxidant capacity of Se on glucose metabolism and insulin sensitivity (Rayman 2000) have raised the public interest in Se supplementation for reducing the risk of T2D, a great contributor to the global burden of disease (Whiting et al. 2011). Because a U-shaped relationship between Se intake/status and health effect was observed in many studies, the degree to which Se supplementation could be beneficial needs to be examined carefully. Large differences in geology, climate, and other factors certainly produce similar differences in food Se concentrations and human Se intakes/status in various areas of world. Therefore, results on the relationship between Se and T2D in the Se-deplete and Se-replete populations might be inconsistent or even conflicting.

Table 17.1 Pro-diabetic potential of high Se intakes or oral administration in animals[a]

Study design	Results and/or conclusion	Sources
Mice (n = 6–7/diet) fed BD, BD+0.1, or BD+0.4 mg Se (as sodium selenite)/kg for 3 months	BD+0.4 mg Se/kg decreased insulin sensitivity and induced hyperinsulinemia compared to BD and BD+0.1 mg Se/kg	Labunskyy et al. (2011)
Male mice (n = 5–7/treatment) fed low- or high-isoflavone diets were subdivided into groups orally receiving water or 3 mg Se (as Se-methylselenocysteine)/kg BW/day for 5 months	Independent of dietary isoflavone concentration, Se supplementation elevated fasting blood glucose and tended to induce glucose intolerance (P = 0.08)	Stallings et al. (2014)
High-fat diet/streptozotocin-induced diabetic mice treated with 2 mg sodium selenite/kg BW/day for 4 weeks via oral gavage	The FPI and HOMA-IR were further increased by oral Se gavage	Zhou et al. (2015a)
Rats (n = 10/group) fed either BD, BD+75, or BD+150 μg Se (sodium selenate)/kg for 8 weeks	Se supplementation elevated BW, liver PTP1B activity, and liver triglyceride concentrations than BD	Mueller et al. (2008)
Rats (n = 7/diet) fed BD, BD+0.2, 1, or 2 mg Se (as selenite and selenate, respectively)/kg for 8 weeks	Compared with BD, Se supplementation increased BW, expression and/or activity of liver Gpx1 and PTP1B, and reduced PTP1B glutathionylation	Mueller et al. (2009b)
Female rats fed BD, BD+0.3, or BD+3 mg Se (as Se-yeast)/kg from 5 weeks before breeding to day 14 postpartum. Offspring (n = 8/diet) of the BD+0.3 and BD+3 mg Se/kg dams were fed with the same respective diet until 112 days old	Compared with BD+0.3 Se/kg, BD+3 mg Se/kg induced hyperinsulinemia, insulin resistance, and glucose intolerance in the dams at late gestation and/or postpartum and in the offspring	Zeng et al. (2012)
Male rats (n = 36/diet) fed 0.25, 0.5, and 2 mg Se (as Se-enriched milk casein)/kg of either low- or high-fat diet for 7 weeks	Hepatic insulin sensitivity was impaired by dietary Se increase	Stahel et al. (2017)
	Increased Se intake impaired the IRS/PI3K/AKT signaling	
Weanling male pigs (n = 8/diet) fed BD, BD+0.3, or BD+3 mg Se (as Se-enriched yeast)/kg for 16 weeks	BD+3 mg Se/kg induced hyperinsulinemia and lowered tissue AKT levels, compared with BD+0.3 mg Se/kg	Liu et al. (2012)
Male pigs fed 0.17 or 0.5 mg Se (as Se-yeast)/kg of diet for 16 weeks	The FPI and cholesterol levels were nonsignificantly increased, and the FPG concentrations and the expression and activity of proteins involved in energy metabolism in major insulin target tissues were not affected by high Se intake	Pinto et al. (2012)

(continued)

Table 17.1 (continued)

Study design	Results and/or conclusion	Sources
Pigs (n = 6/diet) with half males and half females fed 0.3 or 3 mg Se (as Se-rich yeast)/kg for 11 weeks	The 3 mg Se/kg diet increased concentrations of plasma insulin, liver and adipose lipids, and liver and muscle protein. The expression, activity, or both of key factors related to gluconeogenesis, protein synthesis, and energy metabolism in liver were upregulated	Zhao et al. (2016)
Lambs (n = 24/diet) fed BD (0.1 mg Se/kg dry matter) or BD+0.5 mg Se (as sodium selenate)/kg for 8 weeks	The BD+0.5 mg Se/kg significantly increased the mRNA abundances of lipoprotein lipase in liver and muscle and apolipoprotein E in muscle	Juszczuk-Kubiak et al. (2016)
Male chickens were fed 0.15, 3, or 5 mg Se (as sodium selenite)/kg diet for 8 weeks	The 5 mg Se/kg diet intake increased the blood glucose, but decreased the pancreatic antioxidant capacity when compared with the 0.15 or 3 mg Se/kg	Xiang et al. (2017)

[a]*AKT* protein kinase B, *BD* selenium-deficient basal diet, *BW* body weight, *FPG* fasting plasma glucose, *FPI* fasting plasma insulin, *HOMA-IR* homeostasis model assessment of insulin resistance, *IRS* insulin receptor substrate, *PI3K* phosphatidylinositol 3-kinase, *PTP1B* protein-tyrosine phosphatase 1B

Case-Control Observation of Se and T2D

In early case-control studies on population with lower Se status, lower blood Se was observed in diabetic patients compared with healthy controls [64.9 ± 22.8 vs. 74.9 ± 27.3 µg/L in Spain (Navarro-Alarcon et al. 1999), and 59.23 ± 12.2 or 58.23 ± 16.7 vs. 64.2 ± 11.5 µg/L in Croatia (Kljai and Runje 2001)]. However, recent case-control studies in China (Li et al. 2017; Lu et al. 2016; Yuan et al. 2015) and Italy (Cancarini et al. 2017) showed an inverse relationship. A population-based case-control study on a Han Chinese population in Jiangsu Province investigated the association between plasma concentrations of 20 metals and T2D (Li et al. 2017). After adjusting for confounders, plasma Se was associated with diabetes risk. The adjusted odds ratio (OR) values and 95% confidence interval (CI) of diabetes of the third tertile (the highest group) and the second tertile (the middle group) compared with the minimum tertile (the lowest group) for Se were 6.1 (3.0–13) and 8.1 (4.1–16), respectively. A hospital-based case-control study of 847 adults aged more than 40 years old (diabetes: non-diabetes = 1:2) in Northern Taiwan (Lu et al. 2016) showed that the mean serum Se concentration was 88.2 ± 21.2 µg/L. High serum Se levels were associated with increased risk for DM independent of central obesity and insulin resistance. Another matched case-control study including 204 metabolic syndrome (MS) patients and 204 healthy controls was conducted in China (Yuan et al. 2015). The median levels of plasma Se in MS group were 146 (107–199) µg/L, which were significantly higher than those in the control group [127 (95.7–176) µg/L]. Plasma levels of Se were related to the risk of MS in a dose-response manner. Risk of MS was significantly higher in subjects with plasma Se in the highest tertile (T3: $\geq$ 176 µg/L) compared with those in the lowest tertile (T1: < 95.7 µg/L) [OR = 2.4 (1.3, 4.5)]. The plasma levels of Se were positively correlated with fasting plasma glucose (FPG) ($r = 0.27$, $P < 0.001$). Plasma Se at the median (T2: 95.7–176 µg/L) or upper tertile (T3: $\geq$ 176 µg/L) was associated with increased risk of elevated FPG (defined by FPG $\geq$ 6.1 mmol/L) as compared with the lowest tertile (T1: $\leq$ 95.7 µg/L) [T2 vs. T1, OR = 3.5 (1.7, 7.0); T3 vs. T1, OR = 6.2 (3.0, 13)]. In addition, a case-control study in Italy compared the concentrations of several essential and nonessential metallic elements in the tear fluid and serum of patients with T2D and a group of non-diabetic controls (Cancarini et al. 2017), and showed that in both fluids Se concentrations were higher in diabetic patients than in the controls. In contrast, no association between Se and prevalence of T2D could be found in a population-based case-control study in Norway (Simic et al. 2017). The concentrations of Se in whole blood were measured in 267 patients with self-reported T2D and 609 controls selected from the third Nord-Trøndelag Health Survey. Multivariable conditional logistic regression and multivariable linear regression analyses showed no statistical evidence for associations between blood levels of Se and T2D prevalence.

Cross-Sectional Observation on Se and T2D

Most of the cross-sectional studies support a positive association between Se and prevalence of diabetes or fasting blood glucose (Bleys et al. 2007; Laclaustra et al. 2009; Czernichow et al. 2006; Stranges et al. 2011; Obeid et al. 2008; Wang et al. 2017; Su et al. 2016; Zhuo et al. 2004; Gao et al. 2007; Wei et al. 2015; Yin et al. 2015), while there are studies showing no significant (Coudray et al. 1997; Hughes et al. 1997) or negative associations (Rajpathak et al. 2005). In the USA, data from the National Health and Nutrition Examination Survey 1988–1994 (Bleys et al. 2007) and 2003–2004 (Laclaustra et al. 2009) consistently showed positive association between serum Se and prevalence of diabetes when mean serum Se of the US population increased from 127 to 137 µg/L. In France, where Se intake was relatively lower, the Supplementation with Antioxidant Vitamins and Minerals study showed that higher plasma Se levels were associated with higher FPG (Czernichow et al. 2006). In Italy, where the population Se status was also lower, the Olivetti Heart study on 445 adult male participants with average serum Se concentration of 77.5 ± 18.4 µg/L showed that serum Se levels were positively associated with the prevalence of diabetes (Stranges et al. 2011). The study on Lebanese adults supported the positive association as well (Obeid et al. 2008).

However, results from the cross-sectional and nested case-control analyses in another US study showed opposite correlation (Coudray et al. 1997). In Canada, a large population-based study on 2420 subjects without diabetes was carried out to explore the relationship of dietary Se intake with insulin resistance (Wang et al. 2017). High HOMA-IR groups in both males and females had the lowest dietary Se intake, and insulin resistance was decreased with the increase of dietary Se intake in females but not in males after controlling of confounding factors. Higher dietary Se intake was negatively correlated with HOMA-IR after adjusting for other confounding factors in subjects whose dietary Se intake was below 1.6 µg/kg BW/day. However, the negative correlation was no longer significant when dietary Se intake was above 1.6 µg/kg BW/day. Three recent cross-sectional studies in China showed a consistent positive relationship between high Se and diabetes. As a part of the Se and Cognitive Decline Study Cohort (Su et al. 2016), one study recruited 1856 elderly people (≥65 years old) from four Chinese rural counties with different soil Se levels during the 2010–2012 evaluation. The mean nail Se of this population was 0.46 µg/g which was much lower than that of the US population (Zhuo et al. 2004). Results showed that the mean nail Se level was significantly higher in the diabetes than that in the non-diabetes. Comparing with the first quartile group, the adjusted ORs (95% CI) for diabetes were 2.65 (1.48, 4.73), 2.47 (1.37, 4.45), and 3.30 (1.85, 5.88) from the second Se quartile to the fourth quartile, respectively. And the mean serum glucose and HOMA-IR in higher Se quartile groups were significantly higher compared with the lowest quartile group. These cross-sectional findings confirmed the 2002–2003 baseline conclusion according to self-reported diabetes incidence (Gao et al. 2007). Another study evaluated the relationship between dietary Se and diabetes in middle-aged and elderly Chinese adults (Wei et al. 2015). The dietary Se intakes were calculated from the semiquantitative food frequency questionnaire of 5423 subjects during routine health checkups, and diabetes was defined as a fasting blood glucose concentration ≥7.0 mmol/L or currently undergoing drug treatment for control of blood glucose. The average level of dietary Se intake of this urban population was 43.5 µg/day, and the prevalence of diabetes in the study population was 9.7%. The multivariate adjusted OR was 1.52 (1.01, 2.28) for the highest quartile of dietary Se intake in comparison with the lowest quartile. Another population-based, cross-sectional survey of chronic diseases and related risk factors was conducted in Jilin Province of Northeast China (Yin et al. 2015) and showed that hair Se was positively correlated with blood glucose levels ($r = 0.11$, $P = 0.01$).

Longitudinal Observation on Se and T2D

Few longitudinal studies have generated highly conflicting results on the relationship between Se and T2D. In the Epidemiology of Vascular Ageing study, higher baseline plasma Se was found to correlate with lower risk of incident dysglycemia during a 9-year follow-up period in elderly French men (Akbaraly et al. 2010), but no significant relationship in women. This implied a sex-specific effect. Later pooled longitudinal analysis further confirmed that at dietary levels of intake, individuals with higher toenail Se levels were at lower risk for T2D (Park et al. 2012). Although a cohort study in Northern Italy observed increased dietary Se intake associated with an increased risk of T2D (Stranges et al. 2010), a later population-based female cohort nested in this cohort for further exploring the association between baseline toenail Se exposure and incident of diabetes after a median follow-up of 16 years found no association between toenail Se and subsequent development of diabetes (Vinceti et al. 2015). Interestingly, no association between serum Se levels and incidents of diabetes was observed in another Italian longitudinal analysis of Olivetti Heart study (Stranges et al. 2011). In Sweden where the daily dietary intake of Se is still low in spite of decades of nutritional information campaigns (Alehagen et al. 2016), a cohort study on 1925 Swedish men aged 50-year-old without diabetes at baseline in the 1970s was carried out (Gao et al. 2014). The baseline mean serum Se concentration was 75.6 ± 14.3 µg/L. No association between baseline serum Se levels and risk of diabetes during the 20 years of follow-up (OR = 1.06; 95% CI = 0.83–1.38) was observed. Higher Se levels were associated with lower early insulin response at baseline after adjusting for potential confounders, but not with any other measures of β-cell function or insulin sensitivity at baseline or follow-up. However, the association with early insulin response was nonsignificant after taking multiple tests into account, which did not support a role of dietary Se in the development of disturbances in glucose metabolism or diabetes in older individuals. A recent meta-analysis of five previous observational studies (Wang et al. 2016), two cross-sectional studies (Bleys et al. 2007; Laclaustra et al. 2009) and three longitudinal studies (Stranges et al. 2010, 2011; Akbaraly et al. 2010), indicated that there was a significantly higher prevalence of T2D in the highest category of blood Se compared with the lowest (OR = 1.63; 95% CI = 1.04–2.56), and a positive association between serum Se levels and T2D existed in populations with relatively low levels (<97.5 µg/L) and high levels (>133 µg/L) of serum Se, indicating a likely U-shaped nonlinear dose-response relationship between serum Se and T2D.

Se Supplementation and the Risk of T2D

Population-based trials with Se supplementation were supposed to provide more powerful evidence for learning the association between Se and T2D. As reviewed by Rayman and Stranges (2013), of all the randomized controlled trials (RCTs) assessing the effect of Se supplementation on the risk of T2D of subjects without T2D at baseline, none had observed beneficial effect, one had observed adverse effect at the highest baseline of circulating Se tertile (>122 µg/L) (Stranges et al. 2007), and the rest had no effect (Lippman et al. 2009; Rayman et al. 2012; Algotar et al. 2010; Klein et al. 2011). After analyzing the data from 140 men (n = 46, 47, and 47 receiving 0, 200, and 800 µg Se/day, respectively, followed every 3 months for up to 5 years) (Algotar et al. 2010), Algotar et al. (2013) published another study on 699 men (n = 232, 234, and 233 receiving 0, 200, and 400 µg Se/day, respectively, followed every 6 months for up to 5 years). Data from neither study supported the effect of Se supplementation on DM prevention. The newly reported results from the Selenium and Celecoxib (Sel/Cel) Trial showed that Se supplementation might increase the risk of T2D (Thompson et al. 2016). In participants receiving Se, the hazard ratio for new-onset T2D was 1.25 (95% CI: 0.74–2.1), with a statistically significantly increased risk of Se-associated T2D among older participants (rate ratio = 2.21; 95% CI = 1.04–4.67). These findings need to be verified in RCT for assessing the effect of Se supplementation on the risk of T2D in general population.

Mechanism for the Relationship Between Se and DM

Redox Homeostasis and Glucose Metabolism

Insulin is synthesized and stored in the pancreatic β-cells. In these cells, H_2O_2 and other ROS regulate the expression of important transcriptional factors related to insulin synthesis and function including pancreatic duodenal homeobox 1 (PDX1) (Stoffers et al. 1998), nuclear factor kappa B subunit 1 (NF-κB) (Gloire et al. 2006), forkhead box O1a (FOXO1a) (Ponugoti et al. 2012; Klotz et al. 2015), and forkhead box A2 (FOXA2) (Hao et al. 2013) at the epigenetic, transcriptional, and/or post-translational levels. PDX1 is one of the most important transcription factors required for pancreatic development and β-cell differentiation and maturation (Offield et al. 1996). FOXO1a is a transcription factor for multiple genes including two gluconeo-genic enzymes, phosphoenolpyruvate carboxykinase (PEPCK or PCK) and glucose-6-phosphatase (G6P) (Cheng and White 2012), and SELENOP (Speckmann et al. 2008; Walter et al. 2008). Dephosphorylated FOXO1a is the active form that pro-motes expression of its target genes (Cheng and White 2012). FOXA2, a transcrip-tion factor, regulates genes involved in glucose (Wang et al. 2002) and lipid homeostasis (Kanaki and Kardassis 2017) in the liver. FOXA2 is activated under fasting conditions but is inhibited by insulin signaling via phosphatidylinositol 3-kinase (PI3K)/protein kinase B (AKT, a serine/threonine protein kinase) in a phosphorylation-dependent manner, which results in its nuclear exclusion (Howell and Stoffel 2009).

In the glucose-stimulated insulin secretion (GSIS) (Pi et al. 2007), insulin is released from the β-cells and transported to peripheral tissues via circulation. In hepatocytes and adipocytes, binding of insulin to its receptor stimulates a burst of H_2O_2 that temporarily inactivates protein-tyrosine phosphatase 1B (PTP1B or PTPN1: protein-tyrosine phosphatase, non-receptor type 1) and other protein phos-phatases and extends the phosphorylation of insulin receptor (INSR), insulin recep-tor substrate (IRS), and AKT (Mahadev et al. 2001). This H_2O_2-mediated fine regulation of the phosphorylation states of key molecules in the insulin signaling cascade is vitally important for the control of insulin action and sensitivity. Thus, physiological levels of ROS, notably H_2O_2, can play a positive, insulin-mimetic role (Czech et al. 1974). But on the other hand, excessive ROS have been shown to inhibit the insulin-induced tyrosine phosphorylation of the INSR β-subunit in NIH-B cells (Hansen et al. 1999), AKT activation (Gardner et al. 2003), and K(ATP) channel activation in vascular smooth muscle cells (Yasui et al. 2012). Furthermore, in diabetic subjects, sustained high blood glucose may induce oxidation and nonen-zymatic glycation of proteins, thus elevating ROS (Brownlee et al. 1988) and causing further deterioration of the diabetic condition and late complications (Roberts and Sindhu 2009). The dual role of ROS in insulin secretion and signaling might explain the poor success of clinical approaches that have attempted to use antioxidants for the treatment of diabetes (Rains and Jain 2011).

Moreover, an oxidative environment is required in the endoplasmic reticulum (ER) to oxidize thiol groups of cysteine (Cys) residues in newly synthesized proteins to disulfide bonds. Insufficient production of ROS might result in failure in protein folding in the ER, and if the misfolded proteins cannot be degraded due to the deficiency of antioxidants (including the ER-resident selenoproteins), the unfolded-protein response may activate the unfolded protein response or ER-stress. The three well-characterized pathways of ER stress are involved in ER stress of pancreatic β-cells, and were thought to be related to DM (Ariyasu et al. 2017; Watson 2014). Under conditions of obesity and T2D, the unfolded protein response affects both the major insulin target tissues and pancreatic β-cells, contributing to the development of inflammation, insulin resistance, and impaired insulin secretion (Cnop et al. 2012). Apparently, Se may affect the onset or development of DM through the redox-modulating capacity of selenoproteins, in addition to their involvement in the thyroid hormone metabolism (Moura Neto et al. 2016).

Roles of Selenoproteins and Their Related Proteins in Diabetes

Dual Roles of GPX1 as a ROS Scavenger

GPX1 is one of the most Se-sensitive selenoproteins in response to Se deprivation or repletion. Functionally, GPX1 catalyzes the reduction of H_2O_2 and organic hydroperoxides including peroxides of cholesterol, fatty acids, and other lipids (Ladenstein et al. 1979; Arthur 2000). Normal expression of GPX1 is fundamental to support insulin functions, while its absence or overexpression is a risk factor for DM. In the animal liver and/or in the cultured hepatocytes, GPX1 overexpression is somewhat coupled with elevated protein levels of SELENOS, SELENOT, MSRB1 (Labunskyy et al. 2011), and/or SELENOP (Wang et al. 2014), which may contribute partially to the T2D phenotypes. The expression or activity changes of GPX1 were reported in the aforementioned studies (Labunskyy et al. 2011; Mueller et al. 2008, 2009b; Zeng et al. 2012; Liu et al. 2012; Pinto et al. 2012), and its role in linking Se to DM was reviewed previously (Zhou et al. 2013, 2015b; Lei and Vatamaniuk 2016). Briefly, the following mechanisms may be used to explain the dual roles of GPX1 in DM. As pancreatic β-cells produce relatively low levels of GPX, superoxide dismutase (SOD), or catalase (CAT) (Grankvist et al. 1981), GPX1 protects them from being attacked by oxidants. Overexpression of GPX1 over-quenches intracellular ROS or H_2O_2, and thus impairs the insulin signaling pathway by attenuating the inactivation of PTP1B (Mueller et al. 2008, 2009b), suppressing the phosphorylation of INSR and AKT (McClung et al. 2004; Mahadev et al. 2004), and reducing the insulin sensitivity (Loh et al. 2009). The ROS diminished by extra-active GPX1 suppress the expression of glucose transporter 4 and its adenosine monophosphate-activated protein kinase (AMPK)-mediated translocation to the cell membrane to uptake extracellular glucose. Attenuated ROS production caused by the GPX1 over-expression induces the hyperacetylation of H3 and H4 histones in the approximate region of PDX1 promoter (Wang et al. 2008), elevates mRNA and/or protein or activity of PDX1 (Wang et al. 2008; Pepper et al. 2011; Yan et al. 2012), and activates several transcription factors involved in glucose metabolism, such as FOXA2, FOXO1a, peroxisome proliferator-activated receptor-γ coactivator 1α (PGC1α, formally known as PPARGC1A), and forkhead box O3 (Zhou et al. 2015a; Pinto et al. 2011, 2012; Yan et al. 2012).

These changes were concurrent with enhanced ASK1/MKK4/JNK signaling (Zhou et al. 2015a). In islet, overexpression of GPX1 accelerated GSIS and hyperinsulinemia by diminishing mitochondrial uncoupling protein 2 (UCP2), which controls the mitochondria-derived ROS required by GSIS (Wang et al. 2008; Pepper et al. 2011; Arsenijevic et al. 2000; Zhang et al. 2001; Leloup et al. 2009; Pi et al. 2010). In contrast, knockout of GPX1 alone or in combination with SOD1 had the opposite effect on these proteins or events (Loh et al. 2009; Wang et al. 2011).

Several single-nucleotide polymorphisms (SNPs) in the promoter region (rs1987628, rs8179164, and rs3448) and the 3' untranslated region (UTR) (rs9818758) of GPX1 were analyzed to investigate their associations with kidney complications and related oxidative stress in T1D patients. The minor T-allele of rs3448 was found to be associated with kidney complications and higher oxidative stress (Mohammedi et al. 2016). As the SNP is in the promoter region, the finding suggested the implication of GPX1 enzyme activity in the protection against oxidative stress in T1D patients. The missense polymorphism of GPX1 Pro198Leu (rs1050450 C/T) had 1.36 times higher risk of T2DM in North Indian population, and were in linkage disequilibrium with SOD2 Val16Ala (rs4880 T/C) (Vats et al. 2015). In Chinese, the above two SNPs and CAT-262C/T (rs1001179) were also analyzed between the T2D and health population. The combined genotype of TT-CC-CC for SOD2, GPX1, and CAT may contribute to the hypertriglyceridemia in T2D (Chen et al. 2012), which suggests coordination of multiple antioxidant enzymes with the T2D risk.

SELENOP as a Hepatokine Impairing Insulin Signaling

SELENOP possesses 10 to 18 Sec residues depending on the species (Stoytcheva et al. 2006). One Sec located close to its N-terminus accounts for the antioxidant property in extracellular fluids (Saito et al. 1999), and the remaining Sec residues within the C-terminus account for its Se transport function (Saito et al. 2004; Hill et al. 2007; Burk and Hill 2009). SELENOP is of great importance for Se homeostasis in the whole body (Burk and Hill 1994; Himeno et al. 1996) as well as for the Se transportation to the offspring via milk (Hill et al. 2014; Schweizer et al. 2004). Its receptors have been identified in brain (Burk et al. 2007), testis (Olson et al. 2007), kidney (Olson et al. 2008), and muscle (Misu et al. 2017). In circulation, the SELENOP concentration may serve as an indicator of Se nutritional status and it reaches a plateau at an intake of ~105 μg Se/day (Burk and Hill 2009; Xia et al. 2010).

Liver-derived SELENOP has been recognized to play roles in glucose metabolism and insulin sensitivity in a manner of hepatokine (Misu et al. 2017, 2010; Meex and Watt 2017). As a negative regulator of insulin signaling, SELENOP can lower the insulin-stimulated glucose uptake, impair the glucose tolerance, and produce insulin resistance by the counteracting regulation on the proteins in the insulin signaling and glucose metabolism pathway including INSR, AKT, PCK1 (soluble PEPCK), G6P, AMPK, and acetyl-CoA carboxylase 1 (Misu et al. 2010). Having the transcription factors FOXO1a and hepatocyte nuclear factor 4α within its gene promoter, SELENOP is regulated like a gluconeogenic enzyme in the liver of animals or cultured hepatocytes (Speckmann et al. 2008; Walter et al. 2008; Misu et al. 2010), and the co-activator PGC1α was proposed to link glucose metabolism and SELENOP expression (Steinbrenner et al. 2011; Speckmann et al. 2008). The elevated plasma SELENOP might be the result of abnormal glucose metabolism (Mao and Teng 2013; Steinbrenner 2013), and can be decreased by metformin, a drug suppressing hepatic gluconeogenesis and reduce blood glucose levels (Yalakanti and Dolia 2016). While the presence of SELENOP in pancreas has antioxidant protection to islets (Steinbrenner et al. 2013), the knockdown of SELENOP resulted in impaired adipogenesis, attenuated insulin signaling, and dysregulated production of adipokines (Zhang and Chen 2011). Though serum SELENOP levels were increased in adult subjects with either nonalcoholic fatty liver disease or visceral obesity (Choi et al. 2013; Yang et al. 2011), higher serum SELENOP was found in the non-MS children compared with the MS ones (aged 9 years old) (Ko et al. 2014). This suggested a different expression pattern of SELENOP between children and adult in the development of metabolic disorders. Low-density lipoprotein receptor-related protein 1 was identified to be the muscle-specific receptor of SELENOP (Misu et al. 2017) and to mediate its function in the response to exercise of skeletal muscle. Compared with the wild-type mice, *Selenop$^{-/-}$* mice were found to have enhanced responsiveness to regular exercise training with higher glucose-lowering effect of insulin, larger mitochondria in the muscular cells, and elevated expression of genes involved in mitochondrial function and slow-switch-type muscle fibers. While in the acute exercise, *Selenop$^{-/-}$* mice had higher amount of accumulation of oxidative stress and ROS-mediated AMPK phosphorylation, and elevated gene expression of *Ppargc1a* and its downstream genes involved in antioxidant system (*Cat* and *Sod2*) and mitochondrial function (*Ucp3* and estrogen-related receptor alpha) when compared with the wild-type mice. Additionally, SELENOP suppressed the effects of ROS (H_2O_2) on AMPK phosphorylation and *Ppargc1a* gene expression in cultured C2C12 myotubes. Thus, the antioxidant effects of SELENOP on the muscle under exercise condition were strongly suggested (Misu et al. 2017). However, the contribution of the elevated expression of Gpx1 and selenoprotein W needs further examination. Hyperlipidemic condition-induced SELENOP expression was suppressed by salsalate or full-length adiponectin through the activation of AMPK-FOXO1a pathway, resulting in improved glucose intolerance and insulin sensitivity. This implied SELENOP to be a target for salsalate and adiponectin to exhibit their antidiabetic effects (Jung et al. 2013).

Compared with the healthy people, T2D and obese patients had higher circulating SELENOP levels that were positively correlated with FPG (Zhou et al. 2015b; Misu et al. 2010, 2012; Mao and Teng 2013; Yang et al. 2011). But the plasma SELENOP concentration was not higher in GDM women ($n = 35$) than the control ($n = 22$), and was not associated with age, gestational age, prepregnancy body mass index (BMI), hemoglobin A1c, glucose concentrations at oral glucose tolerance test, or serum concentrations of total cholesterol, low-density lipoprotein cholesterol, and triglycerides, but associated with BMI and serum high-density lipoprotein cholesterol (Altinova et al. 2015). Plasma SELENOP concentration in the overweight/obsess subjects ($n = 34$) was higher than that in the lean subjects ($n = 29$), and was associated with insulin resistance. However, the association disappeared after adjusting BMI of subjects. SELENOP mRNA in subcutaneous adipose tissue was negatively correlated with BMI, suggesting a possible tissue-specific regulation. It seems that obesity, rather than insulin resistance, was central to the increase in SELENOP (Yang et al. 2011; Chen et al. 2017). Two highly correlated missense SNPs of rs28919926 (Cys368Arg) and rs146125471 (Ile293Met) were associated with acute insulin response, and the intronic SNP of rs16872779 was with fasting insulin levels, and rs7579 (C/T) in the 3'UTR was with insulin sensitivity index (Hellwege et al. 2014).

SELENOS Related to DM via Inflammation Pathway

SELENOS was firstly identified in Israeli sand rats (*Psammomys obesus*), and named as Tanis (Walder et al. 2002; Liu et al. 2009) or VIMP (valosin-containing protein/p97-interacting membrane protein) (Ye et al. 2004). SELENOS is a single-transmembrane protein, located at the ER membrane (Ye et al. 2004) and the plasma membrane (Gao et al. 2003). The early studies suggested SELENOS to be a glucose-regulated protein. In diabetic animals or cultured cells, its gene expression was inhibited by glucose or insulin, but was increased by fasting or glucose deficiency (Walder et al. 2002; Gao et al. 2004). While in human studies, SELENOS mRNA levels were increased in adipocytes isolated from obese or T2D adults after insulin treatment (Olsson et al. 2011; Karlsson et al. 2004), and were positively correlated with fasting serum insulin levels and HOMA-IR (Olsson et al. 2011; Du et al. 2008). These two parameters were also positively correlated with the 5227GG polymorphism [rs4965373, depending on alternative splicing is either in intron 6 or 3'UTR (Martinez et al. 2008)] (Olsson et al. 2011).

Being a target of the transcriptional factor NF-κB (Gao et al. 2003; Rock and Moos 2009) and a putative receptor for the acute-phase protein serum amyloid A (SAA) (Walder et al. 2002), SELENOS has been proposed to be associated with diabetes risk, possibly through inflammatory signaling pathways (Walder et al. 2002; Curran et al. 2005; Gao et al. 2006; Zhang et al. 2011). Hepatic mRNA levels of SELENOS and SAA were significantly elevated in rats that developed insulin resistance from ingesting a high-fat diet, compared with lean control rats and rosiglitazone-treated insulin-resistant rats (Liu et al. 2009). Human study also found

SELENOS mRNA level to be positively correlated with serum SAA (Du et al. 2008). Furthermore, the minor allele of rs4965373 polymorphism was associated with high plasma cytokine (serum IL-1β), while the minor alleles of −105G/A (rs28665122) in the promoter and the +3705G/A (rs4965814) in an intron were associated with elevated serum TNFα, IL-6, and IL-1β (Curran et al. 2005).

Through inflammatory signaling pathways, overexpression of SELENOS lowered glucose uptake and glycogen biosynthesis in hepatocytes, and attenuated the inhibition of insulin on PEPCK gene expression. It promoted gluconeogenesis, but had no effect on the insulin-stimulated phosphorylation of INSR (Gao et al. 2003). A recent review has given more detailed discussion on SELENOS and DM (Yu and Du 2017). Furthermore, a recent study reported that, in cultured neuronal cells, increased expression of SELENOS mediated the effect of selenate to reduce the ER-stress-induced-phosphorylation of tau protein and had the potential to mitigate the pathologic reaction of Alzheimer's disease (Rueli et al. 2017), which was referred to as "type 3 diabetes" featuring the overlap with both T1D and T2D at the molecular and biochemical levels (de la Monte and Wands 2008).

Other Selenoproteins and DM

DIOs

Predominantly expressed in thyroid, liver, and kidney, DIO1 activates 3,5,3′,5′-tetraiodothyronine (T4) to the bioactive 3,5,3′-triiodothyronine (T3) by 5′-deiodination. A functional defect of DIO1 presumably impairs energy metabolism, and its correlation with glucose metabolism has been reported (Bos et al. 2017). In addition to DIO1, the ER membrane-residing DIO2 catalyzes the conversion of T4 to T3 in thyroid and some other peripheral tissues (e.g., brain, pituitary gland, brown adipose tissues, muscle, etc.) (Arrojo and Bianco 2011). In humans, a polymorphism in the coding region of the DIO2 gene (Thr92Ala, rs225014) was linked to insulin resistance, as Ala/Ala homozygotes exhibited a higher risk for T2D (Mentuccia et al. 2002; Canani et al. 2005; Dora et al. 2010). The 92Ala homozygous variant was associated with lower levels of DIO2, T3/T4 ratio, and paraoxonase activity (Yalakanti and Dolia 2016). Elevated FPG and insulin resistance were observed in $Dio2^{-/-}$ mice. Being fed a high-fat diet, these mice were more obese and glucose intolerant (Marsili et al. 2011), and had higher hepatic deposition of triglycerides (Castillo et al. 2011) than wild-type mice. Hypothyroidism was associated with insulin resistance that could be improved with the thyroid hormone treatment (Rochon et al. 2003). However, serum T3 was not lower in $Dio2^{-/-}$ mice than in wild-type mice (Marsili et al. 2011). Thus, the mechanism of DIO2 deletion on glucose metabolism dysregulation requires further exploration. DIO3 inactivates T4 to inactive reverse T3 or T3 to reverse T2, and is highly expressed (as mRNA and protein) in embryonic and adult pancreatic islets, predominantly in β-cells in both humans and mice (Medina et al. 2011). Knockout of $Dio3$ io in adult mice led to reduced mass, function, and key gene expressions in β-cells, and subsequently impaired insulin secretion and glucose homeostasis.

GPX3

GPX3 is expressed in various tissues as an extracellular selenoprotein. Kidney is probably the predominant source of plasma GPX3 (Avissar et al. 1994; Malinouski et al. 2012), which accounts for nearly all the GPX activity in the plasma (Olson et al. 2010). Accumulating evidences have suggested an association between GPX3 expression/activity and T2D. The expression of GPX3 was changed in a tissue-dependent manner under conditions of T2D or obesity. Lee et al. (2008) reported that *Gpx3* expression was decreased in serum and the adipose tissue, but was increased slightly in the kidneys of ob/ob and db/db mice. Also, *Gpx3* expression in the adipose tissue was remarkably decreased in the high-fat diet-induced obese mice. In line with this, the plasma GPX3 protein levels and the total plasma GPX activity were substantially diminished in obese human subjects (Lee et al. 2008). Moreover, Chung et al. (2009) have shown that plasma GPX3 concentrations were decreased in newly diagnosed, drug-naïve diabetic patients compared with subjects with normal or impaired glucose tolerance, and Gpx3 mRNA levels in the skeletal muscle were lower in db/db or high-fat diet-induced obese mice than in normal mice.

Lee et al. (2008) have further investigated the regulatory role of adipose GPX3 in glucose metabolism. They have shown that GPX3 overexpression in adipocytes improved high glucose-induced insulin resistance and attenuated inflammatory gene expression, whereas GPX3 neutralization in adipocytes promoted expression of proinflammatory genes. Moreover, the antioxidant N-acetyl cysteine and the anti-diabetic drug rosiglitazone increased adipose *Gpx3* expression in obese and diabetic db/db mice. Consistently, troglitazone-mediated activation of peroxisome proliferator-activated receptor gamma (PPARγ, PPARG in GenBank) in human skeletal muscle cells induced gene expression of GPX3, and GPX3 overexpression reduced glucose oxidase-induced extracellular H_2O_2 levels and insulin resistance in these cells (Chung et al. 2009). In contrast, inhibition of GPX3 expression by short interfering RNA prevented the antioxidant effects of troglitazone on insulin action in oxidative stress-induced insulin-resistant cells, suggesting that GPX3 was required for the regulation of PPARγ-mediated antioxidant effects. Taken together, these results have suggested GPX3 as a promising drug target for T2D therapy.

SELENOM

SELENOM is localized in the ER and is involved in the thiol-disulfide exchange through its thioredoxin-like domain (Ferguson et al. 2006). SELENOM was shown to regulate calcium signaling and protect against oxidative stress in vitro (Reeves et al. 2010). Intriguingly, knockout of *Selenom* in mice resulted in adult-onset BW gain and increased adiposity, suggesting that SELENOM might play an important role in obesity. This hypothesis was further supported by high expression of SELENOM in the paraventricular nucleus and the arcuate nucleus of the hypothalamus, which were implicated in energy homeostasis. The arcuate nucleus contains neurons expressing the leptin receptor, which is activated by leptin (Ozcan et al. 2009), and in turn activates the JAK2-STAT3 Jak2-Stat3 pathway. Leptin resistance in the hypothalamus leads to dysregulation of energy metabolism and consequent metabolic disease. Whole-body knockout of Selenom in mice resulted in elevated circulating leptin levels and diminished phosphorylated STAT3 levels in the hypothalamus, indicating a state of leptin resistance (Pitts et al. 2013).

Accordingly, SELENOM may play its role in energy metabolism through regulating leptin signaling. Because ER stress is implicated in hypothalamic leptin resistance (Ozcan et al. 2009), SELENOM, as an ER-resident protein, may promote leptin signaling by protecting against ER stress.

SELENOT

SELENOT is ubiquitously expressed throughout embryonic development and in adulthood of rats, with high expression in pituitary, pancreas, testis, and thyroid (Tanguy et al. 2011), and mainly localized in ER membrane through a hydrophobic domain in all hormone-producing pituitary cell types (Hamieh et al. 2017). As a target gene of the pituitary adenylate cyclase-activating polypeptide (PACAP) in neuroendocrine cells including pancreatic β-cells, SELENOT is upregulated by PACAP coupling Ca^{2+} and induces hormone secretion (Grumolato et al. 2008). Moreover, SELENOT is a novel subunit of the A-type oligosaccharyltransferase, indispensable for its integrity and for ER homeostasis, and exerting a pivotal adaptive function that allows endocrine cells to properly achieve the maturation and secretion of hormones. This may also be a mechanism for its roles in insulin production. When SELENOT was deleted in human and murine pancreatic β-cells, impaired glucose tolerance due to a defect in insulin production/secretion was present (Prevost et al. 2013).

It is noteworthy that DIO2, SELENOM, SELENOS, and SELENOT are all located in the ER. Alterations of the later three members are potentially able to shift the redox status or functional integrity of the ER (Ye et al. 2004; Ozcan et al. 2009; Lilley and Ploegh 2004; Boukhzar et al. 2016). In addition, the blood glucose level and pancreatic function are also associated with pancreatic redox homeostasis via a modulated selenotranscriptome in chickens (Xiang et al. 2017). Even without affecting the mRNA abundances of GPX1 and SELENOP, supranutrition of Se and high-fat diet decreased the expressions (as mRNA and/or protein) of IRS1, IRS2, and PGC1α; attenuated IRS/PI3K/AKT signaling; and impaired insulin sensitivity (Stahel et al. 2017). Likely, there are other selenoproteins to be unraveled for the pro-diabetic effect of Se.

Selenoprotein Synthesis/Metabolism and DM

Key proteins involved in the selenoprotein synthesis and mentalism are also related to DM.

An overall selenoprotein deficiency caused by overexpressing an i(6)A(−) mutant Sec tRNA promoted glucose intolerance and led to a T2D-like phenotype in mice (Labunskyy et al. 2011). However, severely decreased synthesis of multiple selenoproteins and a multisystem disorder caused by a mutation in the gene for the Sec insertion sequence-binding protein 2 in humans enhanced systemic and cellular insulin sensitivity (Schoenmakers et al. 2010). In the Sec lyase (Scly, an enzyme required for Sec decomposition) knockout mice, phenotypes of MS and DM were observed either when selenoprotein level and circulating Se status were maintained by adequate Se supply or when hepatic GPX1 and SELENOS production and circulating SELENOP levels were diminished by Se restriction. Moreover, Scly disruption elevated levels of insulin-signaling inhibitor PTP1B (Seale et al. 2012).

Conclusion and Perspective

Data from both animal and human studies seem to be consistent in supporting a relationship between the Se intake/status and the diabetic risk. Our understanding of the Se role in diabetes has evolved from the view of Se as an insulin mimic to a dual-etiological factor of the diabetes onset and development. Limited human data indicate a pro-diabetic potential of Se supplementation to subjects with high baseline of Se status. After the discovery of T2D-like phenotypes in the GPX1 overexpression mice, involvements of SELENOP, GPX3, SELENOS, SELENOM, SELENOT, DIO1, DIO2, and a couple of selenoprotein synthesis and metabolism-related factors in diabetes, insulin resistance, obesity, and (or) MS have been studied using various gene knockout or overexpressing mouse models. Impacts of these selenoproteins on diabetes may be mediated through regulations of redox status, ER stress, inflammation, and thyroid hormones. Meanwhile, polymorphism of selenoprotein genes such as GPX1 and SELENOP in humans has offered clues to the mechanism for the association of Se/selenoproteins and diabetic risk. Apparently, novel mechanisms and more selenoproteins remain to be revealed for the complete role of Se in the onset and development of diabetes.

Because the optimal dietary intakes of Se for the general population and appropriate Se status for individuals to prevent or treat diabetes are far from clear, the current emphasis on improving Se status for maximal antioxidant defense may expose the public to the risk of stepping close to a dangerous border of overdosing of this micronutrient with dual role in diabetes. Due to confounding factors associated with cross-sectional and longitudinal observational human studies (Rayman and Stranges 2013; Ogawa-Wong et al. 2016), well-designed and long-term RCT is needed to determine the direct effect and optimal intake of Se for glucose homeostasis for subjects of different age, gender, and health condition.

Acknowledgments Research in the authors' laboratories was supported in part by NIH DK53018 and NSFC Projects 30628019, 30700585, 30871844, 31320103920, 81172669, 81372993, and 31270870. No conflict of interest is claimed by all the authors.

References

Agbor GA, et al. Effect of selenium- and glutathione-enriched yeast supplementation on a combined atherosclerosis and diabetes hamster model. J Agric Food Chem. 2007;55(21):8731–6.

Akbaraly TN, et al. Plasma selenium and risk of dysglycemia in an elderly French population: results from the prospective Epidemiology of Vascular Ageing Study. Nutr Metab (Lond). 2010;7:21.

Alehagen U, et al. Relatively high mortality risk in elderly Swedish subjects with low selenium status. Eur J Clin Nutr. 2016;70(1):91–6.

Algotar AM, et al. No effect of selenium supplementation on serum glucose levels in men with prostate cancer. Am J Med. 2010;123(8):765–8.

Algotar AM, et al. Selenium supplementation has no effect on serum glucose levels in men at high risk of prostate cancer. J Diabetes. 2013;5(4):465–70.

Altinova AE, et al. Selenoprotein P is not elevated in gestational diabetes mellitus. Gynecol Endocrinol. 2015;31(11):874–6.

Ariyasu D, Yoshida H, Hasegawa Y. Endoplasmic reticulum (ER) stress and endocrine disorders. Int J Mol Sci. 2017;18(2):E382.

Arrojo EDR, Bianco AC. Type 2 deiodinase at the crossroads of thyroid hormone action. Int J Biochem Cell Biol. 2011;43(10):1432–41.

Arsenijevic D, et al. Disruption of the uncoupling protein-2 gene in mice reveals a role in immunity and reactive oxygen species production. Nat Genet. 2000;26(4):435–9.

Arthur JR. The glutathione peroxidases. Cell Mol Life Sci. 2000;57(13–14):1825–35.

Asayama K, Kooy NW, Burr IM. Effect of vitamin E deficiency and selenium deficiency on insulin secretory reserve and free radical scavenging systems in islets: decrease of islet manganosuperoxide dismutase. J Lab Clin Med. 1986;107(5):459–64.

Avissar N, et al. Human kidney proximal tubules are the main source of plasma glutathione peroxidase. Am J Phys. 1994;266(2 Pt 1):C367–75.

Ayaz M, et al. Protective effect of selenium treatment on diabetes-induced myocardial structural alterations. Biol Trace Elem Res. 2002;89(3):215–26.

Aydemir-Koksoy A, Turan B. Selenium inhibits proliferation signaling and restores sodium/potassium pump function of diabetic rat aorta. Biol Trace Elem Res. 2008;126(1–3):237–45.

Battell ML, Delgatty HL, McNeill JH. Sodium selenate corrects glucose tolerance and heart function in STZ diabetic rats. Mol Cell Biochem. 1998;179(1–2):27–34.

Becker DJ, et al. Oral selenate improves glucose homeostasis and partly reverses abnormal expression of liver glycolytic and gluconeogenic enzymes in diabetic rats. Diabetologia. 1996;39(1):3–11.

Berg EA, et al. Insulin-like effects of vanadate and selenate on the expression of glucose-6-phosphate dehydrogenase and fatty acid synthase in diabetic rats. Biochimie. 1995;77(12):919–24.

Bleys J, Navas-Acien A, Guallar E. Serum selenium and diabetes in U.S. adults. Diabetes Care. 2007;30(4):829–34.

Bos MM, et al. Thyroid Signaling, Insulin Resistance, and 2 Diabetes Mellitus: A Mendelian Randomization Study. J Clin Endocrinol Metab. 2017;102(6):1960–70.

Boukhzar L, et al. Selenoprotein T exerts an essential oxidoreductase activity that protects dopaminergic neurons in mouse models of parkinson's disease. Antioxid Redox Signal. 2016;24(11):557–74.

Brigelius-Flohe R, Flohe L. Selenium and redox signaling. Arch Biochem Biophys. 2017;617:48–59.

Brownlee M, Cerami A, Vlassara H. Advanced glycosylation end products in tissue and the biochemical basis of diabetic complications. N Engl J Med. 1988;318(20):1315–21.

Bunk MJ, Combs GF Jr. Relationship of selenium-dependent glutathione peroxidase activity and nutritional pancreatic atrophy in selenium-deficient chicks. J Nutr. 1981;111(9):1611–20.

Burk RF, Hill KE. Selenoprotein P. A selenium-rich extracellular glycoprotein. J Nutr. 1994;124(10):1891–7.

Burk RF, Hill KE. Selenoprotein P-expression, functions, and roles in mammals. Biochim Biophys Acta. 2009;1790(11):1441–7.

Burk RF, et al. Deletion of apolipoprotein E receptor-2 in mice lowers brain selenium and causes severe neurological dysfunction and death when a low-selenium diet is fed. J Neurosci. 2007;27(23):6207–11.

Campbell SC, et al. Selenium stimulates pancreatic beta-cell gene expression and enhances islet function. FEBS Lett. 2008;582(15):2333–7.

Can B, et al. Selenium treatment protects diabetes-induced biochemical andultrastructural alterations in liver tissue. Biol Trace Elem Res. 2005;105(1–3):135–50.

Canani LH, et al. The type 2 deiodinase A/G (Thr92Ala) polymorphism is associated with decreased enzyme velocity and increased insulin resistance in patients with type 2 diabetes mellitus. J Clin Endocrinol Metab. 2005;90(6):3472–8.

Cancarini A, et al. Trace elements and diabetes: assessment of levels in tears and serum. Exp Eye Res. 2017;154:47–52.

Castillo M, et al. Disruption of thyroid hormone activation in type 2 deiodinase knockout mice causes obesity with glucose intolerance and liver steatosis only at thermoneutrality. Diabetes. 2011;60(4):1082–9.

Chen H, et al. Polymorphic variations in manganese superoxide dismutase (MnSOD), glutathione peroxidase-1 (GPX1), and catalase (CAT) contribute to elevated plasma triglyceride levels in Chinese patients with type 2 diabetes or diabetic cardiovascular disease. Mol Cell Biochem. 2012;363(1–2):85–91.

Chen M, et al. Selenoprotein P is elevated in individuals with obesity, but is not independently associated with insulin resistance. Obes Res Clin Pract. 2017;11(2):227–32.

Cheng Z, White MF. The AKTion in non-canonical insulin signaling. Nat Med. 2012;18(3):351–3.

Choi HY, et al. Increased selenoprotein p levels in subjects with visceral obesity and nonalcoholic Fatty liver disease. Diabetes Metab J. 2013;37(1):63–71.

Chung SS, et al. Glutathione peroxidase 3 mediates the antioxidant effect of peroxisome proliferator-activated receptor gamma in human skeletal muscle cells. Mol Cell Biol. 2009;29(1):20–30.

Cnop M, Foufelle F, Velloso LA. Endoplasmic reticulum stress, obesity and diabetes. Trends Mol Med. 2012;18(1):59–68.

Coudray C, et al. Lipid peroxidation level and antioxidant micronutrient status in a pre-aging population; correlation with chronic disease prevalence in a French epidemiological study (Nantes, France). J Am Coll Nutr. 1997;16(6):584–91.

Curran JE, et al. Genetic variation in selenoprotein S influences inflammatory response. Nat Genet. 2005;37(11):1234–41.

Czech MP, Lawrence JC Jr, Lynn WS. Evidence for electron transfer reactions involved in the Cu2+ −dependent thiol activation of fat cell glucose utilization. J Biol Chem. 1974;249(4):1001–6.

Czernichow S, et al. Antioxidant supplementation does not affect fasting plasma glucose in the Supplementation with Antioxidant Vitamins and Minerals (SU.VI.MAX) study in France: association with dietary intake and plasma concentrations. Am J Clin Nutr. 2006;84(2):395–9.

Division for Nutrition, D.V.a.F.A. Safe upper intake levels for vitamins and minerals. 2006.

Dora JM, et al. Association of the type 2 deiodinase Thr92Ala polymorphism with type 2 diabetes: case-control study and meta-analysis. Eur J Endocrinol. 2010;163(3):427–34.

Douillet C, et al. Effect of selenium and vitamin E supplements on tissue lipids, peroxides, and fatty acid distribution in experimental diabetes. Lipids. 1998;33(4):393–9.

Du JL, et al. Association of SelS mRNA expression in omental adipose tissue withHoma-IR and serum amyloid A in patients with type 2 diabetes mellitus. Chin Med J. 2008;121(13):1165–8.

Erbayraktar Z, et al. Effects of selenium supplementation on antioxidant defense and glucose homeostasis in experimental diabetes mellitus. Biol Trace Elem Res. 2007;118(3):217–26.

Ezaki O. The insulin-like effects of selenate in rat adipocytes. J Biol Chem. 1990;265(2):1124–8.

Fairweather-Tait SJ, et al. Selenium in human health and disease. Antioxid Redox Signal. 2011;14(7):1337–83.

Ferguson AD, et al. NMR structures of the selenoproteins Sep15 and SelM reveal redox activity of a new thioredoxin-like family. J Biol Chem. 2006;281(6):3536–43.

Furnsinn C, et al. Insulin-like vs. non-insulin-like stimulation of glucose metabolism by vanadium, tungsten, and selenium compounds in rat muscle. Life Sci. 1996;59(23):1989–2000.

Gao Y, et al. Elevation in Tanis expression alters glucose metabolism and insulin sensitivity in H4IIE cells. Diabetes. 2003;52(4):929–34.

Gao Y, et al. Regulation of the selenoprotein SelS by glucose deprivation and endoplasmic reticulum stress - SelS is a novel glucose-regulated protein. FEBS Lett. 2004;563(1–3):185–90.

Gao Y, et al. Activation of the selenoprotein SEPS1 gene expression by pro-inflammatory cytokines in HepG2 cells. Cytokine. 2006;33(5):246–51.

Gao S, et al. Selenium level and cognitive function in rural elderly Chinese. Am J Epidemiol. 2007;165(8):955–65.

Gao H, et al. Serum selenium in relation to measures of glucose metabolism and incidence of Type 2 diabetes in an older Swedish population. Diabet Med. 2014;31(7):787–93.

Gardner CD, et al. Hydrogen peroxide inhibits insulin signaling in vascular smooth muscle cells. Exp Biol Med (Maywood). 2003;228(7):836–42.

Gloire G, Legrand-Poels S, Piette J. NF-kappaB activation by reactive oxygen species: fifteen years later. Biochem Pharmacol. 2006;72(11):1493–505.

Grankvist K, Marklund SL, Taljedal IB. CuZn-superoxide dismutase, Mn-superoxide dismutase, catalase and glutathione peroxidase in pancreatic islets and other tissues in the mouse. Biochem J. 1981;199(2):393–8.

Grumolato L, et al. Selenoprotein T is a PACAP-regulated gene involved in intracellular Ca2+ mobilization and neuroendocrine secretion. FASEB J. 2008;22(6):1756–68.

Hamieh A, et al. Selenoprotein T is a novel OST subunit that regulates UPR signalingand hormone secretion. EMBO Rep. 2017;18(11):1935–46.

Hansen LL, et al. Insulin signaling is inhibited by micromolar concentrations of H(2)O(2). Evidence for a role of H(2)O(2) in tumor necrosis factor alpha-mediated insulin resistance. J Biol Chem. 1999;274(35):25078–84.

Hao Y, et al. Pyocyanin-induced mucin production is associated with redox modification of FOXA2. Respir Res. 2013;14:82.

Hei YJ, et al. Stimulation of MAP kinase and S6 kinase by vanadium and selenium in rat adipocytes. Mol Cell Biochem. 1998;178(1–2):367–75.

Hellwege JN, et al. Genetic variants in selenoprotein P plasma 1 gene (SEPP1) are associated with fasting insulin and first phase insulin response in Hispanics. Gene. 2014;534(1):33–9.

Hill KE, et al. The selenium-rich C-terminal domain of mouse selenoprotein P is necessary for the supply of selenium to brain and testis but not for the maintenance of whole body selenium. J Biol Chem. 2007;282(15):10972–80.

Hill KE, et al. Selenoprotein P is the major selenium transport protein in mouse milk. PLoS One. 2014;9(7):e103486.

Himeno S, Chittum HS, Burk RF. Isoforms of selenoprotein P in rat plasma. Evidence for a full-length form and another form that terminates at the second UGA in the open reading frame. J Biol Chem. 1996;271(26):15769–75.

Howell JJ, Stoffel M. Nuclear export-independent inhibition of Foxa2 by insulin. J Biol Chem. 2009;284(37):24816–24.

Huang JQ, et al. The selenium deficiency disease exudative diathesis in chicks is associated with downregulation of seven common selenoprotein genes in liver and muscle. J Nutr. 2011;141(9):1605–10.

Hughes K, et al. Central obesity, insulin resistance, syndrome X, lipoprotein(a), and cardiovascular risk in Indians, Malays, and Chinese in Singapore. J Epidemiol Community Health. 1997;51(4):394–9.

Hwang D, et al. Selenium acts as an insulin-like molecule for the down-regulation of diabetic symptoms via endoplasmic reticulum stress and insulin signalling proteins in diabetes-induced non-obese diabetic mice. J Biosci. 2007;32(4):723–35.

Jung TW, et al. Salsalate and adiponectin improve palmitate-induced insulin resistance via inhibition of selenoprotein P through the AMPK-FOXO1alpha pathway. PLoS One. 2013;8(6):e66529.

Juszczuk-Kubiak E, et al. Effect of inorganic dietary selenium supplementation on selenoprotein and lipid metabolism gene expression patterns in liver and loin muscle of growing lambs. Biol Trace Elem Res. 2016;172(2):336–45.

Kanaki M, Kardassis D. Regulation of the human lipoprotein lipase gene by the forkhead box transcription factor FOXA2/HNF-3beta in hepatic cells. Biochim Biophys Acta. 2017;1860(3):327–36.

Karlsson HK, et al. Relationship between serum amyloid A level and Tanis/SelS mRNA expression in skeletal muscle and adipose tissue from healthy and type 2 diabetic subjects. Diabetes. 2004;53(6):1424–8.

Klein EA, et al. Vitamin E and the risk of prostate cancer: the selenium and vitamin E cancer prevention trial (SELECT). JAMA. 2011;306(14):1549–56.

Kljai K, Runje R. Selenium and glycogen levels in diabetic patients. Biol Trace Elem Res. 2001;83(3):223–9.

Klotz LO, et al. Redox regulation of FoxO transcription factors. Redox Biol. 2015;6:51–72.

Ko BJ, et al. Levels of circulating selenoprotein P, fibroblast growth factor (FGF) 21 and FGF23 in relation to the metabolic syndrome in young children. Int J Obes. 2014;38(12):1497–502.

Kryukov GV, et al. Characterization of mammalian selenoproteomes. Science. 2003;300(5624):1439–43.

de la Monte SM, Wands JR. Alzheimer's disease is type 3 diabetes-evidence reviewed. J Diabetes Sci Technol. 2008;2(6):1101–13.

Labunskyy VM, et al. Both maximal expression of selenoproteins and selenoprotein deficiency can promote development of type 2 diabetes-like phenotype in mice. Antioxid Redox Signal. 2011;14(12):2327–36.

Laclaustra M, et al. Serum selenium concentrations and diabetes in U.S. adults: National Health and Nutrition Examination Survey (NHANES) 2003-2004. Environ Health Perspect. 2009;117(9):1409–13.

Ladenstein R, et al. Structure analysis and molecular model of the selenoenzyme glutathione peroxidase at 2.8 A resolution. J Mol Biol. 1979;134(2):199–218.

Lee YS, et al. Dysregulation of adipose glutathione peroxidase 3 in obesity contributes to local and systemic oxidative stress. Mol Endocrinol. 2008;22(9):2176–89.

Lei XG, Vatamaniuk MZ. Two tales of antioxidant enzymes on beta cells and diabetes. Antioxid Redox Signal. 2011;14(3):489–503.

Lei XG, Vatamaniuk M. Glutathione peroxidase 1: models for diabetes and obesity. In: Hatfield DL, et al., editors. Selenium: its molecular biology and role in human health. New York: Springer; 2016. p. 587–94.

Leloup C, et al. Mitochondrial reactive oxygen species are obligatory signals for glucose-induced insulin secretion. Diabetes. 2009;58(3):673–81.

Li X, et al. Inhibition of islet amyloid polypeptide fibril formation by selenium-containing phycocyanin and prevention of beta cell apoptosis. Biomaterials. 2014;35(30):8596–604.

Li XT, et al. Association between plasma metal levels and diabetes risk: a case-control study in China. Biomed Environ Sci. 2017;30(7):482–91.

Lilley BN, Ploegh HL. A membrane protein required for dislocation of misfolded proteins from the ER. Nature. 2004;429(6994):834–40.

Lippman SM, et al. Effect of selenium and vitamin E on risk of prostate cancer and other cancers: the Selenium and Vitamin E Cancer Prevention Trial (SELECT). JAMA. 2009;301(1):39–51.

Liu J, et al. Upregulation of Tanis mRNA expression in the liver is associated with insulin resistance in rats. Tohoku J Exp Med. 2009;219(4):307–10.

Liu Y, et al. Prolonged dietary selenium deficiency or excess does not globally affect selenoprotein gene expression and/or protein production in various tissues of pigs. J Nutr. 2012;142(8):1410–6.

Loh K, et al. Reactive oxygen species enhance insulin sensitivity. Cell Metab. 2009;10(4):260–72.

Lu CW, et al. High serum selenium levels are associated with increased risk for diabetes mellitus independent of central obesity and insulin resistance. BMJ Open Diabetes Res Care. 2016;4(1):e000253.

Mahadev K, et al. Insulin-stimulated hydrogen peroxide reversibly inhibits protein-tyrosine phosphatase 1b in vivo and enhances the early insulin action cascade. J Biol Chem. 2001;276(24):21938–42.

Mahadev K, et al. The NAD(P)H oxidase homolog Nox4 modulates insulin-stimulated generation of H2O2 and plays an integral role in insulin signal transduction. Mol Cell Biol. 2004;24(5):1844–54.

Malinouski M, et al. High-resolution imaging of selenium in kidneys: a localizedselenium pool associated with glutathione peroxidase 3. Antioxid Redox Signal. 2012;16(3):185–92.

Mao J, Teng W. The relationship between selenoprotein P and glucosemetabolism in experimental studies. Nutrients. 2013;5(6):1937–48.

Marsili A, et al. Mice with a targeted deletion of the type 2 deiodinase are insulin resistant and susceptible to diet induced obesity. PLoS One. 2011;6(6):e20832.

Martinez A, et al. Polymorphisms in the selenoprotein S gene: lack of association with autoimmune inflammatory diseases. BMC Genomics. 2008;9:329.

McClung JP, et al. Development of insulin resistance and obesity in mice overexpressing cellular glutathione peroxidase. Proc Natl Acad Sci U S A. 2004;101(24):8852–7.

McNeill JH, Delgatty HL, Battell ML. Insulinlike effects of sodium selenate in streptozocin-induced diabetic rats. Diabetes. 1991;40(12):1675–8.

Medina MC, et al. The thyroid hormone-inactivating type III deiodinase is expressed in mouse and human beta-cells and its targeted inactivation impairs insulin secretion. Endocrinology. 2011;152(10):3717–27.

Meex RCR, Watt MJ. Hepatokines: linking nonalcoholic fatty liver disease and insulin resistance. Nat Rev Endocrinol. 2017;13(9):509–20.

Mentuccia D, et al. Association between a novel variant of the human type 2deiodinase gene Thr92Ala and insulin resistance: evidence of interaction with the Trp64Arg variant of the beta-3-adrenergic receptor. Diabetes. 2002;51(3):880–3.

Misu H, et al. A liver-derived secretory protein, selenoprotein P, causes insulin resistance. Cell Metab. 2010;12(5):483–95.

Misu H, et al. Inverse correlation between serum levels of selenoprotein P and adiponectin in patients with type 2 diabetes. PLoS One. 2012;7(4):e34952.

Misu H, et al. Deficiency of the hepatokine selenoprotein P increases responsiveness to exercise in mice through upregulation of reactive oxygen species and AMP-activated protein kinase in muscle. Nat Med. 2017;23(4):508–16.

Mohammedi K, et al. Glutathione peroxidase-1 gene (GPX1) variants, oxidative stress and risk of kidney complications in people with type 1 diabetes. Metabolism. 2016;65(2):12–9.

Moura Neto A, et al. Relation of thyroid hormone abnormalities with subclinical inflammatory activity in patients with type 1 and type 2 diabetes mellitus. Endocrine. 2016;51(1):63–71.

Mueller AS, Pallauf J. Compendium of the antidiabetic effects of supranutritional selenate doses. In vivo and in vitro investigations with type II diabetic db/db mice. J Nutr Biochem. 2006;17(8):548–60.

Mueller AS, Pallauf J, Rafael J. The chemical form of selenium affects insulinomimetic properties of the trace element: investigations in type II diabetic dbdb mice. J Nutr Biochem. 2003;14(11):637–47.

Mueller AS, et al. Redox regulation of protein tyrosine phosphatase 1B by manipulation of dietary selenium affects the triglyceride concentration in rat liver. J Nutr. 2008;138(12):2328–36.

Mueller AS, et al. Selenium and diabetes: an enigma? Free Radic Res. 2009a;43(11):1029–59.

Mueller AS, et al. Regulation of the insulin antagonistic protein tyrosine phosphatase 1B by dietary Se studied in growing rats. J Nutr Biochem. 2009b;20(4):235–47.

Mukherjee B, et al. Novel implications of the potential role of selenium on antioxidant status in streptozotocin-induced diabetic mice. Biomed Pharmacother. 1998;52(2):89–95.

Navarro-Alarcon M, et al. Serum and urine selenium concentrations as indicators of body status in patients with diabetes mellitus. Sci Total Environ. 1999;228(1):79–85.

NCD-RisC. Worldwide trends in diabetes since 1980: a pooled analysis of 751 population-based studies with 4.4 million participants. Lancet. 2016;387(10027):1513–30.

NRC. Nutrient requirements of laboratory animals. 4th ed. Washington, DC: National Academy Press; 1995.

Obeid O, et al. Plasma copper, zinc, and selenium levels and correlates with metabolic syndrome components of lebanese adults. Biol Trace Elem Res. 2008;123(1–3):58–65.

Offield MF, et al. PDX-1 is required for pancreatic outgrowth and differentiation of the rostral duodenum. Development. 1996;122(3):983–95.

Ogawa-Wong AN, Berry MJ, Seale LA. Selenium and metabolic disorders: an emphasis on type 2 diabetes risk. Nutrients. 2016;8(2):80.

Olson GE, et al. Apolipoprotein E receptor-2 (ApoER2) mediates selenium uptake from selenoprotein P by the mouse testis. J Biol Chem. 2007;282(16):12290–7.

Olson GE, et al. Megalin mediates selenoprotein P uptake by kidney proximal tubule epithelial cells. J Biol Chem. 2008;283(11):6854–60.

Olson GE, et al. Extracellular glutathione peroxidase (Gpx3) binds specifically to basement membranes of mouse renal cortex tubule cells. Am J Physiol Ren Physiol. 2010;298(5):F1244–53.

Olsson M, et al. Expression of the selenoprotein S (SELS) gene in subcutaneous adipose tissue and SELS genotype are associated with metabolic risk factors. Metabolism. 2011;60(1):114–20.

Ozcan L, et al. Endoplasmic reticulum stress plays a central role in development of leptin resistance. Cell Metab. 2009;9(1):35–51.

Ozdemir S, et al. Effect of selenite treatment on ultrastructural changes in experimental diabetic rat bones. Biol Trace Elem Res. 2005;107(2):167–79.

Papp LV, et al. From selenium to selenoproteins: synthesis, identity, and their role in human health. Antioxid Redox Signal. 2007;9(7):775–806.

Park K, et al. Toenail selenium and incidence of type 2 diabetes in U.S. men and women. Diabetes Care. 2012;35(7):1544–51.

Pepper MP, et al. Impacts of dietary selenium deficiency on metabolic phenotypes of diet-restricted GPX1-overexpressing mice. Antioxid Redox Signal. 2011;14(3):383–90.

Pi J, et al. Reactive oxygen species as a signal in glucose-stimulated insulin secretion. Diabetes. 2007;56(7):1783–91.

Pi J, et al. ROS signaling, oxidative stress and Nrf2 in pancreatic beta-cell function. Toxicol Appl Pharmacol. 2010;244(1):77–83.

Pillay TS, Makgoba MW. Enhancement of epidermal growth factor (EGF) and insulin-stimulated tyrosine phosphorylation of endogenous substrates by sodium selenate. FEBS Lett. 1992;308(1):38–42.

Pinto A, et al. Delaying of insulin signal transduction in skeletal muscle cells by selenium compounds. J Inorg Biochem. 2011;105(6):812–20.

Pinto A, et al. Supranutritional selenium induces alterations in molecular targets related to energy metabolism in skeletal muscle and visceral adipose tissue of pigs. J Inorg Biochem. 2012;114:47–54.

Pitts MW, et al. Deletion of selenoprotein M leads to obesity without cognitive deficits. J Biol Chem. 2013;288(36):26121–34.

Ponugoti B, Dong G, Graves DT. Role of forkhead transcription factors in diabetes-induced oxidative stress. Exp Diabetes Res. 2012;2012:939751.

Prevost G, et al. The PACAP-regulated gene selenoprotein T is abundantly expressed in mouse and human beta-cells and its targeted inactivation impairs glucose tolerance. Endocrinology. 2013;154(10):3796–806.

Rains JL, Jain SK. Oxidative stress, insulin signaling, and diabetes. Free Radic Biol Med. 2011;50(5):567–75.

Rajpathak S, et al. Toenail selenium and cardiovascular disease in men withdiabetes. J Am Coll Nutr. 2005;24(4):250–6.

Rasekh HR, et al. Effect of selenium on plasma glucose of rats: role of insulin and glucocorticoids. Toxicol Lett. 1991;58(2):199–207.

Rayman MP. The importance of selenium to human health. Lancet. 2000;356(9225):233–41.

Rayman MP. Selenium and human health. Lancet. 2012;379(9822):1256–68.

Rayman MP, Stranges S. Epidemiology of selenium and type 2 diabetes: can we make sense of it? Free Radic Biol Med. 2013;65:1557–64.

Rayman MP, Infante HG, Sargent M. Food-chain selenium and human health: spotlight on speciation. Br J Nutr. 2008;100(2):238–53.

Rayman MP, et al. A randomized trial of selenium supplementation and risk of type-2 diabetes, as assessed by plasma adiponectin. PLoS One. 2012;7(9):e45269.

Reddi AS, Bollineni JS. Selenium-deficient diet induces renal oxidative stress and injury via TGF-beta1 in normal and diabetic rats. Kidney Int. 2001;59(4):1342–53.

Reeves MA, Bellinger FP, Berry MJ. The neuroprotective functions of selenoprotein M and its role in cytosolic calcium regulation. Antioxid Redox Signal. 2010;12(7):809–18.

Roberts CK, Sindhu KK. Oxidative stress and metabolic syndrome. Life Sci. 2009;84(21–22): 705–12.

Rochon C, et al. Response of glucose disposal to hyperinsulinaemia in human hypothyroidism and hyperthyroidism. Clin Sci (Lond). 2003;104(1):7–15.

Rock C, Moos PJ. Selenoprotein P regulation by the glucocorticoid receptor. Biometals. 2009;22(6):995–1009.

Rueli RH, et al. Selenoprotein S Reduces Endoplasmic Reticulum Stress-Induced Phosphorylation of Tau: Potential Role in Selenate Mitigation of Tau Pathology. J Alzheimers Dis. 2017;55(2):749–62.

Saito Y, et al. Selenoprotein P in human plasma as an extracellular phospholipid hydroperoxide glutathione peroxidase. Isolation and enzymatic characterization of human selenoprotein p. J Biol Chem. 1999;274(5):2866–71.

Saito Y, et al. Domain structure of bi-functional selenoprotein P. Biochem J. 2004;381(Pt 3): 841–6.

Schoenmakers E, et al. Mutations in the selenocysteine insertion sequence-binding protein 2 gene lead to a multisystem selenoprotein deficiency disorder in humans. J Clin Invest. 2010;120(12):4220–35.

Schweizer U, et al. Efficient selenium transfer from mother to offspring in selenoprotein-P-deficient mice enables dose-dependent rescue of phenotypes associated with selenium deficiency. Biochem J. 2004;378(Pt 1):21–6.

Seale LA, et al. Disruption of the selenocysteine lyase-mediated selenium recycling pathway leads to metabolic syndrome in mice. Mol Cell Biol. 2012;32(20):4141–54.

Sheng XQ, Huang KX, Xu HB. Influence of alloxan-induced diabetes and selenite treatment on blood glucose and glutathione levels in mice. J Trace Elem Med Biol. 2005;18(3):261–7.

Simic A, et al. Trace element status in patients with type 2 diabetes in Norway: the HUNT3 survey. J Trace Elem Med Biol. 2017;41:91–8.

Souness JE, Stouffer JE, Chagoya de Sanchez V. The effect of selenium-deficiency on rat fat-cell glucose oxidation. Biochem J. 1983;214(2):471–7.

Speckmann B, et al. Selenoprotein P expression is controlled through interaction of the coactivator PGC-1alpha with FoxO1a and hepatocyte nuclear factor 4alpha transcription factors. Hepatology. 2008;48(6):1998–2006.

Stahel P, et al. Supranutritional selenium intake from enriched milk casein impairs hepatic insulin sensitivity via attenuated IRS/PI3K/AKT signaling and decreased PGC-1alpha expression in male Sprague-Dawley rats. J Nutr Biochem. 2017;41:142–50.

Stallings MT, et al. A high isoflavone diet decreases 5′ adenosine monophosphate-activated protein kinase activation and does not correct selenium-induced elevations in fasting blood glucose in mice. Nutr Res. 2014;34(4):308–17.

Stapleton SR. Selenium: an insulin-mimetic. Cell Mol Life Sci. 2000;57(13–14):1874–9.

Stapleton SR, et al. Selenium: potent stimulator of tyrosyl phosphorylation and activator of MAP kinase. Biochim Biophys Acta. 1997;1355(3):259–69.

Steinbrenner H. Interference of selenium and selenoproteins with the insulin-regulated carbohydrate and lipid metabolism. Free Radic Biol Med. 2013;65:1538–47.

Steinbrenner H, et al. High selenium intake and increased diabetes risk: experimental evidence for interplay between selenium and carbohydrate metabolism. J Clin Biochem Nutr. 2011;48(1):40–5.

Steinbrenner H, et al. Localization and regulation of pancreatic selenoprotein P. J Mol Endocrinol. 2013;50(1):31–42.

Stoffers DA, Stanojevic V, Habener JF. Insulin promoter factor-1 gene mutation linked to early-onset type 2 diabetes mellitus directs expression of a dominant negative isoprotein. J Clin Invest. 1998;102(1):232–41.

Stoytcheva Z, et al. Efficient incorporation of multiple selenocysteines involves an inefficient decoding step serving as a potential translational checkpoint and ribosome bottleneck. Mol Cell Biol. 2006;26(24):9177–84.

Stranges S, et al. Effects of long-term selenium supplementation on the incidence of type 2 diabetes: a randomized trial. Ann Intern Med. 2007;147(4):217–23.

Stranges S, et al. A prospective study of dietary selenium intake and risk of type 2 diabetes. BMC Public Health. 2010;10:564.

Stranges S, et al. Associations of selenium status with cardiometabolic risk factors: an 8-year follow-up analysis of the Olivetti Heart study. Atherosclerosis. 2011;217(1):274–8.

Su LQ, et al. Nail selenium level and diabetes in older people in rural China. Biomed Environ Sci. 2016;29(11):818–24.

Sunde RA, Raines AM. Selenium regulation of the selenoprotein andnonselenoprotein transcriptomes in rodents. Adv Nutr. 2011;2(2):138–50.

Tanguy Y, et al. The PACAP-regulated gene selenoprotein T is highly induced in nervous, endocrine, and metabolic tissues during ontogenetic and regenerative processes. Endocrinology. 2011;152(11):4322–35.

Thompson JN, Scott ML. Impaired lipid and vitamin E absorption related to atrophy of the pancreas in selenium-deficient chicks. J Nutr. 1970;100(7):797–809.

Thompson PA, et al. Selenium supplementation for prevention of colorectal adenomas and risk of associated type 2 diabetes. J Natl Cancer Inst. 2016;108(12):djw152.

Ulusu NN, Turan B. Beneficial effects of selenium on some enzymes of diabetic rat heart. Biol Trace Elem Res. 2005;103(3):207–16.

Vats P, et al. Association of Superoxide dismutases (SOD1 and SOD2) andGlutathione peroxidase 1 (GPx1) gene polymorphisms with type 2 diabetes mellitus. Free Radic Res. 2015;49(1):17–24.

Vinceti M, et al. Toenail selenium and risk of type 2 diabetes: the ORDET cohort study. J Trace Elem Med Biol. 2015;29:145–50.

Walder K, et al. Tanis: a link between type 2 diabetes and inflammation? Diabetes. 2002;51(6):1859–66.

Walter PL, et al. Stimulation of selenoprotein P promoter activity in hepatoma cells by FoxO1a transcription factor. Biochem Biophys Res Commun. 2008;365(2):316–21.

Wang H, et al. Foxa2 (HNF3beta) controls multiple genes implicated in metabolism-secretion coupling of glucose-induced insulin release. J Biol Chem. 2002;277(20):17564–70.

Wang XD, et al. Molecular mechanisms for hyperinsulinaemia induced by overproduction of selenium-dependent glutathione peroxidase-1 in mice. Diabetologia. 2008;51(8):1515–24.

Wang X, et al. Knockouts of SOD1 and GPX1 exert different impacts on murine islet function and pancreatic integrity. Antioxid Redox Signal. 2011;14(3):391–401.

Wang X, et al. High selenium impairs hepatic insulin sensitivity through opposite regulation of ROS. Toxicol Lett. 2014;224(1):16–23.

Wang XL, et al. Association between serum selenium level and type 2 diabetes mellitus: a non-linear dose-response meta-analysis of observational studies. Nutr J. 2016;15(1):48.

Wang Y, et al. High dietary selenium intake is associated with less insulin resistance in the Newfoundland population. PLoS One. 2017;12(4):e0174149.

Watson JD. Type 2 diabetes as a redox disease. Lancet. 2014;383(9919):841–3.

Wei J, et al. The association between dietary selenium intake and diabetes: a cross-sectional study among middle-aged and older adults. Nutr J. 2015;14:18.

Whiting DR, et al. IDF diabetes atlas: global estimates of the prevalence of diabetes for 2011 and 2030. Diabetes Res Clin Pract. 2011;94(3):311–21.

Xia Y, et al. Optimization of selenoprotein P and other plasma selenium biomarkers for the assessment of the selenium nutritional requirement: a placebo-controlled, double-blind study of selenomethionine supplementation in selenium-deficient Chinese subjects. Am J Clin Nutr. 2010;92(3):525–31.

Xiang LR, et al. The supranutritional selenium status alters blood glucose and pancreatic redox homeostasis via a modulated selenotranscriptome in chickens (Gallus gallus). RSC Adv. 2017;7(39):24438–45.

Yalakanti D, Dolia PB. Association of type II 5' monodeiodinase Thr92Ala single nucleotide gene polymorphism and circulating thyroid hormones among type 2 diabetes mellitus patients. Indian J Clin Biochem. 2016;31(2):152–61.

Yan X, et al. Dietary selenium deficiency partially rescues type 2 diabetes-like phenotypes of glutathione peroxidase-1-overexpressing male mice. J Nutr. 2012;142(11):1975–82.

Yang SJ, et al. Serum selenoprotein P levels in patients with type 2 diabetes and prediabetes: implications for insulin resistance, inflammation, and atherosclerosis. J Clin Endocrinol Metab. 2011;96(8):E1325–9.

Yasui S, et al. Hydrogen peroxide inhibits insulin-induced ATP-sensitive potassium channel activation independent of insulin signaling pathway in cultured vascular smooth muscle cells. J Med Investig. 2012;59(1–2):36–44.

Ye Y, et al. A membrane protein complex mediates retro-translocation from the ER lumen into the cytosol. Nature. 2004;429(6994):841–7.

Yin Y, et al. Identification of risk factors affecting impaired fasting glucose and diabetes in adult patients from Northeast China. Int J Environ Res Public Health. 2015;12(10):12662–78.

Yu SS, Du JL. Selenoprotein S: a therapeutic target for diabetes and macroangiopathy? Cardiovasc Diabetol. 2017;16(1):101.

Yuan Z, et al. High levels of plasma selenium are associated with metabolic syndrome and elevated fasting plasma glucose in a Chinese population: a case-control study. J Trace Elem Med Biol. 2015;32:189–94.

Zeng J, Zhou J, Huang K. Effect of selenium on pancreatic proinflammatory cytokines in streptozotocin-induced diabetic mice. J Nutr Biochem. 2009;20(7):530–6.

Zeng MS, et al. A high-selenium diet induces insulin resistance in gestating rats and their offspring. Free Radic Biol Med. 2012;52(8):1335–42.

Zhang Y, Chen X. Reducing selenoprotein P expression suppresses adipocyte differentiation as a result of increased preadipocyte inflammation. Am J Physiol Endocrinol Metab. 2011;300(1):E77–85.

Zhang CY, et al. Uncoupling protein-2 negatively regulates insulin secretion and is a major link between obesity, beta cell dysfunction, and type 2 diabetes. Cell. 2001;105(6):745–55.

Zhang N, et al. Molecular characterization and NF-kappaB-regulated transcription of selenoprotein S from the Bama mini-pig. Mol Biol Rep. 2011;38(7):4281–6.

Zhao Z, et al. High dietary selenium intake alters lipid metabolism and protein synthesis in liver and muscle of pigs. J Nutr. 2016;146(9):1625–33.

Zhou J, Huang K, Lei XG. Selenium and diabetes—evidence from animal studies. Free Radic Biol Med. 2013;65:1548–56.

Zhou J, et al. Selenite exacerbates hepatic insulin resistance in mouse model of type 2 diabetes through oxidative stress-mediated JNK pathway. Toxicol Appl Pharmacol. 2015a;289(3):409–18.

Zhou JC, et al. Multifaceted and intriguing effects of selenium and selenoproteins on glucose metabolism and diabetes. In: Brigelius-Flohe R, Sies H, editors. Diversity of selenium functions in health and disease. Boca Raton, FL: CRC Press; 2015b. p. 217–46.

Zhuo H, Smith AH, Steinmaus C. Selenium and lung cancer: a quantitative analysis of heterogeneity in the current epidemiological literature. Cancer Epidemiol Biomark Prev. 2004;13(5):771–8.

Chapter 18
Uncovering the Importance of Selenium in Muscle Disease

Alain Lescure, Mireille Baltzinger, and Ester Zito

Abstract A connection between selenium bioavailability and development of muscular disorders both in humans and livestock has been established for a long time. With the development of genomics, the function of several selenoproteins was shown to be involved in muscle activity, including SELENON, which was linked to an inherited form of myopathy. Development of animal models has helped to dissect the physiological dysfunction due to mutation in the *SELENON* gene; however the molecular activity remains elusive and only recent analysis using both in vivo and in vitro experiment provided hints toward its function in oxidative stress defence and calcium transport control. This review sets out to summarise most recent findings for the importance of selenium in muscle function and the contribution of this information to the design of strategies to cure the diseases.

Keywords Selenium · Selenoproteins · Muscle disease · Oxidative stress · Calcium transport · RYR · SERCA

Introduction

Two decades ago, priority in the selenium field was the identification of the exhaustive list of selenium-containing proteins or selenoproteins, believed to be the main biological active form of selenium. Discovery of the selenoproteome based on the peculiarity of the selenocysteine translation machinery was an important milestone showing that selenium is present in a limited number of proteins, 25 in humans,

A. Lescure (✉) · M. Baltzinger
Université de Strasbourg, CNRS, Architecture et Réactivité de l'ARN, IBMC-15, Strasbourg, France
e-mail: a.lescure@ibmc-cnrs.unistra.fr

E. Zito (✉)
Dulbecco Telethon Institute at IRCCS-Istituto di Ricerche Farmacologiche Mario Negri, Milan, Italy
e-mail: ester.zito@marionegri.it

© Springer International Publishing AG, part of Springer Nature 2018
B. Michalke (ed.), *Selenium*, Molecular and Integrative Toxicology,
https://doi.org/10.1007/978-3-319-95390-8_18

reflecting its specialised function in living organisms. To gain further insight into selenium's biological role, many laboratories have been involved in unveiling the function of the newly discovered proteins, contributing to the description of their localisation, expression, structure, or cellular partners. However, though our understanding of the biochemistry and catalysis of the principal members of the selenoprotein family has made considerable progresses, membrane-bound selenoproteins still lag behind (Liu and Rozovsky 2015). Among these, the selenoprotein N or SELENON appeared as a priority, since it was shown shortly after its discovery that mutations in its gene were the causative condition for a class of inherited muscle diseases, referred as SELENON-related myopathy. This indicated the first connection between a gene translated in a selenoprotein and an inherited disease and pointed to many observations indicating an important link between selenium and muscle activity or maintenance. SELENON was identified among a group of endoplasmic reticulum-resident selenoproteins controlling calcium signalling and oxidoreductive homeostasis (Pitts and Hoffmann 2017).

Selenium-Related Muscle Disorders in Human and Livestock

Among the diseases related to selenium, selenium deficiency was identified as a risk factor for different muscular malfunctions both in humans and animals. In animals, nutritional muscular dystrophy is an acute condition affecting cardiac and skeletal muscles, caused by limited selenium supply, also sometimes associated with vitamin E deficiency. These muscle diseases have been seen to be epidemically abundant in young animals reared in places with selenium-deficient soil (Oldfield 2002; Yao et al. 2013; Thompson and Scott 1969; Delesalle et al. 2017). These disorders have been characterised in different species, including lambs, pigs or chicken, with different presentations and so-called nutritional myopathy, rigid syndrome, white muscle disease or exudative diathesis. Skeletal muscle degeneration linked to muscle weakness or stiffness, postural instability or walking disability is usually accompanied by a pale discoloration of the muscle tissue, intramuscular oedema and white streaks corresponding to bands of coagulation necrosis, fibrosis and calcification (Hefnawy and Tortora-Perez 2010; Thompson and Scott 1969). Cardiac muscle necrosis was associated with respiratory distress, cardiac arrhythmia and ultimately sudden death.

Selenium and vitamin E supplementation appeared to be sufficient to prevent the symptoms and the progression of the disease, reducing myocardial degeneration and skeletal muscle wasting (Değer et al. 2008; Beytut et al. 2002; Streeter et al. 2012; Sharp et al. 1972; Combs et al. 1975). However, the pathogenic mechanism remains elusive, and it is not clear whether the muscle degeneration is caused by increased oxidative stress due to a reduced expression of selenoproteins in general or low activity of a subset of selenoenzymes.

Selenoprotein expression was examined in a selenium-deficient broiler chicks model, where several selenoprotein genes were down-regulated in muscle and liver tissues, promoting increased oxidative stress and inducing activation of a p53- and p38-dependent MAPK/JNK/ERK signalling pathway (Yao et al. 2013; Huang et al.

2011, 2015). Selenium supply has been proposed as beneficial for mitigating oxidative muscle damage in exercised horses. The cooperative effect of selenium and vitamin E supplementation to alleviate the muscle disorders suggests convergence in a common antioxidant process that reduces lipid peroxidation (White et al. 2016). Accordingly, a study by Fujihara and Orden (2014) showed that higher consumption of vitamin E resulted in lower selenium accumulation in various organs in rats, indicating the involvement of the two compounds in a common or similar process.

In humans, Keshan disease is an endemic cardiomyopathy that develops in individuals with low selenium status in different areas of eastern China (Beck et al. 2003; Bor et al. 1999; Manar et al. 2001). Necrotic lesions, inflammatory areas and calcification throughout the myocardium are characteristics of this disease (Gu et al. 1983; Burke and Opeskin 2002). A mouse model revealed a dual aetiology of the pathological mechanism of the disease where there is a combination of lack in selenium and infection by the enterovirus *Coxsackie*. The primary infectious virus strain is not harmful per se, but increased oxidative stress in the selenium-deficient host can introduce mutations in the viral genome, increasing its virulence and resulting in the cardiac disease (Beck et al. 1995).

A relation between selenium deprivation and muscle pain or weakness was initially described in patients under prolonged parenteral nutrition (Brown et al. 1986; Kelly et al. 1988; van Rij et al. 1979; Baptista et al. 1984). The characteristic features in the myocardial muscle of these patients are reminiscent of Keshan disease. The hypothesis of selenium as a contributing or aggravating factor in other inherited forms of muscular dystrophies, such as myotonic or Duchenne muscular dystrophies, was therefore investigated. However, no evidence for beneficial effects of selenium could be found (Orndahl et al. 1994; Backman and Henriksson 1990; Gamstorp et al. 1986; Backman et al. 1988; Jackson et al. 1989). Several studies reported a significantly lower serum level in selenium in elderly patients with sarcopenia, a muscle disorder causing muscle weakness and loss of skeletal muscle mass (Lauretani et al. 2007; Beck et al. 2007; Chen et al. 2014), but no supplementation trial was conducted to confirm the importance of selenium in this condition.

A definitive connection between selenium's role and muscle formation and maintenance was finally provided by the identification of mutations in one selenoprotein, the SELENON coding gene being the cause of several congenital muscle disorders.

Selenoproteins in Muscle Disorders

Selenium is incorporated into proteins as part of its main biological active form, the organic amino acid selenocysteine (Sec). The proteins containing selenium in the form of Sec are called selenoproteins. The selenoprotein N or SELENON (previously called SELN or SEPN) is the first member of this protein family to be characterised as the origin of an inherited disorder; in two different studies, genomic screening in patients presenting clinical manifestations of either rigid spine muscular dystrophy (RSMD) or classic forms of multiminicore disease (MmD) detected mutations in the *SELENON* gene at multiple loci (Moghadaszadeh et al. 2001; Ferreiro et al. 2002a, b). Later reassessment of the nosological classification of these disorders, besides the linkage of *SELENON* to desmin-related myopathy with Mallory body-like inclusions (MB-DRM) (Ferreiro et al. 2004) and congenital fibre-type disproportion (CFTD) (Clarke et al. 2006), led to their redefinition under a novel broader entity named *SELENON*-related myopathy (*SELENON*-RM).

SELENON-RM is a congenital disorder originating from heterogeneous mutations in the *SELENON* gene; it affects the muscular system with a wide spectrum of phenotypes and different onset of clinical manifestations, all characterised by muscle weakness mainly affecting neck and trunk muscles, and general muscle atrophy, leading to spine rigidity, severe scoliosis and life-threatening respiratory malfunction requiring assisted ventilation, with relative preservation of limb muscles and ambulation (Cagliani et al. 2011; Scoto et al. 2011). Insulin resistance was also reported in several patients (Clarke et al. 2006), but more systematic analyses are required to address whether this is a general feature of the disease. The clinical pattern, combined with muscle magnetic resonance imaging, provides the basis for the diagnosis of *SELENON*-RM. The histological description of the abnormalities associated with the disease is unusually broad, including enlarged endomysial extracellular matrix, changes in the number and size of muscle fibre types and intracellular lesions such as disorganised bands of sarcomeres, also called minicores, or aggregates of proteins. Since these microscopic features are not systematically observed, they are likely to represent different cellular evolution states of the diseases. A list of nonsense and missense mutations has been identified to date in the *SELENON* gene that cause loss of function of the protein and result in myopathies with an autosomal recessive pattern (see Castets et al. 2012). No direct genotype-phenotype correlation has been established between the mutation and the myopathic phenotype.

Myopathic symptoms with fatigue and weakness affecting neck, proximal and axial muscles were reported in several patients with mutations in the gene coding for the Sec-specific translation factor SECISBP2 (reviewed in Schoenmakers et al. 2016). Patients with mutations in the *SECISBP2* gene present a multi-systemic disorder with abnormal metabolism of thyroid hormones, secondary to loss of activity of the three Sec-containing deiodinase enzymes, together with low plasma selenium. Therefore many *SECISBP2* cases have different degrees of developmental delay affecting mainly the musculoskeletal system. The muscular phenotype described in a subgroup of *SECISBP2* patients is predicted to be related to SELENON deficiency (Schoenmakers et al. 2010). At the mechanistic level, *SECISBP2* mutations result in impaired synthesis and low expression of many selenoproteins. However, some expression is preserved, as functional activity of selenoproteins is still detectable (Schoenmakers et al. 2016). The nature of the mutation occurring in *SECISBP2* is expected to differently affect the set of non-translated selenoproteins that may or may not include SELENON, related to the severity of the muscular symptoms. However, perturbed thyroid hormone metabolism has been recognised as having severe adverse effects on muscle function as well (reviewed in

Marsili et al. 2016). Recent data show that both the local inactivation of thyroid hormone by deiodinase type 3, induced by muscle injury, and deiodinase 2-mediated T4 activation during muscle regeneration control satellite cell proliferation and differentiation, two successive steps essential for proper muscle repair (Dentice et al. 2010, 2014).

Selenoprotein W or SELENOW activity was originally linked to a muscular disorder, since its expression was reduced in muscle from animals with white muscle disease (WMD) (Whanger 2000). The sarcoplasmic reticulum of WMD animals is defective in calcium sequestration, resulting in calcification of both cardiac and skeletal muscle. SELENOW is a cytoplasmic selenoprotein, particularly abundant in skeletal muscle and brain. Based on sequence alignment and NMR studies, SELENOW together with five other selenoproteins (SELENOM, SELENOF, SELENOV, SELENOT and SELENOH), was seen to be part of the Rdx family of proteins. Rdx proteins display a thioredoxin-like fold structure and a conserved CxxC or UxxC (C stands for cysteine and U for selenocysteine) motif located in an exposed loop similar to the redox-active site in thioredoxin (Dikiy et al. 2007; Aachmann et al. 2007). SELENOW was shown to be highly expressed in proliferating myoblasts, and to induce cell proliferation-differentiation transition in skeletal muscle cells (Jeon et al. 2014). SELENOW interacts with the signalling protein 14-3-3, preventing its interaction with other cellular target proteins, such as the cell cycle progression/differentiation controllers CDC25B, Rictor and TAZ. Binding of SELENOW to 14-3-3 protein promotes the translocation of TAZ from the cytoplasm to the nucleus, which is required for its interaction with several transcription factors including MyoD, a key regulator for muscle cell differentiation. In addition, the Sec residue of SELENOW is directly involved in its interaction with 14-3-3 and this complex formation is sensitive to the intracellular redox environment (Jeon et al. 2016).

Molecular Description of SELENON Gene and Protein: Expression and Cell Localisation

SELENON was first identified by a bioinformatic screen then characterised by an in vitro assay; this study showed that *SELENON* mRNA contains the common features for grouping in the selenoprotein family, including a SECIS element within the 3'-UTR that redefines an in-frame UGA codon into a Sec residue (Lescure et al. 1999). The human *SELENON* gene was mapped to chromosome 1 p36-11 and is composed of 13 exons (Fig. 18.1). Genomic studies predicted that *SELENON* gene encodes for two RNA isoforms differing in the alternative splicing of exon 3. However, this additional exon 3 appeared to be primate specific and later analyses indicated that the second isoform, in which exon 3 is spliced out, is the most abundant in cells and the only one to be translated into protein (Petit et al. 2003). Screening for *SELENON* mRNA revealed its expression in many tissues, including

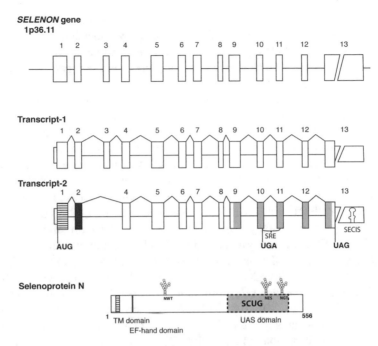

Fig. 18.1 Schematic representation of the human SELENON gene, the two SelenoN transcripts and the SELENON protein. The human *SELENON* gene spans an 18 kb region on the short (p) arm of chromosome 1 at position 36.11. It contains 13 exons (white boxes, upper panel). Exons 3, which corresponds to a primate-specific Alu sequence, is alternatively spliced, giving rise to two different mRNAs in human and other primates (middle panel). Only transcript 2 is translated into a protein. Exons 1 and 13 of transcript 2 contain the 5′- and 3′-UTR of the mRNA, respectively (small white boxes at both ends). Exons 10–11 and exon 13 contain the SRE and SECIS elements, two RNA motifs required for reprograming and selenocysteine insertion at the UGA codon. SELENON is a 556 amino acid long protein (lower panel) and is schematically represented with its functional transmembrane domain at the N-terminal end, allowing it to insert into the membrane of the endoplasmic reticulum (hatched box). Bioinformatic inspection by BLAST of the amino acid sequence identified an EF-hand domain (black line), a compact helix-loop-helix structural motif predicted to bind calcium. In the C-terminal part, a UAS conserved domain (grey box) includes the predicted catalytic site illustrated by the SCUG sequence (U = selenocysteine). SELENON is glycosylated at three different sites (NWT, NES and NGT) depicted in the scheme

skeletal and cardiac muscles, though at different levels (Lescure et al. 1999; Castets et al. 2009; Zhang et al. 2012).

The *SELENON* gene encodes for a 556-amino acid protein with a predicted mass of 62 kDa. However, when fractionated on a SDS-PAGE, SELENON migrated at a higher position, suggesting post-translational modifications, and glycosylation of the protein was experimentally validated (Petit et al. 2003). Inspection of the amino acid sequence revealed a stretch of hydrophobic residues at the N-terminus corresponding to a transmembrane domain (Fig. 18.1).

The cellular localisation of SELENON showed that it is an endoplasmic reticulum (ER)-resident protein, and that the sequence of the first exon was sufficient to address the protein in the ER compartment. Protease protection assay showed that the protein contains a single N-terminal transmembrane domain and that most of the protein, including the catalytic site—predicted from the position of the Sec residue—is located within the lumen of the ER. Amino acid sequence homology identified a classical EF-hand motif, a calcium-binding domain in the N-terminal part of SELENON and a UAS domain in the C-terminal part (Fig. 18.1). UAS is a domain of unknown function conserved in a subgroup of the UBXD protein family: UBXD7, UBXD8 (FAF2) and UBXD12 (FAF1). UBXD proteins are mainly associated with the ER and contribute to the positive or negative regulation of the ER-associated degradation machinery or ERAD (Rezvani 2016). The UAS domain of UBXD8 and UBXD12 binds long-chain unsaturated fatty acids and mediates polymerisation of the proteins (Kim et al. 2013). The Sec residue of SELENON, which is a landmark for the catalytic centre, is located within the UAS domain and is present in a SCUG motif that resembles the active GCUG sequence of thioredoxin reductases (TXNRD), suggesting oxido-reductase activity. In the three TXNRD, this motif, located at the C-terminal of the proteins, is directly involved in reduction of the thioredoxin substrate (Arnér and Holmgren 2000).

Deciphering SELENON Activity

Both zebrafish and mouse animal models were designed to decipher the underlying molecular and physiological dysfunctions arising from *SELENON* gene mutations. The data collected from these models addressing the role of SELENON activity in muscle development and maintenance, as well as during muscle regeneration, were reviewed elsewhere (Castets et al. 2012; Lescure et al. 2016). Here we are focusing on the analysis and combination of information resulting from studies of in vitro, ex vivo and in vivo models.

Defence Against Oxidative Stress in the Endoplasmic Reticulum (ER)

The biochemical activity of SELENON is still unknown, but there are many clues pointing to its important role in the defence against hyperoxidation in the ER, namely the ER stress response. A putative ER stress-responsive element (ERSE) was identified in the promoter region of the *SELENON* gene (Arbogast and Ferreiro 2010), and *SELENON* induction was detected after in vitro treatment with ER stress inducers such as tunicamycin and thapsigargin (Marino et al. 2015). Furthermore, cells devoid of SELENON displayed higher levels of oxidised glutathione (Marino et al. 2015) and were more susceptible to H_2O_2 treatment (Arbogast et al. 2009). This increased susceptibility to oxidative species was rescued by pretreatment with the reductant N-acetyl-cysteine (NAC). Altogether, these data indicate that *SELENON* expression is responsive to ER stress and that SELENON activity is involved in ER defence against oxidative insults.

These two characteristics of SELENON recall a connection with the homeostatic unfolded protein response (UPR), a mechanism which aims at restoring ER fitness after an ER hyperoxidation-induced stress (Ron and Walter 2007; Walter and Ron 2011). The UPR effector, ER oxidoreductin 1 (ERO1), is the main ER protein disulphide oxidase involved in oxidative protein folding, but since its activity is related to production of H_2O_2, it also burdens the ER cell compartment with potentially toxic reactive oxygen species (ROS) (Tu and Weissman 2002; Gross et al. 2004; Zito 2015). The relationship between oxidative protein folding in the ER and oxidative stress is supported by the fact that UPR activity, together with ERO1, also activates genes that combat oxidative stress. Protein kinase R(PKR)-like endoplasmic reticulum kinase (PERK) signalling accounts for a substantial part of this gene expression programme, and compromising signalling in this branch of the UPR markedly increases ROS levels in ER-stressed cells (Harding et al. 2003). A similar process may also exist in yeast, in which unusual high levels of ER stress are coupled with increased oxidative stress (Haynes et al. 2004). Experiments conducted in *C. elegans* confirmed that ERO1 activity contributes to ROS production as knockdown of *ero-1* reduced the levels of endogenous peroxides in ER-stressed tissues (Harding et al. 2003). These findings were consistent with the simple hypothesis that the combination of an ERO1 up-regulation and an inefficient antioxidant response during UPR may compromise cell viability in yeast. In mammalian cells, SELENON expression level paralleled that of ERO1, and *SELENON* hypomorphic myoblasts were hypersensitive to ERO1 overexpression. These two observations suggested the co-regulation of ERO1 and SELENON expression, and that SELENON may have evolved to be part of an UPR-dependent antioxidant response in higher eukaryotes (Marino et al. 2015).

Due to its high metabolic activity, skeletal muscle tissue has a propensity to be exposed to ER stress and produce ROS; therefore it may need to mount an adequate antioxidative response. The UPR is one of the primary processes triggered in skeletal muscle by environmental challenges such as long-distance running or dietary alteration. This signalling activates the skeletal muscle ER-stress pathway and generates ROS; ROS are also produced by skeletal muscle contraction and long periods of muscle immobilisation (Powers et al. 2011; Wu et al. 2011). Clues for an alteration of this signalling pathway in SELENON-deficient individuals were provided by the study of animal models. Unlike in humans and in a zebrafish model, in which *SELENON* loss of function gave rise to an overt muscle phenotype (Deniziak et al. 2007; Jurynec et al. 2008), *SelenoN* knockout (KO) mouse limb muscles were somehow protected and showed no major alterations in their histological or physiological presentation (Rederstorff et al. 2011; Moghadaszadeh et al. 2013). This protection may be provided by the activity of redundant pathways controlling redox balance, and/or the limited muscle activity restraining ER stress and oxidative insults (Rayavarapu 2012). In line with this, *SelenoN* KO mice compared to wild type showed a significant reduction in normalised muscle force after ERO1 overexpression in the gastrocnemius muscle, a symptom that recalls the intrinsic muscle fibre abnormalities and muscle weakness associated with the human phenotype of *SELENON*-related myopathies (Pozzer et al. 2017). These data support the hypothesis that SELENON plays a role in protecting skeletal muscle from the negative consequences of ERO1 overexpression.

In support with the hypothesis that SELENON plays a role in defending skeletal muscle against hyperoxidation, studies showed that removing or reducing the dietary intake of the antioxidants vitamin E or vitamin C worsens the muscle phenotype in *SelenoN* KO mice. Studies from Beggs' laboratory showed that muscle exercise combined with restricted dietary vitamin E led to extensive accumulation of core lesions in the muscle fibre that are reminiscent of the dense minicores described in patients carrying *SELENON* mutations (Moghadaszadeh et al. 2013). Interestingly, zebrafish depleted in SELENON activity by Morpholino injection (Deniziak et al. 2007) showed an overt muscle phenotype and, like humans, zebrafish are auxotroph for vitamin C or ascorbic acid (AA) (Toyohara et al. 1996). AA reductant activity and ER localisation may be perfectly suited to cope with the lack of SELENON. Mice producing their own AA may be more protected against a pathological muscle mechanism. On the basis of these observations, Zito's laboratory has generated a *SelenoN* KO mice model that is dependent on exogenous AA supply, and studied the possible connection between muscle AA levels and a pathological *SELNON*-related muscle phenotype. Supplying a high AA dose in drinking water (corresponding to an average of 20 ng/mg of muscle, a concentration comparable with the average AA level in wild-type or *SelenoN* KO muscles) did not lead to any histologically or physiologically detectable muscle dysfunction, but providing a medium dose (corresponding to an average of 8 ng/mg of muscle) led to muscle ER stress, as well as a myopathic reduction in normalised muscle force and appearance of minicores. Furthermore, a low dose (corresponding to an average of 4 ng/mg of muscle) led to muscle ER stress, more severe muscle atrophy and a reduction in absolute muscle force. In brief, the severity of the progressive muscle defect was inversely proportional to the muscle concentration of AA, suggesting a protective role for AA in the *SelenoN* KO mouse muscle (Pozzer et al. 2017).

SELENON and Calcium Transport: RYR1 and SERCA2

Aside of newly synthetised protein folding, another important ER function controlled by redox status is the flux of calcium between the ER compartment and the cytosol (Appenzeller-Herzog and Simmen 2016). Several transporters determine the homeostatic cytosolic calcium concentration that is essential to control skeletal muscle excitation/contraction coupling. Regulation of calcium handling by these channels is conferred by modification of redox-sensitive cysteines located on both sides of the ER membrane.

Ryanodine receptors (RyRs) are calcium channels located in the membrane of the sarcoplasmic/endoplasmic reticulum (SR/ER), where they mediate the release of calcium ions in order to tune cytosolic calcium concentrations (Lanner et al. 2010). Most of the RyR1 mutations studied so far show a gain-of-function phenotype in which channel opening is facilitated, with a consequent leakage of calcium to the cytoplasm (Dirksen et al. 2002; Ducreux et al. 2006). The overlapping of some histological and clinical signs between patients affected by *SELENON*-related myopathies and the core myopathies associated with RYR1 mutations fuelled studies on a functional link between SELENON and RyRs (Ferreiro et al. 2002a, b).

SELENON protein was immunoprecipitated from rabbit muscle homogenate with an antiserum that recognises all of the RyR isoforms, thus indicating that SELENON and RyRs are present in the same complex. In addition, a functional analysis of equilibrium binding indicated diminished RyR-ryanodine binding capacity in SELENON-depleted tissue, which suggested that SELENON may modulate RyR activity. More strikingly, the reintroduction of SELENON into SELENON-depleted tissue restored the ability of ryanodine binding to respond to changes in redox potential, thus suggesting that SELENON modulates RyR channel behaviour at the level of redox-sensitive residues (Jurynec et al. 2008). However, further functional redox studies aimed at identifying RyR1 cysteines that are sensitive to redox-dependent SELENON activity were hampered by the large number of cysteines represented in RyRs (more than 80 cysteines/protomer) (Xu et al. 1998). More recently, the finding of a characteristic redox-active CU, motif similar to the catalytic site of thioredoxin reductases (TXNRD) on the ER side of the SELENON sequence, suggests an ER reductase activity for SELENON (Castets et al. 2012). Given the electron transfer mechanism of the active catalytic site of TXNRD formed by the C and U residues, it was hypothesised that SELENON may attack and form a covalent bond with an oxidised proteinaceous target via its nucleophilic U.

An unbiased mass spectrometry approach was subsequently used to identify redox proteinaceous interactors of SELENON, among which the sarco/endoplasmic reticulum Ca^{2+}-ATPase (SERCA2) was prominently identified (Marino et al. 2015). SERCAs are multipass transmembrane proteins of the ER/SR importing calcium from the cytosol to the ER; their activity determines the resting cytosolic calcium concentration that is crucial for skeletal muscle excitation/contraction coupling. The importance of SERCA function in skeletal muscle diseases is exemplified by the fact that SERCA1 loss-of-function mutations give rise to Brody myopathy (Stammers et al. 2015; Guglielmi et al. 2013). Two isoforms of SERCA2 have been described: SERCA2a is expressed in the slow-twitch fibres of skeletal muscle and in cardiac muscle, whereas its C-terminally extended isoform, SERCA2b, is ubiquitously expressed in muscle and non-muscle tissues (Baba-Aissa et al. 1998). Redox-active SELENON was shown to co-immunoprecipitate both SERCA2a and SERCA2b.

Early studies suggested the presence of two regulatory cysteines on the ER side of the SERCA2b pump whose redox state influences pump activity (Li and Camacho 2004) and, on the basis of this model, it was shown that the interaction between SELENON and SERCA2 depends on the two redox-active CU amino acids of SELENON and the two cysteines in the L4 domain of SERCA2. Functional experiments investigating the ER calcium concentration in primary *SelenoN* KO mouse embryonic fibroblasts (MEFs) showed reduced calcium levels not only at steady state, but also during maximum calcium uptake, a status in which calcium exit and buffering are negligible and ER calcium level mainly depends on SERCA activity. This result indicated a less active SERCAs in *SelenoN*-depleted MEFs, and normal activity was restored by expression of active SELENON including the selenocysteine (Marino et al. 2015). In contrary to the study of Jurynec et al. (2008), there was no difference in ER calcium exit, thus raising the question as to whether SELENON influences calcium exit from the ER by modulating ER calcium channels/receptors. However, no RyRs were expressed in the analysed cells, and calcium exit was mainly controlled by inositol triphosphate (IP3) receptors.

Very recently, the laboratories of Zito and Blaauw measured SERCA and RyR activity in the more physiological environment of muscle fibres extracted from the flexor digitorum brevis (FDB) of *SelenoN* KO mice. SERCA activity was evaluated by measuring relaxation time after an electrical input, and RYR activity was tested after challenging the muscle fibres with caffeine, a RyR agonist. The relaxation time of *SelenoN* KO fibres was longer, which is consistent with reduced SERCA activity. However, no difference was observed between caffeine-treated wild-type and *SelenoN* KO fibres, indicating once again that SELENON controls ER calcium entry rather than exit. The same laboratories also compared the FDB muscle fibres of *SelenoN* KO mice with those extracted from mice carrying a RyR1-Y522S mutation, a mutation leading to RyR1 leakage. These analyses confirmed that the absence of SELENON influences ER calcium entry, whereas the RyR1 mutant affects calcium exit.

In conclusion, this is a new mammal model based on the functional interaction between SELENON and SERCA2 in which SELENON modulates the SERCA calcium pumping activity into the ER. However, although the interaction between SELENON and the SERCA2a isoform could explain the selective hypotrophy of slow-twitch muscle fibres described in the SELENON loss-of-function zebrafish model (Jurynec et al. 2008), it is still to early to exclude the possibility of interactions between SELENON and other SERCA isoforms.

Other Possible Function for SELENON

It is worth mentioning that SELENON expression is not restricted to muscle tissue, actually being expressed in most tissues. In addition, phylogenetic studies identified an orthologue of the *SELENON* gene in many animal species, both vertebrate and invertebrate; it was shown that *SELENON* is more ancient than previously appreciated and that this gene is already part of the ancestral parazoa and eumetazoa gene repertoire, including primitive organisms such as sponges or cnidarians, which are lacking organised muscle structures. Therefore, it is likely that SELENON original function may have been unrelated to muscle differentiation and maintenance, and that it may have additional functions that remain to be characterised. Interestingly, studies investigating the function of the microRNA miR-193-3p, a microRNA suppressor of breast cancer cell proliferation, identified *SELENON* mRNA as one the five targeted mRNAs (Tsai et al. 2016). Real-time PCR experiments confirmed the down-regulation of *SELENON* gene expression in miR193-3p mimic transfected cells, and knockdown of *SELENON*-suppressed cell growth similar to miR193-3p overexpression in breast cancer cells. In agreement with this observation, SELENON was shown to be highly expressed in proliferative fibroblast, but to be down-regulated during the differentiation into myoblast (Petit et al. 2003). These results point to a function of SELENON in cell proliferation control.

Exploring Therapeutic Strategies for SELENON-Related Myopathies: NAC and Vitamin C

From the therapeutic point of view, more studies are needed in order to clarify whether SERCA hypoactivity is the only factor that accounts for the *SELENON* KO muscle phenotype or whether SELENON has multiple targets, which would mean that rescuing reduced SERCA activity may only partially recover the muscle function.

The function of SELENON has not yet been fully characterised, but there are many indications that it is related to redox reactions and oxidative stress defence. It is therefore not surprising that the therapeutic approaches to *SELENON*-related myopathies have so far been based on this assumption.

Three antioxidants (the flavonoid fisetin, the carotenoid astaxanthin and the glutathione precursor NAC) were tested in the ex vivo pretreated cells taken from patients with *SELENON*-related myopathies in order to evaluate their protective effect against the detrimental consequences of oxidative H_2O_2 (Arbogast et al. 2009), but only NAC was found to improve the fitness of H_2O_2-challenged cells. In addition, it has been found that NAC improves the muscle histology of relatively relaxed (ryr) zebrafish, although no improvement in the muscle contractile properties was detected (Dowling et al. 2012). In another study, NAC was also shown to prevent mutated desmin aggregation in an in vitro cellular model for the desmin-related myopathy (Segard et al. 2013).

The existence of a significant clinical overlap with RYR1-related myopathies, and the fact that NAC, which had already been approved for human use, can counteract muscle fatigue without giving rise to any serious side effects (Reid et al. 1994) represented the proof of concept for the first, and still ongoing, NAC therapeutic trial in patients with *SELENON*-related myopathies. However, in vivo evidences for NAC protective benefits are still missing.

Working along the same lines, ex vivo *SELENON* KO MEFs were treated with low concentrations of EN460, an inhibitor of ERO1 (Blais et al. 2010) that has been shown to protect cells from the deleterious effects of the ER stressor tunicamycin, and may therefore inhibit ERO1 activity in SELENON-devoid cells during conditions of ER stress (Marino et al. 2015). Indeed, SELENON KO cells challenged with EN460 are protected from cell death induced by ER stress. However, the use of EN460 in *SELENON* KO animal models is hampered by its toxicity, and chemical modification studies are currently under way in order to make ERO1 inhibition more selective and to reduce the toxic effects.

As an abundant ER-resident reductant (Lamande et al. 1999), AA stands out among the normally present cellular antioxidants that may counteract the lack of SELENON. A pulse-chase experiment showed that it may be involved in oxidative stress defence in SELENON-deficient cells (Pozzer et al. 2017). Taken together with the fact that reduced AA concentrations in *SELENON* KO skeletal muscle aggravate the pathological *SELENON*-related muscle phenotype, the relative innocuity of AA suggests that it deserves evaluation in a therapeutic trial for *SELENON*-related myopathy. However, it is worth pointing out that, although some positive results have been obtained in mouse models for several human diseases, many clinical trials using AA failed to show any clear improvement (Noto 2015; Passage et al. 2004). Bearing in mind that unlike humans who rely on dietary intake mice produce their own AA, this situation may reflect differences in tissue concentration for this reductant between the two species. It is also important to take into account the differences in the pharmacokinetics of orally or intravenously administered AA: oral administration leads to tightly controlled plasma concentrations, whereas only intravenous administration can lead to the high plasma concentrations that may provide supra-nutritional health effects (Padayatty et al. 2004), which indicates the need to test intravenous AA in any clinical trial.

Acknowledgments This work was supported by a grant from the Meyer Foundation to A.L., a Telethon career award (TDEZ00112T), ERC Cariplo (2014-1856) and biomedical science for young scientist Cariplo (2014-1075) to E.Z.

References

Aachmann FL, Fomenko DE, Soragni A, Gladyshev VN, Dikiy A. Solution structure of selenoprotein W and NMR analysis of its interaction with 14-3-3 proteins. J Biol Chem. 2007;282:37036–44.

Appenzeller-Herzog C, Simmen T. ER-luminal thiol/selenol-mediated regulation of Ca^{2+} signalling. Biochem Soc Trans. 2016;44:452–9.

Arbogast S, Beuvin M, Fraysse B, Zhou H, Muntoni F, Ferreiro A. Oxidative stress in SEPN1-related myopathy: from pathophysiology to treatment. Ann Neurol. 2009;65:677–86.

Arbogast S, Ferreiro A. Selenoproteins and protection against oxidative stress: selenoprotein N as a novel player at the crossroads of redox signaling and calcium homeostasis. Antioxid Redox Signal. 2010;12:893–904.

Arnér E, Holmgren A. Physiological functions of thioredoxin and thioredoxin reductase. Eur J Biochem. 2000;267:6102–9.

Baba-Aissa F, Raeymaekers L, Wuytack F, Dode L, Casteels R. Distribution and isoform diversity of the organellar Ca2+ pumps in the brain. Mol Chem Neuropathol. 1998;33:199–208.

Backman E, Nylander E, Johansson I, Henriksson KG, Tagesson C. Selenium and vitamin E treatment of Duchenne muscular dystrophy: no effect on muscle function. Acta Neurol Scand. 1988;78:429–35.

Backman E, Henriksson KG. Effect of sodium selenite and vitamin E treatment in myotonic dystrophy. J Intern Med. 1990;228:577–81.

Baptista RJ, Bistrian BR, Blackburn GL, Miller DG, Champagne CD, Buchanan L. Suboptimal selenium status in home parenteral nutrition patients with small bowel resections. J Parenter Enter Nutr. 1984;8:542–5.

Beck MA, Shi Q, Morris VC, Levander OA. Rapid genomic evolution of a non-virulent coxsackievirus B3 in selenium-deficient mice results in selection of identical virulent isolates. Nat Med. 1995;1:433–6.

Beck MA, Levander OA, Handy J. Selenium deficiency and viral infection. J Nutr. 2003;133:1463S–7S.

Beck J, Ferrucci L, Sun K, Walston J, Fried LP, Varadhan R, Guralnik JM, Semba RD. Low serum selenium concentrations are associated with poor grip strength among older women living in the community. Biofactors. 2007;29:37–44.

Beytut E, Karatas F, Beytut E. Lambs with white muscle disease and selenium content of soil and meadow hay in the region of Kars, Turkey. Vet J. 2002;163:214–7.

Blais JD, Chin KT, Zito E, Zhang Y, Heldman N, Harding HP, Fass D, Thorpe C, Ron D. A small molecule inhibitor of endoplasmic reticulum oxidation 1 (ERO1) with selectively reversible thiol reactivity. J Biol Chem. 2010;285:20993–1003.

Bor MV, Cevìk C, Uslu I, Güneral F, Düzgün E. Selenium levels and glutathione peroxidase activities in patients with acute myocardial infarction. Acta Cardiol. 1999;54:271–6.

Brown MR, Cohen HJ, Lyons JM, Curtis TW, Thunberg B, Cochran WJ, Klish WJ. Proximal muscle weakness and selenium deficiency associated with long term parenteral nutrition. Am J Clin Nutr. 1986;43:549–54.

Burke MP, Opeskin K. Fulminant heart failure due to selenium deficiency cardiomyopathy (Keshan disease). Med Sci Law. 2002;42:10–3.

Cagliani R, Fruguglietti ME, Berardinelli A, D'Angelo MG, Prelle A, Riva S, Napoli L, Gorni K, Orcesi S, Lamperti C, Pichiecchio A, Signaroldi E, Tupler R, Magri F, Govoni A, Corti S, Bresolin N, Moggio M, Comi GP. New molecular findings in congenital myopathies due to selenoprotein N gene mutations. J Neurol Sci. 2011;300:107–13.

Castets P, Maugenre S, Gartioux C, Rederstorff M, Krol A, Lescure A, Tajbakhsh S, Allamand V, Guicheney P. Selenoprotein N is dynamically expressed during mouse development and detected early in muscle precursors, BMC Dev. Biol. 2009;9:46.

Castets P, Lescure A, Guicheney P, Allamand V. Selenoprotein N in skeletal muscle: from diseases to function. J Mol Med. 2012;90:1095–107.

Chen Y-L, Yang KC, Chang HH, Lee LT, Lu CW, Huang KC. Low serum selenium level is associated with low muscle mass in the community-dwelling elderly. J Am Med Dir Assoc. 2014;15:807–11.

Clarke NF, Kidson W, Quijano-Roy S, Estournet B, Ferreiro A, Guicheney P, Manson JI, Kornberg AJ, Shield LK, North KN. SEPN1: associated with congenital fiber-type disproportion and insulin resistance. Ann Neurol. 2006;59:546–52.

Combs GF Jr, Cantor AH, Scott ML. Effects of dietary polychlorinated biphenyls on vitamin E and selenium nutrition in the chick. Poult Sci. 1975;54:1143–52.

Değer Y, Mert H, Mert N, Yur F, Kozat S, Yörük IH, Sel T. Serum selenium, vitamin E, and sialic acids concentrations in lambs with white muscle disease. Biol Trace Elem Res. 2008;121:39–43.

Delesalle C, de Bruijn M, Wilmink S, Vandendriessche H, Mol G, Boshuizen B, Plancke L, Grinwis G. White muscle disease in foals: focus on selenium soil content. A case series. BMC Vet Res. 2017;13:121.

Deniziak M, Thisse C, Rederstorff M, Hindelang C, Thisse B, Lescure A. Loss of selenoprotein N function causes disruption of muscle architecture in the zebrafish embryo. Exp Cell Res. 2007;313:156–67.

Dentice M, Marsili A, Ambrosio R, Guardiola O, Sibilio A, Paik JH, Minchiotti G, DePinho RA, Fenzi G, Larsen PR, Salvatore D. The FoxO3/type 2 deiodinase pathway is required for normal mouse myogenesis and muscle regeneration. J Clin Invest. 2010;120:4021–30.

Dentice M, Ambrosio R, Damiano V, Sibilio A, Luongo C, Guardiola O, Yennek S, Zordan P, Minchiotti G, Colao A, Marsili A, Brunelli S, Del Vecchio L, Larsen PR, Tajbakhsh S, Salvatore D. Intracellular inactivation of thyroid hormone is a survival mechanism for muscle stem cell proliferation and lineage progression. Cell Metab. 2014;20:1038–48.

Dikiy A, Novoselov SV, Fomenko DE, Sengupta A, Carlson BA, Cerny RL, Ginalski K, Grishin NV, Hatfield DL, Gladyshev VN. SelT, SelW, SelH, and Rdx12: genomics and molecular insights into the functions of selenoproteins of a novel thioredoxin-like family. Biochemistry. 2007;46:6871–82.

Dirksen RT, Avila G. Altered ryanodine receptor function in central core disease: leaky or uncoupled ca(2+) release channels? Trends Cardiovasc Med. 2002;12:189–97.

Dowling JJ, Arbogast S, Hur J, Nelson DD, McEvoy A, Waugh T, Marty I, Lunardi J, Brooks SV, Kuwada JY, Ferreiro A. Oxidative stress and successful antioxidant treatment in models of RYR1-related myopathy. Brain. 2012;135:1115–27.

Ducreux S, Zorzato F, Ferreiro A, Jungbluth H, Muntoni F, Monnier N, Müller CR, Treves S. Functional properties of ryanodine receptors carrying three amino acid substitutions identified in patients affected by multi-minicore disease and central core disease, expressed in immortalized lymphocytes. Biochem J. 2006;395:259–66.

Ferreiro A, Quijano-Roy S, Pichereau C, Moghadaszadeh B, Goemans N, Bönnemann C, Jungbluth H, Straub V, Villanova M, Leroy JP, Romero NB, Martin JJ, Muntoni F, Voit T, Estournet B, Richard P, Fardeau M, Guicheney P. Mutations of the selenoprotein N gene, which is implicated in rigid spine muscular dystrophy, cause the classical phenotype of multiminicore disease: reassessing the nosology of early-onset myopathies. Am J Hum Genet. 2002a;71:739–49.

Ferreiro A, Monnier N, Romero NB, Leroy JP, Bönnemann C, Haenggeli CA, Straub V, Voss WD, Nivoche Y, Jungbluth H, Lemainque A, Voit T, Lunardi J, Fardeau M, Guicheney P. A recessive form of central core disease, transiently presenting as multi-minicore disease, is associated with a homozygous mutation in the ryanodine receptor type 1 gene. Ann Neurol. 2002b;51:750–9.

Ferreiro A, Ceuterick-de Groote C, Marks JJ, Goemans N, Schreiber G, Hanefeld F, Fardeau M, Martin JJ, Goebel HH, Richard P, Guicheney P, Bönnemann CG. Desmin-related myopathy with Mallory body-like inclusions is caused by mutations of the selenoprotein N gene. Ann Neurol. 2004;55:676–86.

Fujihara T, Orden EA. The effect of dietary vitamin E level on selenium status in rats. J Anim Physiol Anim Nutr. 2014;98:921–7.

Gamstorp I, Gustavson KH, Hellström O, Nordgren B. A trial of selenium and vitamin E in boys with muscular dystrophy. J Child Neurol. 1986;1:211–4.

Ghany Hefnawy El A, Tortora-Perez JL. The importance of selenium and the effects of its deficiency in animal health. Small Rumin Res. 2010;89:185.

Gross E, Kastner DB, Kaiser CA, Fass D. Structure of Ero1p, source of disulfide bonds for oxidative protein folding in the cell. Cell. 2004;117:601–10.

Gu BQ. Pathology of Keshan disease. A comprehensive review. Chin Med J. 1983;96:251–61.

Guglielmi V, Vattemi G, Gualandi F, Voermans NC, Marini M, Scotton C, Pegoraro E, Oosterhof A, Kósa M, Zádor E, Valente EM, De Grandis D, Neri M, Codemo V, Novelli A, van Kuppevelt TH, Dallapiccola B, van Engelen BG, Ferlini A, Tomelleri G. SERCA1 protein expression in muscle of patients with Brody disease and Brody syndrome and in cultured human muscle fibers. Mol Genet Metab. 2013;110:162–9.

Harding HP, Zhang Y, Zeng H, Novoa I, Lu PD, Calfon M, Sadri N, Yun C, Popko B, Paules R, Stojdl DF, Bell JC, Hettmann T, Leiden JM, Ron D. An integrated stress response regulates amino acid metabolism and resistance to oxidative stress. Mol Cell. 2003;11:619–33.

Haynes CM, Titus EA, Cooper AA. Degradation of misfolded proteins prevents ER-derived oxidative stress and cell death. Mol Cell. 2004;15:767–76.

Huang JQ, Li DL, Zhao H, Sun LH, Xia XJ, Wang KN, Luo X, Lei XG. The selenium deficiency disease exudative diathesis in chicks is associated with downregulation of seven common selenoprotein genes in liver and muscle. J Nutr. 2011;141:1605–10.

Huang JQ, Ren FZ, Jiang YY, Xiao C, Lei XG. Selenoproteins protect against avian nutritional muscular dystrophy by metabolizing peroxides and regulating redox/apoptotic signaling. Free Radic Biol Med. 2015;83:129–38.

Jackson MJ, Coakley J, Stokes M, Edwards RH, Oster O. Selenium metabolism and supplementation in patients with muscular dystrophy. Neurology. 1989;39:655–9.

Jeon YH, Park YH, Lee JH, Hong JH, Kim IY. Selenoprotein W enhances skeletal muscle differentiation by inhibiting TAZ binding to 14-3-3 protein. Biochim Biophys Acta. 2014;1843:1356–64.

Jeon YH, Ko KY, Lee JH, Park KJ, Jang JK, Kim IY. Identification of a redox-modulatory interaction between selenoprotein W and 14-3-3 protein. Biochim Biophys Acta. 2016;1863:10–8.

Jurynec MJ, Xia R, Mackrill JJ, Gunther D, Crawford T, Flanigan KM, Abramson JJ, Howard MT, Grunwald DJ. Selenoprotein N is required for ryanodine receptor calcium release channel activity in human and zebrafish muscle. Proc Natl Acad Sci U S A. 2008;105:12485–90.

Kelly DA, Coe AW, Shenkin A, Lake BD, Walker-Smith JA, et al. Symptomatic selenium deficiency in a child on home parenteral nutrition. J Pediatr Gastroenterol Nutr. 1988;7:783–6.

Kim H, Zhang H, Meng D, Russell G, Lee JN, Ye J, et al. UAS domain of Ubxd8 and FAF1 polymerizes upon interaction with long-chain unsaturated fatty acids. J Lip Res. 2013;54:2144–52.

Lamandé SR, Bateman JF. Procollagen folding and assembly: the role of endoplasmic reticulum enzymes and molecular chaperones. Semin Cell Dev Biol. 1999;10:455–64.

Lanner JT, Georgiou DK, Joshi AD, Hamilton SL. Ryanodine receptors: structure, expression, molecular details, and function in calcium release. Cold Spring Harb Perspect Biol. 2010;2:a003996.

Lauretani F, Semba RD, Bandinelli S, Ray AL, Guralnik JM, Ferrucci L. Association of low plasma selenium concentrations with poor muscle strength in older community-dwelling adults: the InCHIANTI study. Am J Clin Nutr. 2007;86:347–52.

Lescure A, Gautheret D, Carbon P, Krol A. Novel selenoproteins identified in silico and in vivo by using a conserved RNA structural motif. J Biol Chem. 1999;274:38147–54.

Lescure A, Briens M, Ferreiro A. What do we know about selenium contributions to muscle physiology? In: Hatfield D, Schweizer U, Tsuji PA, Gladyshev V, editors. Selenium, its molecular biology and role in human health. 4th ed. New York: Springer; 2016. p. 475–86.

Li Y, Camacho P. Ca2+−dependent redox modulation of SERCA 2b by ERp57. J Cell Biol. 2004;164:35–46.

Liu J, Rozovsky S. Membrane-bound selenoproteins. Antioxid Redox Signal. 2015;23:795–813.

Manar MJ, MacPherson GD, Mcardle F, Jackson MJ, Hart CA. Selenium status, kwashiorkor and congestive heart failure. Acta Paediatr. 2001;90:950–2.

Marino M, Stoilova T, Giorgi C, Bachi A, Cattaneo A, Auricchio A, Pinton P, Zito E. SEPN1, an endoplasmic reticulum-localized selenoprotein linked to skeletal muscle pathology, counteracts hyperoxidation by means of redox-regulating SERCA2 pump activity. Hum Mol Genet. 2015;24:1843–55.

Marsili A, Larsen PR, Zavacki AM. Tissue-specific regulation of thyroid status by Selenodeiodinases. In: Hatfield D, Schweizer U, Tsuji PA, Gladyshev V, editors. Selenium, its molecular biology and role in human health. 4th ed. New York: Springer; 2016. p. 487–98.

Moghadaszadeh B, Petit N, Jaillard C, Brockington M, Quijano Roy S, Merlini L, Romero N, Estournet B, Desguerre I, Chaigne D, Muntoni F, Topaloglu H, Guicheney P. Mutations in SEPN1 cause congenital muscular dystrophy with spinal rigidity and restrictive respiratory syndrome. Nat Genet. 2001;29:17–8.

Moghadaszadeh B, Rider BE, Lawlor MW, Childers MK, Grange RW, Gupta K, Boukedes SS, Owen CA, Beggs AH. Selenoprotein N deficiency in mice is associated with abnormal lung development. FASEB J. 2013;27:1585–99.

Noto Y. Ascorbic acid and Charcot-Marie-tooth disease. Brain Nerve. 2015;67:1241–6.

Oldfield JE. A brief history of selenium research: from alkali disease to prostate cancer (from poison to prevention). Am Soc Anim Sci. 2002;11:1–3.

Orndahl C, Grimby G, Grimby A, Johansson G, Wilhelmsen L. Functional deterioration and selenium-vitamin E treatment in myotonic dystrophy. A placebo-controlled study. J Intern Med. 1994;235:205–10.

Padayatty SJ, Sun H, Wang Y, Riordan HD, Hewitt SM, Katz A, Wesley RA, Levine M. Vitamin C pharmacokinetics: implications for oral and intravenous use. Ann Intern Med. 2004;140:533–7.

Passage E, Norreel JC, Noack-Fraissignes P, Sanguedolce V, Pizant J, Thirion X, Robaglia-Schlupp A, Pellissier JF, Fontés M. Ascorbic acid treatment corrects the phenotype of a mouse model of Charcot-Marie-tooth disease. Nat Med. 2004;10:396–401.

Petit N, Lescure A, Rederstorff M, Krol A, Moghadaszadeh B, Wewer UM, Guicheney P. Selenoprotein N: an endoplasmic reticulum glycoprotein with an early developmental expression pattern. Hum Mol Genet. 2003;12:1045–53.

Pitts MW, Hoffmann PR. Endoplasmic reticulum-resident selenoproteins as regulators of calcium signaling and homeostasis. Cell Calcium. 2017;70:S0143–4160.

Powers SK, Nelson WB, Hudson MB. Exercise-induced oxidative stress in humans: cause and consequences. Free Radic Biol Med. 2011;51:942–50.

Pozzer D, Favellato M, Bolis M, Invernizzi RW, Solagna F, Blaauw B, Zito E. Endoplasmic reticulum oxidative stress triggers tgf-beta-dependent muscle dysfunction by accelerating ascorbic acid turnover. Sci Rep. 2017;7:40993.

Rayavarapu S, Coley W, Nagaraju K. Endoplasmic reticulum stress in skeletal muscle homeostasis and disease. Curr Rheumatol Rep. 2012;14:238–43.

Rederstorff M, Castets P, Arbogast S, Lainé J, Vassilopoulos S, Beuvin M, Dubourg O, Vignaud A, Ferry A, Krol A, Allamand V, Guicheney P, Ferreiro A, Lescure A. Increased muscle stress-sensitivity induced by selenoprotein N inactivation in mouse: a mammalian model for SEPN1-related myopathy. PLoS One. 2011;6:e23094.

Reid MB, Stokić DS, Koch SM, Khawli FA, Leis AA. N-acetylcysteine inhibits muscle fatigue in humans. J Clin Invest. 1994;94:2468–74.

Rezvani K. UBXD proteins: a family of proteins with diverse functions in cancer. Int J Mol Sci. 2016;17:1724.

Ron D, Walter P. Signal integration in the endoplasmic reticulum unfolded protein response. Nat Rev Mol Cell Biol. 2007;8:519–29.

Schoenmakers E, Agostini M, Mitchell C, Schoenmakers N, Papp L, Rajanayagam O, Padidela R, Ceron-Gutierrez L, Doffinger R, Prevosto C, Luan J, Montano S, Lu J, Castanet M, Clemons N, Groeneveld M, Castets P, Karbaschi M, Aitken S, Dixon A, Williams J, Campi I, Blount M, Burton H, Muntoni F, O'Donovan D, Dean A, Warren A, Brierley C, Baguley D, Guicheney P, Fitzgerald R, Coles A, Gaston H, Todd P, Holmgren A, Khanna KK, Cooke M, Semple R, Halsall D, Wareham N, Schwabe J, Grasso L, Beck-Peccoz P, Ogunko A, Dattani M, Gurnell M, Chatterjee K. Mutations in the selenocysteine insertion sequence-binding protein 2 gene lead to a multisystem selenoprotein deficiency disorder in humans. J Clin Invest. 2010;120:4220–35.

Schoenmakers E, Schoenmakers N, Chatterjee K. Mutations in humans that adversely affect the selenoprotein synthesis pathway. In: Hatfield D, Schweizer U, Tsuji PA, Gladyshev V, editors. Selenium, its molecular biology and role in human health. 4th ed. New York: Springer; 2016. p. 523–38.

Scoto M, Cirak S, Mein R, Feng L, Manzur AY, Robb S, Childs AM, Quinlivan RM, Roper H, Jones DH, Longman C, Chow G, Pane M, Main M, Hanna MG, Bushby K, Sewry C, Abbs S, Mercuri E, Muntoni F. SEPN1-related myopathies: clinical course in a large cohort of patients. Neurology. 2011;76:2073–8.

Segard BD, Delort F, Bailleux V, Simon S, Leccia E, Gausseres B, Briki F, Vicart P, Batonnet-Pichon S. N-acetyl-L-cysteine prevents stress-induced desmin aggregation in cellular models of desminopathy. PLoS One. 2013;8:e76361.

Sharp BA, Young LG, Van Dreumel AA. Effect of supplemental vitamin E and selenium in high moisture corn diets on the incidence of mulberry heart disease and hepatosis dietetica in pigs. Can J Comp Med. 1972;36:393–7.

Stammers AN, Susser SE, Hamm NC, Hlynsky MW, Kimber DE, Kehler DS, Duhamel TA. The regulation of sarco(endo)plasmic reticulum calcium-ATPases (SERCA). Can J Physiol Pharmacol. 2015;93:843–54.

Streeter RM, Divers TJ, Mittel L, Korn AE, Wakshlag JJ. Selenium deficiency associations with gender, breed, serum vitamin E and creatine kinase, clinical signs and diagnoses in horses of different age groups: a retrospective examination 1996-2011. Equine Vet J Suppl. 2012;43:31–5.

Tsai KW, Leung CM, Lo YH, Chen TW, Chan WC, Yu SY, Tu YT, Lam HC, Li SC, Ger LP, Liu WS, Chang HT. Arm selection preference of MicroRNA-193a varies in breast Cancer. Sci Rep. 2016;6:28176.

Thompson JN, Scott ML. Role of selenium in the nutrition of the chick. J Nutr. 1969;97:335–42.

Toyohara H, Nakata T, Touhata K, Hashimoto H, Kinoshita M, Sakaguchi M, Nishikimi M, Yagi K, Wakamatsu Y, Ozato K. Transgenic expression of l-Gulono-γ-lactone oxidase in medaka (Oryzias latipes), a teleost fish that lacks this enzyme necessary for l-ascorbic acid biosynthesis. Biochem Biophys Res Commun. 1996;223:650–3.

Tu BP, Weissman JS. The FAD- and O(2)-dependent reaction cycle of Ero1-mediated oxidative protein folding in the endoplasmic reticulum. Mol Cell. 2002;10:983–94.

van Rij AM, Thomson CD, McKenzie JM, Robinson MF. Selenium deficiency in total parenteral nutrition. Am J Clin Nutr. 1979;32:2076–85.

Walter P, Ron D. The unfolded protein response: from stress pathway to homeostatic regulation. Science. 2011;334:1081–6.

Whanger PD. Selenoprotein W: a review. Cell Mol Life Sci. 2000;57:1846–52.

White SH, Johnson SE, Bobel JM, Warren LK. Dietary selenium and prolonged exercise alter gene expression and activity of antioxidant enzymes in equine skeletal muscle. J Anim Sci. 2016;94:2867–78.

Xu L, Eu JP, Meissner G, Stamler JS. Activation of the cardiac calcium release channel (ryanodine receptor) by poly-S-nitrosylation. Science. 1998;279:234–7.

Wu J, Ruas JL, Estall JL, Rasbach KA, Choi JH, Ye L, Boström P, Tyra HM, Crawford RW, Campbell KP, Rutkowski DT, Kaufman RJ, Spiegelman BM. The unfolded protein response mediates adaptation to exercise in skeletal muscle through a PGC-1α/ATF6α complex. Cell Metab. 2011;13:160–9.

Yao HD, Wu Q, Zhang ZW, Zhang JL, Li S, Huang JQ, Ren FZ, Xu SW, Wang XL, Lei XG. Gene expression of endoplasmic reticulum resident selenoproteins correlates with apoptosis in various muscles of se-deficient chicks. J Nutr. 2013;143:613–9.

Zhang J, Li J, Zhang Z, Sun B, Wang R, Jiang Z, Li S, Xu S. Ubiquitous expression of selenoprotein N transcripts in chicken tissues and early developmental expression pattern in skeletal muscles. Biol Trace Elem Res. 2012;146:187–91.

Zito E. ERO1: a protein disulfide oxidase and H2O2 producer. Free Radic Biol Med. 2015;83:299–304.

Chapter 19
Selenium in Immune Response and Intensive Care

Roland Gärtner

Abstract The pathogenesis of systemic inflammatory response syndrome as well as severe sepsis and septic shock are still not well understood. But there had been increasing evidence from preclinical and clinical studies that an imbalance of the redox system may play a key role, especially within the early phase of severe inflammation. It had been shown that in septic patients the selenium plasma levels were low, and correlated inversely with the severity of the disease. Selenoenzymes are involved in the regulation of the redox homeostasis in all compartments of the body, and therefore it had been supposed that an early selenium supplementation might ameliorate the course of the disease or even reduces mortality. The outcome of these clinical trials is not conclusive, which might be due to the fact that critically ill patients are heterogeneous in many aspects, from underlying, disease, source of infection, concomitant treatments, organ failures and even time between first signs of systemic inflammatory response to treatment. Furthermore the modes of selenium supplementation as well as the dosages needed are unknown. Moreover it still is not clear whether the low selenium levels are a consequence or at least in part the cause of the systemic immune response and organ failure.

Keywords Sepsis · Inflammation · Critically ill patients · Low selenium levels · Organ failure

Introduction

Sepsis is still the leading cause of mortality in intensive care units throughout the world (Tillmann and Wunsch 2018). The efforts of the international societies to give recommendations for diagnosis and treatment (Rhodes et al. 2017) struggle with many problems, first of all, that the pathophysiology of sepsis is poorly understood

R. Gärtner (✉)
Klinikum der Universität München—Medizinische Klinik und Polyklinik IV, Endokrinologie, Munich, Germany
e-mail: Roland.Gaertner@med.uni-muenchen.de

© Springer International Publishing AG, part of Springer Nature 2018
B. Michalke (ed.), *Selenium*, Molecular and Integrative Toxicology,
https://doi.org/10.1007/978-3-319-95390-8_19

(Hotchkiss et al. 2009; Ward 2009). In addition good controlled randomized studies that should underlie the single recommendations are scarce, with the consequence that these recommendations mainly are expert's opinions (Rhodes et al. 2017; Vincent and Grimaldi 2018). Nevertheless these are essential to obtain some progress in the recognition of diagnosis and optimizing patient's care. Sepsis now has been considered as a medical emergency compared to myocardial infarction or stroke. In contrast to those diseases we do not have any FDA-approved treatment for the systemic inflammatory response syndrome (SIRS) and sepsis (Rhodes et al. 2017).

Sepsis induces vasodilatation in the arterial and venous vessels, left ventricular failure, capillary leak syndrome with oedema in all organs including the lung, followed by respiratory distress syndrome, and consecutive tissue hypoxemia, acidosis and kidney failure. Immediate and appropriate hemodynamic resuscitation using vasopressors and careful fluid supplementation beneath the early identification of the underlying infection or non-infectious trigger is important for the survival in septic patients (Rivers et al. 2001). A "surviving sepsis campaign" had been established and updated recommendations had been published from 2004 up to the last 2016 (Rhodes et al. 2017). However, despite the advances made with these recommendations for monitoring and treatment of sepsis and septic shock, many patients develop a multiple organ dysfunction syndrome (MODS) and do not survive; the overall mortality still is around 20–30% despite optimized patient care. This might be due to the fact that besides the early and effective treatment with antibiotics and mechanical resuscitation a specific metabolic resuscitation would be beneficial (Pool et al. 2018).

Within the last decades the theory of an uncontrolled inflammatory response to a pathogen came up as the early event initiating the SIRS. Several studies could demonstrate an increased oxidative stress and reduced antioxidant defence in critically illness, and the worse outcome might be associated with the loss of the redox balance (Brealey et al. 2002; Wu et al. 2017; Melley et al. 2005; Brigelius-Flohe et al. 2004). Oxidative stress is defined as a situation, where the amount of free oxygen species (ROS) such as hydrogen peroxide and superoxide exceeds the capacity of antioxidant defence (Kolls 2006).

ROS and reactive nitrogen-oxygen species (RNOS) have been shown to modulate cell signalling, proliferation, apoptosis and cell protection (Brealey et al. 2002; Wu et al. 2017). The selenium-dependent glutathione peroxidases (GPX) as well as thioredoxin reductases are important compounds responsible for the maintenance of the redox system in a variety of cells including the immune-competent cells. The activities of these enzymes are to our present knowledge regulated mainly by the selenium supplementation (Schomburg et al. 2004). Therefore the requirement of selenium might be increased to cope with the severe oxidative stress in sepsis or septic shock. In most, but not all, studies, patients with SIRS, sepsis and septic shock have a low selenium and plasma GPX activity, which is negatively correlated with the severity of the diseases (Hawker et al. 1990; Maehira et al. 2002; Sakr et al. 2007). The selenium excretion in the urine is not elevated. Moreover, during the course of the disease, the plasma selenium levels increase without supplementation in those patients recovering but remain low or even decrease in those who decease

(Forceville et al. 1998). This makes a shift from plasma to cells/organs more likely than the previous hypothesis that individuals with low selenium are more prone for developing SIRS or sepsis. As about 70% of plasma selenium is bound to selenium-binding protein (SELENOP), it had been hypothesized that SELENOP is binding to the activated endothelium of the vessels (Mostert and Selenoprotein 2000). An association of SELENOP with the vascular endothelium, a prime target of peroxynitrite toxicity, was shown in vitro (Burk et al. 1997). Therefore it seems to be likely that the disappearance of SELENOP from plasma in patients with SIRS or sepsis is the cause for low plasma selenium in these patients. But in a recent trial it had been shown that the erythrocyte selenium concentration, which is considered as a long-term indicator of the nutritional status, is a predictor for ICU and hospital mortality in sepsis (Costa et al. 2014). This would suggest that a better selenium status might reduce the possibility for the development of a severe sepsis after an infection. The final proofs that an adjuvant selenium supplementation will ameliorate the deleterious events leading to multi-organ failure or even death are still in clinical trials.

Clinical Intervention Trials with Selenium Supplementation

Based on the emerging insights about the disturbed redox equilibrium in experimental and clinical severe illness, prospective intervention trials had been initiated. As the best way of selenium application is intravenous sodium selenite, most of the studies had been done on parenteral sodium selenite. Over the last two decades more than 20 randomized clinical trials (RCTs) had been conducted to evaluate whether sodium selenite alone or in combination with other antioxidant micronutrients in critically ill patients might reduce mortality (Manzanares et al. 2016). This ambitious goal is the "golden standard" that has to be achieved to be accepted for general recommendations even as an adjuvant intervention (Rhodes et al. 2017). Because good preclinical trials had been missing, different experimental protocols had been used, either with selenium alone or in combination with other antioxidants. Unfortunately, no dose-finding studies ever were performed, because clinical trials in ICU settings and in accordance with the Helsinki declaration are expensive and difficult without sufficient support.

In one of the first controlled studies, 42 consecutive patients admitted to the ICU and fulfilled the criteria of SIRS and sepsis and had an APACHE II (acute physiological and chronic health evaluation) score of ≥ 15 (expected mortality around 50%) were included. As soon as inclusion criteria were fulfilled, they received either 500 µg sodium selenite parenteral per day for the first 3 days, followed by 250 µg per day for 3 days and 125 µg per day for further 3 days or placebo (Angstwurm et al. 1999). Endpoint of the study was the mortality within 28 days and the treatment was blinded to the physicians and nurses. All patients received a basal selenium supplementation of 35 µg selenite per day. The overall 28-day mortality was 52% in the placebo group and 33% in the selenium group, which is not significant, due to the small numbers. However, a subgroup analysis of the most critically ill patients defined as those with an APACHE II score above the median of all patients (APACHE II >20) revealed a significantly reduced mortality. Most of these patients had been suffering from severe pneumonia with acute respiratory stress syndrome (ARDS). From these 20 patients 4/11 in the selenium group versus 8/9 in the placebo group deceased and this effect hold on for 80 days. Despite the low dose of altogether 2625 µg sodium selenite the plasma selenium was normalized at day 3 as well as the GPX3 activity which both had been low at day 1 (Angstwurm et al. 1999). This obviously suggests that in the most severely ill patients, selenium substitution seems to be most effective concerning mortality rate.

Another prospective but open-labelled placebo-controlled study has been performed with patients after surgery or trauma (Zimmermann et al. 1997). Inclusion criteria were APACHE II score ≥14 and clinical and laboratory signs for infection. Forty patients were included; the observation time was 28 days. Endpoint of the study was mortality rate. The patients received a bolus injection of sodium selenite 1000 µg on the first day and continuous 24-h sodium selenite 1000 µg infusions for 14 days. Most of the patients were suffering from peritonitis. The mortality rate was 40% in control patients and 15% in selenium-treated patients. This result failed statistical significance, but showed a trend to reduced overall mortality in the selenium-treated group of patients. A sub-analysis has not been performed, and also no monitoring of plasma selenium.

In the same time, two small placebo-controlled blinded studies have been published, investigating the effect of selenium together with other trace elements or antioxidative vitamins on the infection rate in patients after major burns or trauma. In one study (Berger et al. 1998) the effect of a cocktail of trace element supplementation (selenium 2.9 µmol/day, Cu 40.4 µmol/day and Zn 406 µmol/day) ($n = 10$) was compared with standard trace element substitution (selenium 0.4 µmol/day, Cu 20 µmol/day and Zn 100 µmol/day) ($n = 10$). Endpoint of the study was the incidence of infections. The infection rate in patients after severe burn could significantly be reduced from 3.1 to 1.9 infections per patient.

In the other small study (Porter et al. 1999) selenomethionine 200 µg/day together with vitamin C (300 mg/day), vitamin E (1200 IU/day) and *N*-acetylcystein (32 g/day) or no antioxidants were substituted in patients after very severe polytrauma. Forty-one patients were enrolled but 23 deceased within the first 24 h; therefore only 18 patients were enrolled in the study. In the substitution group, the infectious complications could be reduced from 18 to 8 and multi-organ failure could be reduced significantly from 9 to 0. None of the patients died during the observation period.

These first trials stimulated the attention to selenium as a possible adjuvant intervention in the treatment of critically ill patients (Berger and Shenkin 2006).

However, in 2004, a Cochrane systemic review of seven randomized trials from critically ill patients (Avenell et al. 2004) found no effect of selenium administration on mortality. In contrast, a meta-analysis from 2005 (Heyland et al. 2005) reported at least a trend towards lower mortality, especially in studies using higher doses (>500 µg/day) of selenium.

One of the main questions was whether an initially high bolus injection followed by a continuous infusion of sodium selenite might be dangerous or even beneficial. High-dose intravenous sodium selenite might have pro-oxidative effects (Spallholz 1997; Stewart et al. 1999) and increase the initial oxidative stress in the early phase of SIRS. In an artificial peritonitis sheep model, it could be demonstrated that a 2 mg bolus injection of sodium selenite followed by a continuous infusion resulted in a delayed hypotension with better maintained cardiac index, delayed hyperlactatemia, fewer sepsis-induced microvascular alterations and a prolonged survival time (Wang et al. 2009). There was no sign for toxicity and obviously the pro-oxidative effect of sodium selenite is not deleterious. The same group consequently initiated a phase II placebo-controlled randomized trial in patients with severe septic shock due to an infection (Forceville et al. 2007). The protocol was a bolus injection with 4000 μg sodium selenite, followed by 1000 μg/day continuous infusion for 9 days. The primary endpoint was the time to vasopressor therapy withdrawal. Second endpoints were duration of mechanical ventilation and mortality rate. Sixty patients could be enrolled. There was however no effect on the time for need of vasopressor therapy and also not on mechanical ventilation time. Also the 28- or 360-day mortality rate was identical in both groups. The critical points might be the small number of patients, heterogeneous diseases and no selection of the severity of the disease like APACHE or SOFA score. Furthermore, the onset of selenium intervention started around 48 h after ICU admission, because positive blood culture was an inclusion criterion. This might be too long for an intervention, designed to interfere with the acute deleterious immune response. This also was in contrast to the animal trial (Wang et al. 2009), where the bolus injection was administered after 9 h after induction of artificial peritonitis. There were no serious adverse events caused by this highest dose of sodium selenite ever used in this setting in humans. Obviously, this even very high bolus of sodium selenite was not toxic (Forceville et al. 2007).

In the same year the results of the largest trial that had been done till then were published, the German SIC (selenium in intensive care) study (Angstwurm et al. 2007). It was designed as a phase III, multicentre, double-blind and randomized placebo-controlled trial. Eleven independent intensive care units participated in the trial including internal medicine, surgical or anaesthetic ICUs. Recruitment time was between 1999 and 2004. Inclusion criteria were patients with severe SIRS, sepsis and septic shock and an APACHE III score >70 who corresponded to an expected mortality rate of around 50%. The study group received 1000 μg sodium selenite within 30 min intravenously followed by 1000 μg sodium selenite over 24 h continuously for 14 days; thus the total amount of selenium was 15 mg within 14 days. The placebo group received sodium chloride 0.9% in the same regimen. Additional selenium supplementation up to 100 μg selenium per day, together with other trace elements during parenteral nutrition, was allowed in all patients. The patients otherwise were treated according to the best medical practice. Primary endpoint was the 28-day mortality; secondary endpoints were survival time, clinical course of APACHE III and LODS scores. In addition, selenium levels in serum, whole blood and urine as well as serum GPX-3 activity were measured. Initially 249 patients were included; however, 11 had to be excluded, because they did not fulfil the inclusion criteria. The intention-to-treat analysis of the remaining 238 patients revealed a mortality of 50.0% in the placebo group, and 39.7% in the selenium-treated group ($p = 0.109$; OR 0.66, CI 0.39–1.1). Further 49 patients had to be excluded before the final analysis because of severe violations of the study protocol. In the per-protocol analysis, 92 patients of the selenium group versus 97 patients of the placebo group could be analysed. The 28-day mortality was significantly reduced to 42.4% by adjuvant selenium treatment compared to 56.7% ($p = 0.049$, OR 0.56; CI 0.32–1.00) without selenium. In the predefined subgroup analyses, the mortality was significantly reduced in patients with septic shock ($n = 67, p = 0.018$) as well as in the most critically ill patients with an APACHE III score ≥ 102 (>75% quartile) ($n = 54, p = 0.040$) or in patients with more than three organ dysfunctions ($n = 83, p = 0.039$, mortality reduction 22.6%). Whole blood selenium concentrations and GPX-3 activity were within the upper normal range during selenium treatment, whereas it remained significantly low in the placebo group. There were no side effects observed due to high sodium selenite treatment. There was a clear and significant relation between the whole blood selenium concentration and outcome. If the whole blood selenium was <1.75 μmol/L on the second day, the mortality rate was 50%, and if it was >1.75 μmol/L it was only 21.9% in the selenium-treated group. If selenium in the placebo group was below 0.88 μmol/L, the mortality rate was 62%; above this cut-off value it was 19.6%. This clearly suggests that higher selenium concentrations within the first days of severe sepsis and septic shock are significantly related to the incidence of mortality.

In a recent systemic review and meta-analysis of parenteral selenium supplementation in critically ill patients (Huang et al. 2013) 12 trials were included and meta-analysis included 9 trials with severe sepsis. A total of 965 patients could be analysed; the mortality was 30.7% in the selenium-treated and 37.3% in the control group. Parenteral adjuvant selenium treatment reduced the all-cause mortality significantly (relative risk 0.83, 95% CI 0.70–0.99, $p = 0.04$). The SIC study was judged to have the highest impact on this result, because of the highest number of included patients and the positive outcome. The administration schedule of selenium had an important impact on mortality risk, like loading bolus on day 1 (>500 μg), longer duration (>10 days) and higher dosages (>500 μg).

The results of the SIC study emphasized the initiation of a large German multi-centre study, the so-called SISPCT study (Bloos et al. 2016). In this trial both the effect of selenium and the influence of a procalcitonin (PCT)-guided antimicrobial therapy in severe septic patients should be evaluated. PCT is a very fast and specific marker for bacterial, especially Gram-negative, infection. Many studies suggested that measurement of PCT improves the diagnosis of sepsis by differentiating between infectious and non-infectious causes of SIRS. Furthermore PCT should be an indicator for the duration of antimicrobial therapy. Since unexpectedly there is an interaction between PCT and selenium, the trial had been designed as a two-by-two factorial trial. The hypothesis was that both selenium and PCT-guided antimicrobial therapy would reduce mortality. The number of patients needed to obtain significant results was calculated from the outcome of the SIC study.

Inclusion criteria were adult patients with SIRS caused by infection combined with acute organ dysfunction or with septic shock defined as sepsis with the need for vasopressors despite fluid resuscitation. Randomization should be started no longer than 24 h after diagnosis. Exclusion criteria were as usual. Intervention was either 1000 μg bolus followed by 1000 μg continuous daily infusion, like in the SIC study, but duration was until discharge from the ICU but no longer than 21 days. Primary endpoint was 28-day mortality, secondary endpoint all-cause 90-day mortality, intervention-free days, antibiotic-free days and secondary infections. It was possible to include 1089 patients with severe sepsis and septic shock into the intention-to-treat analysis. The four intervention groups were equally distributed, comprising 267–273 patients.

The 28-day mortality was 28.3% in the selenium group versus 25.5% in the placebo group. The PCT-guided therapy also had no significant effect on mortality.

This negative trial with the largest sample size was disappointing and it will be difficult to encourage another trial, despite the profound limitations. The observed 28-day mortality was significantly lower than expected, especially in the SIC study where the selenium supplementation was effective. Therefore, the number of included patients was too low. The lower overall mortality might be due to the fact that the included patients were less severely ill, or the supporting treatment modalities of patients had been improved according to the updated "survival sepsis campaign" (Rhodes et al. 2017). It had been assumed that there is no interaction interference between the two treatment factors. This however was not the case; there was a significant ($p < 0.001$) less antibiotic exposure in the selenium-PCT-guided group and also the selenium-only group had a significantly shorter ventilator time and renal replacement requirement. Furthermore, there was no subgroup analysis comparing the most severely ill patients to less ill patients according to clinical scores.

This study had been recently included into the last systematic review and meta-analysis (Manzanares et al. 2016) and of course there was no significant effect of selenium on clinical outcomes anymore. However, there was a significant effect of selenium on infectious complications in those studies with an initial bolus treatment and a similar effect in trials with nonseptic patients. In none of the trials, selenium treatment was associated with negative side effects.

Conclusion Drawn from Clinical Trials

It can be concluded from all the clinical trials that only high doses and administration of i.v. sodium selenite as fast as possible seem to have an effect on the outcome of patients with severe sepsis and septic shock. The significant effect on specific subgroups of critically ill patients, like those with an expected mortality rate >50%, severe capillary leak syndrome and disseminated coagulation (DIC) or more than three organ failures had only been seen in one study (Angstwurm et al. 2007) and needs confirmation. Because of this low quality of evidence the "survival sepsis campaign" (Rhodes et al. 2017) strongly recommended against the i.v. use of selenium in patients with sepsis and septic shock. However, despite the attainment of the resuscitation goals recommended the mortality rate in these patients is still up to 20–30% (Tillmann and Wunsch 2018). Therefore, a metabolic resuscitation is still an additional and promising option (Leite and de Lima 2016). Further clinical trials with specific groups of patients in cooperation with basic research on metabolomics are necessary.

The initial naive hypothesis that increasing the selenium plasma levels with the aim to restore the disturbed redox balance and improve the outcome in critical illness finally failed evidence in the clinical trials (Manzanares et al. 2016). The good answer however is that routine application of high-dose sodium selenite in these patients is not toxic, and does not make any harm (Forceville et al. 2007).

More preclinical studies are necessary to obtain more insight into the possible mechanisms on parenteral sodium selenite administration. Furthermore, it has to be evaluated whether other selenium compounds or a combination with other antioxidants might be more effective.

References

Angstwurm MWA, Schottdorf J, Schopohl J, Gaertner R. Selenium replacement in patients with severe systemic inflammatory response syndrome improves clinical outcome. Crit Care Med. 1999;27:1807–13.

Angstwurm MW, Engelmann L, Zimmermann T, et al. Selenium in intensive care (SIC): results of a prospective randomized, placebo controlled, multicentre study in patients with severe systemic response syndrome, sepsis and septic shock. Crit Care Med. 2007;35:118–26.

Avenell A, Noble DW, Barr J, Engelhardt T. Selenium supplementation for critically ill adults. Cochrane Database Syst Rev. 2004;(4):CD003703.

Berger MM, Shenkin A. Update on clnical microntreint supplementation studies in the critical ill. Curr Opin Clin Nutr Metab Care. 2006;9:711–6.

Berger MM, Spertini F, Shenkin A, et al. Trace element supplementation modulates pulmonary infection rates after major burns: a double-blind, placebo-controlled trial. Am J Clin Nutr. 1998;68:365–71.

Bloos F, Trips E, Nierhaus A, et al. Effect of sodium selenite administration and procalcitonin-guided therapy on mortality in patients with severe sepsis or septic shock: a randomized clinical trial. JAMA Intern Med. 2016;176:1266–76.

Brealey D, Brand M, Hargreaves I, et al. Association between mitochondrial dysfunction and severity and outcome of septic shock. Lancet. 2002;360:219–23.

Brigelius-Flohe R, Banning A, Kny M, Bol GF. Redox events in interleukin-1 signaling. Arch Biochem Biophys. 2004;423:66–73.

Burk R, Hill K, Boeglin ME, et al. Selenoprotein P associates with endothelial cells in rat tissues. Histochem Cell Biol. 1997;108:11–5.

Costa NA, Gut AL, Pimentel JAC, et al. Erythrocyte selenium concentration predicts intensive care unit and hospital mortality in patients with septic: a prospective observational study. Crit Care. 2014;18:R92.

Forceville X, Vitoux D, Gauzit R, et al. Selenium, systemic immune response syndrome, sepsis, and outcome in critically ill patients. Crit Care Med. 1998;26:1536–44.

Forceville X, Laviolle B, Annane D, et al. Effects of high doses of selenium, as sodium selenite, in septic shock: a placebo-controlled, randomized, double blind, phase II study. Crit Care. 2007;11:R73.

Hawker FH, Stewart PM, Snitch PJ. Effects of acute illness on selenium homeostasis. Crit Care Med. 1990;18:442–6.

Heyland DK, Dhaliwal R, Sucher U, Berger MM. Antioxidant nutrients: a systemic review of trace elements and vitamins in the critically ill. Intensive Care Med. 2005;31:321–37.

Hotchkiss RS, Coopersmith CM, McDunn JE, Ferguson TA. Tilting towards immunosuppression. Nat Med. 2009;15:496–7.

Huang TS, Shyu YC, Chen HY, et al. Effect of parenteral selenium supplementation in critically ill patients: a systemic review and meta-analysis. PLoS One. 2013;8(1):e54431.

Kolls JK. Oxidative stress in sepsis: a redox redux. J Clin Invest. 2006;116:984–95.

Leite HP, de Lima LF. Metabolic resuscitation in sepsis: a necessary step beyond the hemodynamic ? J Thorac Dis. 2016;8:E552–7.

Maehira F, Luyo GA, Miyagi I, et al. Alterations of serum selenium concentrations in the acute phase of pathological conditions. Clin Chim Acta. 2002;316:137–46.

Manzanares W, Lermieux M, Elke G, et al. High-dose intravenous selenium does not improve clinical outcomes in the critical ii: a systemic review and meta-analysis. Crit Care. 2016;20:356.

Melley DD, Evans TW, Quinlan GJ. Redox regulation of neutrophil apoptosis and the systemic inflammatory response syndrome. Clin Sci (Lond). 2005;108:413–24.

Mostert V, Selenoprotein P. Properties, functions, and regulation. Arch Biochem Biophys. 2000;15(376):433–8.

Pool R, Gomez H, Kellum JA. Mechanisms of organ dysfunction in sepsis. Crit Care Clin. 2018;34:63–80.

Porter JM, Ivatury RR, Azimuddin K, Swami R. Antioxidant therapy in the prevention of organ dysfunction syndrome and infectious complications after trauma: early results of a prospective randomized study. Am Surg. 1999;65:478–83.

Rhodes A, Evans LE, Alhazzani W, et al. Surviving sepsis campaign: international guidelines for management of sepsis and septic shock: 2016. Intensive Care Med. 2017;43:304–77.

Rivers E, Nguyen B, Havstad S, et al. Early goal-directed therapy in the treatment of severe sepsis and septic shock. N Engl J Med. 2001;345:1368–77.

Sakr Y, Reinhart K, Bloos F, et al. Time course and relationship between plasma selenium concentrations, systemic inflammatory response syndrome, sepsis, and multiorgan failure. Br J Anaesth. 2007;98:775–84.

Schomburg L, Schweizer U, Kohrle J. Selenium and selenoproteins in mammals: extraordinary, essential, enigmatic. Cell Mol Life Sci. 2004;61:1988–95.

Spallholz JE. Free radical generation by selenium compounds and their prooxidant toxicity. Biomed Environ Sci. 1997;10:260–70.

Stewart MS, Spallholz JE, Neldner KH, et al. Selenium compounds have disparate abilities to impose oxidative stress and induce apoptosis. Free Radic Biol Med. 1999;26:42–8.

Tillmann B, Wunsch H. Epidemiology and outcomes. Crit Care Clin. 2018;34:15–27.

Vincent JL, Grimaldi D. Novel interventions: what's new and the future. Crit Care Clin. 2018;34:161–73.

Wang Z, Forceville X, Van Antwerpen P, et al. A large-bolus injection, but not continuous infusion of sodium selenite improves outcome in peritonitis. Shock. 2009;32:140–6.

Ward PA. Seeking a heart salve. Nat Med. 2009;15:497–4978.

Wu DD, T L, Ji XY. Dendritic cells in sepsis: pathological alterations and therapeutic implications. J Immunol Res. 2017;2017:3591248.

Zimmermann T, Albrecht S, Kuhne H, et al. Selenium administration in patients with sepsis syndrome. A prospectice randomized study. Med Klin. 1997;92(Suppl 3):3–4.

Chapter 20
Selenium and Toxicological Aspects: Cytotoxicity, Cellular Bioavailability, and Biotransformation of Se Species

Franziska Ebert, Sandra M. Müller, Soeren Meyer, and Tanja Schwerdtle

Abstract This book chapter reviews the current literature regarding the cytotoxicity, bioavailability, and biotransformation of the diet-relevant selenium species selenite, Se-methylselenocysteine, selenomethionine, as well as selenium excretion metabolites trimethylselenonium and selenosugar 1 in cultured mammalian cells. Limitations as well as potentialities are summarized. In case of no cytotoxic response, it is needful to ensure that the respective selenium species are bioavailable to the respective cellular models before concluding that they exert no toxicity in vitro. To further understand selenium species metabolism in vitro but also to unveil potential causes for the differing cytotoxic potencies of selenium species, a combined quantification of free selenium species in cell lysates and total cellular selenium quantification is recommended. Finally, in vitro approaches are reviewed that helped to identify new selenium species metabolites and thus contributed to our understanding of the role of these metabolites in the detoxification or toxification of selenium species.

Keywords In vitro · Viability · Cellular bioavailability and biotransformation · Selenium speciation · Selenite · Selenomethionine · Se-methylselenocysteine · Trimethylselenonium · Selenosugar 1

F. Ebert · S. M. Müller · S. Meyer
Department of Food Chemistry, Institute of Nutritional Science, University of Potsdam, Potsdam, Germany

T. Schwerdtle (✉)
Department of Food Chemistry, Institute of Nutritional Science, University of Potsdam, Potsdam, Germany

TraceAge—DFG Research Unit on Interactions of Essential Trace Elements in Healthy and Diseased Elderly, Potsdam-Berlin-Jena, Germany
e-mail: tanja.schwerdtle@uni-potsdam.de

© Springer International Publishing AG, part of Springer Nature 2018
B. Michalke (ed.), *Selenium*, Molecular and Integrative Toxicology,
https://doi.org/10.1007/978-3-319-95390-8_20

Introduction

In the last decades the ambivalent role of selenium has been an important subject of ongoing research. Selenium is essential for various systemic functions but is also well known to induce adverse effects at elevated uptake. This is true for both the entire multicellular organisms and single cells. Apart from the selenium dosage and the baseline status of the organism the administered form of selenium has a decisive impact on the respective outcome. Whereas overall the essential functions of selenium are quite well understood, its toxicity after overexposure still awaits further clarification.

Following the guiding 3R principle for more ethical use of animals in toxicity testing, in vitro models have recently also been successfully used to characterize and compare the toxicity of various selenium species in mammalian cells. Moreover, in vitro models enable to explore fundamental roots of the strongly species-dependent effects under cytotoxic conditions. One likely reason is the biotransformation of the respective selenium species to different metabolites, which might either enhance (toxification) or diminish (detoxification) the toxicity of the original applied selenium species.

This book chapter gives an overview about the cytotoxic potencies of five selenium species (Fig. 20.1). Based on the available recent literature, this book chapter in addition demonstrates that speciation studies in mammalian cell models may help to further understand the toxic mode of action of the respective selenium species.

The five selenium species have been selected since they either represent relevant selenium species in our diet or have been identified as important excretion metabolites. As one important dietary source selenomethionine (SeMet) ubiquitously occurs in proteins, in which it is nonspecifically incorporated instead of methionine. Se-methylselenocysteine (MeSeCys) is a plant metabolite, occurring especially in *Allium* and *Brassica* plants. In contrast to inorganic selenite, SeMet and selenium-enriched yeast, which may contain up to 10% organic selenium species other than

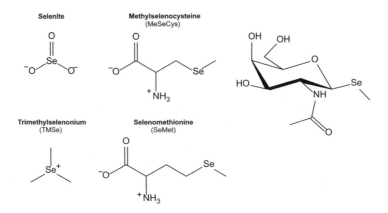

Fig. 20.1 Structures of the selenium species discussed in this book chapter

SeMet (including MeSeCys), MeSeCys is so far not authorized as selenium supplement in the European Union (2015). Excess selenium is mainly excreted via urine as methyl-2-acetamido-2-deoxy-1-seleno-ß-D-galactopyranoside (selenosugar 1) and, depending on genetic polymorphism, as trimethylselenonium ion (TMSe) (Kuehnelt et al. 2015; Gammelgaard et al. 2011).

Cellular Toxicity of Selenium Species: Cytotoxicity

Cytotoxicity of Selenite

Studies in various mammalian cells have shown that low micromolar concentrations of selenite decrease cell number as well as cellular dehydrogenase activity as frequently assessed by the MTT (3-(4,5-dimethylthiazol-2-yl)-2,5-diphenyltetrazolium bromide) assay (Table 20.1). Most studies have been carried out in human cancer cell lines. Here, an increase in reactive oxygen species (ROS), a decrease in cellular GSH, and an increase in cellular GSSG have been detected as well as apoptosis (Shen et al. 1999; Stewart et al. 1997; Xiang et al. 2009). The observed induction of DNA single- and double-strand breaks indicates that selenite can exert in vitro genotoxicity at the beginning cytotoxic concentration (Shen et al. 1999; Lu et al. 1995, 1994). This is likely to be caused by a threshold-linked process, e.g. induction of oxidative stress.

Cytotoxicity of Selenomethionine (SeMet)

In most in vitro studies, SeMet exerted no or low cytotoxicity in the high micromolar to millimolar concentration range (Table 20.2). This low cytotoxic potential might relate to the unspecific incorporation of SeMet in proteins in vitro. It was also hypothesized in literature that, because of limited methionase activity in vitro, SeMet is hardly metabolized to methylselenol (MeSeH), which is known to increase the cellular ROS level and to induce apoptosis (Zhao et al. 2006; Spallholz et al. 2004). On the other hand, SeMet has been shown to cause p53-dependent growth inhibition by inducing apoptosis and a G2/M cell cycle arrest in human colon cancer cells (Goel et al. 2006). Because of the limited studies, a conclusion whether selenomethionine overexposure could cause genotoxic effects is not yet possible. The observed increase of yH2AX foci in human bladder cancer cells upon selenomethionine exposure could indicate for both double-strand breaks and stalled replication forks (Rezacova et al. 2016) (Table 20.2).

Table 20.1 Cytotoxicity and related endpoints of selenite in mammalian cells

Cells	Assay/endpoint	Treatment	Result	Comment	References
Primary human (h.) fibroblasts of normal Caucasian females and of *xeroderma pigmentosum* (XP) patients	Colony forming ability	0, 20–3000 μM; 1.5 h		No SD and no significance given for colony-forming ability; incubation with S9 mix increased capacity of selenite to induce chromosomal aberrations. Response of DNA repair-deficient XP fibroblasts to selenite is comparable to that of control cells	Lo et al. (1978)
		With S-9 activation	≥200 μM		
		Without S-9 activation	≥1000 μM		
Mouse leukemia cells L1210	Trypan blue exclusion	0, 5–20 μM; 24 h	≥10 μM	Selenite induced single- and double-strand breaks at concentrations ≥5 μM; indications for apoptosis are presented	Lu et al. (1994)
	Colony-forming ability		≥5 μM		
Mouse mammary epithelial tumor cells	Cell number Cell membrane integrity	0, 1–10 μM; 4/24 h	≥5 μM	Values for 24 h not shown, after 24 h incubation ≥1 μM single- and double-strand breaks	Lu et al. (1995)
h. colon adenocarcinoma cells HT29	Cell number	0, 0.1–100 μM; 96 h	≥5 μM	A decrease in GSH was assessed	Stewart et al. (1997)
	Apoptosis (TUNEL)		≥5 μM		
h. hepatoma cells HepG2	LDH leakage	0, 1–25 μM; 12/24/48 h	≥1 μM (48 h) ≥5 μM (24 h) 25 μM (12 h)	Selenite induced strand breaks as detected by the comet assay (≥5 μM, 24 h), increased the cellular level of ROS, decreased cellular GSH, and increased cellular GSSG	Shen et al. (1999)
	TUNEL assay	0, 1–25 μM; 12/24 h	≥5 μM (12/24 h)		
h. hepatoma cells HepG2	WST-8 Dehydrogenase activity	0, 0.01–10 mM; 48 h	>0.002 mM	Selenosugar 2 exerted cytotoxicity in similar concentrations	Kuehnelt et al. (2005)

Cell type	Assay	Concentration; exposure	Results	Notes	Reference
h. prostate cancer cells LNCaP	MTT assay Apoptotic bodies	0, 0.5–2.5 µM; 120 h	≥1.5 µM 2.5 µM, 18 h	Selenite induced cell death and apoptosis was accompanied by	Xiang et al. (2009)
	Mitochondrial membrane potential, caspase 9 and 3 activity		2.5 µM, 4 h	superoxide radical production; effects were inhibited by overexpression of MnSOD	
h. colorectal cancer cells HT29	WST-1 XTT MTT Protein content Neutral red	0, 1–256 µM; 48 h	>256 µM 256 µM ≥1 µM ≥1 µM ≥4 µM	WST-1, XTT, and MTT were applied to assess metabolic activity	Schroterova et al. (2009)
h. colorectal cancer cells SW480	WST-1 XTT MTT Protein content Neutral red	0, 1–256 µM; 48 h	256 µM 256 µM ≥1 µM ≥32 µM ≥16 µM		
h. colorectal cancer cells SW620	WST-1 XTT MTT Protein content Neutral red	0, 1–256 µM; 48 h	>256 µM 256 µM ≥16 µM ≥32 µM ≥16 µM		
h. hepatoma cells HepG2	MTT assay	0, 0.1 nM–1.0 mM, 24–72 h	IC_{50} 11 µM (24 h) IC_{50} 5.5 µM (48 h) IC_{50} 1.9 µM (72 h)	100 nM Selenite (72 h) substantially increased SEPP concentration in culture medium	Hoefig et al. (2011)
h. lung adenocarcinoma epithelial cells A549	MTT assay	5 µM; 24–72 h	5 µM, 24 h	Selenium metabolism was studied in parallel	Weekley et al. (2011a)

(continued)

Table 20.1 (continued)

Cells	Assay/endpoint	Treatment	Result	Comment	References
h. colon adenocarcinoma cells HT29	Propidium iodide-positive cells	0, 5–100 µM; 24 h	≥10 µM	Selenate (5–100 µM) exerted no cytotoxicity; metabolism was studied in parallel	Lunoe et al. (2011)
h. prostate carcinoma cells PC-3			≥5 µM		
Acute T-cell leukemia cells Jurkat E6-1			≥5 µM		
h. prostate cancer cells LNCaP	MTT assay	0, 0.5–50 µM; 48 h	IC$_{50}$ 4.5 µM	Selenium biomarkers were studied in parallel	Hendrickx et al. (2013)
h. prostate cancer cells PC3			IC$_{50}$ 79 µM		
h. prostate cancer cells DU145			IC$_{50}$ 3.5 µM		
h. hepatoma cells HepG2	MTT assay	0, 0.05–200 µM, 72 h	IC$_{50}$ 2.3 µM	Selenite substantially increased biomarkers of Se status including GPx and TrxR activity, SePW1, SePH, SeP1.5	Kipp et al. (2013)
h. colorectal cancer cells HT29			IC$_{50}$ 2.5 µM		
Mouse colon cells YAMC			IC$_{50}$ 0.8 µM		
h. lung adenocarcinoma epithelial cells A549	Cell growth	0, 0.5–3.0 mM; 24–96 h	≥1.5 mM, 24 h ≥0.5 mM, 48 h	Microtubule and microfilament structures were affected	Villavicencio et al. (2014)
h. breast cancer cells MCF-7	MTS assay (cell proliferation)	0, 2.5–15 µM; 48 h	≥12.5 µM ≥5 µM	Forced expression of GPX1 increased selenite cytotoxicity through downregulation of selenium-binding protein 1 (SBP1); SBP1 reduction resulted in an increase of oxidative stress and triggered apoptosis	Wang et al. (2015)
h. colon cancer cells HCT116					

Cell type	Assay	Treatment	Results	Comments	Reference
h. astrocytoma cells CCF-STTG1	Cell number, Dehydrogenase activity	0, 2–50 µM; 48 h	Not assessed ≥5 µM	Cellular Se as well as Se speciation was carried out in parallel to study cellular selenite metabolism	Marschall et al. (2016)
h. hepatoma cells HepG2	Cell number, Dehydrogenase activity		≥5 µM ≥7.5 µM		
h. urothelial cells UROtsa	Cell number, Dehydrogenase activity		IC_{50} 2.4 µM IC_{50} 4.3 µM		
h. hepatoma cells HepG2	MTT assay	0, 0.1–15 µM; 24–72 h	$IC_{50 (24 h)}$ > 15 µM $IC_{50 (48 h)}$ 4.2 µM $IC_{50 (72 h)}$ 3.0 µM	The addition of nonessential amino acids to medium decreased selenite-induced cytotoxicity in HepG2 and T24 cells; selenosulfate exerted its cytotoxic effects in similar concentrations like selenite; stronger cytotoxicity in T24 as compared to HepG2 cells was accompanied by higher cellular Se levels in T24 cells	Hinrichsen and Planer-Friedrich (2016)
h. bladder carcinoma cells T24		0, 0.1–15 µM; 24–72 h	$IC_{50 (24 h)}$ 3.5 µM $IC_{50 (48/72 h)}$ 1 µM		
h. malignant melanoma cells A375		0, 0.1–15 µM; 24 h	$IC_{50 (24 h)}$ > 4.7 µM		
h. colon cancer cells Caco-2	Viability via mitochondrial respiratory activity	0, 0.4–80 µg Se/mL; 6 h	≥8 µg Se/mL ≥63 µM selenite		Takahashi et al. (2017)
h. hepatoma cells HepG2		0, 0.4–80 µg Se/mL; 24/48 h	≥0.8 µg Se/mL ≥6.3 µM selenite		

Cytotoxicity of Se-Methylselenocysteine (MeSeCys)

Studies investigating cytotoxicity and related endpoints of MeSeCys are summarized in Table 20.3. In cultured human cells, MeSeCys caused stronger cytotoxic effects as compared to SeMet, but less pronounced cytotoxicity as compared to selenite (Marschall et al. 2016, 2017; Hoefig et al. 2011; Kipp et al. 2013). In contrast to SeMet, MeSeCys is not unspecifically incorporated in proteins, which might account for its higher cytotoxicity in comparison to SeMet. In human cancer cells, MeSeCys has been shown to release MeSeH in the presence of β-lyase. Whether MeSeH is responsible for the ROS and apoptosis induction upon incubation with MeSeCys in human cancer cells and whether this mechanism is only specific for cancer cells is not yet fully understood (Whanger 2004). Genotoxic effects of MeSeCys in cultured mammalian cells are not characterized (Table 20.3).

Cytotoxicity of TMSe and Selenosugar 1

So far the cytotoxicity of TMSe and selenosugar 1 has been studied in human hepatoma (HepG2), astrocytoma (CCF), colon cancer (Caco-2), as well as urothelial cells (UROtsa) (Marschall et al. 2016, 2017; Takahashi et al. 2017; Kuehnelt et al. 2005) and failed to induce cytotoxic effects even though being incubated in the high micromolar concentration range (Table 20.4). No studies were identified investigating the genotoxicity of TMSe or selenosugar 1.

Taken together, regarding the selenium species discussed in this book chapter only selenite shows substantial cytotoxicity, whereas the organic selenium species exerted rather low (in high micromolar concentrations) or no toxicity in mammalian cells. This is in accordance with what is known for selenite, SeMet and MeSeCys from toxicity studies in experimental animals. The toxicity of TMSe and selenosugar 1 has yet not been characterized in experimental animals (Table 20.4).

Cellular Bioavailability and Biotransformation

In case of no cytotoxic response, it is needful to ensure that the respective selenium species are bioavailable to the respective cellular models before concluding that they exert no toxicity in vitro. For TMSe and selenosugar 1 it has been concluded that they are not cytotoxic despite being cellular bioavailable to the respective cell lines as quantified by inductively coupled plasma tandem mass spectrometry (ICP-QQQ-MS) (Marschall et al. 2016, 2017). Nevertheless, for prostate cancer, urothelial, colon cancer, leukemia, and hepatoma cells, no direct interspecies correlation between total cellular selenium and potencies of cytotoxic effects was found for selenite, SeMet, MeSeCys, TMSe, or selenosugar 1 (Marschall et al. 2016, 2017; Lunoe et al. 2011).

Table 20.2 Cytotoxicity and related endpoints of selenomethionine (SeMet) in mammalian cells

Cells	Assay/endpoint	Treatment	Result	Comment	References
h. prostate cancer cells LNCaP (wtp53) h. prostate cancer cells PC3 (p53-null)	MTT assay	0, 0.5–5 µM	No significant effects on viability	A coincubation with methionase strongly enhanced cellular toxicity as measured by MTT and apoptosis-related endpoints	Zhao et al. (2006)
h. colon cancer cells HCT116 (wtp53) h. colon cancer cells HCT116 (p53KO) h. colon cancer cells RKO h. colon cancer cells Caco-2	MTT assay	0, 25–100 µM; 24–72 h	$IC_{50} > 100$ µM	Data indicate that SeMet exerts p53-dependent growth inhibitory effects by inducing apoptosis and G2/M cell cycle arrest	Goel et al. (2006)
h. colorectal cancer cells HT29	WST-1 XTT MTT Protein content Neutral red	0, 1–256 µM; 48 h	>256 µM 256 µM ≥1 µM ≥64 µM ≥1 µM	WST-1, XTT, and MTT were applied to assess metabolic activity	Schroterova et al. (2009)
h. colorectal cancer cells SW480	WST-1 XTT MTT Protein content Neutral red	0, 1–256 µM; 48 h	≥16 µM ≥64 µM ≥1 µM ≥64 µM ≥4 µM		
h. colorectal cancer cells SW620	WST-1 XTT MTT Protein content Neutral red	0, 1–256 µM; 48 h	≥32 µM ≥128 µM ≥16 µM ≥64 µM ≥8 µM		

(continued)

Table 20.2 (continued)

Cells	Assay/endpoint	Treatment	Result	Comment	References
h. hepatoma cells HepG2	MTT assay	0, 0.1 nM–1.0 mM, 24–72 h	>1 mM	100 nM SeMet (72 h) increased SEPP concentration in culture medium	Hoefig et al. (2011)
h. lung adenocarcinoma epithelial cells A549	MTT assay	Concentration range not given; 72 h	IC_{50} 500 ± 200 μM	No data or graphs shown; the only value given is the IC_{50}	Weekley et al. (2011a)
h. prostate cancer cells LNCaP	MTT assay	0, 0.5–200 μM; 48 h	IC_{50} 400 μM	IC_{50} values were only estimated from lower concentrations; selenium biomarkers were studied in parallel	Hendrickx et al. (2013)
h. prostate cancer cells PC3			IC_{50} > 800 μM		
h. prostate cancer cells DU145			IC_{50} 300 μM		
h. hepatoma cells HepG2 h. colorectal cancer cells HT29 Mouse colon cells YAMC	MTT assay	0, 0.05–200 μM, 72 h	IC_{50} 165.8 μM IC_{50} 148.5 μM IC_{50} 99.5	SeMet (≥200 nM) increased GPx and TrxR activity	Kipp et al. (2013)
h. lung adenocarcinoma epithelial cells (A549)	Cell growth	0, 0.5–3.0 mM; 24–96 h	≥1.5 mM, 48 h ≥0.5 mM, 72 h	Microtubule and microfilament structures were affected	Villavicencio et al. (2014)
h. bladder cancer cells RT-112	Cell number	0, 1–100 μM; 24–72 h	≥10 μM, 24 h ≥2.5 μM, 48/72 h	Mitochondrial production of superoxide peaked between 3 and 6 h; simultaneously the number of γH2AX foci increased indicating DNA damage	Rezacova et al. (2016)
	ATP decrease Mitochondrial membrane potential	10 μM, 3–24 h	≥6 h		

Cell type	Method	Concentration; time	Effect level	Comment	Reference
h. astrocytoma cells CCF-STTG1	Cell number / Dehydrogenase activity	0, 25–1000 µM; 48 h	Not assessed / ≥1000 µM	Cellular Se as well as Se speciation was carried out in parallel to study cellular selenite metabolism	Marschall et al. (2016)
h. hepatoma cells HepG2	Cell number / Dehydrogenase activity		≥100 µM / ≥200 µM		
h. urothelial cells UROtsa	Cell number / Dehydrogenase activity		≥250 µM / ≥500 µM		
h. hepatoma cells HepG2	Cell number	0, 150, 200 µM; 48/96 h	≥150 µM	Se speciation was carried out in parallel to study cellular SeMet metabolism	Marschall et al. (2017)
h. colon cancer cells Caco-2	Viability via mitochondrial respiratory activity	0, 0.4–80 µg Se/mL; 6 h	>80 µg Se/mL / 408 µM SeMet	After 6 (80 µg Se/mL) and 24 h (≥8 µg Se/mL) SeMet increased cell viability	Takahashi et al. (2017)
h. hepatoma cells HepG2		0, 0.4–80 µg Se/mL; 48 h	≥40 µg Se/mL / 204 µM SeMet		

Table 20.3 Cytotoxicity and related endpoints of Se-Methylselenocysteine (MeSeCys) in mammalian cells

Cells	Assay/endpoint	Treatment	Result	Comment	References
h. colorectal cancer cells HT29	WST-1 XTT MTT Protein content Neutral red	0, 1–256 μM; 48 h	256 μM 256 μM ≥32 μM ≥32 μM ≥32 μM	WST-1, XTT, and MTT were applied to assess metabolic activity	Schroterova et al. (2009)
h. colorectal cancer cells SW480	WST-1 XTT MTT Protein content Neutral red	0, 1–256 μM; 48 h	>256 μM 256 μM ≥64 μM ≥64 μM ≥32 μM		
h. colorectal cancer cells SW620	WST-1 XTT MTT Protein content Neutral red	0, 1–256 μM; 48 h	256 μM ≥128 μM ≥64 μM ≥64 μM ≥8 μM		
h. hepatoma cells HepG2	MTT assay	0, 0.1 nM–1.0 mM, 24–72 h	$IC_{50(24h)}$ 235 μM $IC_{50(48h)}$ 164 μM $IC_{50(72h)}$ 177 μM	100 nM Selenite (72 h) substantially increased SEPP concentration in culture medium	Hoefig et al. (2011)
h. promyelotic leukemia cells HL-60	Cell viability (WST-1)	0, 10–200 μM; 24 h	IC_{50} 50 μM	ROS formation (DCF fluorescence) was observed after 30-min incubation with ≥25 μM; ≥25 μM induced caspase 3 and ≥25 μM caspase 9 activity after 8–24 h and 18 h, respectively	Jung et al. (2001)
	Apoptosis (DNA fragmentation)		≥10 μM		
	Apoptosis (SubG1)		≥25 μM		
h. lung adenocarcinoma epithelial cells A549	MTT assay	Concentration range not given; 72 h	IC_{50} 100 ± 20 μM	No data or graphs shown; the only value given is the IC_{50}	Weekley et al. (2011a)

Cells	Assay	Treatment	Result	Comments	Reference
h. prostate cancer cells LNCaP	MTT assay	0, 0.5–200 µM; 48 h	IC_{50} 175.6 µM	Selenium biomarkers were studied in parallel	Hendrickx et al. (2013)
h. prostate cancer cells PC3			IC_{50} 606.3 µM		
h. prostate cancer cells DU145			IC_{50} 141.7 µM		
h. hepatoma cells HepG2 h. colorectal cancer cells HT29 Mouse colon cells YAMC	MTT assay	0, 0.05–200 µM, 72 h	≥200 µM IC_{50} 49.8 µM IC_{50} 32.0 µM	MeSeCys (≥200 nM) increased GPx and TrxR activity	Kipp et al. (2013)
h. astrocytoma cells CCF-STTG1	Cell number Dehydrogenase activity	0, 25–1000 µM; 48 h	Not assessed ≥350 µM	Cellular Se as well as Se speciation was carried out in parallel to study cellular selenite metabolism	Marschall et al. (2016)
h. hepatoma cells HepG2	Cell number Dehydrogenase activity		≥100 µM ≥200 µM		
h. urothelial cells UROtsa	Cell number Dehydrogenase activity		IC_{50} 39.5 µM IC_{50} 90.0 µM		
h. hepatoma cells HepG2	Cell number	0, 500 µM, 48 h; 96 h	>500 µM	Se speciation was carried out in parallel to study cellular SeMet metabolism	Marschall et al. (2017)
h. colon cancer cells Caco-2	Viability via mitochondrial	0, 0.4–80 µg Se/mL; 6 h	>80 µg Se/mL, 439 µM	After 6 (≥0.8 µg Se/mL), 24 h (≥40 µg Se/mL) and 48 h (≥8 µg Se/mL) MeSeCys increased cell viability	Takahashi et al. (2017)
h. hepatoma cells HepG2	Respiratory activity	0, 0.4–80 µg Se/mL; 24/48 h	≥40 µg Se/mL; 48 h 220 µM		

Table 20.4 Cytotoxicity and related endpoints of selenosugar 1 or trimethylselenonium (TMSe) in mammalian cells

Cells	Assay/endpoint	Treatment	Result	Comment	References
h. hepatoma cells HepG2	WST-8 Dehydrogenase activity	Selenosugar 1 0, 0.001–10 mM; 48 h	≥10 mM	Selenosugar 2 exerted cytotoxicity in similar concentrations	Kuehnelt et al. (2005)
h. astrocytoma cells CCF-STTG1	Cell number Dehydrogenase activity	Selenosugar 1 or TMSe 0, 100–500, 1000 µM, 48 h	Not assessed >1000 µM	Se speciation was carried out in parallel to study cellular SeMet metabolism	Marschall et al. (2016)
h. hepatoma cells HepG2	Cell number Dehydrogenase activity		>500 µM >1000 µM		
h. urothelial cells UROtsa	Cell number Dehydrogenase activity		>500 µM >1000 µM		
h. colon cancer cells Caco-2	Viability via mitochondrial respiratory activity	Selenosugar 1 or TMSe 0, 0.4–80 µg Se/mL; 6 h	>80 µg Se/mL Selenosugar 1268 µM TMSe 645 µM		Takahashi et al. (2017)
h. hepatoma cells HepG2		Selenosugar 1 or TMSe 0, 0.4–80 µg Se/mL; 24/48 h	>80 µg Se/mL Selenosugar 1268 µM TMSe 645 µM		

To further understand selenium species metabolism in vitro but also to unveil potential causes for the differing cytotoxic potencies of selenium species a combined quantification of free selenium species in cell lysates and total cellular selenium quantification has been carried out in some studies (Marschall et al. 2016, 2017; Lunoe et al. 2011; Gabel-Jensen and Gammelgaard 2010).

Biotransformation of Selenite in Mammalian Cells

After 4 h incubation of isolated rat hepatocytes with selenite, the majority of selenite was metabolized. In the cell lysates, only traces of selenite and two unknown metabolites were observed by liquid chromatography inductively coupled plasma mass spectrometry (LC-ICP-MS). The authors concluded that the limited amount of small selenium species in the cell lysates as well as the respective culture media indicate that the more important metabolic pathway of selenite isolated rat hepatocytes may be related to interaction with proteins (Gabel-Jensen and Gammelgaard

2010). LC-ICP-MS analysis of a lysate of human prostate carcinoma PC-3 cells incubated for 4 h with selenite revealed only selenite itself, while size-exclusion chromatography (SEC)-ICP-MS indicated that selenite was bound to proteins to a substantial amount (Lunoe et al. 2011).

Applying X-ray absorption spectroscopy, Weekley et al. (2011a) showed that selenite was rapidly metabolized by cultured human A549 lung adenocarcinoma cells to the extent that within 1 h of incubation no selenite was detected in the cells. Within 4 h of treatment, selenodiglutathione (GSSeSG) and elemental Se were detected, with GSSeSG accounting for 25% of the cellular selenium species. This presence of GSSeSG is in accordance with the proposed reductive metabolism of selenite by GSH and GSH reductase in vivo. Additionally, selenocystine (CysSeSeCys) and selenocysteine (SeCys) were identified. In doing so, the authors concluded that the identification of cellular SeCys may reflect the presence of selenoproteins rather than free SeCys. The substantial formation of diselenide species between 24 and 48 h indicates intracellular oxidizing conditions which is in agreement with the generation of superoxide radical anion as a cytotoxic mode of action of selenite. Accordingly, after 24–48 h selenite incubation cell viability declined (Weekley et al. 2011a).

Anan et al. identified selenocyanate as new selenite metabolite after 24 h selenite incubation of human hepatoma HepG2 cells by electrospray ionization mass spectrometry (ESI-MS) and ESI quadrupole time-of-flight mass spectrometry (ESI-Q-TOF-MS) (Anan et al. 2015). Since incubated selenocyanate was less toxic to HepG2 cells than selenite or cyanide, the authors hypothesize that selenite was metabolized to selenocyanate to temporarily ameliorate its toxicity and to serve as an intrinsic selenium pool in cultured cells in case of selenite overexposure. In human urothelial UROtsa cells after 48 h incubation with selenite, cellular selenite as well as one unknown metabolite were detected by means of LC-ICP-QQQ-MS (Marschall et al. 2016).

Biotransformation of SeMet in Mammalian Cells

Studies published for SeMet biotransformation in cultured mammalian cells are very much in accordance with each other. After SeMet incubation of isolated rat hepatoytces (Gabel-Jensen and Gammelgaard 2010), human prostate PC-3 cancer cells, human HT-29 colon cancer cells, and human leukemia Jurkat E6-1 cells (Lunoe et al. 2011) as well as human urothelial UROtsa and hepatoma HepG2 cells (Marschall et al. 2016, 2017) SeMet entered the cells in large amounts. As analyzed by LC-ICP-(QQQ)-MS SeMet was the primary cellular selenium species found in addition to two species. One of these peaks is likely to be oxidized SeMet (SeOMet), a sample preparation artifact (Marschall et al. 2016, 2017; Lunoe et al. 2011). The second peak has not been identified yet. An analytical method based on direct headspace GC-MS indicated no formation of the volatile selenium species MeSeH, dimethylselenide (DMeSe) and dimethyldiselenide (DMeDSe) in human leukemia

Jurkat cells after 24 h incubation with SeMet (Gabel-Jensen et al. 2010). X-ray absorption spectroscopy of human A549 lung adenocarcinoma cells treated with SeMet for 24 h showed that selenium was found exclusively in carbon-bound forms (Weekley et al. 2011b).

Biotransformation of MeSeCys in Mammalian Cells

When human leukemia Jurkat cells were incubated for 24 h with MeSeCys, the only volatile selenium species detected via headspace GC-MS in traces was DMeSe, indicating that in this in vitro system MeSeH is not formed as a MeSeCys metabolite (Gabel-Jensen et al. 2010). Full recovery of applied selenium was observed when isolated rat hepatocytes were incubated with MeSeCys for 4 h and LC-ICP-MS measurements indicated no MeSeCys metabolism in these primary rat hepatocytes (Gabel-Jensen and Gammelgaard 2010). LC-ICP-MS measurements of lysates from MeSeCys-incubated human prostate PC-3 cancer cells, human HT-29 colon cancer cells, and human leukemia Jurkat E6-1 cells revealed no apparent transformation of MeSeCys in these cell lines. The authors concluded that the lack of substantial cytotoxicity of MeSeCys in these cell lines may thus be explained by lacking of ß-lyase, which is known to convert MeSeCys to cytotoxic MeSeH in vivo. After 24 h incubation of human A549 lung adenocarcinoma cells with MeSeCys carbon-bound selenium species but also a diselenide species were identified by X-ray absorption spectroscopy. X-ray absorption and X-ray fluorescence spectroscopy both demonstrated that the selenium content of MeSeCys-treated cells was much lower as compared to SeMet-incubated cells, with selenium being homogeneously distributed throughout the MeSeCys-incubated cells (Weekley et al. 2011b). A 48 h incubation of human urothelial UROtsa cells with MeSeCys at cytotoxic concentrations showed cellular MeSeCys and two unknown metabolites (Marschall et al. 2016). These two additional metabolites have not been seen before after 24 h incubation with subcytotoxic MeSeCys, concentrations in human prostate PC-3 cancer cells, human HT-29 colon cancer cells, human leukemia Jurkat E6-1 cells, or human hepatoma HepG2 cells. In lysates of HepG2 cells treated with MeSeCys for 4 days, the incubated species was detected in its intact form. Additionally, two MeSeCys metabolites were detected in the lysates and identified as γ-glutamyl-Se-Methylselenocysteine (γ-glutamyl-MeSeCys) and Se-methylselenoglutathione (MeSeGSH) by means of LC-electrospray-ionization-Orbitrap-MS. Furthermore, a small amount of volatile DMeSe was detected in the lysates. γ-Glutamyl-MeSeCys was only detected in the cytotoxic concentration range of MeSeCys and in comparison to cellular MeSeCys γ-glutamyl-MeSeCys increased over proportionally in its cellular concentrations. This might suggest that y-glutamyl-MeSeCys is involved in the cytotoxicity, either as a cause or a consequence (Marschall et al. 2017).

Biotransformation of TMSe and Selenosugar 1 in Mammalian Cells

TMSe and selenosugar 1 were bioavailable to human urothelial UROtsa cells, but LC-ICP-QQQ-MS analysis of cell lysates indicated that both species were not significantly metabolized after 48 h incubation (Marschall et al. 2016). Likewise in HepG2 cells, after 4 days of incubation both species were not metabolized. Thus, when comparing the cellular TMSe and selenosugar 1 concentrations (quantified via isotope dilution (ID)-LC-ICP-QQQ-MS) with the total cellular selenium concentration, nearly quantitative recoveries were obtained (Marschall et al. 2017).

Taken together, despite being taken up, TMSe and selenosugar 1 are noncytotoxic in human urothelial and hepatoma cells, most likely because they are not metabolically activated. This absent in vitro toxicity of TMSe and selenosugar 1 up to high supraphysiological concentrations supports their importance as metabolites for Se detoxification in vivo.

Concluding Remarks

Toxicity studies in mammalian cells are increasingly used to assess and compare the toxic potential of selenium species. Nevertheless, the limitations of these models should be taken into account when aiming to conclude on the in vitro toxic potential of selenium species. This can be partly achieved by quantifying in parallel cytotoxicity, cellular bioavailability, as well as cellular metabolism of the respective selenium species as reviewed in this book chapter. Finally, in vitro approaches could help to identify new selenium species metabolites and can contribute to our understanding of the role of these metabolites in the detoxification or toxification of selenium species.

References

Anan Y, Kimura M, Hayashi M, Koike R, Ogra Y. Detoxification of selenite to form selenocyanate in mammalian cells. Chem Res Toxicol. 2015;28(9):1803–14. https://doi.org/10.1021/acs.chemrestox.5b00254.

European Union. Directive 2002/46/EC of the European Parliament and the Council of 10 June 2002 on the approximation of the laws of the member states relating to food supplements. 2015.

Gabel-Jensen C, Gammelgaard B. Selenium metabolism in hepatocytes incubated with selenite, selenate, selenomethionine, Se-methylselenocysteine and methylseleninc acid and analysed by LC-ICP-MS. J Anal At Spectrom. 2010;25(3):414–8. https://doi.org/10.1039/b921365a.

Gabel-Jensen C, Lunoe K, Gammelgaard B. Formation of methylselenol, dimethylselenide and dimethyldiselenide in in vitro metabolism models determined by headspace GC-MS. Metallomics. 2010;2(2):167–73. https://doi.org/10.1039/b914255j.

Gammelgaard B, Jackson MI, Gabel-Jensen C. Surveying selenium speciation from soil to cell-forms and transformations. Anal Bioanal Chem. 2011;399(5):1743–63. https://doi.org/10.1007/s00216-010-4212-8.

Goel A, Fuerst F, Hotchkiss E, Boland CR. Selenomethionine induces p53 mediated cell cycle arrest and apoptosis in human colon cancer cells. Cancer Biol Ther. 2006;5(5):529–35. https://doi.org/10.4161/cbt.5.5.2654.

Hendrickx W, Decock J, Mulholland F, Bao Y, Fairweather-Tait S. Selenium biomarkers in prostate cancer cell lines and influence of selenium on invasive potential of PC3 cells. Front Oncol. 2013;3:239. https://doi.org/10.3389/fonc.2013.00239.

Hinrichsen S, Planer-Friedrich B. Cytotoxic activity of selenosulfate versus selenite in tumor cells depends on cell line and presence of amino acids. Environ Sci Pollut Res Int. 2016;23(9):8349–57. https://doi.org/10.1007/s11356-015-5960-y.

Hoefig CS, Renko K, Kohrle J, Birringer M, Schomburg L. Comparison of different selenocom-pounds with respect to nutritional value vs. toxicity using liver cells in culture. J Nutr Biochem. 2011;22(10):945–55. https://doi.org/10.1016/j.jnutbio.2010.08.006.

Jung U, Zheng X, Yoon SO, Chung AS. Se-methylselenocysteine induces apoptosis mediated by reactive oxygen species in HL-60 cells. Free Radic Biol Med. 2001;31(4):479–89. https://doi.org/10.1016/S0891-5849(01)00604-9.

Kipp AP, Frombach J, Deubel S, Brigelius-Flohe R. Selenoprotein W as biomarker for the efficacy of selenium compounds to act as source for selenoprotein biosynthesis. Methods Enzymol. 2013;527:87–112. https://doi.org/10.1016/B978-0-12-405882-8.00005-2.

Kuehnelt D, Kienzl N, Traar P, Le NH, Francesconi KA, Ochi T. Selenium metabolites in human urine after ingestion of selenite, L-selenomethionine, or DL-selenomethionine: a quantita-tive case study by HPLC/ICPMS. Anal Bioanal Chem. 2005;383(2):235–46. https://doi.org/10.1007/s00216-005-0007-8.

Kuehnelt D, Engstrom K, Skroder H, Kokarnig S, Schlebusch C, Kippler M, Alhamdow A, Nermell B, Francesconi K, Broberg K, Vahter M. Selenium metabolism to the trimethyl-selenonium ion (TMSe) varies markedly because of polymorphisms in the indolethylamine N-methyltransferase gene. Am J Clin Nutr. 2015;102(6):1406–15. https://doi.org/10.3945/ajcn.115.114157.

Lo LW, Koropatnick J, Stich HF. The mutagenicity and cytotoxicity of selenite, "activated" selenite and selenate for normal and DNA repair-deficient human fibroblasts. Mutat Res. 1978;49(3):305–12. https://doi.org/10.1016/0027-5107(78)90103-3.

Lu J, Kaeck M, Jiang C, Wilson AC, Thompson HJ. Selenite induction of DNA strand breaks and apoptosis in mouse leukemic L1210 cells. Biochem Pharmacol. 1994;47(9):1531–5. https://doi.org/10.1016/0006-2952(94)90528-2.

Lu J, Jiang C, Kaeck M, Ganther H, Vadhanavikit S, Ip C, Thompson H. Dissociation of the genotoxic and growth inhibitory effects of selenium. Biochem Pharmacol. 1995;50(2):213–9. https://doi.org/10.1016/0006-2952(95)00119-K.

Lunoe K, Gabel-Jensen C, Sturup S, Andresen L, Skov S, Gammelgaard B. Investigation of the selenium metabolism in cancer cell lines. Metallomics. 2011;3(2):162–8. https://doi.org/10.1039/c0mt00091d.

Marschall TA, Bornhorst J, Kuehnelt D, Schwerdtle T. Differing cytotoxicity and bioavailability of selenite, methylselenocysteine, selenomethionine, selenosugar 1 and trimethylselenonium ion and their underlying metabolic transformations in human cells. Mol Nutr Food Res. 2016;60(12):2622–32. https://doi.org/10.1002/mnfr.201600422.

Marschall TA, Kroepfl N, Jensen KB, Bornhorst J, Meermann B, Kuehnelt D, Schwerdtle T. Tracing cytotoxic effects of small organic Se species in human liver cells back to total cellular Se and Se metabolites. Metallomics. 2017;9(3):268–77. https://doi.org/10.1039/c6mt00300a.

Rezacova K, Canova K, Bezrouk A, Rudolf E. Selenite induces DNA damage and specific mito-chondrial degeneration in human bladder cancer cells. Toxicol In Vitro. 2016;32:105–14. https://doi.org/10.1016/j.tiv.2015.12.011.

Schroterova L, Kralova V, Voracova A, Haskova P, Rudolf E, Cervinka M. Antiproliferative effects of selenium compounds in colon cancer cells: comparison of different cytotoxicity assays. Toxicol In Vitro. 2009;23(7):1406–11. https://doi.org/10.1016/j.tiv.2009.07.013.

Shen HM, Yang CF, Ong CN. Sodium selenite-induced oxidative stress and apoptosis in human hepatoma HepG2 cells. Int J Cancer. 1999;81(5):820–8. https://doi.org/10.1002/(SICI)1097-0215(19990531)81:5<820::AID-IJC25>3.0.CO;2-F.

Spallholz JE, Palace VP, Reid TW. Methioninase and selenomethionine but not Se-methylselenocysteine generate methylselenol and superoxide in an in vitro chemiluminescent assay: implications for the nutritional carcinostatic activity of selenoamino acids. Biochem Pharmacol. 2004;67(3):547–54. https://doi.org/10.1016/j.bcp.2003.09.004.

Stewart MS, Davis RL, Walsh LP, Pence BC. Induction of differentiation and apoptosis by sodium selenite in human colonic carcinoma cells (HT29). Cancer Lett. 1997;117(1):35–40. https://doi.org/10.1016/S0304-3835(97)00212-7.

Takahashi K, Suzuki N, Ogra Y. Bioavailability comparison of nine bioselenocompounds in vitro and in vivo. Int J Mol Sci. 2017;18(3) https://doi.org/10.3390/ijms18030506.

Villavicencio LLF, Cruz-Jimenez G, Barbosa-Sabanero G, Kornhauser-Araujo C, Mendoza-Garrido ME, de la Rosa G, Sabanero-Lopez M. Human lung cancer cell line A-549 ATCC is differentially affected by supranutritional organic and inorganic selenium. Bioinorg Chem Appl. 2014;2014:923834. https://doi.org/10.1155/2014/923834.

Wang Y, Fang W, Huang Y, Hu F, Ying Q, Yang W, Xiong B. Reduction of selenium-binding protein 1 sensitizes cancer cells to selenite via elevating extracellular glutathione: a novel mechanism of cancer-specific cytotoxicity of selenite. Free Radic Biol Med. 2015;79:186–96. https://doi.org/10.1016/j.freeradbiomed.2014.11.015.

Weekley CM, Aitken JB, Vogt S, Finney LA, Paterson DJ, de Jonge MD, Howard DL, Witting PK, Musgrave IF, Harris HH. Metabolism of selenite in human lung cancer cells: X-ray absorption and fluorescence studies. J Am Chem Soc. 2011a;133(45):18272–9. https://doi.org/10.1021/ja206203c.

Weekley CM, Aitken JB, Vogt S, Finney LA, Paterson DJ, de Jonge MD, Howard DL, Musgrave IF, Harris HH. Uptake, distribution, and speciation of selenoamino acids by human cancer cells: X-ray absorption and fluorescence methods. Biochemistry. 2011b;50(10):1641–50. https://doi.org/10.1021/bi101678a.

Whanger PD. Selenium and its relationship to cancer: an update. Br J Nutr. 2004;91(1):11–28. https://doi.org/10.1079/Bjn20031015.

Xiang N, Zhao R, Zhong W. Sodium selenite induces apoptosis by generation of superoxide via the mitochondrial-dependent pathway in human prostate cancer cells. Cancer Chemother Pharmacol. 2009;63(2):351–62. https://doi.org/10.1007/s00280-008-0745-3.

Zhao R, Domann FE, Zhong W. Apoptosis induced by selenomethionine and methioninase is superoxide mediated and p53 dependent in human prostate cancer cells. Mol Cancer Ther. 2006;5(12):3275–84. https://doi.org/10.1158/1535-7163.MCT-06-0400.

Chapter 21
Selenium Nanoparticles: Biomedical Applications

Ivana Vinković Vrček

Abstract Nanotechnology has introduced nanoparticulate form of selenium for a wide variety of applications. Due to exceptional catalytic, photoreactive, biocidal, anticancer, and antioxidant properties, selenium nanoparticles (SeNPs) attract considerable interest for use in antimicrobial coatings, nutritional supplements, nanotherapeutics, diagnostics, and medical devices, as well as in other applications such as rectifiers, photocopiers, xerography, and solar cells. Preparation and synthesis of SeNPs may be conducted following different physical, chemical, or biological techniques. Depending on the selected synthetic route, physicochemical properties of final SeNPs can be controlled by careful setup of experimental conditions including reactant concentrations, reaction temperature and pH, time for preparation, addition of catalysts, coating agent for surface stabilization, etc. Any application of SeNPs should be ascertained by the risk versus benefit ratio profiling. Implementation of safe-by-design concept, which is designed to ensure safety for humans and the environment, would help in timely identification of all risks related to the innovation processes and value chain of SeNPs.

Keywords Nanoparticles · Synthesis · Anticancer · Drug resistance · Antimicrobial · Antioxidant · Safe-by-design

Introduction

Selenium in the form of nanoparticles (NPs) has attracted considerable interest a decade ago for a wide variety of applications due to its exceptional properties (Eswarapriya and Jegatheesan 2015). However, nanoformulation of selenium (Se) does not represent absolute novelty. Biologically derived elemental Se exists always in the nanoform (Buchs et al. 2013). Natural Se cycle involves formation of selenium nanoparticles (SeNPs) in oxygen-limited conditions or during bioreduction

I. Vinković Vrček (✉)
Institute for Medical Research and Occupational Health, Zagreb, Croatia
e-mail: ivinkovic@imi.hr

© Springer International Publishing AG, part of Springer Nature 2018
B. Michalke (ed.), *Selenium*, Molecular and Integrative Toxicology,
https://doi.org/10.1007/978-3-319-95390-8_21

393

of selenite and selenate by microorganisms (Buchs et al. 2013; Mal et al. 2017). In addition, in situ bioremediation and treatment of Se-contaminated waters involve process of conversion of selenite and selenate to colloidal SeNPs, i.e., SeNPs (Nancharaiah and Lens 2015).

Nanotechnology, as one of the six key enabling technologies (KETs), boosted the development and application of engineered SeNPs like for many other nanomaterials (e.g., carbon nanotubes, fullerenes). Although nanotechnological development started in 1970s, production of materials by the reduction of their size to the level of nanometers has been known since ancient times (Sengupta et al. 2014). Thus, NPs have been applied in the Ayurvedic medicine revealing that roots of nanotechnology emanate since the origin of therapeutics (Paul and Chugh 2011). For example, gold ash known as Swarna Bhasma belongs to the most potent therapeutics of Ayurvedic medicine, which was used for healing of rheumatoid arthritis and tuberculosis (Richards et al. 2002). The basic principles of nanotechnology have been established by Richard Feynman in 1959. In his talk "There's Plenty of Room at the Bottom," he brought the scientific concept of nanotechnology when he described the possibility of material production through direct manipulation at the atomic level. The first formal term "nanotechnology" had been introduced by Norio Taniguchi in 1974 (Kazlev 1998). Development of innovative NPs is the promising approach to meet unmet human needs by controlling shape and size of structures, devices, and systems at nano level during their design, production, and application. In this way, NP properties including reactivity, strength, and electrical characteristics are significantly different from the bulk materials. The most critical factors that provoke these differences are the increased relative surface area and the quantum effects (Emerich and Thanos 2003). Nowadays, nanotechnology deals with many different tools for preparation of NPs. Wide range of specific and peculiar optoelectronic, magnetic, mechanical, photoresponsive, catalytic properties make NPs a promising approach also for diverse biomedical applications including drug and gene delivery, biosensor development, bioimaging, tissue engineering, bioelectronics, and tissue regeneration (Kapur et al. 2017). Among many different types of nanomaterials, metallic NPs are very attractive owing to their simple synthesis and facile surface chemistry that supports a wide variety of functionalization features (Zheng and Chen 2012). Among many different metal-based NPs, SeNPs have appeared remarkable for biomedical applications concerning their degradability in vivo and low toxicity (Zheng and Chen 2012). Due to their excellent catalytic, photoreactive, biocidal, anticancer, and antioxidant properties, SeNPs are increasingly designed for application in a wide range of antimicrobial coatings, nutritional supplementation formulas for food and feed, nanotherapeutics, diagnostic, and other medical devices (Husen and Siddiqi 2014). The search on the SeNPs performed on 27th October 2017 in all databases of the ISI Web of Science (WoS) showed 3473 publications altogether (Fig. 21.1). According to this analysis, almost a quarter of all published studies reported synthetic routes for preparation of SeNPs, while 10% of papers presented different medical aspects of SeNPs. Most papers described applications of SeNPs in the drug delivery systems (44% of all medical publications), while antimicrobial and anticancer activities of SeNPs were evaluated by

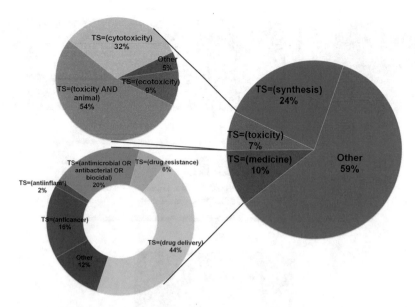

Fig. 21.1 Number of publication in the ISI Web of Science on selenium nanoparticles. Search was performed on 27.10.2017 using the main search term "selenium AND nano," whereas all other search terms indicated as data labels were combined with the main search term using AND option

similar number of studies. Due to the large and still increasing number of newly developed SeNPs, a full risk assessment of their use and subsequent release into the environment is of utmost importance. According to the results of ISI WoS search (Fig. 21.1), toxicity evaluation of SeNPs was performed in only 7% of all publications.

Final fate of the most innovative ideas in the biomedical field is usually just publication in the high-ranked international scientific journals, while technology transfer is suffering from the translational gaps associated with the safety concerns and socioeconomic uncertainties (Rösslein et al. 2017). Thus, current innovation processes and risk management for SeNPs have to be enhanced by quality, efficacy, and safety (QES) management applying safe-by-design (SbD) concept (Micheletti et al. 2017; Ahonen et al. 2017). This concept, developed within the European research projects NANoREG, ProSafe, and NanoReg2, encourages as early as possible identification of uncertainties and risks related to their production and use (Ahonen et al. 2017).

Synthesis of SeNPs

Utilization of SbD approach should start at the level of SeNP preparation, which requires precise control of all factors that directly affect physicochemical properties of SeNPs. Depending on the selected synthesis method, all parameters should be

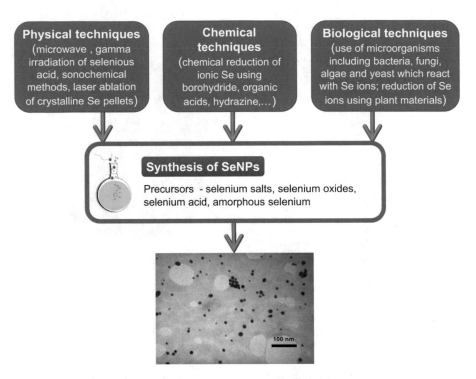

Fig. 21.2 Strategies for synthesis of selenium nanoparticles (SeNPs)

carefully tested and defined including reactant concentrations, reaction temperature and pH, time for preparation, addition of catalysts, coating agent for surface stabilization or functionalization, etc. Three different synthetic approaches can be used for SeNP synthesis: (1) physical, (2) chemical, or (3) biological techniques (Fig. 21.2) (Skalickova et al. 2017; Dobias et al. 2011).

The most common physical methods for the SeNP synthesis are microwave or gamma irradiation of selenious acid, sonochemical methods, and laser ablation of crystalline Se pellets (Skalickova et al. 2017). Physical methods have some advantage over chemical ones including the lack of contamination with reagents and substances present during chemical or biological synthesis, low-cost equipment, rapid reactions, and easy separation and purification of SeNPs (Shahbazi et al. 2015; Panahi-Kalamuei et al. 2014).

Chemical approach to SeNPs synthesis mostly relies on the reduction of selenium ions to elemental Se. Different reducing agents can be employed including borohydride, hydrazine, thiosulfate, and range of organic acids such as ascorbic, folic, citric, acetic, oxalic, benzoic, and gallic acids (Skalickova et al. 2017; Dhand et al. 2015). Interesting chemical approach for SeNP preparation is hydrothermal method that employs a nucleation-dissolution-recrystallization growth mechanism (Xi et al. 2006). In this method, heating time is the main parameter that determines the size and shape of formed SeNPs. Compared to physical approach, chemical methods result in smaller, homogeneous, and more stable SeNPs. As this approach permits dispersion in aqueous media and further modification of SeNPs with different functional or stabilizing agents, it is favored for SeNP preparation in biomedical applications.

All above-mentioned physical and chemical techniques are usually expensive or hazardous. Therefore, green biotechnological methods have gained popularity and great interest due to their cost-effectiveness, widely available raw material, lower toxicity of prepared SeNPs, and great potential in pharmacology (Maiyo and Singh 2017; Ramamurthy et al. 2013). These eco-friendly and energy-efficient techniques use mainly microorganisms including bacteria, fungi, algae, and yeast which react differently with metal ions (Maiyo and Singh 2017; Ramamurthy et al. 2013). Many different microorganisms can be used. For example, *Bacillus licheniformis* cultivated under sodium selenite stress converted toxic selenite ions into nontoxic SeNPs (Husen and Siddiqi 2014). Live biomass of the rhizobacterium *Azospirillum brasilense* Sp7 was used in the process of selenite reduction to yield monodisperse SeNPs (Kamnev et al. 2017). In a fermentation procedure, alginate and alginate/chitosan microspheres containing SeNPs were produced using probiotic yogurt bacteria *Lactobacillus casei* (Cavalu et al. 2017). Gram-negative bacterial strain *Escherichia coli* ATCC 35218 was tested in the biosynthetic method for the preparation of SeNPs from sodium selenite under ambient temperature and pressure (Kora and Rastogi 2017). Anoxygenic photosynthetic bacteria *Rhodobacter sphaeroides* YL75, tolerant to selenite, was used in adsorption reduction process under anaerobic condition for preparation of red SeNPs (Xiao et al. 2017). Bacteria *Enterococcus faecalis* were applied for reduction of sodium selenite yielding SeNPs that were efficient against *Staphylococcus aureus* infections (Shoeibi and Mashreghi 2017). Biologically synthesized SeNPs by nonpathogenic, economic, and easy-to-handle bacterium *Ralstonia eutropha* showed excellent antimicrobial activity against *Pseudomonas aeruginosa, Staphylococcus aureus, Escherichia coli*, and *Streptococcus pyogenes*, and antifungal activity against *Aspergillus clavatus* (Srivastava and Mukhopadhyay 2015). Many other biosynthetic procedures for SeNPs have been reported using, for example, *Lactobacillus acidophilus, Streptococcus thermophilus* and *Lactobacillus casei* (Eszenyi et al. 2011), *Staphylococcus carnosus* (Estevam et al. 2017), *Zooglea ramigera* (Srivastava and Mukhopadhyay 2013), *Pseudomonas alcaliphila* (Zhang et al. 2011), or *Pseudomonas putida* KT2440 (Avendaño et al. 2016). In all these methods, intra- or extracellular formation of SeNPs is involved, whereas various biological agents and different biomolecules are responsible for the process of SeNP genesis (Husen and Siddiqi 2014). Besides all benefits of applying the optimum growth condition including pH, temperature, and nutrients in these biogenic methods with microorganisms, extraction and purification of SeNPs after synthetic are usually difficult and time consuming (Maiyo and Singh 2017; Ramamurthy et al. 2013).

Rapid procedures using plant materials have also showed a great potential for SeNP biosynthesis (Maiyo and Singh 2017). Biomolecules from plants, like those from microorganisms, enable both reduction and stabilization of SeNPs. Methods using plant extracts are less expensive and do not require any special conditions as compared to biosynthesis by microorganisms. For example, fruit extract prepared from dried *Vitis vinifera* was used for SeNP synthesis from selenous acid (Sharma et al. 2014). Bioreductive capacity of a leaf extract from plant *Terminalia arjuna* was utilized for preparation of SeNPs that showed protective effect against arsenite-induced cell death and DNA damage (Prasad and Selvaraj 2014). Other examples include stabilization of SeNPs with hydrolyzed arabic gum using selenium dioxide as precursor in the synthesis (Kong et al. 2014), or sodium selenite reduction with lemon leaf extract (Prasad et al. 2013).

Great advantages of described biosynthetic procedures include accessibility of raw material for SeNP production, applicability in various fields, and relevance for bioremediation of naturally occurring toxic selenium compounds.

Regardless to the synthetic method applied for SeNP preparation, control over the size, dispersity state, and stability of NPs is always challenging (Maiyo and Singh 2017). During synthesis, nucleation and growth of NPs are affected by various experimental factors including the concentration of precursors and reducing agents used, temperature, reaction rate, pH, and presence or absence of agents used for stabilization and functionalization of NPs (Maiyo and Singh 2017). For any biomedical application, SeNPs must satisfy certain criteria to be useful in biomedicine. They must maintain colloidal stability under physiological conditions. NPs are usually functionalized in order to prevent their agglomeration in the matrix structure or to bind the NPs to the matrix or to improve their physicochemical properties (Nowack et al. 2011). They should outperform the conventional agents while inducing minimal toxicity, avoiding nonspecific interactions with plasma proteins (opsonization) or premature release of specific deliver, and either evading or allowing uptake by the reticuloendothelial system depending on the application (Thanh and Green 2010). For example, in order for SeNPs to be internalized by target cells, they have to be weakly positively charged or neutral, as the outer cell membrane is negatively charged, while the intracellular membrane is hydrophobic (Thanh and Green 2010). The functionalized SeNPs may differ greatly from the nonfunctionalized SeNPs, while the selection of a stabilization mechanism depends on the final application. Functionalization may reduce toxicity of Se in the nanoform or may result in system functionalized with different biomolecules on the surface of SeNPs (Kapur et al. 2017). For targeted delivery, attachment of antibodies, organic ligands, or aptamers to the SeNP surface will result in very flexible surface chemistry (Fig. 21.3).

Functionalization during chemical synthesis has been usually performed by "one-pot synthesis" in which Se ions are reduced in the presence of a stabilizing agent. Different NP functionalization strategies have been reviewed extensively over the years (Kapur et al. 2017). It is important to highlight that synthetic procedures should be carefully planned following safe-by-design approach (Micheletti et al. 2017). For achieving the best risk/benefit ratio, a range of physicochemical properties of SeNPs should be defined including chemical composition, NP size and size distribution, NP shape and crystal structure, purity, and stability of SeNPs under conditions relevant for the application of SeNPs as recommended by the NanoCommission (EC 2017).

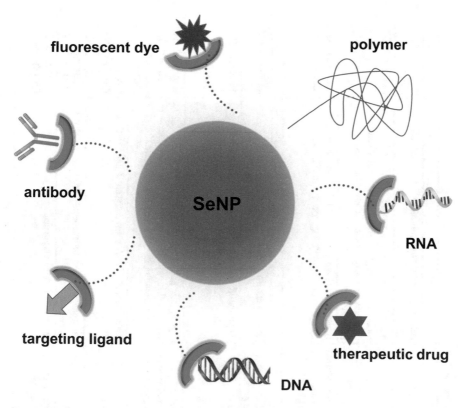

Fig. 21.3 Functionalization strategies of selenium nanoparticle SeNP

Biomedical Applications of SeNPs

Application field of SeNPs has been growing dramatically during recent years owing to its essential role in cellular metabolism. According to the WoS search (Fig. 21.1), 10% of all published papers on SeNPs describe their biomedical applications. SeNPs exhibit excellent optical, photoelectric, and photoconductive properties. Their high reactivity with other inorganic elements has often been exploited for the production of advanced functional materials, like quantum dots (QD) used in imaging and diagnostic techniques (Dobias et al. 2011; Ferrari et al. 2006). Due to favorable optoelectronic properties Se in nanoform has broad applications in different types of rectifiers, photocopiers, photographic exposure meters, xerography, and solar cells (Jiang et al. 2017). However, search of WoS database (Fig. 21.1) revealed that almost half of all research studies (44%) were focused on SeNPs in drug delivery systems, 20% on biocidal activity, more than 15% on their anticancer activity, while other studies presented antioxidative, anti-inflammatory, optical applications, or SeNPs as possible agents to overcome multidrug resistance (MDR). Today, targeted drug delivery, anticancer therapy, biocidal activities, and antioxidant actions represent the major biomedical applications of SeNPs as presented in Table 21.1.

Table 21.1 Examples of biomedical applications of selenium nanoparticles (SeNPs)

SeNP type	Type of application	Mechanism of action	References
Transferrin-conjugated SeNPs	Doxorubicin delivery system for mammalian breast cancer cell line MCF-7	Apoptosis and growth inhibition of cancer cell	Huang et al. (2013)
5-Fluorouracil surface-functionalized SeNPs	Delivery of 5-fluorouracil	Selectivity between cancer and normal cells; induction of apoptosis in A375 human melanoma cells; chemopreventive and chemotherapeutic activity	Liu et al. (2012)
Chemically synthesized SeNPs	Chemotherapy-preventive agent to protect against toxicities of anticancer drug irinotecan and synergistically enhance the antitumor treatment effect in vitro and in vivo	Increased cytotoxic effect with HCT-8 tumor cells by apoptosis; inhibited tumor growth in vivo	Gao et al. (2014a, b)
Cyclic peptide-capped SeNPs	Delivery of doxorubicin, gemcitabine, clofarabine, etoposide, camptothecin, irinotecan, epirubicin, fludarabine, dasatinib, and paclitaxel	The antiproliferative activities of several anticancer drugs were improved	Kumar et al. (2014)
SeNPs modified with G2-PAMAM and poly(allylamine hydrochloride) citraconic anhydride	Delivery of siRNA to silence the tumor vascularization and metastasis	Suppressed tumor growth and reduced microvessel density, indicating decreased tumor vascularization	Yu et al. (2014)
PAMAM (G5)-modified SeNPs	Multidrug resistance; mdr1 siRNA and the chemotherapeutic drug cisplatin were delivered to the drug-resistant human lung adenocarcinoma cell line, A549	Synergistic activity of the drug with siRNA; confirmed in vivo in mice treated with the dual carrier, showing a 75% reduction in tumor size	Kapse-Mistry et al. (2014), Zheng et al. (2016)
Chiral SeNPs modified with luminescent ruthenium (II) complexes	MDR–siRNA delivery	Protection of pDNA from enzymatic degradation	Chen et al. (2015)
SeNPs enriched lactobacillus	Anitcancer activity	Antigiogenic and antimetastatic effect in mice with breast tumors	Yamada et al. (2015)
Ruthenium (II)- and polypyridyl-functionalized SeNPs	Anticancer activity against human hepatoma cancer cells (HepG2)	Antiangiogenesis inhibition	Yamada et al. (2015)

Folic acid-conjugated SeNPs	Cancer-targeted drug delivery	Multidrug resistance in liver cancer; improved selectivity between cancer and normal cells	Jabr-Milane et al. (2008)
Chemically synthesized SeNPs	Delivery of chemotherapeutic agent Adriamycin	Inhibition of proliferation in cancer Bel7402 cells	Tan et al. (2009)
SeNPs modified with sialic acid	Anticancer activity in HeLa human cervical carcinoma cells	Induction of apoptosis and DNA damage	Skalickova et al. (2017)
SeNPs modified with folate-chitosan	Multidrug resistance and targeting cancer cells	Oxidative damage and promoted apoptosis	Yu et al. (2014)
Se coated titanium disc	Antibacterial activity	Decreased bacterial adhesion of *Staphylococcus aureus* and *Staphylococcus epidermidis*	Eswarapriya and Jegatheesan (2015)
SeNPs synthesized by Gram-negative *Stenotrophomonas maltophilia* and Gram-positive *Bacillus mycoides*	Antibacterial activity	Activity against a number of clinical isolates of *Pseudomonas aeruginosa*	Cremonini et al. (2016)
Chemically synthesized SeNPs	Antibacterial activity	Activity against *Staphylococcus aureus*	Chudobova et al. (2014), Tran and Webster (2011), Cihalova et al. (2015)
SeNPs synthesized by *Lactobacillus acidophilus*	Antibacterial activity	Activity against 50 antibiotic resistance strains from 436 samples (80% *Escherichia coli* and 20% *Acinetobacter*)	Beladi et al. (2015)
SeNPs stabilized by polysorbate 20	Antibacterial activity	Activity against common biofilm-forming gram-positive bacteria *Staphylococcus aureus* and *Staphylococcus epidermidis*	Bartůněk et al. (2015)
Biogenically produced SeNPs	Antibacterial activity	Activity against the biofilm produced by clinically isolated strains of *Staphylococcus aureus*, *Pseudomonas aeruginosa*, and *Proteus mirabilis*	Shakibaie et al. (2015)

As important part of many enzymes involved in cellular protection against oxidative damages, Se is involved in many vital functions of human body. Thus, many different selenium compounds have been designed to be used as antioxidants, immunomodulatory agents, and antitumor and anti-infective agents (Parnham and Graf 1991). Nanotechnology and its impact on nanomedicine have opened innovative and promising ways for the production of more efficient and safer Se-based products (Emerich and Thanos 2003). Similar to other metallic NPs, Se in nanoform has a huge potential to improve the field of disease prevention, diagnosis, treatment, and control.

Many authors claim that SeNPs exhibit less toxicity, higher bioavailability, and stronger biological activities than inorganic or organic selenium compounds (Wang et al. 2007; Gao et al. 2000). This is one of the main reasons why SeNPs attracted huge interest in nanomedicine (Maiyo and Singh 2017). Anticancer activity of SeNPs derived from diverse mechanisms of actions including modification of thiol compounds, binding of chromatin (Maiyo and Singh 2017), and triggering of apoptosis by depletion of mitochondrial membrane potential and overproduction of reactive oxygen species (ROS) (Wei et al. 2011). Accumulation of ROS inside the cells is caused by interaction of SeNPs with intracellular proteins and enzymes that have cysteine in their active site such as glutathione peroxidase, superoxide dismutase, or catalase (Yang et al. 2012). Cancer cells are characterized by higher level of these enzymes due to their increased metabolic activity and mitochondrial respiration. This may explain higher toxicity of SeNPs for cancer cells compared to normal cells. Selenium by itself is well known for cancer-protective action in breast, lung, prostate, and colon cancers (Weekley and Harris 2013; Sanmartín et al. 2012). Small size of SeNPs allows their efficient internalization into tumor cells which is ideal for passive targeting (Emerich and Thanos 2003). In some cases, differences in tumor porosity may reduce drug accumulation and activity, while application of nanoformulation enhances permeability and retention of drugs at the tumor site. In addition, attachment of different moieties and active molecules, including antibodies, aptamers, or peptides (Fig. 21.3), that will be recognized by specific receptors of the tumor cells, enables active targeting (Emerich and Thanos 2003; Maiyo and Singh 2017). SeNPs are increasingly being employed as nanocarriers due to their biocompatibility, simple preparation procedures, low toxicity, in vivo degradability, and favorable antioxidant activity (Liu et al. 2012; Huang et al. 2013).

Preclinical studies showed that SeNPs reduced systemic toxicities of conventional chemotherapeutic drugs when used as carrier for these drugs, while worked synergistically improving their efficacy (Maiyo and Singh 2017). The drug can be physically dispersed in SeNP colloidal solution or even chemically bound to the SeNP surface. Use of Se-nanodelivery system may enhance drug solubility and availability while providing concomitant protection from degradation and systemic toxicities (Nicolas et al. 2013). For example, efficient deliveries of doxorubicin, cisplatin, and 5-fluorouracil using SeNPs to cancer cells were described (Huang et al. 2013). Polymeric nanoformulation of selenium has also been described in controlled drug- or gene-release system employing responsive stimuli such as temperature, pH, light, and redox state (Xu et al. 2016; Zhou et al. 2017). In such nano-Se systems, Se–Se bonds are weaker and more cleavable in an oxidative environment than S–S, C–C, and C–Se bonds which lead to more favorable drug/gene release (Xu et al. 2013). Synergistic effect and less side effects were also shown for SeNPs conjugated with transferrin and loaded with doxorubicin (Wei et al. 2011) or for hyaluronic acid attached to the SeNPs (Yang et al. 2012). Furthermore, multifunctional properties of SeNPs are useful for dual drug delivery or co-delivery by binding and transporting different therapeutic cargoes to various destinations in the body (Maiyo and Singh 2017). Such systems have been showed as an innovative strategy not just in targeted therapy, but also in imaging, diagnosis, and combating multidrug resistance (MDR). Causes of MDR may be both cellular and noncellular mechanisms, and may involve acquired and multiple multidrug-resistant mechanisms. Usually, MDR is a result of the expression of drug efflux pumps, upregulation of antiapoptotic proteins, and increase in regulators of drug metabolism (Liu et al. 2015). For prevention of drug resistance and adaptation ability of the cancer cells, different chemotherapeutic agents are usually combined in cancer patients, but MDR is often inevitable (Gottesman 2002; Jabr-Milane et al. 2008). Targeted delivery systems are employed to improve stimuli-triggered drug release and to minimize the side effects of drugs if released to normal cells (Liu et al. 2015). One of the very promising strategies to combat MDR is inactivation of MDR-associated genes through siRNA targeting (Kapse-Mistry et al. 2014). Although the potential of SeNPs is still not fully exploited, SeNPs have been successfully employed for co-delivery of chemotherapeutic agents and siRNA to reverse MDR (Kapse-Mistry et al. 2014). The use of Se is still a novel and largely unexplored biomedical field especially for the gene delivery. Most studies described development of SeNP-based multifunctional therapeutic vehicles for delivery of siRNA as a powerful gene-silencing tool (Liu et al. 2015; Zheng et al. 2015).

Another very important biomedical application of SeNPs is associated with the development of novel biocidal agents due to the emergence of antimicrobial resistance (AMR). AMR is a consequence of overuse of antibiotics either for human use or extensive agricultural usage of antibiotics in livestock as a growth supplement. Such practice inevitably leads to AMR and increases the threat of bacterial infections and biofilm-associated infections (Tor and Fair 2014; Ahonen et al. 2017). Multidrug-resistant bacteria are one of the important factors for mortality increase and costs in the healthcare sector. It has been estimated that AMR-derived infections are responsible for 25,000 deaths every year only in the European Union (Renwick et al. 2016; Tor and Fair 2014). The most serious concerns are related to the methicillin-resistant *Staphylococcus aureus* (MRSA), vancomycin-resistant *Enterococcus faecium* (VRE), drug-resistant *Streptococcus pneumoniae*, multidrug-resistant *Acinetobacter baumannii* (MRAB), carbapenem-resistant Enterobacteriaceae (CRE), and *Pseudomonas aeruginosa* (Tor and Fair 2014). Another huge problem in the healthcare sector comprising up to 80% of all human bacterial infections is represented by biofilm-related infections including chronic wounds, urinary tract infections, and infections related to the use of medical devices (Michael et al. 2014; Ahonen et al. 2017; Bjarnsholt 2013; Michael et al. 2014). Nanotechnology can provide innovative solutions to fight against AMR microorganisms. Nanoparticles can be designed as targeted and combinatorial delivery systems for antibiotics; they may provide biocidal activity by themselves, or they may be used as adjuvants and delivery vehicles in vaccines (Gao et al. 2014a, b). For SeNPs, 20% of all published studies are related to their biocidal activity as can be seen in Fig. 21.1. Representative antibacterial activities of SeNPs as published recently are given in Table 21.1. The commonly accepted mechanism of biocidal activity of SeNPs is the release of the Se ions into the bacterial cell after close interaction of SeNPs with the bacterial surface, similar as has been ascribed to the biocidal activity of silver NPs (Grant and Hung 2013; Cremonini et al. 2016; Sondi and Salopek-Sondi 2004). Internalization of ionic Se induces a cascade of damaging pathways for bacterial cells including oxidation stress, inhibition of protein synthesis, or DNA mutation. In addition to antibacterial mode of actions, SeNPs have been shown also as effective antifungal agents (Eswarapriya and Jegatheesan 2015).

Besides chemotherapeutic, vehicle, and biocidal properties, SeNPs are characterized by high antioxidant activity exhibiting a range of preventive and protective actions in vitro and in vivo (Forootanfar et al. 2014; Huang et al. 2003). There are many promising reports on preventive abilities of SeNPs such as radical scavenging efficiency, protective actions against different toxicants or radiation, and immunomodulatory activities (Huang et al. 2003; Boostani et al. 2015; Cai et al. 2012; Hu et al. 2012; Ungvári et al. 2014). For example, antioxidative activity of SeNPs was demonstrated in rats exposed to oxidative stress by treatment with tert-butyl hydroperoxide (Nasirpour et al. 2017) and in rats treated with cisplatin and gamma-radiation (Fahmy et al. 2016). Furthermore, the antidiabetic potency of SeNPs delivered in liposomes was demonstrated in adult female Wistar rats (Ahmed et al. 2017). Supplementation with SeNPs preserved the integrity of pancreatic beta cells, increased insulin secretion, suppressed oxidative stress, and consequently inhibited pancreatic inflammation. In rats exposed to lead, SeNPs inhibited the adverse effects of such intoxication by exhibiting antioxidant activity and protecting immune system function (Dehkordi et al. 2017). Along with antioxidative activity, SeNPs demonstrated a range of anti-inflammatory potential modulating pro/anti-inflammation cytokine secretion profiles (Wang et al. 2014). Due to its antioxidant, anti-inflammatory, and anti-apoptotic properties, SeNPs are attractive for inventive food supplementation. Indeed, innovations that promote sustainable agriculture and food technology increasingly apply SeNPs for improved food safety, processing, nutrition, and enhanced packaging (El-Ramady et al. 2014).

Safety Aspects of Biomedical Applications of SeNPs

Any biomedical application of NPs should be ascertained by the risk versus benefit ratio profiling. Due to the unique physicochemical characteristics at the nanolevel, NPs differ largely from traditional chemicals although sharing the same chemical composition. Thus, their interaction with biological system and subsequent safety and toxicity profile should be considered completely different from their bulk form.

In spite of huge number of reports and studies published on different aspects of nanomaterials and enormous investments in nanotechnology, there is still gap between application and safety assessment of NPs. This gap exists for three reasons: (1) the scientific research required to develop nanotechnology does not yield adequate data to assess the risks of those products; (2) scientific research data are not robust and adequate enough for the regulatory agencies to conduct risk assessments; and (3) research on the environmental health and safety of NPs receives less than 5% of the funding spent to develop new nanomaterials (Sengupta et al. 2014; Klaine et al. 2012; Rösslein et al. 2017). On the other hand, final fate of the most ideas in the field of nanomedicine, irrespective of how innovative, ingenious, and effective they are, is usually just publication in the high-ranked international scientific journals characterized by low translational success of innovative ideas to the market. Only few of innovative nanoproducts have entered any routine clinical application due to the significant translational gaps associated with the safety concerns and socioeconomic uncertainties (Rösslein et al. 2017). The search in WoS database showed that only 7% of all results obtained for the term "selenium AND nano" is related also to the term "toxicity" (Fig. 21.1). Most toxicity data were reported for SeNP toxicity effects in animal experiments (>50%), while results on cytotoxicity of SeNPs were reported in ca. 30% of all published "toxicity" papers (Fig. 21.1).

For SeNPs, one could expect nanotoxicity due to the essential role of selenium in the body, its antioxidative properties, and importance in nutrition and medicine. However, Se has one of the smallest gaps between dietary deficiency and toxic levels. Thus, lower limit of daily intake for Se is 40 µg for an adult healthy person, while toxicity effects are exhibited already at ten times higher concentration. Toxicity of Se is mainly attributed to its inorganic form (selenite), while selenomethionine and selenocysteine are less toxic. Selenite and other inorganic Se compounds readily react with biological thiols with subsequent ROS formation. Another possible mechanism of Se toxicity is inhibition of thiol-containing proteins and enzymes due to similarity of Se with sulfur, which may result in nonspecific replacement of sulfur in proteins (Tinggi 2003). Typical symptoms of Se toxicity in humans, also called selenosis, include garlic breath, hair and nail loss, thickened and brittle nails, teeth deformation, skin lesions, and decrease in hemoglobin (Tinggi 2003). Many studies have claimed lower toxicity of Se in the nanoparticulate form (Sengupta et al. 2014). For example, folate-conjugated SeNPs exhibited significant selectivity in growth inhibition between cancer and normal cells and almost three-fold lower acute liver toxicity than selenite or selenomethionine in treated mice (Liu et al. 2015).

Other researchers showed higher bioavailability of SeNPs and their increased potency to increase the activity of selenoenzyme peroxidase and thioredoxin reductase compared to bulk Se compounds (Skalickova et al. 2017). Similarly, comparable efficacy in upregulating seleno-enzymes along with lower toxicity in vivo has been reported for SeNPs as compared with selenomethionine (Wang et al. 2007). Studies of absorption, distribution, metabolism, and excretion (ADME) pattern of albumin-coated SeNPs using rats as animal model revealed their ADME similar to selenite (Loeschner et al. 2014). By the detection of the metabolites Se-methylseleno-

N-acetylgalactosamine and trimethylselenonium ion in urine samples of treated rats, similar excretion patterns were proven for SeNPs and selenite. However, administration of high doses resulted in significantly higher level of elemental Se in liver and kidney compared to the low doses, which indicated that the natural ADME pattern of Se was exhausted at the high doses (Loeschner et al. 2014). At the same time, upregulation of blood biomarker selenoprotein P was similar for both ionic and nanoparticulate forms of Se in rats treated with high doses (Loeschner et al. 2014). This study, as many other studies on SeNPs fate in vivo, did not demonstrate detailed mechanism of SeNP ADME. Thus, extensive safety assessment of SeNPs is still lacking.

For environmental risk assessment of SeNPs, information deficiency is even larger. Less than 10% of all publication on toxicity of SeNPs was focused on their ecotoxicity and environmental effects (Fig. 21.1). Thus, very few studies reported the effect of SeNPs on aquatic organisms which represent the most sensitive and weak link in the environment. Study on Medaka fish showed efficient bioaccumulation and subsequent clearance of both SeNPs and selenite in fish livers, gills, muscles, and whole bodies, but hyper-accumulation of SeNPs in liver was sixfold higher than for selenite (Li et al. 2008). Clearance from whole bodies and muscles of medaka fish was similar for both SeNPs and selenite (Li et al. 2008). Contrary to the effect reported for rodents, stronger toxicity and oxidative stress response were observed for medaka fish treated with SeNPs compared to selenite (Li et al. 2008). In another study using zebrafish embryos as ecotoxicity model, the toxicity of biogenically synthesized SeNPs was compared with that of chemically prepared SeNPs and selenite (Joyabrata et al. 2016). This study has evidenced toxicity of both types of SeNPs with biogenically prepared SeNPs being less toxic than selenite and chemically obtained SeNPs (Mal et al. 2016). Furthermore, authors of this study demonstrated that mechanism of SeNPs toxicity was quite complicated highlighting the necessity for further supportive and extensive investigation on the investigation of the risks versus benefits of SeNP applications (Mal et al. 2016).

Due to limited information on biotransformation behavior, ADME pattern, and toxicity of SeNPs in vivo, it is wise to implement precautionary principle as issued by the European Commission in a Communication on the precautionary principle (EC 2000) in overcoming existing uncertainties for risk and exposure assessment of SeNPs, as for others engineered nanomaterials. The possible proactive approach to follow this principle is the implementation SbD concept, which is designed to ensure safety for humans and the environment by identifying timely all risks related to the innovation processes and value chain of nanomaterials (Micheletti et al. 2017). A common SbD approach, as presented in Fig. 21.4, is characterized by safe production, safe products, and safe use. Safe production provides knowledge and methodology for control of industrial processes along the production chain. Safe products are enabled by design of less hazardous NPs using combination of non-testing predictions together with high-throughput screening tools. Safe use encompasses evaluation of exposure risk for workers, consumers, and environment by identifying actions for risk mitigation such as life cycle assessment and cost versus benefit analysis.

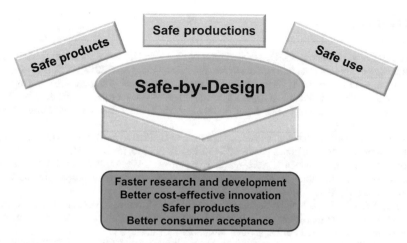

Fig. 21.4 Safe-by-design approach for metal-based nanomaterials

Key issues of SbD approach (Ahonen et al. 2017) include (a) characterization of NPs providing the key characteristics that influence the release, exposure, behavior, effects, and subsequent environmental and human risks of NPs; (b) transformation pattern of NPs encompassing the conditions, extent, and rate of change of NP structure and stability throughout the different stages of their life cycle; (c) dose metrics that define a particular response of NPs in certain biological or environmental systems; (d) detailed information on physicochemical characteristics, exposure, and/or hazard of different forms, types, and sizes of NPs for read across and/or grouping within the risk assessment of nanomaterials; (e) fate of NPs in certain biological or environmental compartments governed by their interaction with different components of these compartments that change the identity of NPs. Thus, risk/benefit ratio assessment of NPs should involve researchers from a wide range of disciplines (chemists, physics, material scientists, microbiologist, toxicologists, etc.), producers, end users (healthcare institutions, industry, etc.), governmental and nongovernmental organizations (regulatory agencies, environmental and chemical agencies), and also media.

Conclusion

Nanotechnology introduced a novel conception of function and usage of selenium. The flexibility of SeNPs for diverse functionalization and modifications enables prospective and innovative wide range of possibilities for usage in human diet and disease treatment. However, safety issue of SeNPs should be carefully considered for any successful biomedical application.

References

Ahmed HH, Abd El-Maksoud MD, Abdel Moneim AE, Aglan HA. Pre-clinical study for the anti-diabetic potential of selenium nanoparticles. Biol Trace Elem Res. 2017;177(2):267–80.

Ahonen M, Kahru A, Ivask A, Kasemets K, Kõljalg S, Mantecca P, Vinković Vrček I, Keinänen-Toivola M, Crijns F. Proactive approach for safe use of antimicrobial coatings in healthcare settings: opinion of the COST action network AMiCI. Int J Environ Res Public Health. 2017;14:366–89.

Avendaño R, Chaves N, Fuentes P, Sánchez E, Jiménez JI, Chavarría M. Production of selenium nanoparticles in Pseudomonas putida KT2440. Sci Rep. 2016;15(6):37155.

Bartůněk V, Junková J, Šuman J, Kolářová K, Rimpelová S, Ulbrich P, Sofer Z. Preparation of amorphous antimicrobial selenium nanoparticles stabilized by odor suppressing surfactant polysorbate 20. Mater Lett. 2015;152:207–9.

Beladi M, Sepahi AA, Mehrabian S, Esmaeili A, Sharifnia F. Antibacterial activities of selenium and selenium nano-particles (products from Lactobacillus acidophilus) on nosocomial strains resistant to antibiotics. J Pure App Microbiol. 2015;9(4):2843–51.

Bjarnsholt T. The role of bacterial biofilms in chronic infections. APMIS Suppl. 2013;136:1–51.

Boostani A, Sadeghi AA, Mousavi SN, Chamani M, Kashan N. Effects of organic, inorganic, and nano-Se on growth performance, antioxidant capacity, cellular and humoral immune responses in broiler chickens exposed to oxidative stress. Livest Sci. 2015;178:330–6.

Buchs B, Evangelou MW, Winkel LH, Lenz M. Colloidal properties of nanoparticular biogenic selenium govern environmental fate and bioremediation effectiveness. Environ Sci Technol. 2013;47:2401–7.

Cai SJ, Wu CX, Gong LM, Song T, Wu H, Zhang LY. Effects of nano-selenium on performance, meat quality, immune function, oxidation resistance, and tissue selenium content in broilers. Poult Sci. 2012;91(10):2532–9.

Cavalu S, Prokisch J, Laslo V, Vicas S. Preparation, structural characterisation and release study of novel hybrid microspheres entrapping nanoselenium, produced by green synthesis. IET Nanobiotechnol. 2017;11(4):426–32.

Chen Q, Yu Q, Liu Y, Bhavsar D, Yang L, Ren X, Sun D, Zheng W, Liu J, Chen LM. Multifunctional selenium nanoparticles: chiral selectivity of delivering MDR–siRNA for reversal of multidrug resistance and real-time biofluorescence imaging. Nanomedicine. 2015;11(7):1773–84.

Chudobova D, Cihalova K, Dostalova S, Ruttkay-Nedecky B, Rodrigo MA, Tmejova K, Kopel P, Nejdl L, Kudr J, Gumulec J, Krizkova S, Kynicky J, Kizek R, Adam V. Comparison of the effects of silver phosphate and selenium nanoparticles on Staphylococcus aureus growth reveals potential for selenium particles to prevent infection. FEMS Microbiol Lett. 2014;351(2):195–201.

Cihalova K, Chudobova D, Michalek P, Moulick A, Guran R, Kopel P, Adam V, Kizek R. Staphylococcus aureus and MRSA growth and biofilm formation after treatment with antibiotics and SeNPs. Int J Mol Sci. 2015;16(10):24656–72.

Cremonini E, Zonaro E, Donini M, Lampis S, Boaretti M, Dusi S, Melotti P, Lleo MM, Vallini G. Biogenic selenium nanoparticles: characterization, antimicrobial activity and effects on human dendritic cells and fibroblasts. J Microbial Biotechnol. 2016;9(6):758–71.

Dehkordi A, Jafari Mohebbi AN, Aslani MR, Ghoreyshi SM. Evaluation of nanoselenium (Nano-Se) effect on hematological and serum biochemical parameters of rat in experimentally lead poisoning. Hum Exp Toxicol. 2017;36(4):421–7.

Dhand C, Dwivedi N, Loh XJ, Ying ANJ, Verma NK, Beuerman RW, Lakshminarayanan R, Ramakrishna S. Methods and strategies for the synthesis of diverse nanoparticles and their applications: a comprehensive overview. RSC Adv. 2015;5(127):105003–37.

Dobias J, Suvorova EI, Bernier-Latmani R. Role of proteins in controlling selenium nanoparticle size. Nanotechnology. 2011;22(19):195605.

EC (European Commission). Commission of the European Communities. 2 February 2000 Communication from the Commission on the Precautionary Principle. 2000.

EC (European Commission). 2017.; http://cordis.europa.eu/nanotechnology/actionplan.htm. Accessed 5 Oct 2017.

El-Ramady H, Domokos-Szabolcsy É, Abdalla NA, Alshaal TA, Shalaby TA, Sztrik A, Prokisch J, Fári M. Selenium and nano-selenium in agroecosystems. Environ Chem Lett. 2014;12(4):495–510.

Emerich DF, Thanos CG. Nanotechnology and medicine. Expert Opin Biol Ther. 2003;3(4):655–63.

Estevam EC, Griffin S, Nasim MJ, Denezhkin P, Schneider R, Lilischkis R, Dominguez-Alvarez E, Witek K, Latacz G, Keck C, Schäfer KH, Kieć-Kononowicz K, Handzlik J, Jacob C. Natural selenium particles from Staphylococcus carnosus: hazards or particles with particular promise? J Hazard Mater. 2017;324(Pt A):22–30.

Eswarapriya B, Jegatheesan K. Antifungal activity of biogenic selenium nanoparticles. Synthesized from Electronic Waste. Int J PharmTech Res. 2015;8(3):383–6.

Eszenyi P, Sztrik A, Babka B, Prokisch J. Production of Lactomicrosel (R) and nanosize (100–500 NM) selenium spheres by probiotic lactic acid bacteria. In: Food Engineering and Biotechnology. Edited by Wu KJ. 2011;9:97-101.

Fahmy HA, Azim AS, Gharib OA. Protective effects of omega-3 fatty acids and/or nano- selenium on cisplatin and ionizing radiation induced liver toxicity in rats. Indian J Pharm Educ Res. 2016;50(4):649–56.

Ferrari M, Ravera F, Rao S, Liggieri L. Surfactant adsorption at superhydrophobic surfaces. Appl Phys Lett. 2006;89:053104.

Forootanfar H, Adeli-Sardou M, Nikkhoo M, Mehrabani M, Amir-Heidari B, Shahverdi AR, Shakibaie M. Antioxidant and cytotoxic effect of biologically synthesized selenium nanoparticles in comparison to selenium dioxide. J Trace Elem Med Biol. 2014;28(1):75–9.

Gao XY, Zhang JS, Zhang LD, Zhu MX. Nano-Se has a 7-fold lower acute toxicity than sodium selenite in mice. China Public Health. 2000;16:42.

Gao F, Yuan Q, Gao L, Cai P, Zhu H, Liu R, Wang Y, Wei Y, Huang G, Liang J, Gao X. Cytotoxicity and therapeutic effect of irinotecan combined with selenium nanoparticles. Biomaterials. 2014a;35(31):8854–66.

Gao W, Thamphiwatana S, Angsantikul P, Zhang L. Nanoparticle approaches against bacterial infections: nanoparticle against bacterial infections. Wiley Interdiscip Rev Nanomed Nanobiotechnol. 2014b;6(6):532–47.

Gottesman MM. Mechanisms of cancer drug resistance. Annu Rev Med. 2002;53:615–27.

Grant SS, Hung DT. Persistent bacterial infections, antibiotic tolerance, and the oxidative stress response. Virulence. 2013;4:273–83.

Hu CH, Li YL, Xiong L, Zhang HM, Song J, Xia MS. Comparative effects of nano elemental selenium and sodium selenite on selenium retention in broiler chickens. Anim Feed Sci Technol. 2012;177(3-4):204–10.

Huang B, Zhang JS, Hou JW, Chen C. Free radical scavenging efficiency of nano-Se in vitro. Free Radic Biol Med. 2003;35(7):805–13.

Huang Y, He L, Liu W, Fan C, Zheng W, Wong YS, Chen T. Selective cellular uptake and induction of apoptosis of cancer-targeted selenium nanoparticles. Biomaterials. 2013;34(29):7106–16.

Husen A, Siddiqi KS. Plants and microbes assisted selenium nanoparticles: characterization and application. J Nanobiotechology. 2014;12:28.

Jabr-Milane LS, van Vlerken LE, Yadav S, Amiji MM. Multi-functional chnanocarriers to overcome tumor drug resistance. Cancer Treat Rev. 2008;34:592–602.

Jiang F, Cai W, Tan G. Facile synthesis and optical properties of small selenium nanocrystals and nanorods. Nanoscale Res Lett. 2017;12:401.

Kamnev AA, Manchenkova PV, Yu A, Dyatlova AV, Tugarova AV. FTIR spectroscopic studies of selenite reduction by cells of the rhizobacterium Azospirillum brasilense Sp7 and the formation of selenium nanoparticles. J Mol Struct. 2017;1140:106–12.

Kapse-Mistry S, Govender T, Srivastava R, Yergeri M. Nanodrug delivery in reversing multidrug resistance in cancer cells. Front Pharmacol. 2014;5:159.

Kapur M, Soni K, Kohli K. Green synthesis of selenium nanoparticles from broccoli, characterization, application and toxicity. Adv Tech Biol Med. 2017;5:198.

Kazlev AM. History of nanotechnology. 1998. http://www.kheper.net/topics/nanotech/nanotech-history.htm. Accessed 25 Nov 2017.

Klaine S, Koelmans AA, Horne N, Carley S, Handy RD, Kapustka L, Nowack B, von der Kammer F. Paradigms to assess the environmental impact of manufactured nanomaterials. Environ Toxicol Chem. 2012;31:3–14.

Kong H, Yang J, Zhang Y, Fang Y, Nishinari K, Phillips GO. Synthesis and antioxidant properties of gum arabic-stabilized selenium nanoparticles. Int J Biol Macromol. 2014;65:155–62.

Kora AJ, Rastogi L. Bacteriogenic synthesis of selenium nanoparticles by Escherichia coli ATCC 35218 and its structural characterisation. IET Nanobiotechnol. 2017;11(2):179–84.

Kumar A, Beni YA, Parang K. Cyclic peptide – selenium nanoparticles as drug transporters. Mol Pharm. 2014;11:3631–41.

Li H, Zhang J, Wang T, Luo W, Zhou Q, Jiang G. Elemental selenium particles at nano-size (Nano-Se) are more toxic to Medaka (Oryzias latipes) as a consequence of hyper-accumulation of selenium: a comparison with sodium selenite. Aquat Toxicol. 2008;89:251–6.

Liu W, Li X, Wong YS, Zheng W, Zhang Y, Cao W, Chen T. Selenium nanoparticles as a carrier of 5-fluorouracil to achieve anticancer synergism. ACS Nano. 2012;6:6578–91.

Liu T, Zeng L, Jiang W, Fu Y, Zheng W, Chen T. Rational design of cancer-targeted selenium nanoparticles to antagonize multidrug resistance in cancer cells. Nanomedicine. 2015;11(4):947–58.

Loeschner K, Hadrup N, Hansen M, Pereira SA, Gammelgaard B, Møller LH, Mortensen A, Lam HR, Larsen EH. Absorption, distribution, metabolism and excretion of selenium following oral administration of elemental selenium nanoparticles or selenite in rats. Metallomics. 2014;6(2):330–7.

Maiyo F, Singh M. Selenium nanoparticles: potential in cancer gene and drug delivery. Nanomedicine (Lond). 2017;12(9):1075–89.

Mal J, Veneman WJ, Nancharaiah JV, van Hullebusch ED, Peijnenburg WJ, Vijver MG, Lens PN. A comparison of fate and toxicity of selenite, biogenically, and chemically synthesized selenium nanoparticles to zebrafish (Danio rerrio) embryogenesis. Nanotoxicology 2017;11(1):87–97.

Mal J, Veneman WJ, Nancharaiah YV, van Hullebusch ED, Peijnenburg WJ, Vijver MG, Lens PN. A comparison of fate and toxicity of selenite, biogenically and chemically synthesized selenium nanoparticles to zebrafish (Danio rerio) embryogenesis. Nanotoxicology. 2016;11(1):87–97.

Michael CA, Dominey-Howes D, Labbate M. The antimicrobial resistance crisis: causes, consequences, and management. Front Public Health. 2014;2(145):1–8.

Micheletti C, Roman M, Tedesco E, Olivato I, Benetti F. Implementation of the NANoREG safe-by-design approach for different nanomaterial applications. J Phys Conf Ser. 2017;838:012019.

Nancharaiah YV, Lens PNL. Selenium biomineralization for biotechnological applications. Trends Biotechnol. 2015;33:323–30.

Nasirpour M, Sadeghi AA, Chamani M. Effects of nano-selenium on the liver antioxidant enzyme activity and immunoglobolins in male rats exposed to oxidative stress. J Livestock Sci. 2017;8:81–7.

Nicolas J, Mura S, Brambilla D, Mackiewicz N, Couvreur P. Design, functionalization strategies and biomedical applications of targeted biodegradable/biocompatible polymer-based nanocarriers for drug delivery. Chem Soc Rev. 2013;42(3):1147–235.

Nowack B, Ranville JF, Diamond S, Alberto Gallego-Urrea A, Metcalfe C, Rose J, Horne N, Koelmans AA, Klaine SJ. Potential scenarios for nanomaterial release and subsequent alteration in the environment. Environ Toxicol Chem. 2011;31:50–9.

Panahi-Kalamuei M, Salavati-Niasari M, Hosseinpour-Mashkani SM. Facile microwave synthesis, characterization, and solar cell application of selenium nanoparticles. J Alloy Compd. 2014;617:627–32.

Parnham MJ, Graf E. Pharmacology of synthetic organic selenium compounds. Prog Drug Res. 1991;36:9–47.

Paul S, Chugh A. Assessing the role of Ayurvedic 'Bhasmas' as Ethno- nanomedicine in the metal based nanomedicine patent regime. J Intellect Pro Rig. 2011;16:509–15.

Prasad KS, Selvaraj K. Biogenic synthesis of selenium nanoparticles and their effect on As(III)-induced toxicity on human lymphocytes. Biol Trace Elem Res. 2014;157(3):275–83.

Prasad KS, Patel H, Patel T, Patel K, Selvaraj K. Biosynthesis of Se nanoparticles and its effect on UV-induced DNA damage. Colloids Surf B Biointerfaces. 2013;103:261–6.

Ramamurthy C, Sampath KS, Arunkumar P, Kumar MS, Sujatha V, Premkumar K, Thirunavukkarasu C. Green synthesis and characterization of selenium nanoparticles and its augmented cytotoxicity with doxorubicin on cancer cells. Bioprocess Biosyst Eng. 2013;36(8):1131–9.

Renwick MJ, Brogan DM, Mossialos E. A systematic review and critical assessment of incentive strategies for discovery and development of novel antibiotics. J Antibiot (Tokyo). 2016;69(2):73–88.

Richards DG, McMillin DL, Mein EA, Nelson CD. Gold and its relationship to neurological/glandular conditions. Int J Neurosci. 2002;112:31–53.

Rösslein M, Liptrott N, Owen A, Boisseau P, Wick P, Herrmann IK. Sound understanding of environmental, health and safety, clinical, and market aspects is imperative to clinical translation of nanomedicines. Nanotoxicology. 2017;11(2):147–9.

Sanmartín C, Plano D, Sharma AK, Palop JA. Selenium compounds, apoptosis and other types of cell death: an overview for cancer therapy. Int J Mol Sci. 2012;13(8):9649–72.

Sengupta J, Ghosh S, Datta P, Gomes A, Gomes A. Physiologically important metal nanoparticles and their toxicity. J Nanosci Nanotechnol. 2014;14(1):990–1006.

Shahbazi B, Taghipour M, Rahmani H, Sadrjavadi K, Fattahi A. Preparation and characterization of silk fibroin/oligochitosan nanoparticles for siRNA delivery. Colloids Surf B Biointerfaces. 2015;136:867–77.

Shakibaie M, Forootanfar H, Golkari Y, Mohammadi-Khorsand T, Shakibaie MR. Anti-biofilm activity of biogenic selenium nanoparticles and selenium dioxide against clinical isolates of Staphylococcus aureus, Pseudomonas aeruginosa, and Proteus mirabilis. J Trace Elem Med Biol. 2015;29:235–41.

Sharma G, Sharma AR, Bhavesh R, Park J, Ganbold B, Nam JS, Lee SS. Biomolecule-mediated synthesis of selenium nanoparticles using dried Vitis vinifera (raisin) extract. Molecules. 2014;19(3):2761–70.

Shoeibi S, Mashreghi M. Biosynthesis of selenium nanoparticles using Enterococcus faecalis and evaluation of their antibacterial activities. J Trace Elem Med Biol. 2017;39:135–9.

Skalickova S, Milosavljevic V, Cihalova K, Horky P, Richtera L, Adam V. Perspective of selenium nanoparticles as a nutrition supplement. Nutrition. 2017;33:83–90.

Sondi I, Salopek-Sondi B. Silver nanoparticles as antimicrobial agent: a case study on E. coli as a model for gram-negative bacteria. J Colloid Interface Sci. 2004;275(1):177–82.

Srivastava N, Mukhopadhyay M. Biosynthesis and structural characterization of selenium nanoparticles mediated by Zooglea ramigera. Powder Technol. 2013;244:26–9.

Srivastava N, Mukhopadhyay M. Green synthesis and structural characterization of selenium nanoparticles and assessment of their antimicrobial property. Bioprocess Biosyst Eng. 2015;38(9):1723–30.

Tan L, Jia X, Jiang X, Zhang Y, Tang H, Yao S, Xie Q. In vitro study on the individual and synergistic cytotoxicity of adriamycin and selenium nanoparticles against Bel7402 cells with a quartz crystal microbalance. Biosens Bioelectron. 2009;24(7):2268–72.

Thanh NTK, Green LAW. Functionalisation of nanoparticles for biomedical applications. Nano Today. 2010;5:213–30.

Tinggi U. Essentiality and toxicity of selenium and its status in Australia: a review. Toxicol Lett. 2003;137:103–10.

Tor Y, Fair R. Antibiotics and bacterial resistance in the 21st century. Perspect Medicin Chem. 2014;6:25–64.

Tran PA, Webster TJ. Selenium nanoparticles inhibit Staphylococcus aureus growth. Int J Nanomedicine. 2011;6:1553–8.

Ungvári É, Monori I, Megyeri A, Csiki Z, Prokisch J, Sztrik A, Jávor A, Benkő I. Protective effects of meat from lambs on selenium nanoparticle supplemented diet in a mouse model of polycyclic aromatic hydrocarbon-induced immunotoxicity. Food Chem Toxicol. 2014;64:298–306.

Wang H, Zhang J, Yu H. Elemental selenium at nano size possesses lower toxicity without compromising the fundamental effect on selenoenzymes: comparison with selenomethionine in mice. Free Radic Biol Med. 2007;42:1524–33.

Wang J, Zhang Y, Yuan Y, Yue T. Immunomodulatory of selenium nano-particles decorated by sulfated Ganoderma lucidum polysaccharides. Food Chem Toxicol. 2014;68:183–9.

Weekley CM, Harris HH. Which form is that? The importance of selenium speciation and metabolism in the prevention and treatment of disease. Chem Soc Rev. 2013;42(23):8870–94.

Wei A, Pan L, Huang W. Recent progress in the ZnO nanostructure-based sensors. Mater Sci Eng B. 2011;176:1409–21.

Xi GC, Xiong K, Zhao QB, Zhang R, Zhang HB, Qian YT. Nucleation-dissolution-recrystallization: a new growth mechanism for t-selenium nanotubes. Cryst Growth Des. 2006;6(2):577–82.

Xiao X, Zhao C, Yang S, Guo S. Characteristics of nano-selenium synthesized by Se(IV) adsorption and reduction with anoxygenic photosynthetic bacteria. Digest J Nanomat Biostruct. 2017;12(1):205–14.

Xu H, Cao W, Zhang X. Selenium-containing polymers: promising biomaterials for controlled release and enzyme mimics. Acc Chem Res. 2013;46(7):1647–58.

Xu Q, He C, Xiao C, Chen X. Reactive oxygen species (ROS) responsive polymers for biomedical applications. Macromol Biosci. 2016;16(5):635–46.

Yamada M, Foote M, Prow TW. Therapeutic gold, silver, and platinum nanoparticles. Wiley Interdiscip Rev Nanomed Nanobiotechnol. 2015;7:428–45.

Yang F, Tang Q, Zhong X, Bai Y, Chen T, Zhang Y, Li Y, Zheng W. Surface decoration by Spirulina polysaccharide enhances the cellular uptake and anticancer efficacy of selenium nanoparticles. Int J Nanomedicine. 2012;7:835–44.

Yu B, Li XL, Zheng WJ, Feng YX, Wong YS, Chen TF. pH-responsive cancer-targeted selenium nanoparticles: a transformable drug carrier with enhanced theranostic effects. J Mater Chem B. 2014;2(33):5409–18.

Zhang W, Chen Z, Liu H, Zhang L, Gao P, Li D. Biosynthesis and structural characteristics of selenium nanoparticles by Pseudomonas alcaliphila. Colloids Surf B Biointerfaces. 2011;88(1):196–201.

Zheng Y, Chen T. Targeting nanomaterials: future drugs for cancer chemotherapy. Int J Nanomedicine. 2012;7:3939–49.

Zheng W, Cao C, Liu Y, Yu Q, Zheng C, Sun D, Ren X, Liu J. Multifunctional polyamidoamine-modified selenium nanoparticles dual-delivering siRNA and cisplatin to A549/DDP cells for reversal multidrug resistance. Acta Biomater. 2015;11:368–80.

Zheng W, Yin T, Chen Q, Qin X, Huang X, Zhao S, Xu T, Chen L, Liu J. Co-delivery of Se nanoparticles and pooled SiRNAs for overcoming drug resistance mediated by P-glycoprotein and class III β-tubulin in drug-resistant breast cancers. Acta Biomater. 2016;31:197–210.

Zhou W, Wang L, Li F, Zhang W, Huang W, Huo F, Xu H. Selenium-containing polymer@metal-organic frameworks nanocomposites as an efficient multiresponsive drug delivery system. Adv Funct Mater. 2017;27:1605465.

Chapter 22
Selenium Interactions with Other Trace Elements, with Nutrients (and Drugs) in Humans

Josiane Arnaud and Peter van Dael

Abstract Selenium is both a toxic and an essential trace element. Both deficiency and overload are reported in humans due to geographical variability in soil concentrations. Selenium metabolically interacts with numerous nutrients and toxic substances. These interrelationships may be synergistic or antagonistic, and involve different biological pathways with opposite effects and a complex interplay of interactions involving numerous substances, lifestyle, and health status. The complexity of these interactions may contribute to inter-individual variability in the susceptibility to various chronic diseases. This review is focused on the interactions of selenium with heavy metals in the top ten chemicals of major public health concern (arsenic, cadmium, fluoride, mercury, and lead) and with the most common and widespread deficiencies in the world (iodine, iron, zinc, and vitamin A) according to the World Health Organization. The principal mechanisms of action and a summary of different studies in humans are briefly presented. More information is available in the reference listed.

Keywords Selenium · Interaction · Heavy metal · Essential trace elements · Vitamins

Selenium (Se) is an essential nutrient which metabolically interacts with other nutrients, in particular trace elements and vitamins as well as non-nutrient substances, in particular heavy metals, toxic substances, and medications. The complexity of the human biological system and the variability of nutritional and environmental factors complicate these interactions as well as their implications to human. As shown in Fig. 22.1, Se interactions are a complex interplay of interactions involving

J. Arnaud (✉)
Institute of Biology and Pathology, University Hospital of Grenoble and Alpes,
Grenoble, France
e-mail: JArnaud@chu-grenoble.fr

P. van Dael
DSM Nutritional Products, Kaiseraugst, Switzerland
e-mail: peter.van-dael@dsm.com

© Springer International Publishing AG, part of Springer Nature 2018
B. Michalke (ed.), *Selenium*, Molecular and Integrative Toxicology,
https://doi.org/10.1007/978-3-319-95390-8_22

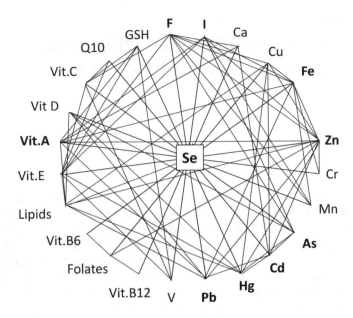

Fig. 22.1 Complex interplay between Se, nutrients, and toxic metals. In bold characters, the metals and micronutrients identified by the World Health Organization (WHO) as major public health problems

numerous substances, lifestyle, and health status. The complexity of these interactions may explain, at least in part, the inter-individual differences in the susceptibility to various chronic diseases.

The interactions between Se and heavy metals are of particular importance. Human exposure to toxic elements such as arsenic (As), cadmium (Cd), chromium (Cr), cobalt (Co), mercury (Hg), nickel (Ni), and lead (Pb) is no longer limited to occupational exposure. Indeed, these elements are contaminants or pollutants and therefore are ingested and/or breathed daily. As, Cd, Hg, Pb, as well as fluoride (F) are in the top ten chemicals of major public health concern according to the World Health Organization (WHO). Exposure to these heavy metals increases the risk of chronic diseases and may be associated to a reduced essential trace element status (Afridi et al. 2014; Wadhwa et al. 2015). These interrelationships may be synergistic or antagonistic and depend on numerous factors (Table 22.1). The understanding of the heavy metal–Se interactions is a prerequisite for the development of risk reduction or dietary management approaches to the exposure to or poisoning with heavy metals. However our knowledge of these interactions remains limited as different metabolic pathways are or may be involved with opposite effects. The major metabolic pathways are mentioned in Table 22.2.

Although many studies have been conducted in animals and in vitro, this review primarily focuses on human studies. The first part of this review summarizes the principal mechanisms of action and the second deals with the specific interactions between Se and the overloads (As, Cd, F, Hg, and Pb) or deficiencies (Fe, I, Zn, and vitamin A) identified by the WHO as major public health problems. Recent human

Table 22.1 Factors affecting the interactions between Se and other inorganic elements or vitamins

Age, gender, body mass index
Se status
Lifestyle, income such as smoking, nutrition
Single-nucleotide polymorphisms in selenoprotein genes
Other genetic polymorphisms
Chemical form and oxidation state of Se and the interactive substances
Solubility of the substances
Concentration ratios of the interactive substances
Duration of exposure/ supplementation/deficiency
Administration route of the interactive substances

Table 22.2 Principal mechanisms involved in the interactions between Se and other inorganic elements or vitamins

Modulation of absorption, transport, distribution, excretion, and status
Formation of complexes
Redox imbalance
Immune and inflammatory processes
Methylation pathway
Cellular signaling
Modulation of gene expression and epigenetic
Modulation of selenoprotein synthesis and activities

studies are summarized in Tables 22.3, 22.4, 22.5, and 22.6. The reader will find more information in reviews referenced in this chapter.

Principal Mechanisms of Interactions

Modulation of Absorption, Transport, Distribution, Excretion, and Status (See Chap. 5)

Se status is determined by its absorption and excretion characteristics as well as by Se transport and distribution in the human body. Some elements such as As, calcium (Ca), Fe, and Pb have been reported to decrease the absorption of Se (Mehdi et al.

Table 22.3 Selenium interactions: summary of some case—control studies conducted in humans

Population studied	Measured parameters	Main results	References
849 adults >18 years 303 patients with As-related skin lesions, Bangladesh	As in blood, urine, water Se in blood	Inverse associations between blood Se and skin lesions whatever the adjustment factors; Se in blood and As in urine No association between Se and As in blood	Chen et al. (2007)
Subjects exposed to As 20 with skin lesions 43 controls China	As in water, duplicated diet, urine, and serum Se in duplicate diet, urine and serum Speciation of As in urine and serum	Inverse associations between Se and inorganic As in serum; Se and MMA/DMA ratio or MMA in urine; Se in serum and skin lesions Positive associations between DMA and Se in urine; As/Se ratio in serum or urine and skin lesions	Huang et al. (2008)
138 patients with skin lesions divided in 2 groups: High As High As+Se (blood Se > 1.27 μmol/L) 76 controls divided in 2 groups (control and high Se) China	As and Se in blood, urine and hair Vitamin C, SOD, GPX, CAT, MDA in serum 8-OHdG in urine HO-1, OGG1 mRNA, and protein in mononuclear blood cells	Inverse associations between As in blood and Se in hair or blood Enzyme activities and OGG1 (mRNA and protein) ↓; MDA and 8-OHdG ↑ in the high As group compared to the other groups HO-1 mRNA and protein levels ↑ in high Se and high Se + As groups compared to control and high As groups, control group being the lowest	Xue et al. (2010)

(continued)

Table 22.3 (continued)

Population studied	Measured parameters	Main results	References
100 patients with fluorosis, 28–68 years: 50 living in high Se + F area (21 men, 29 women) and 50 in high F area (22 men, 28 women) 20 healthy people living in high Se area (9 men, 11 women) 46 control subjects (20 men, 26 women) China	F in spot urine and serum Se in hair MDA, GPX, SOD, CAT in serum HSP70 and β-actin expression in mononuclear blood cells	Compared to control group: SOD and GPX activity ↓ and MDA ↑ in high F group CAT and HSP70/β-actin ↑, GPX and MDA ↓ in high F + Se group: SOD, CAT, HSP70/β-actin ↑ and GPX and MDA ↓ in high Se group Compared to high F group: GPX, SOD, CAT, HSP70 mRNA and HSP70 ↑and MDA ↓ in high F + Se and high Se groups	Chen et al. (2009)
30 patients with fluorosis living in high Se + F area (16 men, 14 women) 30 patients with fluorosis living in high F area (14 men, 16 women) 30 control subjects not exposed to F (15 men, 15 women) China	Se in hair F in serum and urine P38 MAKP, NF-κB p65, p53, and caspase 3 expression in mononuclear blood cells	Expression of p38 MAKP, NF-κB p65, and caspase 3 ↑ in high F compare to high F + Se or control groups Expression of p53 ↑ in high F + Se compared to high F or control groups	Chen et al. (2010)
25 miners and 12 residents from Hg-contaminated area 35 residents from a non-contaminated area China	Se and Hg in serum and urine GPX and MDA in serum Se speciation	Se retention ↑ in Hg-exposed people Positive correlation between Hg and Se in urine GPX ↑ in miners compared to control Selenoproteins may bind Hg through selenol group and act as antioxidant	Chen et al. (2006)
215 thyroid cancers 331 controls French Polynesia	Se and I in fingernails	No association between thyroid cancer and Se in fingernails; I and Se in fingernails	Ren et al. (2014)

(continued)

Table 22.3 (continued)

Population studied	Measured parameters	Main results	References
136 children, mean age = 11.1 years, with goiter (90 girls, 46 boys) 38 control, mean age = 11.5 years (19 girls, 19 boys) Poland	Se in blood, GPX, TSH, fT4 in plasma I in urine Sonography of thyroid	Se, GPX, and I ↓ in patients compared to control Negative association between GPX and thyroid volume divided by age-adjusted upper limit of normal thyroid volume No association between Se and thyroid hormones In girls with the lowest blood Se, ↑ fT4 and TSH	Zagrodzki et al. (2000)
25 smelters (9 were reexamined after 10 months) 25 controls	Pb in blood Se in plasma Alanine amino transferase, γ glutamyl transpeptidase, uric acid	Pb ↑and Se ↓ in smelters compared to controls Negative association between Pb and Se After 10 months Pb ↑ but Se remains similar	Gustafson et al. (1987)
63 workers (steel factory) 7 controls Japan	Pb, Zn protoporphyrin; δ aminolevulinic acid dehydratase in blood Ag, As, Bi, Cd, Co, Cr, Cs, Cu, Fe, Ga, Ge, Hg, In, K, Mn, Mo, Ni, Pb, Pd, Pt, Rb, Sb, Sn, Sr, Te, Th, Tl, V, U, Zn, and Zr in plasma and erythrocytes GPX in erythrocytes SOD, CAT, GPX in plasma δ aminolevulinic acid in urine	When Pb ↑, plasma CAT and K and erythrocyte Se ↑, erythrocyte Mg ↓, antioxidant enzymes are not modify except ↑ CAT	Chiba et al. (1996)
25 patients with multinodular goiter, 29–65 years (21 women, 4 men), mildly I deficient 20 healthy subjects, 30–60 years (16 women, 4 men) Turkey	TSH, fT4, fT3, Cu, Zn, Mn, Se, Fe in plasma I in urine	No difference in Se between groups No association between Se and thyroid hormone or urinary I	Giray et al. (2010)

(continued)

Table 22.3   (continued)

Population studied	Measured parameters	Main results	References
14 pregnant women with neural tube defect fetus 14 controls Turkey	Pb in blood Cu, Zn, Se in serum	Zn and Se ↓ and Cu and Pb ↑ in cases compared to controls No association between Pb and other elements Positive correlation between Zn and Se Negative correlation between Cu and Se	Cengiz et al. (2004)

MMA monomethyl As, *DMA* dimethyl As, *GPX* glutathione peroxidase, *CAT* catalase, *SOD* superoxide dismutase, *8OHdG* 8hydroxy-2'deoxyguanosine, *MDA* malondialdehyde, *HO-1* heme oxygenase 1, *OGG1* 8-oxoguanine DNA glycosylase 1, *HSP70* heat-shock protein 70, *p38 MAPK* p38 mitogen-activated protein kinase, *NF-κB p65* nuclear factor kappa B p65, *TSH* thyroid-stimulating hormone, *fT4* free thyroxine, *fT3* free triiodothyronine

Table 22.4   Selenium interactions: summary of some prospective studies conducted in humans

Population studied	Measured parameters	Main results	References
93 pregnant women, 18–45 years Chile	Se and As in water and urine As speciation in urine	Inverse association between inorganic As and Se in urine Positive associations between total As or DMA and Se after adjustments	Christian et al. (2006)
287 adult men and women Bangladesh	Folate, vitamin B12, homocysteine, and Se in plasma As in water Total As and As speciation in urine and blood Genomic methylation of leukocyte DNA	Inverse association between plasma Se and genomic DNA methylation, total urinary As, total blood As, blood MMA Positive association between blood DMA and plasma Se whatever the adjustments	Pilsner et al. (2010)

MMA monomethyl As, *DMA* dimethyl As, *DNA* deoxyribonucleic acid

2013). Decrease in Se absorption has been reported to affect the inflammatory and immune responses and to increase oxidative stress (Mocchegiani et al. 2014). In contrast, vitamin D has been found to facilitate the absorption and assimilation of Se (Schwalfenberg and Genuis 2015), but also the uptake of toxic elements such as aluminum (Al), As, Co, Pb, and strontium (Sr). Antioxidants such as vitamin E, A, and C have been demonstrated to promote Se absorption in animals and their intakes modulate the recommended daily Se intake (Rayman 2008). Se status of mother may modify the concentration of bromine (Br), Cd, Pb, and Zn in human milk (Perrone et al. 1994).

Status markers of Se and other nutrients have been found to be associated in humans (Bates et al. 2002a, b). Se is strongly linked with thyroid functioning

Table 22.5 Selenium interactions: summary of some observational and cross-sectional studies conducted in humans

Population studied	Measured parameters	Main results	References
129 men, 15–99 years Germany	Cd and Se in postmortem prostate, liver, kidney, and urine	In prostate: ↑ Cd tends to be associated with ↓ Se No association between Se and Cd in the liver and kidney (Cd sequestration by metallothioneins) Se/Cd ratios ↓ more rapidly and consistently with age in smokers than in nonsmokers	Drasch et al. (2005), Schöpfer et al. (2010)
250 mothers and newborns Saudi Arabia	Cd and comet assay in mother and cord blood Se and MDA in mother and cord serum 8-OHdG, cotinine, and creatinine in mother urine Se and Cd in placenta Gestational age, birth height and weight, head circumference, ponderal index, cephalization index, apgar score at 1 and 5 min Placental weight and thickness and cord length	No association between cord serum Se and cord blood Cd or placental Cd; mother serum Se and Cd in placenta, cord, and mother blood Negative associations between cord serum Se and mother blood Cd; cord Cd/Se ratio and birth weight or placenta thickness; placenta Cd/Se ratio and placenta weight Positive association between cord Cd/Se ratio and cephalization index No antagonistic mechanism between Cd and Se	Al-Saleh et al. (2015)
Pregnant women, 18–45 years, at full-term delivery Hawaii	Hg and Se in cord blood and placenta mRNA and selenoproteins in placenta Seafood intake	↑ cord blood and placenta Hg but not Se with ↑ seafood intake No difference in selenoprotein expression, placenta GPX, and Txnrd activities according to fish consumption	Gilman et al. (2015)

(continued)

Table 22.5 (continued)

Population studied	Measured parameters	Main results	References
135 patients who had first (35 men, 23 women), second (25 men, 15 women), or third (23 men, 14 women) myocardial ischemia attack 107 controls (51 men, 56 women) Pakistan	Hg and Se in blood, urine, and hair Anthropometry, blood pressure, history of diabetes, hyperlipidemia, and hypertension Coronary angiogram	↓ Se in blood and hair and Se/Hg ratio, ↑ Se in urine and Hg in the 3 biological medium in patient compared to controls Inverse association between Se and degree of myocardial damage Inverse association between Se and Hg stronger in patient at the third stage of myocardial ischemia	Afridi et al. (2014)
250 mothers at delivery Saudi Arabia	Se and Hg in placenta 8-OHdG in urine DNA damage and Hg in cord blood Se and MDA in cord serum Anthropometric measurement at birth Sociodemographic and lifestyle questionnaires	Positive associations between placenta Hg and Se; Se/Hg ratio in cord blood and Se/Hg in placenta or birth height; Se/Hg ratio in placenta and MDA in cord blood and seafood intake Negative associations between Se/Hg ratio and Hg in cord blood and placenta; Se/Hg ratio in placenta and DNA damages in cord blood; Se/Hg ratio in cord blood and crown-heel length, head circumference, and placenta weight No significant interaction between Se and Hg	Al-Saleh et al. (2014)
52 women, 57 men Italy	Se, Zn, T3, T4, fT4, TSH in serum GPX in erythrocytes	GPX, Se ↓ and T4 ↑ with age Positive associations between GPX or Se and T3/T4 ratio	Olivieri et al. (1996)
572 Pregnant women Zaire	Se, TSH, T3, T4 in serum I in urine	Positive association between Se and I No significant relation between Se and thyroid hormones	Ngo et al. (1997)

(continued)

Table 22.5 (continued)

Population studied	Measured parameters	Main results	References
1601 adults 287 children, 8–11 years Exposure to As (water As >10 µg/L) or Mn (water Mn > 500 µg/L) or both vs. non-exposed Bangladesh	As and Se in blood As in urine and water Folate and vitamin B12 in plasma	In adults: Inverse association between blood Se and urinary As whatever the adjustment factors; no association between As and Se in blood In children: Inverse associations between Se and As in blood; blood Se and urinary As whatever the adjustment factors; positive correlation between vitamin B12 and Se	George et al. (2013)
375 children, mean age = 5 years Bangladesh	Cd, As, and Se in urine As speciation Blood pressure, kidney function (kidney volume, eGFR, cystatin c)	Positive associations between urinary Se and urinary Cd or As Stronger inverse association between urinary Cd and eGFR when Se is low	Skröder et al. (2015)
376 healthy low-income children, 3–4.2 years (196 boys, 180 girls), from 7 urban and peri-urban daycare centers Brazil	Ferritin, soluble transferrin receptors, Zn, Se, retinol, vitamin B12, CRP, α 1 glycoprotein in serum Folates in erythrocytes Blood count, hemoglobin variants Stool collection (intestinal parasites)	Positive association between Se and Hb	Lander et al. (2014)
896 inuits, 18–74 years (405 men, 491 women) Canada	Hg, Pb, Se in blood PON1, cholesterol, triglycerides, HDL cholesterol, LDL cholesterol in plasma PUFAs in erythrocyte membranes PON1 single-nucleotide polymorphisms (variants of rs662, rs854560, and rs705379)	Blood Se and plasma PUFAs oppose the effect of Hg on plasma PON1 activity	Ayotte et al. (2011)

(continued)

Table 22.5 (continued)

Population studied	Measured parameters	Main results	References
600 adults from four areas (3 Hg-contaminated area and one control) China	Mn, Fe, Cu, Zn, As, Se, Cd, Hg and MeHg, Pb in blood Se in rice	80.2% of subject at risk of Hg exposure (blood Hg > 5.8 µg/L) Blood As, Se, Hg, and MeHg ↑ in the contaminated area compared to control area No difference in Pb, Zn, Cd, Fe, Cu, ↑ Mn in the area nearest from the mine compared to control Positive associations between Hg, MeHg, and Se in blood Negative associations between Se/Hg ratio and Hg; Se/MeHg and MeHg in blood High concentration of As, Hg, and Se in rice	Li et al. (2016)
154 men, 19–55 years Croatia	Cu, Zn, and Se in serum Pb and Cd in blood δ-Aminolevulinic acid dehydratase in plasma, protoporphyrin in erythrocytes, hematocrit Blood pressure	Positive correlations between serum Se and Zn; systolic and diastolic blood pressure and blood Pb/serum Se ratio Negative correlation between blood Cd and serum Se No association between systolic and diastolic blood pressure and blood Cd/serum Se ratio ↓ Se levels ↑ the effect of blood Pb on blood pressure	Telišman et al. (2001)
792 men, 45–60 years and 1108 women, 35–60 years France	TSH, fT4, Se, Zn, retinol, α-tocopherol, β carotene in serum I and thiocyanate in urine Thyroid volume by ultrasonography Alcohol consumption and smoking history questionnaire Height and weight	Positive correlations between Se and urinary I, α-tocopherol, and retinol Negative associations between Se and thiocyanate; Se and thyroid volume, risk of goiter, hypoechogenicity in women after adjustment for age, TSH, thiocyanate, smoking, body surface No association between Se and nodule occurrence	Derumeaux et al. (2003)

(continued)

Table 22.5 (continued)

Population studied	Measured parameters	Main results	References
500 adults (227 men, 273 women) with newly diagnosed pulmonary tuberculosis Malawi	Hb in blood Erythropoietin, ferritin, carotenoids, retinol, α-tocopherol, Zn, Se, IL6, HIV load in plasma Anthropometric measurements	370 were HIV positive and 130 HIV negative Positive association between plasma Se and Hb after adjustment for BMI, micronutrient concentrations, sex, and age	van Lettow et al. (2005)
503 urban and semi-urban high-income children, 5–15 years New Zealand	Transferrin saturation, ferritin, Zn, Se, 25 hydroxyvitamin D, CRP in serum Blood count Height, weight	Using multilinear regression model, the positive association between Se and Hb comprises a direct effect and an indirect relation mediated by Zn	Houghton et al. (2016)
74 women, 20.5 ± 2.5 years Spain	Se intake Cholesterol, HDL-cholesterol, triglycerides, glucose, insulin in serum Plasma RBP4 Anthropometric measurements, blood pressure Semiquantitative food frequency and lifestyle questionnaires	Negative association between RBP4 and Se intake after adjustment by energy, Zn, vitamin E and C intakes, smoking, and physical activity	Hermsdorff et al. (2009)
Free-living people ≥65 years Long-stay institutionalized UK	Se in plasma GPX in whole blood Wide range of biochemical status analyses	Positive associations between plasma Se and plasma vitamin C, carotenoids, retinol, vitamin E, vitamin D, vitamin B6, Fe, Zn, Ca, serum folate, vitamin B12, ferritin, Hb, and red cell count	Bates et al. (2002b)

(continued)

Table 22.5 (continued)

Population studied	Measured parameters	Main results	References
590 boys and 537 girls, 4–18 years UK	Se in plasma and erythrocytes GPX in plasma and whole blood Wide range of biochemical status analyses	Inverse associations between erythrocyte Se and plasma 25-hydroxyvitamin D (↓ by including season in the model); between GPX and total or LDL cholesterol Positive associations between minerals, fat- and water-soluble vitamins	Bates et al. (2002a)
2092 adults ≥65 years NHANES III USA	Hb Fe, ferritin, folates, vitamin B12, and Se in serum Creatinine clearance	↓ serum Se in anemic compared with non-anemic Positive association between plasma Se and Hb	Semba et al. (2009)
632 women, 70–79 years USA	Blood count, Se, ferritin, folate, vitamin B12, CRP, IL6, CMV antibodies in serum Interview, physical examination, and questionnaires	Prevalence of anemia ↓ with ↑Se even in the absence of Fe, folate, and vitamin B12 deficiencies and after adjustment for demographic factors, chronic diseases, serum ferritin, and IL-6	Semba et al. (2006)
123 healthy adults, 20–60 years (51 men, 72 women) Vietnam	Hb Ferritin, retinol, Cu, Zn, Se, Fe in serum	Se, Fe, and retinol ↓ in anemic subjects Positive association between Se and retinol No association between Se and Zn	Van Nhien et al. (2006)

GPX glutathione peroxidase, *Txnrd* thioredoxin reductase, *8OHdG* 8hydroxy-2'deoxyguanosine, *MDA* malondialdehyde, *DNA* deoxyribonucleic acid, *RNA* ribonucleic acid; *PON1* paraoxonase 1, *TSH* thyroid-stimulating hormone, *fT4* free thyroxine, *fT3* free triiodothyronine, *Hb* hemoglobin, *RBP4* retinol-binding protein 4, *CRP* C-reactive protein, *IL6* interleukin 6, *HDL* high-density lipoprotein, *LDL* low-density lipoprotein, *PUFA* polyunsaturated fatty acids, *BMI* body mass index, *eGFR* estimated glomerular filtration rate, *HIV* human immunodeficiency virus, *CMV* cytomegalovirus

Table 22.6 Selenium interactions: Summary of some intervention studies conducted in humans

Population studied	Supplementation	Measured parameters	Effect of supplementation Main other results	References
54 adults (28 men and 26 women) exposed to As and with skin lesions in Se group vs. 29 (14 men and 15 women) in placebo group Mongolia	Se supplementation as yeast (200 µg/day for 3 months, then 100 µg/day for 3 months; then 200 µg/day for 3 months, and finally 100 µg/day for 5 months)	As and Se in hair and blood skin evaluation (hyperkeratosis, depigmentation, and pigmentation)	↓ blood and hair As Improvement of skin lesions	Yang et al. (2002)
100 patients in Se group vs. 86 in placebo group exposed to As Mongolia	Se supplementation (100–200 µg/day as yeast for 14 months) As free water (<50 µg/L) in both groups	As in water, hair, urine, blood, skin lesions (hyperkeratosis, depigmentation, pigmentation, skin cleft) Clinical examination Liver function test, hepatic ultrasonotomography, electrocardiogram	Higher ↓ As in all the biological fluids Recovery of As skin lesions	Wang et al. (2001)
121 adults with As overload and skin lesions Bangladesh	Supplementation for 6 months with either vitamin E (400 UI), Se (200 µg as SeMet), or vitamin E + Se vs Placebo	As in urine Clinical outcomes Gene expression Protein carbonyl	Upregulation of genes involved in immune functions, oxidative stress, apoptosis, and cell proliferation ↓ urinary As Insignificant ↓ protein carbonyl Insignificant improvement of skin lesions	Verret et al. (2005), Kibriya et al. (2007), Mahata et al. (2007)
22 nonpregnant women, 20–40 years Norway	Se supplementation (400 µg as SeMet ± ≥ 3 fish dinners/week or as selenite + ≥ 3 fish dinners/week) vs. placebo + ≥ 3 fish dinners/week for 15 weeks	Fish diary As and Se in fish consumed T4, T3, thyrotropin, thyroxine-binding-globulin, Se, As, Zn, and Cu in blood collected at week 0, 2, 4, 10 and 15 Se in urine	Se supplementation erases the negative association between As and thyroid hormones No association between Se and As	Meltzer et al. (2002)

(continued)

Table 22.6 (continued)

Population studied	Supplementation	Measured parameters	Effect of supplementation Main other results	References
5 volunteers exposed to Hg China	Se supplementation (100 μg as yeast) for 90 day	Collection of urine before and after 7–15–30–45–60 and 90 days after supplementation. Speciation of Hg and Se in urine	↑ urinary Hg SeCys and inorganic Hg were the major forms in urine Hg is not co-eluted with Se	Li et al. (2007)
103 residents, 18–65 years, living in a polluted Hg area for at least 15 years and with Hg in urine between 10 and 50 μg/L China	Se supplementation (100 μg as yeast) for 90 days vs. placebo	Collection of urine before and after 15–30–45–60–75 and 90 days after supplementation Hg, Se, MDA, and 8 OHdG in urine	↑ urinary Hg and ↓ MDA and 8 OHdG	Li et al. (2012)
35 pregnant women (18 Se supplemented) 17 nonpregnant Se-supplemented women New Zealand	Se supplementation (50 μg Se/day as SeMet) for 18 months vs. placebo	I and Se in urine, Se in plasma and GPX in blood at 2-3-4-5-6-7-8-9 months of pregnancy and at 3–6–12 months postpartum Collection of blood and urine from nonpregnant women at comparable intervals	Modification of Se metabolism during pregnancy Positive association between urinary Se and I	Thomson et al. (2001)
1. Area affected by severe, intermediate and lack of goiter 2. Intervention in 52 children in the severely affected area Zaire	1. Epidemiological study 2. Intervention study Se supplementation (50 μg/day Se as SeMet) for 2 months followed by I supplementation (0.5 mL/day as Lipiodol)	Se, TSH, T3, rT3, T4, and fT4 in serum, GPX in erythrocytes	Progressive ↓ in serum Se, erythrocyte GPX and urinary I associated with ↑ incidence of goiters ↓ T4, fT4, rT3 and no change in T3, TSH after Se supplementation Thyroid hormones return to reference ranges after I supplementation	Thilly et al. (1992), Contempré et al. (1992)

GPX glutathione peroxidase, *SeMet* selenomethionine, *SeCys* selenocysteine, *8OHdG* 8hydroxy-2'deoxyguanosine, *MDA* malondialdehyde, *TSH* thyroid-stimulating hormone, *fT4* free thyroxine, *fT3* free triiodothyronine, *rT3* triiodothyronine reverse

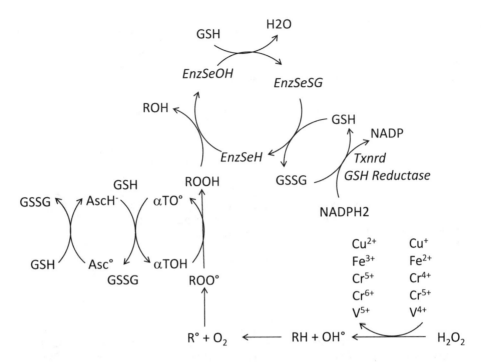

Fig. 22.2 Schematic view of antioxidant interactions to degrade oxygen reactive species: The selenol group (EnzSeH) degrades peroxides (ROOH) to alcohol (ROH). The selenenic acid formed (EnzSeOH) reacts with glutathione (GSH) to produce the selenenyl sulfide (EnzSeSG) which further reacts with second equivalent of GSH to regenerate EnzSeH and produce diglutathione (GSSG). Thioredoxin reductase (Txnrd) or GSH reductase regenerates GSH. Metals (i.e., Cu, Fe, Cr, V) generate hydroxyl radicals (OH°) from hydrogen peroxide (H_2O_2). OH° reacts with non-radical compounds (RH) to generate carbon radical (R°) which further reacts with oxygen (O_2) to generate peroxyl radical (ROO°). Alpha-tocopherol (αTOH) reacts with ROO° to form alpha-tocopherol radical (αTO°) and peroxide (ROOH). Ascorbate ($AscH^-$) or GSH regenerates (αTO°) and produces semi-dehydroascorbate radical (Asc°) and GSSG. GSH regenerates Asc°

(see Chap. 8) and therefore to iodine (I), iron (Fe), manganese (Mn), and zinc (Zn) (Lyons et al. 2004; Schomburg and Köhrle 2008; Duntas 2010; Köhrle 2015).

Redox Imbalance

Most of the interactions between Se and heavy metals, trace elements, or vitamins can be explained, at least in part, by the redox network (Figs. 22.2 and 22.3) which plays a major role in the regulation of cell metabolism and signaling. In addition, Se, similarly to Cu and Zn, affects many genes related to the inflammation and oxidative stress, which in turn affect the intestinal absorption of these micronutrients (Mocchegiani et al. 2014).

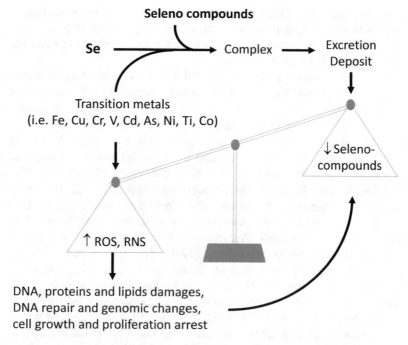

Fig. 22.3 Interactions between toxic elements and Se: Toxic elements generate reactive oxygen (ROS) or nitrogen (RNS) species that damage lipids, proteins, and deoxyribonucleic acid (DNA). Inorganic Se forms complex with transition metals and seleno-compounds that decrease their toxicity. Both complex formation and oxidative damages contribute to decrease seleno-compound concentrations

Exposure to toxic metals is associated with the formation of reactive oxygen species (ROS), reactive nitrogen species (RNS). This oxidative stress damages deoxyribonucleic acids (DNA), proteins, and lipids; interferes with DNA repair systems, resulting in genomic instability; and interrupts cell growth and proliferation via signaling pathways and dysregulation of genes [(Koedrith and Seo 2011), see Chap. 4].

Enzymatic and nonenzymatic antioxidants decrease the adverse effects of ROS and RNS, or both. Glutathione peroxidases (GPXs) and thioredoxine reductases (TxnrdRs) as well as superoxide dismutases and catalase are the principal enzymatic antioxidants. Se, Cu, and Zn are linked in cytosolic defense against ROS and RNS. Cu-Zn–superoxide dismutase catalyzes the conversion of superoxide to oxygen and hydrogen peroxide, which is then reduced to water and oxygen by GPXs (Lyons et al. 2004). Se and other antioxidants such as glutathione (GSH), thioredoxin, vitamin E and C, coenzyme Q10, flavonoids, and some carotenoids cooperate in a complex antioxidant network to avoid the formation of very aggressive species such as hydroxyl, alkoxyl, and peroxinitryl radicals or hypochlorous acid. Interactions between nonenzymatic antioxidants occur based on the order of reactivity of their oxidation-reduction potentials. Some antioxidants act in a hydrophilic environment, others in a hydrophobic environment, and some in both environments.

Some nonenzymatic antioxidants can regenerate other antioxidants and thus restore their function. However, depending on the dose, oxygen concentration, and presence of other anti- and prooxidants, these nonenzymatic antioxidants can become prooxidants and cause damage to cells.

Most of the transition metals, i.e., As, Cd, Co, Cr, copper (Cu), iron (Fe), Ni, titanium (Ti), and vanadium (V), can generate free radicals via Fenton reaction [(Valko et al. 2006), Figs. 22.2 and 22.3] and most of the selenocompounds, i.e., selenocysteine (SeCys), selenomethionine (SeMet), GPXs, TXNRDs, and selenoprotein P (SelenoP), act as enzymatic or nonenzymatic antioxidants [(Koedrith and Seo 2011), see Chap. 4]. They are depleted to counterbalance the damages caused by prooxidant metals through coordination of metal ions with their thiol/selenol groups (Koedrith and Seo 2011; Zwolak and Zaporowska 2012; Zimmerman et al. 2015). GPX isoenzymes are one of the most efficient enzymatic antioxidant families. The efficient catalysis of redox reactions by selenoenzymes is mainly based on two biochemical properties of SeCys: the selenol group is more acidic than the thiol group in cysteine and SeCys is more readily oxidized than cysteine. The selenol group (EnzSeH) degrades peroxides to alcohol and/or water. The selenenic acid formed (EnzSeOH) reacts with GSH to produce the selenenyl sulfide (EnzSeSG) which further reacts with second equivalent of GSH to regenerate the selenol [(Valko et al. 2006; Steinbrenner and Sies 2009), Fig. 22.2]. In addition, SeCys reduces tyrosyl radicals in proteins. SeMet, the selenium analogue of methionine, is oxidized by peroxynitrite to methionine selenoxide, which can be reduced back to SeMet by GSH (Steinbrenner and Sies 2009). SelenoP reduces phospholipid hydroperoxide using GSH or thioredoxin as cosubstrate, and protected plasma proteins against peroxynitrite-induced oxidation and nitration or low-density lipoproteins (LDL) from peroxidation (Steinbrenner and Sies 2009).

GSH is the major intracellular nonenzymatic antioxidant. It reacts with oxidized proteins to form S glutathiolated proteins which are reduced in protein sulfhydryls through glutathione reductase and small proteins such as glutaredoxin or thioredoxin. Glutathione reductase and Txnrd are involved in protection against ROS through the maintenance of a high ratio of reduced to oxidized GSH and thioredoxin. GSH and thioredoxin serve as electron and hydrogen donor for a number of intra- and extracellular antioxidant enzymes such as oxidized peroxiredoxins, methionine sulfoxide reductases, and GPXs (Valko et al. 2006; Steinbrenner and Sies 2009). GSH regenerates tocopherol and ascorbyl radical to vitamin E and ascorbate (Valko et al. 2006). Alpha- and dihydro-lipoic acid couple regenerates GSH, oxidized proteins, ascorbate, and vitamin E and chelate metals such as Cu^{2+}, Cd^{2+}, and Fe^{2+} (Valko et al. 2006).

Alpha-tocopherol protects membranes against lipid peroxidation. During the antioxidant reaction, alpha-tocopherol is converted to an alpha-tocopherol radical and lipid peroxyl radical into lipoperoxide. Ascorbate and GSH regenerate alpha-tocopherol and are transformed in semi-dehydroascorbate radical and oxidized GSH. GSH regenerates ascorbate from dehydroascorbate using glutaredoxin but nicotinamide adenine dinucleotide phosphate (NADPH) regenerates ascorbate using Txnrd. Coenzyme Q10 also reduced tocopheryl and ascorbyl radicals (Chaudière and Ferrari-Iliou 1999). In addition, ascorbic acid reduces metals involved in Fenton reaction. Part of oxidized GSH reacts with thiol groups of proteins.

Nitric oxide radical is an endogenous inhibitor of GPXs and GPX induction occurs in case of peroxide overload.

Formation of Complexes (Fig. 22.3)

The formation of complexes between Se and toxic inorganic elements may decrease the toxicity of heavy metals or metalloids, such as silver (Ag), As, Cd, Cu, Fe, Hg, and Pb. Ag, Cd, Hg, and selenide form metal-Se complexes in the presence of GSH, which then binds to proteins, particularly SelenoP, forming a ternary complex (Jamba et al. 1997; Sasakura and Suzuki 1998). More detailed mechanisms are indicated in the different metal sections below.

Methylation Pathway (Fig. 22.4)

Methionine synthase and betaine homocysteine methyltransferase methylate homocysteine to methionine. The first enzyme is folate dependent and its activity is therefore reduced in case of folate deficiency. Se stimulates the activity of betaine

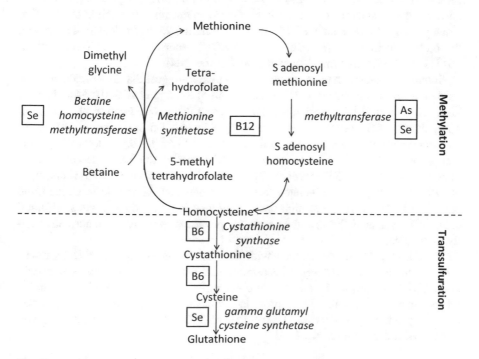

Fig. 22.4 Impact of Se, As, folate, vitamin B6 and B12 on the methylation pathway

homocysteine methyltransferase and Se supplementation can compensate the decrease in methylation. However, Se supplementation decreases cystathionine synthase activity and therefore increases homocysteine and decreases the S-adenosyl methionine (SAM)/S-adenosyl homocysteine (SAH) ratio. Selenium deficiency increases the activity of gamma-glutamylcysteine synthetase and cystathionine synthase and therefore the concentration of glutathione, the increase in cystathionine synthase being more pronounced in case of combined folate and Se deficiencies (Davis and Uthus 2003). In addition, As uses SAM as methyl donor (Sun et al. 2014).

Specific Se Interactions

Se and As Interactions

Millions of people are exposed to As due to ingestion of contaminated water and foods. Inorganic As is reported to be more toxic than organic As, and arsenite (As^{3+}) is more toxic than arsenate (As^{5+}) (Sun et al. 2014). Human studies (Tables 22.3, 22.4, 22.5, and 22.6) suggest that Se may improve the skin lesions and may counteract As accumulation in the human organism (Raie 1996; Wang et al. 2001; Chen et al. 2007; Huang et al. 2008). Low Se status has been reported in some but not all studies (Xue et al. 2010; Kolachi et al. 2011). However, association between Se and As can be either antagonist or synergistic (Sun et al. 2014) depending, at least in part, on their respective concentrations, the chemical form (Christian et al. 2006; Huang et al. 2008; Pilsner et al. 2010), the population studied (George et al. 2013), the biological indices used (Chen et al. 2007; Pilsner et al. 2010; George et al. 2013), and the different mechanisms of action involved.

Studies conducted in cells, animal, and humans suggest that Se protects against oxidative stress induced by As (Verret et al. 2005; Kibriya et al. 2007; Mahata et al. 2007; Xue et al. 2010; Zwolak and Zaporowska 2012; Messarah et al. 2012) via upregulation of the selenoproteins, mainly GPXs and Txnrd (Sun et al. 2014). Se and vitamin E supplementation of subjects exposed to As has been shown to upregulate genes involved in oxidative stress and inflammation that have been downregulated by As exposure (Kibriya et al. 2007). Antioxidant enzyme activities and lipid or DNA damages were associated to the ratio between As and Se in China (Xue et al. 2010). However, Se at high doses may also induce oxidative stress (Vinceti et al. 2009; Sun et al. 2014) and As has been proposed as medicine to cure Se toxicity in the past.

In addition, Se and As interact with the zinc-finger structures of DNA repair protein which may explain its anticarcinogenic properties at low doses (Hartwig et al. 2003). In contrast Se and As have synergistic toxic effects by increasing Zn release from critical zinc-finger proteins which may lead to increased genomic instability at high concentrations (Hartwig et al. 2003; Zeng et al. 2005; Zwolak and Zaporowska 2012; Sun et al. 2014).

Antagonistic effect between Se and As has been reported on cellular signal transduction. Se inhibits As-activated transcription nuclear factor κB (NFκB) and activator protein 1 (AP-1). Similarly, some As species can prevent Se toxicity and even suppress Se-toxic necrotic effect (Zeng et al. 2005; García-Barrera et al. 2012). In addition, organo-seleno compounds counteract the pro-angiogenesis induced by As^{3+} and mediated by mitogen-activated protein kinase (MAPK) and $\alpha\nu\beta 3$ integrin (Mousa et al. 2006).

The formation of selenobis (S-glutathionyl) arsenium ion $[(GS)_2AsSe]^-$ in liver allows Se^{4+} to decrease As^{3+} toxicity (Manley et al. 2006; Gailer 2009). Due to high intracellular concentrations of GSH in hepatocyte, when As and Se enter in the cells simultaneously, the hydroxyl (OH) groups of arsenous acid $(As(OH)_3)$ can be substituted by glutathionyl moieties to form $(GS)_2AsOH$; then hydrogen selenide (HSe^-) which is formed between Se^{4+} and GSH displaces the OH group to form $[(GS)_2AsSe]$. $[(GS)_2AsSe]^-$ is an excretory route for excess ingested As, but not Se, via the hepatobiliary route and fecal elimination. Thus, low-dietary Se intake adversely affects As excretion. On the contrary, Se sufficiency increases the excretion of As (García-Barrera et al. 2012). In addition, when cells are depleted in GSH, detoxification ability is compromised and inorganic As increases in the body (Sun et al. 2014).

Se^{4+} and As^{5+} form insoluble hemi-selenide (As_2Se) deposits by direct interaction in tissues (Zeng et al. 2005) that counteract both As and Se toxicity and contribute to skin pigmentation in arsenicosis. As As_2Se is insoluble, long-time chronic exposure to As-polluted water decreases the availability of Se for protein synthesis and lowers the levels of Se antioxidant compounds.

As^{3+} and selenide (Se^{2-}) use SAM as methyl donor (Fig. 22.4) to form monomethyl arsenic acid (MMA^{5+}) or methyl selenol (Sun et al. 2014). As the SAM concentration in cells is limited, there is a mutual inhibition of their methylation pathways which increases retention and therefore toxicity of both elements (Zeng et al. 2005; Sun et al. 2014). Additionally, Se influences the reduction of MMA^{5+} to monomethyl arsonous acid (MMA^{3+}) by thioredoxin. Because Se deficiency decreases Txnrd activity, the regeneration of thioredoxin is reduced. The second methylation of As to dimethyl arsenic acid (DMA^{5+}), the major metabolite found is urine, is compromised (Pilsner et al. 2010), which as a consequence that increases the toxicity of As due to higher retention of inorganic and/or monomethyl As in tissues. In contrast, high doses of Se^{4+} enhance inorganic As toxicity by inhibiting methylation of As^{3+}. Se changes the structure and inhibits the activity of arsenite methyltransferase through the interaction with cysteine and formation of inactive protein adducts (Walton et al. 2003; Song et al. 2010; Sun et al. 2014). In people exposed to As, high plasma Se concentration has been unexpectedly found to be associated to hypomethylation of lymphocyte DNA (Pilsner et al. 2010). However, arsenite enhances the antitumor effect of selenobetaine possibly by inhibiting Se methylation which suggests that partially methylated forms of Se may be directly involved in the anticarcinogenic action of Se (García-Barrera et al. 2012).

It has been reported that As^{3+} and arsenic trioxide (As_2O_3) but not MMA^{3+} or DMA^{3+} inhibit selenoprotein and particularly Txnrd synthesis (Ganyc et al. 2006;

Talbot et al. 2008). MMA^{3+} inhibits the expression of cellular GPX and small selenoproteins whereas DMA^{3+} stimulates selenoprotein synthesis, particularly cellular GPX (Ganyc et al. 2006). Other selenoenzymes or selenoproteins, such as deiodinases, are inhibited by As (Meltzer et al. 2002).

Se and Cd Interactions

Cd pollutant is widespread and is most often associated with smoking habits and occupational health. Se may counteract the negative health effect of Cd (Wadhwa et al. 2015; Wei et al. 2015) but it is difficult to predict the interactions of Se and Cd due to numerous confounding factors (Tables 22.3 and 22.5) such as age, lifestyle, and measured biological markers (Drasch et al. 2005; Schöpfer et al. 2010; Al-Saleh et al. 2015; Skröder et al. 2015). Interestingly, Zn and Se appear to synergistically reduce the toxicity of Cd in animals (Hammouda et al. 2008; Messaoudi et al. 2009, 2010a, b; Saïd et al. 2010; Banni et al. 2011; García-Barrera et al. 2012).

Cd is unable to perform redox reactions in biological systems, but it stimulates oxidative stress through inhibition of antioxidants (i.e., SelenoP, GPXs, glutathione reductase, catalase, and GSH) through the interaction with their thiol groups (Jamba et al. 1997; Hammouda et al. 2008; Messaoudi et al. 2009, 2010a, b; Banni et al. 2011; Koedrith and Seo 2011; Zwolak and Zaporowska 2012). Se supplementation with inorganic or organic Se compounds has been reported, in animal studies, to decrease oxidative lipid damages in different tissues and organs such as liver, brain, kidney, and testis (Li et al. 2010; Messaoudi et al. 2010a; Zwolak and Zaporowska 2012; Xie et al. 2016), increase catalase and GPX activities, but lower Na$^+$/K$^+$-adenosine triphosphatase activity (Messaoudi et al. 2010a; Xie et al. 2016). In addition, the activity of Se is strongly dependent on the chemical form of Se, with Se^{4+} being efficient against lipid damages generated by Cd, whereas Se^{6+} on the other hand shows no effect (Serafín Muñoz et al. 2007).

Se administration may decrease the nephrotoxicity and hepatotoxicity of Cd in animals (Flora et al. 1982). The toxic effect on heart tissue of Cd and Se when administered individually may be counteracted when both elements are administrated simultaneously (Skowerski et al. 2000). These observations could be related to the formation of a Cd-Se complex as reported in vitro. Cd and selenide, produced from selenite, formed a Cd-Se complex in the presence of GSH, which then bound to proteins, particularly SelenoP, to form a ternary complex (Jamba et al. 1997; Sasakura and Suzuki 1998). However, the sequestration of Cd by Se works only as long as Se is available in excess over Cd, placing smokers with low Se status at higher risk of developing chronic diseases such as cancer (Schrauzer 2009; Wei et al. 2015). The role of Se/Cd ratio in chelation partly explains the discrepancies observed in animal studies.

Se and F Interactions (Table 22.3)

Fluorosis is associated with an increase in oxidative stress and apoptosis (Chen et al. 2009; Basha and Madhusudhan 2010; Feng et al. 2012; Miao et al. 2013). Se can counteract this oxidative stress by modulation of antioxidant enzyme activities, increase in antioxidant capacity, decrease in nitric oxide and nitric oxide synthase activity, induction of HSP70, and decrease in lipid, RNA, and protein oxidation (Chen et al. 2009; Basha and Madhusudhan 2010; Feng et al. 2012). Se and F exhibit antagonist effects on p38 MAPK/caspase 3 signal transduction pathway (Chen et al. 2010; Miao et al. 2013; Zheng et al. 2016). Se reduces the neurotoxicity of F partly due to changes in postsynaptic density protein expression (Qian et al. 2013).

F induces malabsorption and maldigestion of nutrient. In contrast, antioxidants such as Se, Zn, and vitamin E and C are able to increase the elimination of F (Basha and Madhusudhan 2010).

Se and Fe Interactions

Several human studies have reported an association between low Se status and risk of anemia [(Bates et al. 2002b; van Lettow et al. 2005; Semba et al. 2006, 2009, Van Nhien et al. 2006, 2008, 2009; Nhien et al. 2008; Lander et al. 2014; Houghton et al. 2016), Table 22.5]. This relationship may be present even in the absence of Fe, folate, and vitamin B_{12} deficiencies (Semba et al. 2006) and is independent on age (Van Nhien et al. 2006, 2008, 2009; Nhien et al. 2008). The hematopoietic effects of Se could be related to the protection of cell membrane and intracellular organelles by the antioxidant effects of vitamin E and selenoenzymes. In addition, Se deficiency decreases the activity of Txnrd, which in turn upregulates heme oxygenase-1 through AP-1. Heme oxygenase-1 is implicated in the initial step of heme catabolism and the release of Fe^{2+} from the cells (Mostert et al. 2003, 2007; Van Nhien et al. 2008; Nhien et al. 2008; Semba et al. 2009; Houghton et al. 2016). Moreover, experimental studies suggest that Se deficiency limits erythropoiesis (Semba et al. 2009) and availability of Fe for hemoprotein synthesis (Mostert et al. 2007). Organoselenium compounds inhibit Fe-mediated oxidative DNA damages due to metal-binding mechanism as described for Cu (Battin et al. 2011; Zwolak and Zaporowska 2012). The association of serum Se and anemia may also be indirect as GPXs regulate the release and transfer of Zn from metallothionein to Cu-Zn superoxide dismutase (Maret 2000; Houghton et al. 2016).

In addition, Fe may decrease the intestinal absorption of Se by formation of Fe^{+3}-Se complex which cannot be absorbed by the enterocytes (Mehdi et al. 2013). In low-income and elderly populations, the positive associations between anemia, plasma Se concentration, and different micronutrients may reflect the complex multisystem decline related to decreased nutritional intakes, frailty, and associated diseases [(Bates et al. 2002b; Semba et al. 2009), Table 22.5].

Se and Hg Interactions

Chronic exposure to Hg is a major health issue as millions of people are exposed to Hg-contaminated seafood or to industrial Hg sources. The most neurotoxic form of Hg is methyl mercury (MeHg) (Khan and Wang 2009).

Many human studies (Tables 22.3, 22.5, and 22.6) suggest that Se may counteract Hg accumulation in the human organism. However, the effect of Se supplementation largely depends on the Se and Hg species, the way of Hg and Se administration, the relative concentrations of Hg and Se, the time and duration in which the Hg and Se species are administered, and the sensitivity of the animal or the biological material studied (Khan and Wang 2009; Dang and Wang 2011; Branco et al. 2012; García-Barrera et al. 2012; Luque-Garcia et al. 2013; Al-Saleh et al. 2014; Afridi et al. 2014). Synergistic effects of Hg and Se have indeed been reported in birds and in vitro (Brandão et al. 2005; Khan and Wang 2009; Heinz et al. 2012). In addition, the presence of other elements such as As, Zn, fatty acids, or protein and molecules with thiol groups may modify the Se-Hg interaction (Chmielnicka et al. 1983; Cuvin-Aralar and Furness 1991).

Se supplementation has been reported to decrease Hg absorption (Cuvin-Aralar and Furness 1991), increase urinary Hg concentrations in exposed humans (Li et al. 2007, 2012), and decrease brain Hg concentrations (Glaser et al. 2010).

Human exposure to Hg increases lipoperoxides and DNA damage (Kobal et al. 2004; Li et al. 2012). MeHg generates free methyl radicals, inhibits the activities of the complexes I to IV of the respiratory chain and paraoxonase 1, is a strong thiol-binding molecule, causes Se deficiency, and inhibits selenoprotein synthesis and selenoenzyme activities (Watanabe et al. 1999; Kim et al. 2005; Chen et al. 2006; Berry and Ralston 2008; Khan and Wang 2009; Grotto et al. 2009; Ayotte et al. 2011; Koedrith and Seo 2011; Branco et al. 2012; García-Barrera et al. 2012). Se supplementation (Table 22.6) has been reported to alleviate the effects of Hg on selenoproteins such as GPXs, Txnrds, and oxidized GSH; restore mitochondrial function, paraoxonase 1 activity, and biogenesis; and decrease malondialdehyde (MDA) and DNA damage induced by Hg poisoning (dos Santos et al. 2007; Khan and Wang 2009; Grotto et al. 2009; Ayotte et al. 2011; Branco et al. 2012; García-Barrera et al. 2012; Li et al. 2012; Luque-Garcia et al. 2013). However, other studies do not demonstrate significant beneficial effects of Se^{4+} or SeMet on thiobarbituric acid (TBARS) levels, and mitochondrial enzyme activities generated by Hg^{2+} or MeHg (Brandão et al. 2005; Kaur et al. 2009; Glaser et al. 2010; Luque-Garcia et al. 2013). It is important to take into consideration that exposure to Se^{4+} alone can also inhibit the activity of mitochondrial enzymes and increase TBARS (Glaser et al. 2010; Luque-Garcia et al. 2013).

Se and MeHg inversely modify the transcription of key functional classes of genes related to the immune system, cell adhesion, and development (Jayashankar et al. 2011).

Interestingly, Se has been found to protect microorganisms and animals from the toxicity of both inorganic Hg and MeHg even when Hg concentrations in tissues and body fluids continue to increase (dos Santos et al. 2007; Khan and Wang 2009). Accumulations of total Hg and Se have been reported to vary concurrently, generally following a 1:1 molar ratio, in the organs and fluids of animals and humans and regardless of the molecular ratio present in the diet (Khan and Wang 2009; García-Barrera et al. 2012). These accumulations are not associated with signs of Se and Hg toxicity due to the formation of (HgSe)n complexes (Gailer et al. 2000; Yang et al. 2008; Zwolak and Zaporowska 2012). The presence of HgSe(n) granules has been reported in the liver and kidneys of marine mammals and sea birds. As their solubility is low, the concentration of these chemically inert complexes increases with age as a result of their low elimination rate and hence represent a natural protection mechanism against Hg toxicity (Khan and Wang 2009; Luque-Garcia et al. 2013). The complexes are formed easily as the formation constant between MeHg and Se is greater than between MeHg and sulfur (Berry and Ralston 2008; Khan and Wang 2009). Complex formation occurs by a demethylation process via the formation of bis(methylmercuric) selenide, which is unstable at physiological temperature and decomposes to inorganic HgSe(n) or to a direct reaction between Hg^{2+} (or its complexes) and HSe^- (Khan and Wang 2009). However, it seems that when the MeHg concentration is under a threshold value, the demethylation does not occur (Khan and Wang 2009). In addition, Hg^{2+} released after demethylation of MeHg may be highly toxic due to its strong affinity to thiol and selenol groups. The formation of HgSe complexes also decreases the availability of Se for selenoprotein synthesis and may contribute to Se deficiency (Watanabe et al. 1999; Kim et al. 2005; Berry and Ralston 2008; Khan and Wang 2009; Koedrith and Seo 2011; García-Barrera et al. 2012). However inconsistent results have been reported regarding selenoprotein expression and Hg intake (Chen et al. 2006; Gilman et al. 2015). Zn may counteract the formation of HgSe complexes in biological tissues and fluids, despite the fact that the affinity of Se for Hg is higher than for Zn (Chmielnicka et al. 1983). Additionally, Se has been reported to counteract the stimulation of metallothionein synthesis induced by Hg and divert the binding of Hg to higher molecular weight proteins (Burk et al. 1977; Komsta-Szumska and Chmielnicka 1977; Cuvin-Aralar and Furness 1991).

Se and I Interactions (See Chap. 8)

The interaction between I and Se status leads to conflicting results (Tables 22.3, 22.4, 22.5, and 22.6) as the relationship is modulated by other nutrients such as thiocyanate, As, Cu, Fe, Mg, Mn, Zn, and vitamin E and A and other associated factors, i.e., age, gender, fungal toxins, virus infections, and thyroid diseases (Meltzer et al. 2002; Zimmermann and Köhrle 2002; Derumeaux et al. 2003; Lyons et al. 2004; Giray et al. 2010). Although Se and I deficiencies are clearly predisposing factors of Kashin-Beck disease, vitamin E and Zn deficiencies, malnutrition, toxin contamination of foods, or genetic polymorphisms may contribute to this osteochondral disease (Zimmermann and Köhrle 2002; Lyons et al. 2004; Yao et al. 2011; Yu et al. 2016; Wang et al. 2017).

Se is strongly linked with thyroid functioning (Derumeaux et al. 2003; Lyons et al. 2004; Schomburg and Köhrle 2008; Duntas 2010; Köhrle 2015). The content of Se in thyroid is higher than most of the organs and different selenoproteins are expressed (GPX 1, 3, and 4; deiodinase 1 and 2; Txnrd 1 and 2; selenoprotein 15, P, M, and S) (Schomburg and Köhrle 2008; Köhrle 2015). In addition, deiodinases are involved in thyroid hormone turnover and mutation of SeCys incorporation sequence-binding protein 2 (SeCys SBP2) disrupts thyroid hormone metabolism consequently to deficient selenoprotein synthesis. However, the relationship between Se and thyroid hormones largely varies according to studies (Thilly et al. 1992; Contempré et al. 1992; Olivieri et al. 1996; Ngo et al. 1997; Zagrodzki et al. 2000; Meltzer et al. 2002; Derumeaux et al. 2003; Giray et al. 2010; Ren et al. 2014). High I intake decreases thyroid Se content and selenoprotein expression, whereas low I intake is associated with an increase in thyroid Se and selenoproteins (Köhrle 2015).

GPXs as well as Txnrds protect, at least partially, the thyroid gland from oxidative damages particularly in case of I excess (Zimmermann and Köhrle 2002; Lyons et al. 2004). Combination of Se and I deficiencies is involved in the pathogenesis of endemic myxedematous cretinism due to insufficient GPXs and Txnrds to remove H_2O_2 and lipid peroxides and decrease cell defenses, cell necrosis being the result of an additional factor such as intake of thiocyanate or toxins. High thiocyanate intake inhibits the hemoprotein thyroperoxidase activity and I uptake (Contempré et al. 2004; Schomburg and Köhrle 2008; Duntas 2010). In these populations, normalization of I intake is necessary before initiation of Se supplementation in order to avoid exacerbation of hypothyroidism by stimulation of thyroxine metabolism (Contempré et al. 1991; Zimmermann and Köhrle 2002; Lyons et al. 2004). Interestingly, Se analogues of antithyroid drugs protect thyroid cells from H_2O_2 oxidative damage and reversibly inhibit the peroxidase oxidation and iodination by reduction of H_2O_2 (Roy and Mugesh 2008).

Se analogues of antithyroid drugs also react with I to produce diselenide–iodide complexes, which may inhibit thyroid hormones. However, their higher efficiency/toxicity ratio as compared to current antithyroid drugs has not been demonstrated yet (Roy and Mugesh 2008).

The role of Se in immunity and inflammation may contribute to the association between Se status and thyroid diseases, i.e., goiter, autoimmune thyroid disease, or thyroid cancer (Derumeaux et al. 2003; Köhrle 2015).

Se and Pb Interactions

Pb exposure is a widely reported health hazard. No (Chiba et al. 1996; Cengiz et al. 2004), negative (Gustafson et al. 1987), or positive (Perrone et al. 1994; Chiba et al. 1996) association has been reported between Pb and Se depending on population and biological index (Tables 22.3 and 22.5). However, decrease in Se status may increase the deleterious effect of Pb on blood pressure (Telišman et al. 2001).

In experimental models, the administration of Se prior to Pb exposure protects against toxicity of Pb, possibly related to a decrease in oxidative stress (Othman and El Missiry 1998). The formation of a stable Pb-Se complex can also explain the beneficial effect of Se against Pb toxicity (Koedrith and Seo 2011).

Se and Zn Interactions

In humans (Tables 22.3 and 22.5), plasma or serum Se and Zn concentrations are generally positively associated (Telišman et al. 2001; Bates et al. 2002b; Cengiz et al. 2004) although some studies do not report any correlation (Van Nhien et al. 2006). In animals, Se supplementation has been reported to increase Zn concentration in different organs and cells and to decrease Zn excretion by urine and feces (Chmielnicka et al. 1983, 1985, 1986, 1988; Johansson and Lindh 1987). In contrast, Zn supplementation reduces the excretion of urinary Se (Chmielnicka et al. 1988). The Se/Zn interaction can be modulated by the intake of toxic metals such as Cd, Hg, and Pb, and the status of essential trace elements such as Fe and Cu (Chmielnicka et al. 1983, 1985, 1986; Abdulla and Chmielnicka 1989).

Se, through GPXs and GSH, regulates the release of Zn from oxidized metallothionein and suppression of metallothionein synthesis, which in turn activates Cu-Zn superoxide dismutase and controls the available Zn concentration in the cells (Chmielnicka et al. 1983; Maret 2000, 2003; Lyons et al. 2004; Blessing et al. 2004; Mocchegiani et al. 2014; Houghton et al. 2016). In addition, Se and Zn are linked in cytosolic defense against reactive oxygen and nitrogen species. Cu-Zn superoxide dismutase catalyzes the conversion of superoxide to oxygen and hydrogen peroxide, which is then reduced to water and oxygen by GPXs. Moreover, Zn upregulates the GPX gene expression.

Some, but not all, seleno-compounds induce a release of Zn from Zn finger proteins and therefore inhibit Zn finger proteins which in turn affect gene expression, DNA repair, and gene stability and may open new possibilities for chronic disease amelioration (Blessing et al. 2004; Larabee et al. 2009).

Se and Vitamin A Interactions

Vitamin A and retinoids are essential nutrients and which are used in the treatment of dermatological lesions and some types of cancer. However, they are toxic due to redox imbalance and mitochondrial dysfunction (Saied and Hamza 2014). Se may counteract, at least in part, this toxicity. An inverse relationship between retinol or retinyl ester and Se in rat liver (Albrecht et al. 1994) and between Se intakes and retinol-binding protein 4 (RBP4) in human plasma (Hermsdorff et al. 2009) has been reported. This negative association may be related to inflammation (Hermsdorff et al. 2009) and redox imbalance (Albrecht et al. 1994). Co-administration of retinoic acid and Se has been reported to decrease nitric oxide and TBARS in liver and increase the level of GSH and superoxide dismutase (Saied and Hamza 2014). In addition, combined administration of Se and retinyl ester has greater inhibitory effect on carcinogenic process than retinyl acetate alone (Thompson et al. 1981). However, positive association between plasma or serum Se and retinol concentrations has been reported in multi-micronutrient-deficient populations (Bates et al. 2002b; Van Nhien et al. 2006).

References

Abdulla M, Chmielnicka J. New aspects on the distribution and metabolism of essential trace elements after dietary exposure to toxic metals. Biol Trace Elem Res. 1989;23:25–53.

Afridi HI, Kazi TG, Talpur FN, et al. Interaction between essential elements selenium and zinc with cadmium and mercury in samples from hypertensive patients. Biol Trace Elem Res. 2014;160:185–96. https://doi.org/10.1007/s12011-014-0048-y.

Albrecht R, Pélissier MA, Boisset M. Excessive dietary selenium decreases the vitamin A storage and the enzymatic antioxidant defence in the liver of rats. Toxicol Lett. 1994;70:291–7.

Al-Saleh I, Al-Rouqi R, Obsum CA, et al. Mercury (Hg) and oxidative stress status in healthy mothers and its effect on birth anthropometric measures. Int J Hyg Environ Health. 2014;217:567–85. https://doi.org/10.1016/j.ijheh.2013.11.001.

Al-Saleh I, Al-Rouqi R, Obsum CA, et al. Interaction between cadmium (Cd), selenium (Se) and oxidative stress biomarkers in healthy mothers and its impact on birth anthropometric measures. Int J Hyg Environ Health. 2015;218:66–90. https://doi.org/10.1016/j.ijheh.2014.08.001.

Ayotte P, Carrier A, Ouellet N, et al. Relation between methylmercury exposure and plasma paraoxonase activity in inuit adults from Nunavik. Environ Health Perspect. 2011;119:1077–83. https://doi.org/10.1289/ehp.1003296.

Banni M, Chouchene L, Said K, et al. Mechanisms underlying the protective effect of zinc and selenium against cadmium-induced oxidative stress in zebrafish Danio rerio. Biometals. 2011;24:981–92. https://doi.org/10.1007/s10534-011-9456-z.

Basha PM, Madhusudhan N. Pre and post natal exposure of fluoride induced oxidative macromolecular alterations in developing central nervous system of rat and amelioration by antioxidants. Neurochem Res. 2010;35:1017–28. https://doi.org/10.1007/s11064-010-0150-2.

Bates CJ, Thane CW, Prentice A, et al. Selenium status and associated factors in a British National Diet and Nutrition Survey: young people aged 4–18 y. Eur J Clin Nutr. 2002a;56:873–81. https://doi.org/10.1038/sj.ejcn.1601405.

Bates CJ, Thane CW, Prentice A, Delves HT. Selenium status and its correlates in a British National Diet and Nutrition Survey: people aged 65 years and over. J Trace Elem Med Biol. 2002b;16:1–8. https://doi.org/10.1016/S0946-672X(02)80002-5.

Battin EE, Zimmerman MT, Ramoutar RR, et al. Preventing metal-mediated oxidative DNA damage with selenium compounds. Metallomics. 2011;3:503. https://doi.org/10.1039/c0mt00063a.

Berry MJ, Ralston NVC. Mercury toxicity and the mitigating role of selenium. EcoHealth. 2008;5:456–9. https://doi.org/10.1007/s10393-008-0204-y.

Blessing H, Kraus S, Heindl P, et al. Interaction of selenium compounds with zinc finger proteins involved in DNA repair: selenium and zinc finger DNA repair proteins. Eur J Biochem. 2004;271:3190–9. https://doi.org/10.1111/j.1432-1033.2004.04251.x.

Branco V, Canário J, Lu J, et al. Mercury and selenium interaction in vivo: effects on thioredoxin reductase and glutathione peroxidase. Free Radic Biol Med. 2012;52:781–93. https://doi.org/10.1016/j.freeradbiomed.2011.12.002.

Brandão R, Lara FS, Pagliosa LB, et al. Hemolytic effects of sodium selenite and mercuric chloride in human blood. Drug Chem Toxicol. 2005;28:397–407. https://doi.org/10.1080/01480540500262763.

Burk RF, Jordan HE, Kiker KW. Some effects of selenium status on inorganic mercury metabolism in the rat. Toxicol Appl Pharmacol. 1977;40:71–82.

Cengiz B, Söylemez F, Öztürk E, Çavdar AO. Serum zinc, selenium, copper, and lead levels in women with second-trimester induced abortion resulting from neural tube defects: a preliminary study. Biol Trace Elem Res. 2004;97:225–36. https://doi.org/10.1385/BTER:97:3:225.

Chaudière J, Ferrari-Iliou R. Intracellular antioxidants: from chemical to biochemical mechanisms. Food Chem Toxicol. 1999;37:949–62.

Chen C, Yu H, Zhao J, et al. The roles of serum selenium and selenoproteins on mercury toxicity in environmental and occupational exposure. Environ Health Perspect. 2006;114:297–301.

Chen Y, Hall M, Graziano JH, et al. A prospective study of blood selenium levels and the risk of arsenic-related premalignant skin lesions. Cancer Epidemiol Biomark Prev. 2007;16:207–13. https://doi.org/10.1158/1055-9965.EPI-06-0581.

Chen Q, Wang Z, Xiong Y, et al. Selenium increases expression of HSP70 and antioxidant enzymes to lessen oxidative damage in Fincoal-type fluorosis. J Toxicol Sci. 2009;34:399–405.

Chen Q, Wang Z, Xiong Y, et al. Comparative study of p38 MAPK signal transduction pathway of peripheral blood mononuclear cells from patients with coal-combustion-type fluorosis with and without high hair selenium levels. Int J Hyg Environ Health. 2010;213:381–6. https://doi.org/10.1016/j.ijheh.2010.06.002.

Chiba M, Shinohara A, Matsushita K, et al. Indices of lead-exposure in blood and urine of lead-exposed workers and concentrations of major and trace elements and activities of SOD, GSH-Px and catalase in their blood. Tohoku J Exp Med. 1996;178:49–62.

Chmielnicka J, Komsta-Szumska E, Zareba G. Effect of interaction between 65Zn, mercury and selenium in rats (retention, metallothionein, endogenous copper). Arch Toxicol. 1983;53:165–75.

Chmielnicka J, Bem EM, Brzeźnicka EA, Kasperek M. The tissue disposition of zinc and copper following repeated administration of cadmium and selenium to rats. Environ Res. 1985;37:419–24.

Chmielnicka J, Brzeźnicka E, Sniady A. Kidney concentrations and urinary excretion of mercury, zinc and copper following the administration of mercuric chloride and sodium selenite to rats. Arch Toxicol. 1986;59:16–20.

Chmielnicka J, Zareba G, Witasik M, Brzeźnicka E. Zinc-selenium interaction in the rat. Biol Trace Elem Res. 1988;15:267–76.

Contempré B, Vanderpas J, Dumont JE. Cretinism, thyroid hormones and selenium. Mol Cell Endocrinol. 1991;81:C193–5.

Contempré B, Duale NL, Dumont JE, et al. Effect of selenium supplementation on thyroid hormone metabolism in an iodine and selenium deficient population. Clin Endocrinol. 1992;36:579–83.

Contempré B, de Escobar GM, Denef J-F, et al. Thiocyanate induces cell necrosis and fibrosis in selenium- and iodine-deficient rat thyroids: a potential experimental model for myxedematous endemic cretinism in central Africa. Endocrinology. 2004;145:994–1002. https://doi.org/10.1210/en.2003-0886.

Cuvin-Aralar ML, Furness RW. Mercury and selenium interaction: a review. Ecotoxicol Environ Saf. 1991;21:348–64.

Dang F, Wang WX. Antagonistic interaction of mercury and selenium in a marine fish is dependent on their chemical species. Environ Sci Technol. 2011;45:3116–22. https://doi.org/10.1021/es103705a.

Davis CD, Uthus EO. Dietary folate and selenium affect dimethylhydrazine-induced aberrant crypt formation, global DNA methylation and one-carbon metabolism in rats. J Nutr. 2003;133:2907–14.

Derumeaux H, Valeix P, Castetbon K, et al. Association of selenium with thyroid volume and echostructure in 35- to 60-year-old French adults. Eur J Endocrinol. 2003;148:309–15.

dos Santos APM, Mateus ML, Carvalho CML, Batoréu MCC. Biomarkers of exposure and effect as indicators of the interference of selenomethionine on methylmercury toxicity. Toxicol Lett. 2007;169:121–8. https://doi.org/10.1016/j.toxlet.2006.12.007.

Drasch G, Schöpfer J, Schrauzer GN. Selenium/cadmium ratios in human prostates: indicators of prostate cancer risk of smokers and nonsmokers, and relevance to the cancer protective effects of selenium. Biol Trace Elem Res. 2005;103:103–8. https://doi.org/10.1385/BTER:103:2:103.

Duntas LH. Selenium and the thyroid: a close-knit connection. J Clin Endocrinol Metab. 2010;95:5180–8. https://doi.org/10.1210/jc.2010-0191.

Feng P, Wei J, Zhang Z. Influence of selenium and fluoride on blood antioxidant capacity of rats. Exp Toxicol Pathol. 2012;64:565–8. https://doi.org/10.1016/j.etp.2010.11.014.

Flora SJ, Behari JR, Ashquin M, Tandon SK. Time-dependent protective effect of selenium against cadmium-induced nephrotoxicity and hepatotoxicity. Chem Biol Interact. 1982;42:345–51.

Gailer J. Chronic toxicity of AsIII in mammals: the role of (GS)2AsSe–. Biochimie. 2009;91:1268–72. https://doi.org/10.1016/j.biochi.2009.06.004.

Gailer J, George GN, Pickering IJ, et al. Structural basis of the antagonism between inorganic mercury and selenium in mammals. Chem Res Toxicol. 2000;13:1135–42.

Ganyc D, Talbot S, Konate F, et al. Impact of trivalent arsenicals on selenoprotein synthesis. Environ Health Perspect. 2006;115:346–53. https://doi.org/10.1289/ehp.9440.

García-Barrera T, Gómez-Ariza JL, González-Fernández M, et al. Biological responses related to agonistic, antagonistic and synergistic interactions of chemical species. Anal Bioanal Chem. 2012;403:2237–53. https://doi.org/10.1007/s00216-012-5776-2.

George CM, Gamble M, Slavkovich V, et al. A cross-sectional study of the impact of blood selenium on blood and urinary arsenic concentrations in Bangladesh. Environ Health. 2013;12:52. https://doi.org/10.1186/1476-069X-12-52.

Gilman CL, Soon R, Sauvage L, et al. Umbilical cord blood and placental mercury, selenium and selenoprotein expression in relation to maternal fish consumption. J Trace Elem Med Biol. 2015;30:17–24. https://doi.org/10.1016/j.jtemb.2015.01.006.

Giray B, Arnaud J, Sayek İ, et al. Trace elements status in multinodular goiter. J Trace Elem Med Biol. 2010;24:106–10. https://doi.org/10.1016/j.jtemb.2009.11.003.

Glaser V, Nazari EM, Müller YMR, et al. Effects of inorganic selenium administration in methylmercury-induced neurotoxicity in mouse cerebral cortex. Int J Dev Neurosci. 2010;28:631–7. https://doi.org/10.1016/j.ijdevneu.2010.07.225.

Grotto D, Barcelos GRM, Valentini J, et al. Low levels of methylmercury induce DNA damage in rats: protective effects of selenium. Arch Toxicol. 2009;83:249–54. https://doi.org/10.1007/s00204-008-0353-3.

Gustafson A, Schütz A, Andersson P, Skerfving S. Small effect on plasma selenium level by occupational lead exposure. Sci Total Environ. 1987;66:39–43.

Hammouda F, Messaoudi I, El Hani J, et al. Reversal of cadmium-induced thyroid dysfunction by selenium, zinc, or their combination in rat. Biol Trace Elem Res. 2008;126:194–203. https://doi.org/10.1007/s12011-008-8194-8.

Hartwig A, Blessing H, Schwerdtle T, Walter I. Modulation of DNA repair processes by arsenic and selenium compounds. Toxicology. 2003;193:161–9.

Heinz GH, Hoffman DJ, Klimstra JD, Stebbins KR. A comparison of the teratogenicity of methylmercury and selenomethionine injected into bird eggs. Arch Environ Contam Toxicol. 2012;62:519–28. https://doi.org/10.1007/s00244-011-9717-4.

Hermsdorff HHM, Zulet MÁ, Puchau B, et al. Association of retinol-binding protein-4 with dietary selenium intake and other lifestyle features in young healthy women. Nutrition. 2009;25:392–9. https://doi.org/10.1016/j.nut.2008.09.015.

Houghton LA, Parnell WR, Thomson CD, et al. Serum zinc is a major predictor of anemia and mediates the effect of selenium on hemoglobin in school-aged children in a nationally representative survey in New Zealand. J Nutr. 2016;146:1670–6. https://doi.org/10.3945/jn.116.235127.

Huang Z, Pei Q, Sun G, et al. Low selenium status affects arsenic metabolites in an arsenic exposed population with skin lesions. Clin Chim Acta. 2008;387:139–44. https://doi.org/10.1016/j.cca.2007.09.027.

Jamba L, Nehru B, Bansal MP. Redox modulation of selenium binding proteins by cadmium exposures in mice. Mol Cell Biochem. 1997;177:169–75.

Christian WJ, Hopenhayn C, Centeno JA, Todorov T. Distribution of urinary selenium and arsenic among pregnant women exposed to arsenic in drinking water. Environ Res. 2006;100:115–22. https://doi.org/10.1016/j.envres.2005.03.009.

Jayashankar S, Glover CN, Folven KI, et al. Cerebral gene expression in response to single or combined gestational exposure to methylmercury and selenium through the maternal diet. Cell Biol Toxicol. 2011;27:181–97. https://doi.org/10.1007/s10565-010-9180-4.

Johansson E, Lindh U. Interactions of selenium with metal ions at the cellular level. Biol Trace Elem Res. 1987;12:101–8. https://doi.org/10.1007/BF02796668.

Kaur P, Evje L, Aschner M, Syversen T. The in vitro effects of selenomethionine on methylmercury-induced neurotoxicity. Toxicol In Vitro. 2009;23:378–85. https://doi.org/10.1016/j.tiv.2008.12.024.

Khan MAK, Wang F. Mercury–selenium compounds and their toxicological significance: toward a molecular understanding of the mercury–selenium antagonism. Environ Toxicol Chem. 2009;28:1567–77. https://doi.org/10.1897/08-375.1.

Kibriya MG, Jasmine F, Argos M, et al. Changes in gene expression profiles in response to selenium supplementation among individuals with arsenic-induced pre-malignant skin lesions. Toxicol Lett. 2007;169:162–76. https://doi.org/10.1016/j.toxlet.2007.01.006.

Kim YJ, Chai YG, Ryu JC. Selenoprotein W as molecular target of methylmercury in human neuronal cells is down-regulated by GSH depletion. Biochem Biophys Res Commun. 2005;330:1095–102. https://doi.org/10.1016/j.bbrc.2005.03.080.

Kobal AB, Horvat M, Prezelj M, et al. The impact of long-term past exposure to elemental mercury on antioxidative capacity and lipid peroxidation in mercury miners. J Trace Elem Med Biol. 2004;17:261–74. https://doi.org/10.1016/S0946-672X(04)80028-2.

Koedrith P, Seo YR. Advances in carcinogenic metal toxicity and potential molecular markers. Int J Mol Sci. 2011;12:9576–95. https://doi.org/10.3390/ijms12129576.

Köhrle J. Selenium and the thyroid. Curr Opin Endocrinol Diabetes Obes. 2015;22:392–401. https://doi.org/10.1097/MED.0000000000000190.

Kolachi NF, Kazi TG, Wadhwa SK, et al. Evaluation of selenium in biological sample of arsenic exposed female skin lesions and skin cancer patients with related to non-exposed skin cancer patients. Sci Total Environ. 2011;409:3092–7. https://doi.org/10.1016/j.scitotenv.2011.05.008.

Komsta-Szumska E, Chmielnicka J. Binding of mercury and selenium in subcellular fractions of rat liver and kidneys following separate and joint administration. Arch Toxicol. 1977;38:217–28.

Lander RL, Bailey KB, Lander AG, et al. Disadvantaged pre-schoolers attending day care in Salvador, Northeast Brazil have a low prevalence of anaemia and micronutrient deficiencies. Public Health Nutr. 2014;17:1984–92. https://doi.org/10.1017/S1368980013002310.

Larabee JL, Hocker JR, Hanas JS. Mechanisms of inhibition of zinc-finger transcription factors by selenium compounds ebselen and selenite. J Inorg Biochem. 2009;103:419–26. https://doi.org/10.1016/j.jinorgbio.2008.12.007.

van Lettow M, West CE, van der Meer JWM, et al. Low plasma selenium concentrations, high plasma human immunodeficiency virus load and high interleukin-6 concentrations are risk factors associated with anemia in adults presenting with pulmonary tuberculosis in Zomba district, Malawi. Eur J Clin Nutr. 2005;59:526–32. https://doi.org/10.1038/sj.ejcn.1602116.

Li YF, Chen C, Li B, et al. Simultaneous speciation of selenium and mercury in human urine samples from long-term mercury-exposed populations with supplementation of selenium-enriched yeast by HPLC-ICP-MS. J Anal At Spectrom. 2007;22:925. https://doi.org/10.1039/b703310a.

Li JL, Gao R, Li S, et al. Testicular toxicity induced by dietary cadmium in cocks and ameliorative effect by selenium. Biometals. 2010;23:695–705. https://doi.org/10.1007/s10534-010-9334-0.

Li YF, Dong Z, Chen C, et al. Organic selenium supplementation increases mercury excretion and decreases oxidative damage in long-term mercury-exposed residents from Wanshan, China. Environ Sci Technol. 2012;46:11313–8. https://doi.org/10.1021/es302241v.

Li P, Li Y, Feng X. Mercury and selenium interactions in human blood in the Wanshan mercury mining area, China. Sci Total Environ. 2016;573:376–81. https://doi.org/10.1016/j.scitotenv.2016.08.098.

Luque-Garcia JL, Cabezas-Sanchez P, Anunciação DS, Camara C. Analytical and bioanalytical approaches to unravel the selenium–mercury antagonism: a review. Anal Chim Acta. 2013;801:1–13. https://doi.org/10.1016/j.aca.2013.08.043.

Lyons GH, Stangoulis JCR, Graham RD. Exploiting micronutrient interaction to optimize biofortification programs: the case for inclusion of selenium and iodine in the HarvestPlus program. Nutr Rev. 2004;62:247–52.

Mahata J, Argos M, Verret W, et al. Effect of selenium and vitamin E supplementation on plasma protein carbonyl levels in patients with arsenic-related skin lesions. Nutr Cancer. 2007;60:55–60. https://doi.org/10.1080/01635580701761282.

Manley SA, George GN, Pickering IJ, et al. The seleno bis (*S*-glutathionyl) arsinium ion is assembled in erythrocyte lysate. Chem Res Toxicol. 2006;19:601–7. https://doi.org/10.1021/tx0503505.

Maret W. The function of zinc metallothionein: a link between cellular zinc and redox state. J Nutr. 2000;130:1455S–8S.

Maret W. Cellular zinc and redox states converge in the metallothionein/thionein pair. J Nutr. 2003;133:1460S–2S.

Mehdi Y, Hornick J-L, Istasse L, Dufrasne I. Selenium in the environment, metabolism and involvement in body functions. Molecules. 2013;18:3292–311. https://doi.org/10.3390/molecules18033292.

Meltzer HM, Maage A, Ydersbond TA, et al. Fish arsenic may influence human blood arsenic, selenium, and T4:T3 ratio. Biol Trace Elem Res. 2002;90:83–98. https://doi.org/10.1385/BTER:90:1-3:83.

Messaoudi I, El Heni J, Hammouda F, et al. Protective effects of selenium, zinc, or their combination on cadmium-induced oxidative stress in rat kidney. Biol Trace Elem Res. 2009;130:152–61. https://doi.org/10.1007/s12011-009-8324-y.

Messaoudi I, Banni M, Saïd L, et al. Involvement of selenoprotein P and GPx4 gene expression in cadmium-induced testicular pathophysiology in rat. Chem Biol Interact. 2010a;188:94–101. https://doi.org/10.1016/j.cbi.2010.07.012.

Messaoudi I, Hammouda F, El Heni J, et al. Reversal of cadmium-induced oxidative stress in rat erythrocytes by selenium, zinc or their combination. Exp Toxicol Pathol. 2010b;62:281–8. https://doi.org/10.1016/j.etp.2009.04.004.

Messarah M, Klibet F, Boumendjel A, et al. Hepatoprotective role and antioxidant capacity of selenium on arsenic-induced liver injury in rats. Exp Toxicol Pathol. 2012;64:167–74. https://doi.org/10.1016/j.etp.2010.08.002.

Miao K, Zhang L, Yang S, et al. Intervention of selenium on apoptosis and Fas/FasL expressions in the liver of fluoride-exposed rats. Environ Toxicol Pharmacol. 2013;36:913–20. https://doi.org/10.1016/j.etap.2013.08.003.

Mocchegiani E, Costarelli L, Giacconi R, et al. Micronutrient–gene interactions related to inflammatory/immune response and antioxidant activity in ageing and inflammation. A systematic review. Mech Ageing Dev. 2014;136–137:29–49. https://doi.org/10.1016/j.mad.2013.12.007.

Mostert V, Hill KE, Burk RF. Loss of activity of the selenoenzyme thioredoxin reductase causes induction of hepatic heme oxygenase-1. FEBS Lett. 2003;541:85–8.

Mostert V, Nakayama A, Austin LM, et al. Serum iron increases with acute inductionof hepatic heme oxygenase-1 in mice. Drug Metab Rev. 2007;39:619–26. https://doi.org/10.1080/03602530701468342.

Mousa SA, O'Connor L, Rossman TG, Block E. Pro-angiogenesis action of arsenic and its reversal by selenium-derived compounds. Carcinogenesis. 2006;28:962–7. https://doi.org/10.1093/carcin/bgl229.

Ngo DB, Dikassa L, Okitolonda W, et al. Selenium status in pregnant women of a rural population (Zaire) in relationship to iodine deficiency. Trop Med Int Health. 1997;2:572–81.

Nhien NV, Khan NC, Yabutani T, et al. Relationship of low serum selenium to anemia among primary school children living in rural Vietnam. J Nutr Sci Vitaminol (Tokyo). 2008;54:454–9.

Olivieri O, Girelli D, Stanzial AM, et al. Selenium, zinc, and thyroid hormones in healthy subjects: low T3/T4 ratio in the elderly is related to impaired selenium status. Biol Trace Elem Res. 1996;51:31–41. https://doi.org/10.1007/BF02790145.

Othman AI, El Missiry MA. Role of selenium against lead toxicity in male rats. J Biochem Mol Toxicol. 1998;12:345–9.

Perrone L, Di Palma L, Di Toro R, et al. Interaction of trace elements in a longitudinal study of human milk from full-term and preterm mothers. Biol Trace Elem Res. 1994;41:321–30.

Pilsner JR, Hall MN, Liu X, et al. Associations of plasma selenium with arsenic and genomic methylation of leukocyte DNA in Bangladesh. Environ Health Perspect. 2010;119:113–8. https://doi.org/10.1289/ehp.1001937.

Qian W, Miao K, Li T, Zhang Z. Effect of selenium on fluoride-induced changes in synaptic plasticity in rat hippocampus. Biol Trace Elem Res. 2013;155:253–60. https://doi.org/10.1007/s12011-013-9773-x.

Raie RM. Regional variation in As, Cu, Hg, and Se and interaction between them. Ecotoxicol Environ Saf. 1996;35:248–52. https://doi.org/10.1006/eesa.1996.0107.

Rayman MP. Food-chain selenium and human health: emphasis on intake. Br J Nutr. 2008;100:254–68. https://doi.org/10.1017/S0007114508939830.

Ren Y, Kitahara CM, Berrington de Gonzalez A, et al. Lack of association between fingernail selenium and thyroid cancer risk: a case-control study in French Polynesia. Asian Pac J Cancer Prev. 2014;15:5187–94.

Roy G, Mugesh G. Selenium analogues of antithyroid drugs – recent developments. Chem Biodivers. 2008;5:414–39. https://doi.org/10.1002/cbdv.200890042.

Saïd L, Banni M, Kerkeni A, et al. Influence of combined treatment with zinc and selenium on cadmium induced testicular pathophysiology in rat. Food Chem Toxicol. 2010;48:2759–65. https://doi.org/10.1016/j.fct.2010.07.003.

Saied NM, Hamza AA. Selenium ameliorates isotretinoin-induced liver injury and dyslipidemia via antioxidant effect in rats. Toxicol Mech Methods. 2014;24:433–7. https://doi.org/10.3109/15376516.2014.937514.

Sasakura C, Suzuki KT. Biological interaction between transition metals (Ag, Cd and Hg), selenide/sulfide and selenoprotein P. J Inorg Biochem. 1998;71:159–62.

Schomburg L, Köhrle J. On the importance of selenium and iodine metabolism for thyroid hormone biosynthesis and human health. Mol Nutr Food Res. 2008;52:1235–46. https://doi.org/10.1002/mnfr.200700465.

Schöpfer J, Drasch G, Schrauzer GN. Selenium and cadmium levels and ratios in prostates, livers, and kidneys of nonsmokers and smokers. Biol Trace Elem Res. 2010;134:180–7. https://doi.org/10.1007/s12011-010-8636-y.

Schrauzer GN. Selenium and selenium-antagonistic elements in nutritional cancer prevention. Crit Rev Biotechnol. 2009;29:10–7. https://doi.org/10.1080/07388550802658048.

Schwalfenberg GK, Genuis SJ. Vitamin D, essential minerals, and toxic elements: exploring interactions between nutrients and toxicants in clinical medicine. Sci World J. 2015;2015:1–8. https://doi.org/10.1155/2015/318595.

Semba RD, Ferrucci L, Cappola AR, et al. Low serum selenium is associated with anemia among older women living in the community: the Women's health and aging studies I and II. Biol Trace Elem Res. 2006;112:97–108. https://doi.org/10.1385/BTER:112:2:97.

Semba RD, Ricks MO, Ferrucci L, et al. Low serum selenium is associated with anemia among older adults in the United States. Eur J Clin Nutr. 2009;63:93–9. https://doi.org/10.1038/sj.ejcn.1602889.

Serafín Muñoz AH, Wrobel K, Gutierrez Corona JF, Wrobel K. The protective effect of selenium inorganic forms against cadmium and silver toxicity in mycelia of Pleurotus ostreatus. Mycol Res. 2007;111:626–32. https://doi.org/10.1016/j.mycres.2007.03.002.

Skowerski M, Jasik K, Konecki J. Effects of interaction between cadmium and selenium on heart metabolism in mice: the study of RNA, protein, ANP synthesis activities and ultrastructure in mouse heart. Med Sci Monit. 2000;6:258–65.

Skröder H, Hawkesworth S, Kippler M, et al. Kidney function and blood pressure in preschool-aged children exposed to cadmium and arsenic - potential alleviation by selenium. Environ Res. 2015;140:205–13. https://doi.org/10.1016/j.envres.2015.03.038.

Song X, Geng Z, Li C, et al. Transition metal ions and selenite modulate the methylation of arsenite by the recombinant human arsenic (+3 oxidation state) methyltransferase (hAS3MT). J Inorg Biochem. 2010;104:541–50. https://doi.org/10.1016/j.jinorgbio.2010.01.005.

Steinbrenner H, Sies H. Protection against reactive oxygen species by selenoproteins. Biochim Biophys Acta. 2009;1790:1478–85. https://doi.org/10.1016/j.bbagen.2009.02.014.

Sun HJ, Rathinasabapathi B, Wu B, et al. Arsenic and selenium toxicity and their interactive effects in humans. Environ Int. 2014;69:148–58. https://doi.org/10.1016/j.envint.2014.04.019.

Talbot S, Nelson R, Self WT. Arsenic trioxide and auranofin inhibit selenoprotein synthesis: implications for chemotherapy for acute promyelocytic leukaemia. Br J Pharmacol. 2008;154:940–8. https://doi.org/10.1038/bjp.2008.161.

Telišman S, Jurasović J, Pizent A, Cvitković P. Blood pressure in relation to biomarkers of lead, cadmium, copper, zinc, and selenium in men without occupational exposure to metals. Environ Res. 2001;87:57–68. https://doi.org/10.1006/enrs.2001.4292.

Thilly CH, Vanderpas JB, Bebe N, et al. Iodine deficiency, other trace elements, and goitrogenic factors in the etiopathogeny of iodine deficiency disorders (IDD). Biol Trace Elem Res. 1992;32:229–43.

Thompson HJ, Meeker LD, Becci PJ. Effect of combined selenium and retinyl acetate treatment on mammary carcinogenesis. Cancer Res. 1981;41:1413–6.

Thomson CD, Packer MA, Butler JA, et al. Urinary selenium and iodine during pregnancy and lactation. J Trace Elem Med Biol. 2001;14:210–7. https://doi.org/10.1016/S0946-672X(01)80004-3.

Valko M, Rhodes CJ, Moncol J, et al. Free radicals, metals and antioxidants in oxidative stress-induced cancer. Chem Biol Interact. 2006;160:1–40. https://doi.org/10.1016/j.cbi.2005.12.009.

Van Nhien N, Khan NC, Yabutani T, et al. Serum levels of trace elements and Iron-deficiency anemia in adult Vietnamese. Biol Trace Elem Res. 2006;111:1–10. https://doi.org/10.1385/BTER:111:1:1.

Van Nhien N, Khan NC, Ninh NX, et al. Micronutrient deficiencies and anemia among preschool children in rural Vietnam. Asia Pac J Clin Nutr. 2008;17:48–55.

Van Nhien N, Yabutani T, Khan NC, et al. Association of low serum selenium with anemia among adolescent girls living in rural Vietnam. Nutrition. 2009;25:6–10. https://doi.org/10.1016/j.nut.2008.06.032.

Verret WJ, Chen Y, Ahmed A, et al. A randomized, double-blind placebo-controlled trial evaluating the effects of vitamin E and selenium on arsenic-induced skin lesions in Bangladesh. J Occup Environ Med. 2005;47:1026–35.

Vinceti M, Maraldi T, Bergomi M, Malagoli C. Risk of chronic low-dose selenium overexposure in humans: insights from epidemiology and biochemistry. Rev Environ Health. 2009;24:231–48.

Wadhwa SK, Kazi TG, Afridi HI, et al. Interaction between carcinogenic and anti-carcinogenic trace elements in the scalp hair samples of different types of Pakistani female cancer patients. Clin Chim Acta. 2015;439:178–84. https://doi.org/10.1016/j.cca.2014.10.007.

Walton FS, Waters SB, Jolley SL, et al. Selenium compounds modulate the activity of recombinant rat As[III]-methyltransferase and the methylation of arsenite by rat and human hepatocytes. Chem Res Toxicol. 2003;16:261–5. https://doi.org/10.1021/tx025649r.

Wang W, Yang L, Hou S, et al. Prevention of endemic arsenism with selenium. Curr Sci. 2001;81:1215–8.

Wang X, Ning Y, Yang L, et al. Zinc: the other suspected environmental factor in Kashin-Beck disease in addition to selenium. Biol Trace Elem Res. 2017;179:178–84. https://doi.org/10.1007/s12011-017-0964-8.

Watanabe C, Yoshida K, Kasanuma Y, et al. In UteroMethylmercury Exposure Differentially Affects the Activities of Selenoenzymes in the Fetal Mouse Brain. Environ Res. 1999;80:208–14. https://doi.org/10.1006/enrs.1998.3889.

Wei XL, He JR, Cen YL, et al. Modified effect of urinary cadmium on breast cancer risk by selenium. Clin Chim Acta. 2015;438:80–5. https://doi.org/10.1016/j.cca.2014.08.014.

Xie L, Wu X, Chen H, et al. A low level of dietary selenium has both beneficial and toxic effects and is protective against Cd-toxicity in the least killifish Heterandria formosa. Chemosphere. 2016;161:358–64. https://doi.org/10.1016/j.chemosphere.2016.07.035.

Xue W, Wang Z, Chen Q, et al. High selenium status in individuals exposed to arsenic through coal-burning in Shaanxi (PR of China) modulates antioxidant enzymes, heme oxygenase-1 and DNA damage. Clin Chim Acta. 2010;411:1312–8. https://doi.org/10.1016/j.cca.2010.05.018.

Yang L, Wang W, Hou S, et al. Effects of selenium supplementation on arsenism: an intervention trial in inner mongolia. Environ Geochem Health. 2002;24:359–74.

Yang DY, Chen YW, Gunn JM, Belzile N. Selenium and mercury in organisms: interactions and mechanisms. Environ Rev. 2008;16:71–92. https://doi.org/10.1139/A08-001.

Yao Y, Pei F, Kang P. Selenium, iodine, and the relation with Kashin-Beck disease. Nutrition. 2011;27:1095–100. https://doi.org/10.1016/j.nut.2011.03.002.

Yu FF, Zhang YX, Zhang LH, et al. Identified molecular mechanism of interaction between environmental risk factors and differential expression genes in cartilage of Kashin–Beck disease. Medicine (Baltimore). 2016;95:e5669. https://doi.org/10.1097/MD.0000000000005669.

Zagrodzki P, Szmigiel H, Ratajczak R, et al. The role of selenium in iodine metabolism in children with goiter. Environ Health Perspect. 2000;108:67–71.

Zeng H, Uthus EO, Combs GF Jr. Mechanistic aspects of the interaction between selenium and arsenic. J Inorg Biochem. 2005;99:1269–74. https://doi.org/10.1016/j.jinorgbio.2005.03.006.

Zheng X, Sun Y, Ke L, et al. Molecular mechanism of brain impairment caused by drinking-acquired fluorosis and selenium intervention. Environ Toxicol Pharmacol. 2016;43:134–9. https://doi.org/10.1016/j.etap.2016.02.017.

Zimmerman MT, Bayse CA, Ramoutar RR, Brumaghim JL. Sulfur and selenium antioxidants: challenging radical scavenging mechanisms and developing structure–activity relationships based on metal binding. J Inorg Biochem. 2015;145:30–40. https://doi.org/10.1016/j.jinorgbio.2014.12.020.

Zimmermann MB, Köhrle J. The impact of Iron and selenium deficiencies on iodine and thyroid metabolism: biochemistry and relevance to public health. Thyroid. 2002;12:867–78. https://doi.org/10.1089/105072502761016494.

Zwolak I, Zaporowska H. Selenium interactions and toxicity: a review: selenium interactions and toxicity. Cell Biol Toxicol. 2012;28:31–46. https://doi.org/10.1007/s10565-011-9203-9.

Part VIII
Selenium Analytics, Speciation and Biomonitoring

Chapter 23
Biomarkers of Se Status

Kostja Renko

Abstract Even if there is no doubt about the essential role of Se within the mammalian organism and beyond, it is a matter of careful evaluation which indicator within the respective (experimental) model or system can be chosen to gradually define the status between deficiency, sufficiency and toxicity. Respective biomarkers are discussed for human beings, animal models and cell culture with a strong focus on significance and Se dependence to provide practical guidance.

Advantage can be taken from considering more than one biomarker, as the complex "Se status" consists of different pools (e.g. unbound vs. protein bound) with individual kinetics and accessibility for the organism itself.

Keywords Human organism · Animal models · Cell culture · Selenium-dependence · Selenium intake

Introduction

Selenium (Se) status is an artificial concept, as different forms of Se are taken up by the daily nutrition, circulate in blood and are metabolised to specific intermediates in a tissue-specific way. Nevertheless, without a clear definition of Se status, most medical practitioners, scientists and researchers have a more or less clear idea about the meaning of Se status and its importance. As Se is an essential trace element, an insufficient intake leads to a low Se status associated with certain health risks. Moreover, certain diseases adversely affect Se absorption and usage and cause a dysregulated Se metabolism (Forceville et al. 1998). On the other hand, as a biologically active trace element, a surplus intake of Se may cause adverse health effects and signs of selenosis (Nogueira and Rocha 2011). It is therefore of utmost importance to relate these obvious health issues of the insufficient or surplus intake with

K. Renko (✉)
Institut für Experimentelle Endokrinologie, Charité—Universitätsmedizin Berlin,
Berlin, Germany
e-mail: Kostja.Renko@charite.de

© Springer International Publishing AG, part of Springer Nature 2018　　　　　451
B. Michalke (ed.), *Selenium*, Molecular and Integrative Toxicology,
https://doi.org/10.1007/978-3-319-95390-8_23

a measurable parameter that can be quantified precisely and used as a surrogate biomarker of Se status.

This requirement defines a number of prerequisites that need to be met by such a potential biomarker of Se status: (1) the parameter needs to respond to Se intake, (2) the parameter should be accessible to analytical and/or clinical chemistry, (3) the parameter should be associated with diseases that are related to Se supply and (4) the biomarker should be more or less specific in reflecting Se intake and turnover and be largely independent from interfering parameters.

The value of a diagnostic biomarker also depends on the nature of the read-out, which can be of absolute or relative character. Indeed, the majority of potential molecular markers are frequently quantified via immunoblotting or semiquantitative qPCR, which is useful in experimental settings and model systems when directly comparing samples within one experiment, but of limited value to define reference values or to compare two different study groups from separate experimental settings. As an individual read-out in personalised medicine, they are of very little value.

In the following chapters, these requirements will be discussed in view of the current knowledge on Se metabolism and Se intake, different options will be presented and their advantages and disadvantages will be discussed.

Responsiveness to Se Intake

Nutrition is providing Se in different chemical forms, i.e. as the amino acids selenomethionine and selenocysteine, as derivatives of these amino acids, especially from plant sources, and as inorganic selenite or selenate, especially from liquids, plants with high hydration grade, or dietary supplements. Other intake routes except from nutrition or supplementation are not known, which allows a monitoring and balancing of the individual dietary pattern over a certain period of time to allow for assessing the net Se intake. However, the Se content of a given food item is usually not known and moreover varies drastically depending on plant or animal species, area of growth and geographical origin and other unpredictable parameters (Silva Junior et al. 2017; Wiesner-Reinhold et al. 2017). This lack of knowledge makes it nearly impossible to calculate individual daily Se intake just from the pattern of nutritional supply, as evaluated by nutrition frequency questionnaires. However, the highest standard of nutritional monitoring constitutes in preparing double-portion sizes and storing an identical portion of the meals and drinks consumed for later analysis (de Brätter et al. 1995). This method is suitable for very precise albeit also very expensive and laborious clinical studies. The stored mirror portions may then be analysed for Se content after closing the study period for a specific assessment of Se supply and intake over a certain time period. However, on the search for a biomarker, this information would be very useful to mirror Se intake, but it is of little value to determine Se turnover and metabolism, which may differ to some or a considerable extent between separate individuals (Jäger et al. 2016). To conclude, a very precise monitoring of dietary Se intake is possible, albeit at high costs, only in controlled studies or experimental settings, and providing only limited physiological information.

Most proposed biomarkers for Se status reflect, to some degree, intake of all different Se forms derived by the diet. Indeed the degree of correlation not only depends on the total amount of Se, but also on the ingested Se forms and their route of metabolism and/or excretion.

While selenomethionine (SeMet) supplementation can elevate blood Se even in subjects with high Se dietary intake, this is not the case for the inorganic forms.

The amino acid SeMet is of specific interest as it can be included into regular protein biosynthesis in parallel to methionine (Met); therefore it becomes also inserted into circulating albumin and other proteins. As this is an unregulated process without specific limitations regarding the translational incorporation of SeMet, it can elevate total Se concentrations in blood and tissues in an almost linear way, in direct relation to the amount of SeMet taken up. In contrast, inorganic forms of Se are metabolised by the tissues to form functional selenoproteins, e.g. selenoprotein P (SELENOP) as a circulating Se transporter from liver to the other organs. When the upper limits of selenoprotein biosynthesis are reached, a further increase in inorganic Se intake is not anymore adequately reflected by increasing selenoprotein biosynthesis and total Se levels in blood. This difference between the metabolism of SeMet and selenite is of relevance for their potential toxicity during high dietary intakes. It is thus conceivable that a single biomarker might not be fully sufficient to describe the physiological Se status and metabolism.

Availability and Suitability for Analytical Quantification

A useful biomarker needs to be accessible from a given subject in sufficient quantities, frequencies and needs to be detectable by a quantitative technique with a certain degree of precision. Another aspect of a potential biomarker would be the requirement to compare its quantity between experiments, laboratories and published studies. Indeed, intra- and inter-laboratory variations are an unresolved issue for numerous parameters in clinical routine, leading to uncertainties and variations in clinical diagnoses across different countries and even between neighbouring laboratories and hospitals. For these reasons, absolute quantities expressed in SI units are necessary, along with standardised reference materials for allowing cross-lab comparisons. Another important restriction for a routine biomarker of Se status for clinical analyses is given by the limited availability of biosamples, i.e. the matrices that are accessible for analysis. In the clinics, this restriction leads to the few biomaterials (blood, urine, tears, sweat, hair, nail clippings) as the only potential matrices that are available, as tissue samples cannot routinely be obtained (Fig. 23.1).

Biomarkers from tissues or intracellular metabolites and proteins are usually not available from human subjects, severely limiting the choice of potential biomarkers in respective studies. The choices therefore are limited to bodily fluids, hair or nail

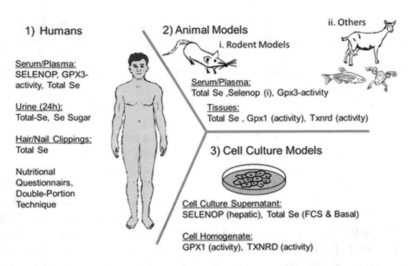

Fig. 23.1 Biomarkers enabling quantitative analyses of Se status. This overview presents potential biomarkers of Se status in human studies (1), animal models (2) and cell culture experiments (3). Only a subset of Se-dependent parameters are suitable for absolute quantification. Data from relative read-outs, e.g. Western blot analyses, which are available for almost each selenoprotein in humans and rodents, can hardly be compared across different studies when not conducted within the same lab or experimental run. Restricted material access is a severe limitation for clinical analyses, whereas studies with model systems or cells in culture can take advantage of the unlimited availability of the biological material and are not restricted to secreted or circulating parameters. The selection presented here represents a personal preference of the author and does not claim completeness

clippings. Hair and nail bear the disadvantage of being exposed to the daily environment and being manipulated for reasons of stability, hygiene or cosmetics. This is especially problematic for hair, as many shampoos used for daily washing and care, artificial colours or dressing sprays or gels are of unknown composition and potential sources of contamination. Similarly, hand and foot nail clippings are of unknown preanalytical history and subject to the same problematic treatments, especially aesthetic manipulations, as mentioned above for hair. Nevertheless, they can be useful tools for a longitudinal analysis of changing Se uptake over time, if due care is taken during study design, sample acquisition, storage and workup (Bermejo Barrera et al. 2000; Harrison et al. 1995; Filippini et al. 2017).

The analytical researcher is therefore mainly left with bodily fluids. Saliva, sweat or tear drops are a potential matrix, of which only tear drops seem to mirror other body compartments and provide a certain degree of constant composition, whereas the compositions of saliva and sweat vary dynamically according to the time of day, external stressors and other unpredictable parameters. Similarly, urine constitutes an amply available, easily collectable and non-invasive matrix. Urine composition is dynamically adapted to the actual metabolism of the organism and varies with time of day, disease and kidney function. A single-spot urine sample does therefore only provide limited information on the Se status of a given subject. Similar to the analytical procedures for iodine status, a 24-h collected urine average sample appears as a more reliable read-out for Se status and nicely mirrors the metabolism of Se at least over a certain period of time (Rodríguez et al. 2009; Thomson et al. 1996; Longnecker et al. 1996).

Alternatively, cerebrospinal fluid (CSF) becomes available under certain medical indications, when the diagnosis of neurological diseases is carried out or when injuries or potential infections of the central nervous system are analysed (Vinceti et al. 2017). During the acquisition of CSF, an invasive procedure called lumbar puncture is performed, which constitutes a potential source of contamination of the usually clear fluid with blood, thereby potentially compromising a reliable trace element analysis (Aasebø et al. 2014).

From all these considerations mentioned above, blood, serum or plasma remain the preferred matrices for Se determination both in research and in the clinics. Blood itself is a heterogeneous matrix consisting of both cells and fluid. The composition of cells again is not uniform, and metabolically active cells bearing a nucleus and nucleus-free erythrocytes are the major cell types present, albeit in dynamically controlled concentrations depending on health state, oxygen demand, nutritional status and other personal characteristics. Nevertheless, full blood is a clearly defined matrix, which can be easily obtained both in the form of small amounts by finger- or ear pricks, or in larger quantity by venous blood drawing. Full blood has the tendency to clot, if no clotting preservatives like heparin, citrate or EDTA are added, which generates a matrix of two major components that can be easily separated by centrifugation, i.e. the cell-rich fraction containing or not the clotted material. The supernatant is called serum if clotting has taken place and the proteins involved in clotting (mainly fibrinogen) are no longer present in the supernating serum, or it is called plasma if clotting was inhibited. Both serum and plasma are typical matrices used in the clinics for assessment of Se status. The Se concentrations of serum and plasma preparations differ marginally when drawn from a given subject (Kasperek et al. 1981). When total Se concentrations are to be determined, both matrices are relatively stable and Se loss by volatilisation or other mechanisms is usually not observed, as long as the sample is sterile. Microbial or fungal contaminations, introduced during the blood drawing or separation processes, may strongly affect the composition of the sample and potentially generate volatile selenocompounds. It is therefore advantageous to store serum or plasma samples in a frozen state, if not analysed within a short time frame.

From a technical point of view, total Se can be measured by analytical chemistry methods, variants of atomic absorption spectrometry (hydride generation-AAS or electrothermal-AAS) or spectrofluorimetry. All the methods require a specific pre-treatment of the samples, including oxidative digestion. As an alternative, total X-ray fluorescence spectrometry (TXRF) has emerged as a convenient technology. The method is relatively robust against matrix effects, enabling a straightforward and uncomplicated pre-analytical preparation of the samples. Furthermore, only minute amounts of tissue or fluids are needed (e.g. ~5 μL of serum or ~5 mg of solid tissue) without compromising quantification quality (Fig. 23.2).

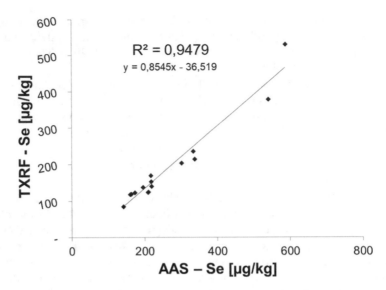

Fig. 23.2 Correlation between GF-AAS and TXRF from liver samples. Tissue samples were taken from sheep liver for GF-AAS (~400 mg) and TXRF (~10 mg, comparable amount as received from liver biopsy), digested and measured in parallel. Both methods show a high degree of correlation, supporting the notion that both techniques are suitable for total Se analysis (Renko and Human-Ziehank, unpublished)

Association with Diseases that Are Related to Se Supply

A useful biomarker in medical research or routine clinical use should show some association with the health status of the subject under investigation (Strimbu and Tavel 2010). This requirement may change the preference of the matrix to be analysed with respect to availability, relevance and nature of the selenocompounds found within the given matrix. Health risk assessment and nutritional status in epidemiological research should ideally rely on a marker that is reflecting a long-term Se supply from an easily available matrix. Selenium intake analyses from nutritional food frequency questionnaires or other more modern or more accurate ways of monitoring the dietary patterns (mobile phone pictures of actual meals and portion sizes, preparing of a mirror portion of meal for analytical purposes, consumption of provided food items with known composition) are a suitable choice if conducted according to high standards (Rusin et al. 2013). However, these analyses provide data on Se intake only. For drawing a balance, the data need to be set in relation to Se excretion via the different routes (urine, faeces, sweat, breath), which appears almost impossible to conduct.

Again, one is left with the quest for a more reliable and accessible biomarker reflecting both intake and loss, thereby reporting on the sufficiency of Se supply for its biological role in different pathways. As discussed above, analysing a 24-h urine sample would be a suitable way if available. However, collection and storage of a 24-h urine sample is tedious and cumbersome and needs to be executed with the due care. Alternatively, nail clippings constitute a non-invasive matrix and reflecting Se availability for biosynthetic purposes over a longer period of time (Longnecker et al. 1996). The only major drawbacks are given by the potential pre-analytical history of the nails, aesthetic manipulations and degree of moisturisation, as a nail sample taken directly after having a shower or bath differs from a dry nail in water content, thereby affecting its density and relation of organic to water mass (Noisel et al. 2010). In addition, the pre-analytical sample workup is more challenging for an inhomogeneous and solid sample than for a liquid and rather uniform matrix.

In the clinics, again serum or plasma samples are most widespread and readily available matrices for analytical purposes. From these two, both total Se concentrations and certain informative selenocompounds can be analysed. Selenium is needed for the biosynthesis of selenoproteins. Two of the 25 selenoprotein genes encode actively secreted, therefore circulating, proteins, i.e. glutathione peroxidase-3 (GPX3) and SELENOP. The former is routinely determined by measuring its activity in coupled optical test procedures (Flohé and Günzler 1984) whereas the latter is available for antibody-based detection measures such as a sandwich ELISA (Hollenbach et al. 2008; Hybsier et al. 2015). Both can also be analysed by more sophisticated speciating techniques relying on chromatographic fractionation and mass-specific detection, which are usually not available in a non-specialised lab environment (Cardoso et al. 2017; Michalke 2016; Vinceti et al. 2015). Comparing these two extracellular selenoproteins, the former (GPX3) is mainly provided by the kidney to the circulation whereas the latter (SELENOP) in serum or plasma is mainly of hepatic origin as a liver-derived protein. Studies with transgenic mice have indicated that the renal Se supply depends on SELENOP, indicating that GPX3 depends on an intact liver, regular SELENOP supply and normal kidney function (Renko et al. 2008; Schomburg et al. 2003). Conversely, SELENOP depends on nutritional Se intake and regular liver function.

One of these two biomarkers may thus yield clinically more relevant insights than the other, depending on the disease symptoms and assumed diagnosis. For example, GPX3 expression becomes strongly dysregulated after treatment with the fungal nephrotoxin orellanine (Nilsson et al. 2008), in renal cell carcinoma (Liu et al. 2015) or ischemia-induced acute kidney injury (Basile et al. 2012). SELENOP on the other hand represents an acute-phase protein, regulated directly by increasing cytokines or hypoxia. Furthermore, hepatic selenoprotein biosynthesis appears to be shifted on the translational level in situations of systemic inflammatory response (SIRS) or sepsis (Forceville et al. 1998), (Renko et al. 2009; Stoedter et al. 2010).

Both markers will appear saturated at some point, when Se supply is sufficiently high. GPX activity reaches its saturated level earlier than SELENOP; therefore the dynamic range as a marker appears to be larger for the latter one (Xia et al. 2010).

Besides these two actively secreted proteins, certain selenoenzymes such as GPX1 and members of the thioredoxin reductase (TXNRD) family are available from circulating cells (Nève et al. 1988). However, these analyses have not found an application as widespread as the two extracellular selenoproteins. GPX activity is found in high quantities in circulation erythrocytes and platelets; therefore contamination in plasma and serum samples by incomplete separation from the cell fraction can result in high variations between different samples because of inconsistent handling issues.

Apart from the procedure of blood processing after sampling, other aspects of sample history need special attention. While SELENOP detection via immunoassay turns out to be robust against freeze-thaw cycles (Hybsier et al. 2015), enzymatic activity of GPX3 will suffer and significantly decrease depending on storage conditions, freezing and handling. Storage at temperatures below −40 °C and tracking of freeze-thaw cycles are mandatory when reliable readings are to be obtained.

Besides selenoproteins as potentially informative biomarkers, also non-protein selenocompounds can be detected in serum or plasma. Among the small selenocompounds, selenosugars have drawn increased attention in recent years as they seem to constitute a form of Se disposal by liver as an indication of Se availability and supply. Unfortunately, the two major Se-containing acetyl-glucosamine derivatives again need elaborate, expensive and very skilled analysis, as they are too small to be quantified by immune-based detection measures (Flouda et al. 2016). It is for this reason, that very few reports on the clinical and diagnostic relevance of these circulating selenocompounds are available. Two more small selenocompounds are characterised as potential indicators of surplus Se supply, i.e., clinical suspicion of selenosis. These are dimethyl-selenide and tri-methyl selenonium. The former is a volatile substance that may be exhaled whereas the latter is water soluble and may be excreted via sweat, urine or saliva (Jackson et al. 2013; Lunøe et al. 2010). Apart from the characteristic smell of exhaled dimethyl-selenide, no routine use of these biomarkers has been established in the clinics.

Collectively, total Se concentrations in serum or plasma, serum or plasma GPX3 activities or cellular GPX1 activity as well as circulating concentrations of the Se transporter SELENOP constitute the biomarkers currently in use for an assessment of Se status in epidemiological analyses with healthy subjects as well as in the clinics.

Specificity of the Biomarker for Se Metabolism and Dependence on Interfering Parameters

Ideally, a biomarker of Se status should be independent from other interfering parameters. On the other hand, it is exactly this dependence that renders a biomarker suitable for medical purposes, as a deviation from the expected level may provide insightful information on any underlying diseases or disease risks. From the biomarkers mentioned above, total Se concentrations in plasma or serum constitute a composite biomarker of small selenocompounds like Se-amino acids and their derivatives and the different selenosugars, other selenometabolites in smaller quantities and the two actively secreted selenoproteins GPX3 and SELENOP. Total Se concentrations are thus a suitable average estimation of Se status, providing little information on specific Se-dependent pathways, and potentially prone to interfering influences from acute Se-rich or Se-poor nutrition. From the pathways controlling Se turnover, it can be expected that a high fraction of SeMet present in circulating proteins indicates an ample supply with Se; otherwise this Se source would be recruited for the support of the biosynthesis of the essential selenoproteins. The specificity of total Se analysis from serum or blood is therefore limited in terms of underlying reasons of deviations, but of high importance for obtaining a general assessment. An analysis of typical selenocompounds associated with potential selenosis is of high specificity as it is known that, e.g., dimethyl selenide is only exhaled in response to toxic Se intake (Wilber 1980). However, there is little value of measuring this selenocompound in terms of general information that can be deduced from dimethyl selenide under regular Se supply.

One is again left with the two circulating selenoproteins GPX3 and SELENOP as relatively specific and informative biomarkers of Se status. This notion applies to regular conditions and healthy subjects. As circulating GPX3 is mainly derived from kidney and SELENOP from liver, diseases with hepatic or renal involvement will affect their biosynthesis. Under these conditions, their value as general biomarkers of Se status is compromised, but on the other hand these proteins become informative and valuable markers for kidney and liver diseases. Among the specific signals, controlling GPX3 and SELENOP biosynthesis are proinflammatory cytokines, explaining some compromised biosynthesis in infection (Renko et al. 2009), hypoxia (Becker et al. 2014), certain medications [aminoglycoside antibiotics (Martitz et al. 2016; Renko et al. 2017), statins (Moosmann and Behl 2004), metformin (Speckmann et al. 2009)] and potentially age, sex and genotype (Combs et al. 2012). As these interfering parameters often work in conjunction affecting the selenoprotein biosynthesis in a coordinated and potentially synergistic manner, further large clinical analyses are needed for obtaining a better and more refined picture on the advantages and disadvantages of the different Se status biomarkers in health and especially in certain diseases.

Summary

The suggested and evaluated biomarkers can be roughly divided into two fractions, the "unspecific" determination of total Se reflecting the current integral amount of Se content of the full organism versus the analysis of fractions permitting a more detailed insight into the various metabolic pathways.

Between all accessible selenoproteins reflecting Se status and saturation of the selenoproteome, GPX3 activity and SELENOP are the most promising biomarkers regarding the initially defined prerequisites:

1. Their concentration/functional read-out shows dependence and dynamic towards changing Se supply, with a higher dynamic for SELENOP.
2. They are accessible via blood samples, which are usually available in respective studies or in the clinical situation. GPX3 is determined via a coupled optical test

(photometric determination of NADPH oxidation), which makes it applicable to almost any mammalian species. SELENOP quantification depends on immuno-detection and is well established for human samples. Due to the high specificity of the antibodies used, a simple transfer to other species is difficult to achieve.

3. & 4. Indeed, both parameters are affected in diseases, which has already been observed for Se-related effects, e.g. cancer or sepsis, and both are regulated in many ways on the level of transcription and translation.

Since these biomarkers give a narrow and focussed view on the status of the selenoproteome, they allow conclusion on the risk for nutritional deficiency and on the degree of saturation of the selenoprotein biosynthesis machinery. Parallel

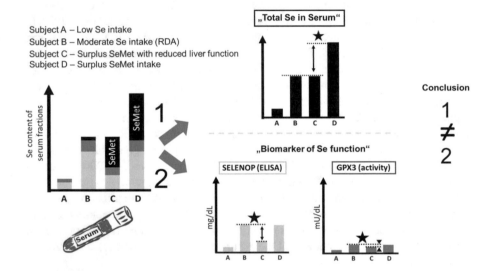

Fig. 23.3 The need for parallel determination of total Se versus functional biomarkers in serum samples. The total pool of all circulating Se forms can roughly be divided into two components. While the "active" form of Se as SeCys is integrated into functional selenoproteins, i.e. GPX3 and SELENOP, synthesised and secreted by kidney and liver, respectively, another fraction is derived by unspecific integration of SeMet into circulating proteins. The latter ones can be utilised by trans-selenation pathways in situations of suboptimal saturation of selenoprotein biosynthesis. While a daily Se intake of ~50 μg/day or ~70 μg/day already leads to a plateau of GPX3 or SELENOP levels, respectively, surplus SeMet supplementation will still raise the totals Se concentration by increase in the unspecifically integrated fraction. Determination of total Se from serum (1) defines the amount of Se that is absorbed and retained by the organism (subject A vs. B vs. D), though it fails to provide specific information about capacity and saturation of the functional Se fraction. Therefore, a parallel assessment of functional biomarkers is needed. While subject B is not distinguishable from subject C via total Se concentration measurements, the reduced capacity of SELENOP biosynthesis in the latter one gives a clear indication for suboptimal total capacity as a result of negatively affected liver function, e.g. secondary to cirrhosis or hepatitis. Because the kidney depends on circulating SELENOP as preferred Se source, GPX3 activity is also reduced. This conclusion can only be drawn by the combination of these three biomarkers, which demonstrates the benefit of this strategy. Diagrams represent stylised patterns for demonstration, inspired by Burk et al. (2001)

determination of total Se measurements from blood yields an insightful information on Se intake (see Fig. 23.3).

The focus of this chapter resulted from practical considerations. Indeed, also other biomarkers can be shortlisted from the literature, but with little impact for clinical approaches and human studies. Some of the suggested parameters might increase in relevance and importance in the future, largely by becoming better detected and quantified, and will then add new aspects to the diagnostic opportunities as the additional read-outs alone. One could imagine that specific activities of less well-characterised selenoenzymes or transcript levels from biomaterial such as isolated buccal cells, which are also easily accessible from patients, will find a more widespread application. Other parameters may gain in importance for the in vivo and in vitro experimental studies with model systems, in basic research, as discussed in the last paragraph. Whether a more detailed analysis and labeling of food items will enable a better Se intake assessment can hardly be predicted.

Biomarkers in Model Systems of Basic Research The former paragraphs are more dedicated to the available biomarkers useful for human subjects in clinical trials or observational studies. The experimental researcher has typically a broader access to biomaterials that can be used for biomarker analysis. In Se research, most of the experimental work is conducted in transgenic or nutritional animal models and cell culture.

Hence availability and type of accessible materials for analysis are fundamentally different and the choice for a Se-dependent biomarker in these models is relying on other limitations. In a mouse experiment with fatal endpoints, all animal tissues are available for analysis. Also here, blood-derived matrices (serum or plasma) are a well-defined and homogeneous starting material for total Se determination. Also Gpx3 and Selenop concentrations can be detected from these sample species. Since Gpx3 activity measurement relies on the same principle in mouse and men, this is a well-established parameter regarding protocols. Selenop quantification on the other hand relies on the availability of specific antibodies and ELISA kits. While for human serum samples the published and commercially available systems have reached a high level of quality needed for clinical application (Hybsier et al. 2015), this is unfortunately not the case for mouse-specific immunodetection kits, yet. As already discussed, liver turns out to be a central authority in Se metabolisation and distribution (Renko et al. 2008). Other organs more or less depend on Selenop as a humoral Se carrier protein; therefore individual Se status of different organs can contribute to a more detailed picture on "central" and "peripheral" Se availability.

Within tissues, Gpx activities are a reliable parameter, together with total Se concentration. Furthermore, Txnrd and, in some tissues, absolute iodothyronine deiodinase (Dio) type 1 activities can be accessed with moderate effort. Due to plasticity of response under changing conditions of Se supply, Gpx is the most promising read-out regarding amplitude and time course of responsiveness, compared to the latter activities. Besides enzymatic activities, various antibodies are available for almost all selenoproteins, which allows relative quantification via

Western blot analysis as a suitable read-out, but this method is not qualified for absolute measurement and quantification. Therefore, also relative transcript concentrations of selenoproteins, which are to some degree regulated by the Se supply (Reszka et al. 2012; Sunde and Raines 2011), e.g. via the nonsense-mediated decay (NMD) mechanism, are possible read-outs, but not preferable biomarkers.

For other animal models, e.g. zebrafish, very little literature is available for a reliable assessment of accessible biomarkers. Here, a determination of total Se from blood species or organs is probably the most comprehensive and defined approach to get data in a comparable manner. Furthermore, enzymatic activities (Gpx, Txnrd, Dio) can be assessed from respective tissues to get a read-out for selenoprotein function and saturation. In livestock industry and veterinary medicine, including large animals (e.g. cattle, pig, sheep), Gpx activity and total Se in blood are the most reliable and best documented parameters (Humann-Ziehank 2016).

In cell culture, the available biomarkers are very much depending upon cell type and culture conditions. For example the frequently used hepatoma cell line HepG2 takes up various forms of Se and is able to produce a high yield of SELENOP, which is, in large quantities, secreted into the medium over time (Hoefig et al. 2011).

Almost all cell lines (this statement limited to lines characterised by the authors' group so far) do express GPX isoenzymes and can be tested by the respective enzymatic activity. As this read-out has a high degree of dynamics in response to changing Se conditions, it is a good starting point to determine Se status of the cultured cells. It has to be taken into account that foetal calf serum (FCS) already contributes Se to the culture medium in poorly defined amounts. Usually, addition of 10% FCS will raise the Se concentration in the media into the nanomolar range, which is usually sufficient to contribute significantly to the intracellular GPX activity. Therefore, the full dynamic of a given cell system requires Se-deficient culture conditions without FCS to define the basal situation.

Determination of total Se within the cells would be the most robust read-out, but its accessibility is technically limited due to the low intracellular concentrations under physiological conditions.

In some cases, a Se-sensitive reporter system might be a helpful tool to monitor intracellular Se status by using, e.g. luciferase or green fluorescent protein as quantitative surrogate marker gene. There are several variants of such systems (Fig. 23.4), all of them following the same paradigm by coupling reporter gene synthesis with an Se-sensitive in-frame Opal codon and a 5′-UTR SECIS element (Martitz et al. 2016; Gupta and Copeland 2007; Kollmus et al. 1996). As a simple approach, an in-frame codon of the reporter is mutated to a TGA codon; thereby a successful recoding of selenocysteine (SeCys) will lead to synthesis of the fully functional reporter protein. In case of termination due to lack of available SeCys-tRNA or impaired insertion machinery, a truncated inactive fragment will appear. In a more complex version of the system, two separate reporters are coupled via a linker sequence containing the TGA codon. Successful recoding leads to a bifunctional reporter-fusion protein, while termination produces a fragment with reporter A activity alone. Using this system, a ratio can be calculated and reporter A activity

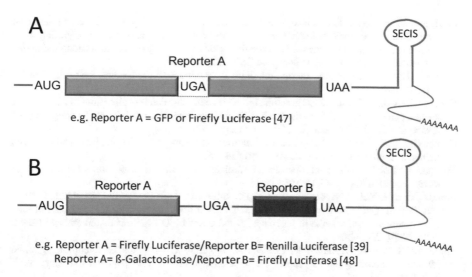

A

Reporter A

—AUG [| UGA | | UAA] —

e.g. Reporter A = GFP or Firefly Luciferase [47]

SECIS

AAAAAAA

B

Reporter A   Reporter B

—AUG [|]—UGA—[| UAA] —

e.g. Reporter A = Firefly Luciferase/Reporter B= Renilla Luciferase [39]
Reporter A= ß-Galactosidase/Reporter B= Firefly Luciferase [48]

SECIS

AAAAAAA

Fig. 23.4 Variants of eukaryotic Se-sensitive reporter systems. As an helpful tool and surrogate marker for endogenous biomarkers in cell culture experiments, Se-sensitive reporter systems are available with the option of transient or stable transfection into the cell of choice. In these constructs, expression of a given reporter gene is coupled to the efficiency of co-translational SeCys insertion by the introduction of an in-frame Opal codon and a respective SECIS sequence in the 5'-UTR

can serve as reference signal for normalisation of cell number, transfection efficiency and general translation.

Sensitivity depends on the read-out itself, but also on the combination of Opal codon context and origin of the SECIS element. Some of these systems are combined with eukaryotic selection markers and can therefore be used to produce stable reporter cell lines. As these systems usually use constitutive and artificial promotor elements, a potential interference with physiological regulations on the transcript level can be avoided to a certain degree.

References

Aasebø E, Opsahl JA, Bjørlykke Y, Myhr K-M, Kroksveen AC, Berven FS. Effects of blood contamination and the rostro-caudal gradient on the human cerebrospinal fluid proteome. PLoS One. 2014;9(3):e90429.

Basile DP, Leonard EC, Beal AG, Schleuter D, Friedrich J. Persistent oxidative stress following renal ischemia-reperfusion injury increases ANG II hemodynamic and fibrotic activity. Am J Physiol Renal Physiol. 2012;302(11):F1494–502.

Becker N-P, et al. Hypoxia reduces and redirects selenoprotein biosynthesis. Metallomics. 2014;6(5):1079.

Bermejo Barrera P, Lorenzo Alonso MJ, Bermejo Barrera A, Cocho de Juan JA, Fraga Bermúdez JM. Selenium determination in mother and child's hair by electrothermal atomic absorption spectrometry. Forensic Sci Int. 2000;107(1):149–56.

de Brätter VEN, Brätter P, Reinicke A, Schulze G, Alvarez WOL, Alvarez N. Determination of mineral and trace elements in total diet by inductively coupled plasma atomic emission spectrometry: comparison of microwave-based digestion and pressurized ashing systems using different acid mixtures. J Anal At Spectrom. 1995;10(7):487–91.

Burk RF, Hill KE, Motley AK. Plasma selenium in specific and non-specific forms. Biofactors. 2001;14(1–4):107–14.

Cardoso BR, et al. Selenium levels in serum, red blood cells, and cerebrospinal fluid of Alzheimer's disease patients: a report from the Australian imaging, biomarker & lifestyle flagship study of ageing (AIBL). J Alzheimers Dis. 2017;57(1):183–93.

Combs GF, et al. Differential responses to selenomethionine supplementation by sex and genotype in healthy adults. Br J Nutr. 2012;107(10):1514–25.

Filippini T, et al. Toenail selenium as an indicator of environmental exposure: a cross-sectional study. Mol Med Rep. 2017;15(5):3405–12.

Flohé L, Günzler WA. Assays of glutathione peroxidase. Methods Enzymol. 1984;105:114–20.

Flouda K, et al. Quantification of low molecular weight selenium metabolites in human plasma after treatment with selenite in pharmacological doses by LC-ICP-MS. Anal Bioanal Chem. 2016;408(9):2293–301.

Forceville X, Vitoux D, Gauzit R, Combes A, Lahilaire P, Chappuis P. Selenium, systemic immune response syndrome, sepsis, and outcome in critically ill patients. Crit Care Med. 1998;26(9):1536–44.

Gupta M, Copeland PR. Functional analysis of the interplay between translation termination, selenocysteine codon context, and selenocysteine insertion sequence-binding protein 2. J Biol Chem. 2007;282(51):36797–807.

Harrison I, Littlejohn D, Fell GS. Determination of selenium in human hair and nail by electrothermal atomic absorption spectrometry. J Anal At Spectrom. 1995;10(3):215–9.

Hoefig CS, Renko K, Köhrle J, Birringer M, Schomburg L. Comparison of different selenocompounds with respect to nutritional value vs. toxicity using liver cells in culture. J Nutr Biochem. 2011;22(10):945–55.

Hollenbach B, et al. New assay for the measurement of selenoprotein P as a sepsis biomarker from serum. J Trace Elem Med Biol. 2008;22(1):24–32.

Humann-Ziehank E. Selenium, copper and iron in veterinary medicine-from clinical implications to scientific models. J Trace Elem Med Biol. 2016;37:96–103.

Hybsier S, et al. Establishment and characterization of a new ELISA for selenoprotein P. Perspect Sci. 2015;3(1–4):23–4.

Jackson MI, Lunøe K, Gabel-Jensen C, Gammelgaard B, Combs GF. Metabolism of selenite to selenosugar and trimethylselenonium in vivo: tissue dependency and requirement for S-adenosylmethionine-dependent methylation. J Nutr Biochem. 2013;24(12):2023–30.

Jäger T, Drexler H, Göen T. Human metabolism and renal excretion of selenium compounds after oral ingestion of sodium selenate dependent on trimethylselenium ion (TMSe) status. Arch Toxicol. 2016;90(1):149–58.

Kasperek K, Kiem J, Iyengar GV, Feinendegen LE. Concentration differences between serum and plasma of the elements cobalt, iron, mercury, rubidium, selenium and zinc determined by neutron activation analysis. Sci Total Environ. 1981;17(2):133–43.

Kollmus H, Flohé L, McCarthy JE. Analysis of eukaryotic mRNA structures directing cotranslational incorporation of selenocysteine. Nucleic Acids Res. 1996;24(7):1195–201.

Liu Q, et al. Frequent epigenetic suppression of tumor suppressor gene glutathione peroxidase 3 by promoter hypermethylation and its clinical implication in clear cell renal cell carcinoma. Int J Mol Sci. 2015;16(5):10636–49.

Longnecker MP, et al. Use of selenium concentration in whole blood, serum, toenails, or urine as a surrogate measure of selenium intake. Epidemiology. 1996;7(4):384–90.

Lunøe K, Skov S, Gabel-Jensen C, Stürup S, Gammelgaard B. A method for analysis of dimethyl selenide and dimethyl diselenide by LC-ICP-DRC-MS. Anal Bioanal Chem. 2010;398(7–8):3081–6.

Martitz J, Hofmann PJ, Johannes J, Köhrle J, Schomburg L, Renko K. Factors impacting the aminoglycoside-induced UGA stop codon readthrough in selenoprotein translation. J Trace Elem Med Biol. 2016;37:104–10.

Michalke B. Capillary electrophoresis-inductively coupled plasma mass spectrometry. Methods Mol Biol. 2016;1483:167–80.

Moosmann B, Behl C. Selenoprotein synthesis and side-effects of statins. Lancet. 2004;363(9412):892–4.

Nève J, Vertongen F, Capel P. Selenium supplementation in healthy Belgian adults: response in platelet glutathione peroxidase activity and other blood indices. Am J Clin Nutr. 1988;48(1):139–43.

Nilsson UA, et al. The fungal nephrotoxin orellanine simultaneously increases oxidative stress and down-regulates cellular defenses. Free Radic Biol Med. 2008;44(8):1562–9.

Nogueira CW, Rocha JBT. Toxicology and pharmacology of selenium: emphasis on synthetic organoselenium compounds. Arch Toxicol. 2011;85(11):1313–59.

Noisel N, Bouchard M, Carrier G. Disposition kinetics of selenium in healthy volunteers following therapeutic shampoo treatment. Environ Toxicol Pharmacol. 2010;29(3):252–9.

Renko K, et al. Hepatic selenoprotein P (SePP) expression restores selenium transport and prevents infertility and motor-incoordination in Sepp-knockout mice. Biochem J. 2008;409(3):741–9.

Renko K, et al. Down-regulation of the hepatic selenoprotein biosynthesis machinery impairs selenium metabolism during the acute phase response in mice. FASEB J. 2009;23(6):1758–65.

Renko K, et al. Aminoglycoside-driven biosynthesis of selenium-deficient selenoprotein P. Sci Rep. 2017;7(1):4391.

Reszka E, Jablonska E, Gromadzinska J, Wasowicz W. Relevance of selenoprotein transcripts for selenium status in humans. Genes Nutr. 2012;7(2):127–37.

Rodríguez REM, Sanz AMT, Díaz RC. Urinary selenium status of healthy people. Clin Chem Lab Med. 2009;33(3):127–34.

Rusin M, Årsand E, Hartvigsen G. Functionalities and input methods for recording food intake: a systematic review. Int J Med Inform. 2013;82(8):653–64.

Schomburg L, Schweizer U, Holtmann B, Flohé L, Sendtner M, Köhrle J. Gene disruption discloses role of selenoprotein P in selenium delivery to target tissues. Biochem J. 2003;370(2):397–402.

Silva Junior EC, et al. Natural variation of selenium in Brazil nuts and soils from the Amazon region. Chemosphere. 2017;188:650–8.

Speckmann B, Sies H, Steinbrenner H. Attenuation of hepatic expression and secretion of selenoprotein P by metformin. Biochem Biophys Res Commun. 2009;387(1):158–63.

Stoedter M, Renko K, Hög A, Schomburg L. Selenium controls the sex-specific immune response and selenoprotein expression during the acute-phase response in mice. Biochem J. 2010;429(1):43–51.

Strimbu K, Tavel JA. What are biomarkers? Curr Opin HIV AIDS. 2010;5(6):463–6.

Sunde RA, Raines AM. Selenium regulation of the selenoprotein and nonselenoprotein transcriptomes in rodents. Adv Nutr. 2011;2(2):138–50.

Thomson CD, Smith TE, Butler KA, Packer MA. An evaluation of urinary measures of iodine and selenium status. J Trace Elem Med Biol. 1996;10(4):214–22.

Vinceti M, et al. Selenium speciation in human serum and its implications for epidemiologic research: a cross-sectional study. J Trace Elem Med Biol. 2015;31:1–10.

Vinceti M, et al. A selenium species in cerebrospinal fluid predicts conversion to Alzheimer's dementia in persons with mild cognitive impairment. Alzheimers Res Ther. 2017;9:100.

Wiesner-Reinhold M, et al. Mechanisms of selenium enrichment and measurement in Brassicaceous vegetables, and their application to human health. Front Plant Sci. 2017;8:1365.

Wilber CG. Toxicology of selenium: a review. Clin Toxicol. 1980;17(2):171–230.

Xia Y, et al. Optimization of selenoprotein P and other plasma selenium biomarkers for the assessment of the selenium nutritional requirement: a placebo-controlled, double-blind study of selenomethionine supplementation in selenium-deficient Chinese subjects1234. Am J Clin Nutr. 2010;92(3):525–31.

Chapter 24
Human Biomonitoring of Selenium Exposure

Thomas Göen and Annette Greiner

Abstract Selenium is one of the most prominent essential trace elements for humans. Generally, the major supply of selenium results from the regular nutrition. In the regular diet almost all selenium exists in the form of organic compounds, e.g. as selenomethionine and other selenoamino acids. In contrast, special exposure by functional food, environmental contamination or occupational exposure may occur partly or mainly in the form of inorganic selenium compounds and elemental selenium, which differ in absorption, distribution, metabolism and elimination compared to the organic compounds.

Because of the small margin between beneficial and adverse effects and because of the different toxicokinetics of the selenium compounds an adequate assessment of the human exposure is of pharmacological and toxicological interest. The most reasonable approach for a reliable assessment of the human exposure is offered by the determination of the selenium concentration in human biological materials (human biomonitoring, HBM). For the assessment of selenium exposure in humans several biomarkers were developed and applied in the past. Their applicability has to be reviewed with regard to their specificity and sensitivity. Moreover, their kinetics and determinants have to be considered for an appropriate sampling design and a correct interpretation of the results. Additionally, a toxicological evaluation of HBM results needs biological limit values, e.g. biological tolerance values (BAT) and biological exposure indices (BEI), which indicate the threshold between the tolerable and non-tolerable internal exposure.

Keywords Selenium · Human biomonitoring · Biological material · Exposure limits · Kinetics

T. Göen (✉) · A. Greiner
Friedrich-Alexander-Universität Erlangen-Nürnberg, Institut und Poliklinik für Arbeits-, Sozial- und Umweltmedizin, Erlangen, Germany
e-mail: thomas.goeen@fau.de; Annette.Greiner@fau.de

© Springer International Publishing AG, part of Springer Nature 2018   467
B. Michalke (ed.), *Selenium*, Molecular and Integrative Toxicology,
https://doi.org/10.1007/978-3-319-95390-8_24

Introduction

Selenium is one of the most prominent essential trace elements for humans. In the form of selenocysteine it is a structural component of multiple enzymes such as glutathione peroxidases, thioredoxin reductase and deiodinases, and thus plays a crucial role in human health. However, selenium and its compounds represent a relatively small therapeutic margin, and adverse health effects may occur after slightly elevated intake of selenium (Navarro-Alarcon and Cabrera-Vique 2008; Glover 1970; Diskin et al. 1979; Vinceti et al. 2001; Stranges et al. 2007).

Generally, the major supply of selenium results from the regular nutrition. In the regular diet almost all selenium exists in the form of organic compounds, e.g. as selenomethionine and other selenoamino acids (Burk and Hill 2015). In contrast, special exposure by functional food, environmental contamination or occupational exposure may occur partly or mainly in the form of inorganic selenium compounds or elemental selenium (Göen et al. 2015), which differ in absorption, distribution, metabolism and elimination compared to the organic compounds (Jäger et al. 2016a, b).

Because of the small margin between beneficial and adverse effects and because of the different toxicokinetics of the selenium compounds an adequate assessment of the human exposure is of pharmacological and toxicological interest. The most reasonable approach for a reliable assessment of the human exposure is offered by the determination of the selenium concentration in human biological materials (human biomonitoring, HBM). For the assessment of selenium exposure in humans several biomarkers were developed and applied in the past. Their applicability has to be reviewed with regard to their specificity and sensitivity. Moreover, their kinetics and determinants have to be considered for an appropriate sampling design and a correct interpretation of the results. Additionally, a toxicological evaluation of HBM results needs biological limit values, e.g. *Biological tolerance values* (BAT) and *Biological exposure indices* (BEI), which indicate the threshold between the tolerable and non-tolerable internal exposure.

Characteristics of the HBM Parameters

Human biomonitoring is performed by measuring selenium, selenium metabolites or their reaction products in human body fluids and tissues. It is crucial for a toxicological risk assessment that a certain HBM parameter reliably reflects the systemic concentration of a substance.

It might be reasonably assumed that selenium in blood and blood compartments should display the status of systemic selenium exposure adequately. Thus, selenium levels in whole blood, in erythrocytes, plasma and serum, respectively, have been established as standard parameters for the selenium status in humans since the 1950s (Nève 1991; Combs et al. 2011). The parameters selenium in the erythrocyte fraction (Se-RBC) and selenium in plasma/serum (Se-P) do differ not only in their levels but also in their toxicokinetics. Therefore a separate review of each of these parameters is required. Another parameter for the systemic exposure to selenium may be the selenium level in saliva (Se-Sal).

Additionally, the determination of selenium in different excretions can serve as HBM parameter of selenium exposure (Gil and Hermández 2015). Potential parameters are selenium in urine (Se-U), selenium in faeces (Se-Faeces), selenium in breast milk (Se-BM), selenium in hair (Se-Hair) and selenium in toenails and fingernails (Se-Nails).

Selenium in Plasma/Serum

There is no clue for a different content and composition of selenium and its compounds in human serum and plasma, which led to a joint review of the results for both matrices (Nève 1991). In human plasma/serum the predominant portion of selenium exists in the form of selenoamino acids which are bond in proteins. The most prominent ones are selenoprotein P (SELENOP), glutathione peroxidase (GPX) and albumin (HSA). Under normal circumstances, the shares of selenium bound in these proteins in the total amount of Se-P are in the range of 52–56% for SELENOP, 19–25% for GPX and 12–23% for HSA (Achouba et al. 2016; Jitaru et al. 2008; Reyes et al. 2003; Letsiou et al. 2010). The appearance of selenium in plasma proteins implies a linkage of total plasma selenium with the generation and fate of the plasma proteins. In most selenoproteins selenium is incorporated via the regular protein synthesis in the form of selenocysteine (Labunskyy et al. 2014). Therefore a metabolic transfer of selenium is required. However, a specific analysis of plasma proteins in human studies with different selenium supplements revealed an uncontrolled placement of selenomethionine instead of methionine in HSA, whereas the supplementation of selenate did not result in an increase of selenium in the HSA fraction (Burk et al. 2001). Moreover, long-term supplementation studies indicated a steady-state term for the selenium level in plasma in the range of 4–10 weeks during selenomethionine supplementation, whereas the equilibrium was reached within 2 weeks during selenate supplementation (Xia et al. 1992; Thomson et al. 1993; Robinson et al. 1997). A follow-up after cessation of supplementation of selenised yeast (60–90% of selenium as selenomethionine) and bread, respectively, revealed that the Se-P level needs more than 10 weeks to reach the background level again (Levander et al. 1983; Reilly 2006). The faster recovery was indicated after a Se-P accretion by selenite supplementation (Robinson et al. 1978; Levander et al. 1983). There are some indications that the net increase of Se-P is inversely correlated to the usual selenium intake, suggesting a homeostatic mechanism above a certain plasma level (Nève 1991). The intra-individual variance of Se-P in the general populations appeared to be low. A study on the selenium level in plasma samples taken in each month during 1 year from 26 healthy adults resided in the Antwerp region revealed intra-individual coefficients of variation between 2.9 and 12.9% (Van Cauwenbergh et al. 2004).

Selenium in Erythrocytes

Whereas selenium in plasma/serum occurs mainly in an extracellular compartment, Se-RBC is attributed to cellular parts exclusively. More than 95% of the RBC-Se is bound in high-mass molecules (>30 kDa), e.g. haemoglobin, the majority of rest in the cell membrane and a marginal share as low-molecular selenium species (Haratake et al. 2008). GPX accounts for approximately 15% of selenium content in the erythrocytes (Nève 1991). Although a minor part of macromolecular bound selenium may be converted to low-molecular species by a haemoglobin-mediated transformation process and may subsequently be released to the plasma (Haratake et al. 2008), the predominant part of Se-RBC remains in the erythrocyte until its apoptosis. In accordance with the average life span of erythrocytes of about 120 days, the steady-state time during long-term supplementation of selenised yeast was found to be 3–5 months (Xia et al. 1992; Thomson et al. 1993). The selenium supplementation by selenate affected the RBC-Se levels only marginally and indicated a shorter steady-state time of 4 weeks (Xia et al. 1992).

The poor responsiveness of erythrocyte selenium as compared to plasma selenium concentration may be partly due to the fact that selenium incorporation into red blood cells is influenced by the rather long time period required for the synthesis of these cells (Nève 1991).

The slower kinetics of the red blood cell compartment was also verified during the post-dosing period as selenium concentrations decreased at slower rates than in the plasma compartment.

Erythrocyte selenium forms may therefore constitute storage sites for the element. Despite the imprecision associated with the calculation of the net increase in plasma and erythrocyte selenium concentrations at the end of the various experiments, the variations were generally lower in erythrocytes than in plasma but roughly parallel in the two compartments.

Selenium in Whole Blood

The selenium level in whole blood shows a kinetic behaviour which is affected by the fate of selenium in both compartments (Se-RBC; Se-P). Consequently, the sloping curve of Se-B during long-term supplementation of selenised yeast showed a merged course of both parameters but did not exhibit a clear steady-state time point (Thomson et al. 1993; Robinson et al. 1978). During selenate supplementation the kinetics of Se-B was almost similar with the course of Se-P (Thomson et al. 1993). Interestingly, the ratio of Se-P/Se-RBC depends on the extent of the selenium exposure. Along with rising selenium concentrations in whole blood, Yang et al. (1989b) found a decrease of the Se-P/Se-RBC ration from 0.89 to 0.24 in population groups of Se-B levels between 30 and 432 µg/L.

Selenium in Saliva

In principle, the selenium level in saliva (Se-Sal) may represent the internal exposure to selenium, because the secretion of the salivary gland is associated to the levels in blood plasma (Michalke et al. 2015). For this parameter several applications in population studies exist (Olmez et al. 1988; Zaichick et al. 1995; Raghunath et al. 2002), but no reports on studies of its kinetic behaviour are available. Nevertheless, it can be assumed that the kinetics of Se-Sal may be comparable with that of Se-P. Several sampling devices for saliva collection are commercially available and different saliva pre-preparation procedures are described by producers and scientists, which result in diverse modifications of the matrix. However, a harmonisation of sampling and pre-preparation procedures is still missing, which precludes comparability of results between different studies (Michalke et al. 2015).

Selenium in Urine

In contrast to the long-term parameter Se-P, Se-RBC, Se-B and Se-Sal, selenium concentration in urine may serve as a parameter for temporary turnover of selenium compounds (Francesconi and Pannier 2004). After single oral administration of selenite, selenised yeast and selenomethionine 5–10%, 11–13% and 7.4% of the applied dose were excreted within 24 h via urine (Jäger et al. 2016b; Griffiths et al. 1976), whereas 28–44% of the applied dose was found after administration of selenate (Jäger et al. 2016a). A higher urinary excretion rate of 52% was found after single oral administration of ^{74}Se-selenite to four young men (Martin et al. 1988). Information on the kinetic behaviour of Se-U exists from single administration and long-term supplemental studies using selenised yeast, selenomethionine, selenate and selenite (Thomson and Stewart 1974; Martin et al. 1988; Robinson et al. 1997; Jäger et al. 2016a, b) as well as during consumption of high-selenised bread (Robinson et al. 1985). The urinary level of total selenium reached the maximal excretion rate within 2–7 h after single oral administration of selenate, selenised yeast and selenite (Jäger et al. 2016a, b; Martin et al. 1988). Consistently, steady state of Se-U is reached directly after starting long-term supplementation with selenite (Martin et al. 1988; Thomson and Stewart 1974), selenomethionine and selenate (Robinson et al. 1997). After single oral administration of selenate, selenite and selenised yeast the urinary selenium concentration decreased from the maximal level with half-life of 2 h, 6 h and 4–7 h, respectively (Griffiths et al. 1976; Jäger et al. 2016a, b). The fast kinetics of urinary selenium was also indicated by the results from individuals periodically supplemented by high-selenised bread consumption (Robinson et al. 1985) and women after a single oral administration of ^{75}Se-selenomethionine (Griffiths et al. 1976).

Further studies on the elimination of selected selenium species in human urine found a high share of low-molecular species in the urinary excreted selenium (Gammelgaard et al. 2003; Gammelgaard and Bendahl 2004; Bendahl and

Gammelgaard 2004; Kuehnelt et al. 2005). The studies indicated selenosugars, e.g. methyl-2-acetamido-2-deoxy-1-seleno-β-D-galacto-pyranoside (SeSug1), methyl-2-acetamido-2-deoxy-1-seleno-β-D-glucosamine (SeSug2) and methyl-2-amino-2-deoxy-1-seleno-β-D-galactopyranoside (SeSug3), as major urinary eliminated metabolites. Another selenium metabolite, which was found in human urine very early, is the trimethyl selenium ion (TMSe) (Nahapetian et al. 1984; Martin et al. 1988; Yang et al. 1989b). However, more recent investigations revealed a predisposition for TMSe excretion in one-fifth of the European population, whereas the majority of the population excreted TMSe physiologically as well as after supplementation only in negligible amounts (Jäger et al. 2013, 2016a, b). This resulted in the definition of TMSe eliminators and non-TMSe eliminators. Further low-molecular selenium species found in the human urine are selenate, selenite, methylselenocysteine (SeMCys) and monomethylseleninic acid (Gammelgaard and Jøns 2000; Ogra et al. 2003; Jäger et al. 2013).

The separate determination of selenium species in urine enables a specific exploration and diagnosis of the selenium exposure. After supplementation of selenate, almost all selenium excreted within the first 24 h via urine could be assigned to the low-molecular-mass species, of which selenate covered 73–95% (Fig. 24.1). Only in TMSe eliminators the TMSe portion in the urine during 24 h after the exposure to selenate reached 17%. Moreover, the experiments revealed a very fast urinary elimination of selenate with half-life of 2 h (Jäger et al. 2016a). After oral supplementation of selenite and selenised yeast, in non-TMSe eliminators SeSug1 represented the main species in 24-h urine post-exposure with shares of 44% and 56%, respectively. In TMSe eliminators the TMSe ion represented the main metabolite, which covered 54% and 25%, respectively, of the total excreted selenium, whereas the second major metabolite SeSug1 covered 36 and 9% in this subpopulation. Moreover, selenate was found in the urine of both groups after selenite exposure with shares

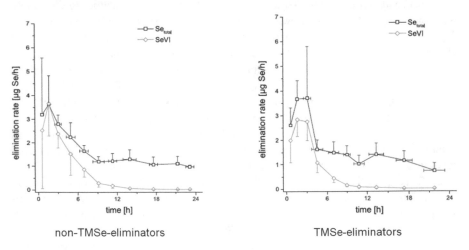

non-TMSe-eliminators   TMSe-eliminators

Fig. 24.1 Urinary elimination of total selenium and selenate (SeVI), respectively, after single oral administration of sodium selenate (from Jäger et al. 2016a)

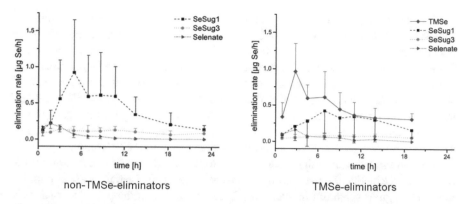

Fig. 24.2 Urinary elimination of selenium species after single oral administration of sodium selenite (from Jäger et al. 2016b)

between 6 and 7%. The elimination half-life of SeSug1 was found between 6.4 and 8.5 h for both groups after selenite exposure and somewhat faster (4.4 h) in non-TMSe eliminators after selenised yeast exposure (Fig. 24.2). The elimination kinetic of TMSe showed a half-life between 5.9 and 6.8 h (Jäger et al. 2016b).

Selenium in Faeces

Faecal excretion within 2 weeks after a single oral administration of ^{75}Se-selenomethionine was 5.3% (Griffiths et al. 1976), but 33–58% within 2 weeks after single administration of ^{75}Se-selenite (Thomson and Stewart 1974). The faecal excretion was almost completed 6 days after ^{75}Se-selenite administration (Thomson and Stewart 1974). During long-term administration both selenite and selenomethionine steady-state level of selenium in faeces was reached within the first week (Robinson et al. 1978).

Selenium in Nails and Hair

The determination of selenium in nails (Se-Nails) is one of the most prominent HBM parameters for selenium status in populations and in epidemiology studies on selenium toxicity, which demands a review of its performance and kinetic behaviour. The selenium concentration in nails is below 1 µg/g in population with regular selenium intake (see Table 24.3), which represents a minor share of nail selenium in the total excretion of selenium. Due to the slow growth of nails, especially of toenails, and the long term for reaching the top point, the parameter provides a time-delayed and, depending on the clipping length, also a time-integrated measure of the selenium excretion, which enables the assessment of past exposure periods (He

2011). Consequently a strong correlation between Se-Nails and Se-P was found in settled populations (Satia et al. 2006). The fingernails showed an average growth rate of approximately 3 mm per month and toenails of about 1 mm per month (Dawber 1970; Geyer et al. 2004; Yaemsiri et al. 2010), which results in a time shift of the assessment period up to 12 months. Consequently, recent exposure can't be assessed by the selenium analysis of the nail tops. Moreover, a significant inter-individual variation of nail growth rate was found depending on age, gender and health status (Yaemsiri et al. 2010; He 2011). Moreover, nail varnishing and other special treatments of the nails can result in a contamination of selenium.

Selenium in hair (Se-Hair) is very similar to selenium in nails concerning excretion rate and kinetics. The selenium concentration in hair is below 1 μg/g in population with regular selenium intake, too (Table 24.1). The parameter also enables a retrospective analysis of the exposure. In settled populations a strong correlation between Se-Hair and Se-P was found likewise (Kvicala et al. 1999). Hair grows at several body sites, but its growth depends on the anatomic location. Scalp hair, the most common specimen, is produced at a rate of approximately 0.6–1.4 cm/month, which indicates that common hair lengths cover a production term between several months and a very few years (Villain et al. 2004; Kempson and Lombi 2011). However, hair growth happens in a series of growing and resting phases. It is estimated that a delay of 2–4 weeks exists between the incorporation of an element in hair and the hair emergence from the skin, which very clear inhibits the assessment of the recent exposure to selenium by its determination in hair, in spite of sampling at the bottom of the hair. Even the assessment of a defined past exposure period requires the sampling of the correct hair section. Significant inter-individual variation of selenium excretion process via hair may depend on many other factors, e.g. hair colour (melanin content), age, gender, ethnicity and hormonal status. Additionally, the effects of hair treatment, e.g. by using selenium-containing hair shampoo and hair-colouring procedures, and external contamination by the ambient air have to be considered in practice of hair analysis (Kempson and Lombi 2011).

Selenium in Breast Milk

Selenium is secreted in breast milk (Se-BM) as organic compounds and its major part is found in the whey fraction as selenoproteins as well as low-molecular selenium species (Dorea 2002). However, the molecular species occurred only as organic compounds, e.g. selenoglutathione, selenomethionine, selenocystein and selenocystamine, but not as inorganic selenium species in pre-concentrated breast milk (Michalke and Schramel 1998). The total concentration of selenium in breast milk depends on the stage of lactation and breastfeeding. In Polish lactating women the selenium level was 22.8 ± 10.1 μg/L in the colostrum, 11.3 ± 3.8 μg/L in the transitional milk and 9.2 ± 3.6 μg/L in the mature milk (Wasowicz et al. 2001). The same trend was observed in the breast milk of different lactation stages in Libyan women, but on a much higher level (Hannan et al. 2005), as well as in breast milk samples of a German woman (Dörner et al. 1990). The results of a study of the

Table 24.1 Characteristics of HBM parameters for selenium exposure

Parameter	Steady-state time	Sensitivity	Specificity	Specific determinates
Se-P	1–3 months	Low, due to homeostatic regulation	Low specificity for composition of Se uptake	
Se-RBC	3–5 months	Low, due to erythrocyte lifetime	Low specificity for composition of Se uptake	
Se-B	Mix of Se-P and Se-RBC	Low	Low specificity for composition of Se uptake	
Se-Sal	– (No data)	Low (depending on Se-P)	Low (depending on Se-P)	Sampling procedure not standardised
Se-U (total)	A few hours	High	High, response depends on Se species uptake	Renal dilution (creatinine standardisation required)
Se-U (species)	A few hours	High	Very high, excreted species correspond with Se species uptake	Renal dilution (creatinine standardisation required)
Se-Faeces	A few days	Medium	Low specificity for composition of Se uptake	
Se-Nails	Several months[a]	Low	Low specificity for composition of Se uptake	Nail growths (age, gender), sampling protocol
Se-Hair	Several months[b]	Low	Low specificity for composition of Se uptake	Hair growth and colour, age, gender, ethnicity, sampling protocol
Se-BM	– (No data)	Not specified	Not specified	Stage of lactation

[a]Period between placing during nail production until reaching top position
[b]2-week minimum period between placing during hair production until sticking out of the skin surface

Se-BM levels in Nigerian women up to 180 days postpartum indicate the ongoing of this trend for a longer period (Arnaud et al. 1993). Moreover, the selenium breast milk level decreases by the number of daily breast milk feeding. In the breast milk of Saudi Arabian women the selenium level was 27.2 ± 18.9 µg/L for daily breast-feedings below 5, 16.9 ± 7.12 µg/L for 5–10 breast milk feeding the day and 15.9 ± 5.77 µg/L for more than 10 breastfeedings per day (Al-Saleh et al. 1997).

Determinants of Selenium Exposure in General Populations

The selenium concentration in diverse biological materials from different general populations worldwide is presented in Tables 24.2 and 24.3. A consistent determinant for the selenium levels in almost all HBM parameters is the geographic

Table 24.2 Selenium levels in blood and blood compartments of general population

Region	Population	Period[a]	Concentration (mean ± standard deviation (range))	References
Selenium in whole blood				
Austria	Adult population (n = 153)	2002–2004	85.9 ± 24.0 μg/L (41.7–183 μg/L)	Gundacker et al. (2006)
Brazil	Amazonian population (n = 236)	2003	362 ± 256 μg/L (142–2030 μg/L)	Lemire et al. (2006)
Brazil	Amazonian population (n = 143)	2006	292 μg/L[b] (132–1500 μg/L)	Lemire et al. (2010)
Canada	Inuit adults	2004	261 μg/L[b]; 869 μg/L[c] (119–3550 μg/L)	Achouba et al. (2016)
China	Pop. in low-Se area (n = 62)	1985	160 ± 30 μg/L	Yang et al. (1989a)
	Pop. in medium-Se area (n = 106)	1985	360 ± 206 μg/L	
	Pop. in high-Se area (n = 100)	1985	1510 ± 500 μg/L	
India	Adults (n = 35)	2000	99.6 ± 1.34 μg/L[d] (32–178 μg/L)	Raghunath et al. (2002)
Norway	Pregnant women (n = 119)	2003–2004	106 μg/L[b]; 141 μg/L[c]; 107 ± 21.4 μg/L	Brantsæter et al. (2009)
USA	Adults, in high-Se area (n = 44)	1985–1986	254 ± 62.4 μg/L (187–555 μg/L)	Swanson et al. (1990)
USA	Pop. in S. Dakota, Wyoming (n = 49)	1985–1986	233 ± 30.0 μg/L (182–344 μg/L)	Longnecker et al. (1991)
	Pop. in seleniferous areas (n = 29)	1995–1996	310 ± 86.1 μg/L (214–570 μg/L)	
	Pop. in seleniferous areas (n = 64)	1996–1997	392 ± 108 μg/L (212–674 μg/L)	
Selenium in plasma/serum				
Australia, southeastern	Adults (n = 140)	2007	100.2 ± 15.4 μg/L (63.0–173 μg/L)	Lymbury et al. (2008)
Belgium, Antwerp	Adults (n = 26)	1991–1992	84.3 ± 9.4 μg/L (51.40–122 μg/L)	Van Cauwenbergh et al. (2004)
Brazil	Children, 3–6 years, Macapá (n = 41)	2014	107 ± 27.2 μg/L (73.0–172 μg/L)	Martens et al. (2015)
	Children, 2–6 years, Belém (n = 88)	2014	83.6 ± 23.3 μg/L (47.0–142 μg/L)	
Canada	Inuit adults	2004	139 μg/L[b]; 170 μg/L[c] (84.5–229 μg/L)	Achouba et al. (2016)

(continued)

Table 24.2 (continued)

Region	Population	Period[a]	Concentration (mean ± standard deviation (range))	References
China, Linxian	Female adults (n = 970)	1985	69.9 µg/L[b]; 92.1 µg/L[c]	Mark et al. (2000)
	Male adults (n = 1171)	1985	71.6 µ/L[b]; 94.4 µg/L[c]	
The Czech Republic	Females in low-Se area (n = 60)	1987–1998	58.4 ± 11.3 µg/L	Kvicala et al. (1999)
	Males in low-Se area (n = 74)	1987–1998	58.1 ± 9.2 µg/L	
	Girls in low-Se area (n = 60)	1987–1998	50.5 ± 11.3 µg/L	
	Boys in low-Se area (n = 59)	1987–1998	51.0 ± 8.8 µg/L	
France, national survey	Female adults (n = 7423)	1994	86.1 ± 15.0 µg/L	Arnaud et al. (2006)
	Male adults (n = 4915)	1994	90.0 ± 15.8 µg/L	
Germany	Adults (n = 24)	1988	66 ± 11 µg/L	Oster and Prellwitz (1990)
Germany	Elderly women (n = 167)	2002	92.4 ± 18.2 µg/L	Wolters et al. (2006)
Germany	Children, 1–5 years (n = 221)	2001	71.1 µg/L[b] (12–135 µg/L)	Muntau et al. (2002)
	Children, 5–18 years (n = 623)	2001	78.2 µg/L[b] (30–130 µg/L)	
Germany	Male adults (n = 20)	2013	76 µg/L[b]; 101 µg/L[c] (52–102 µg/L)	Göen et al. (2015)
Germany	Adults (n = 20)	2017	76.9 µg/L[b] (70.6–115 µg/L)	Greiner et al. (2018)
Hungary	Blood donors (n = 238)	1991	55.3 ± 9.48 µg/L (32.4–93.2 µg/L)	Alfthan et al. (1992)
India	Adults (n = 201)	2000	100 ± 1.33 µg/L[d] (35.8–186 µg/L)	Raghunath et al. (2002)
Iran, Tehran	Children, 1–16 years (n = 54)	2004	84.2 ± 11.0 µg/L (58–105 µg/L)	Safaralizadeh et al. (2005)
	Adolescents and adults (n = 130)	2004	101 ± 12.9 µg/L (74–134 µg/L)	
Iran, Tehran	Children, <4 years (n = 67)	2006	63.7 ± 20.3 µg/L	Safaralizadeh et al. (2007)
	Children, ≥4 years (n = 149)	2006	75.8 ± 13.4 µg/L	

(continued)

Table 24.2 (continued)

Region	Population	Period[a]	Concentration (mean ± standard deviation (range))	References
Italy, northern	Adults ($n = 293$)	1991	115 µg/L[b]; 119 ± 27.2 µg/L	Sesana et al. (1992)
Latvia, Gulf of Riga	Males, low fish intake	1997	54.5 µg/L[b] (23.7–90.0 µg/L)	Hagmar et al. (1998)
	Males, medium fish intake	1997	71.9 µg/L[b] (36.3–116 µg/L)	
	Males, high fish intake	1997	93.2 µg/L[b] (52.1–123 µg/L)	
Poland, northern	Adults ($n = 146$)	2000	72.5 µg/L[b]; 73.3 ± 14.4 µg/L	Ha'c et al. (2002)
Poland	Women in low-Se area ($n = 19$)	1981–1983	95 ± 13 µg/L	Wasowicz et al. (2003)
	Women in low-Se area ($n = 58$)	1990–1991	59 ± 5 µg/L	
	Women in low-Se area ($n = 98$)	1997–1999	54 ± 12 µg/L	
Russia	Pop. in lowest Se region ($n = 27$)	1995	71.9 ± 11.1 µg/L (50.5–107 µg/L)	Golubkina and Alfthan (1999)
	Pop. in highest Se region ($n = 58$)	1991	137 ± 4.7 µg/L (135–145 µg/L)	
Russia, northwestern	Male adults, 19–21 years ($n = 19$)	2004–2005	82.3 ± 11.2 µg/L	Parshukova et al. (2014)
Saudi Arabia	Children, 3–16 years ($n = 513$)	2003–2004	95.1 ± 20.9 µg/L	Al-Saleh et al. (2006)
Singapore	Female adults ($n = 478$)	1993–1995	119 µg/L	Hughes et al. (1998)
	Male adults ($n = 471$)	1993–1995	125 µg/L	
South Korea	Female adults ($n = 50$)	2006	44.8 ± 13.9 µg/L (57.8–192 µg/L)	Kim et al. (2009)
	Male adults ($n = 50$)	2006	45.9 ± 14.7 µg/L (32.6–190 µg/L)	
Spain, southern	Adults ($n = 340$)	1998–2000	82.7 ± 48.3 µg/L	Sánchez et al. (2010)
Taiwan	Adolescents and adults ($n = 2775$)	2003	110.9 ± 21.5 µg/L (40.5–186 µg/L)	Chen et al. (2006)
Tibet, around Lhasa	Children, 4–15 years ($n = 521$)	1995	8.7 µg/L[b] (<5–57 µg/L)	Moreno-Reyes et al. (1998)
Turkey, eastern	Lactating women ($n = 30$)	2007	68.5 ± 3.6 µg/L	Özdemir et al. (2008)

(continued)

Table 24.2 (continued)

Region	Population	Period[a]	Concentration (mean ± standard deviation (range))	References
	Neonates, UC blood (*n* = 30)	2007	120 ± 18.1 µg/L	
United Kingdom	Children, 4–18 years (*n* = 1127)	1997	67.9 µg/L[b]; 68.7 ± 11.8 µg/L	Bates et al. (2002)
United Kingdom	Pregnant women (*n* = 1924)	1997–1999	79.1 µg/L[b]; 107.9 µg/L[c]	Devereux et al. (2007)
United Kingdom	Adults (*n* = 1050)	2000–2001	85.3 µg/L[b] (77.4–94.8 µg/L)[f]	Spina et al. (2013)
USA, national survey	Adults, ≥40 years (*n* = 917)	2003–2004	137.1 ± 19.9 µg/L	Laclaustra et al. (2009)
USA	Pop. in S. Dakota, Wyoming (*n* = 49)	1985–1986	154 ± 15.8 µg/L (123–205 µg/L)	Longnecker et al. (1991)
	Pop. in seleniferous areas (*n* = 29)	1995–1996	193 ± 45.0 µg/L (129–321 µg/L)	
	Pop. in seleniferous areas (*n* = 64)	1996–1997	233 ± 54.5 µg/L (148–363 µg/L)	
USA	Adults in high-Se area (*n* = 44)	1985–1986	166 ± 30.0 µg/L (123–293 µg/L)	Swanson et al. (1990)
USA, northwestern	Adults, partly suppl. (*n* = 220)	2001	161 ± 29 µg/L	Satia et al. (2006)
USA	Adult population (*n* = 261)	2010	143 ± 24.3 µg/L	Combs et al. (2011)
Venezuela	Women in low-Se area (*n* = 44)	1993	229 ± 51 µg/L	Brätter et al. (1997)
	Women in medium-Se area (*n* = 19)	1993	327 ± 80 µg/L	
	Women in high-Se area (*n* = 14)	1993	621 ± 199 µg/L	
Selenium in erythrocytes				
Brazil	Children, 3–6 years, Macapá (*n* = 41)	2014	133 ± 32.2 µg/L (78.0–195 µg/L)	Martens et al. (2015)
	Children, 2–6 years, Belém (*n* = 88)	2014	94.7 ± 18.6 µg/L (67.0–150 µg/L)	
Germany	Adults (*n* = 20)	2017	53.3 µg/L blood (38.3–89.9 µg/L blood)	Greiner et al. (2018)
United Kingdom	Children, 4–18 years (*n* = 1127)	1997	116 µg/L[b]; 119 ± 23.7 µg/L	Bates et al. (2002)

(continued)

Table 24.2 (continued)

Region	Population	Period[a]	Concentration (mean ± standard deviation (range))	References
United Kingdom	Adults (n = 1050)	2000–2001	128 µg/L[b] (109–151 µg/L)[f]	Spina et al. (2013)
Venezuela	Women in low-Se area (n = 29)	1993	344 ± 100 µg/L	Brätter et al. (1997)
	Women in medium-Se area (n = 8)	1993	429 ± 125 µg/L	
	Women in high-Se area (n = 11)	1993	1270 ± 50 µg/L	

[a]Year before submission of the publication, if assessment period was not stated
[b]Median
[c]95th percentile
[d]Geometric mean ± geometric standard deviation
[e]90th percentile
[f]1st quantile-third quantile

location of the population, which is derived from the selenium content in the soil of the region and the resultant selenium burden of the regional food. Regions with high soil selenium levels are North and South America and the most regions in Asia, whereas especially regions in East Europe and Australia exhibit low selenium levels. Moreover, the composition of the diet can affect the internal selenium exposure. An example is the high selenium content in Brazil nuts, which resulted in a high exposure of populations consuming this foodstuff frequently (Lemire et al. 2010; Martens et al. 2015). A second example is the increase of the internal selenium levels by the elevated frequency of seafish consumption, which was demonstrated in Latvian fishmen (Hagmar et al. 1998). Another general determinant of the internal selenium level is the chemical species of the selenium intake. Organic selenium forms (selenised yeast, selenomethionine, food Se) show better performance in terms of the net increase as compared with inorganic species. Differences in absorption and excretion rates may significantly contribute to this effect (Griffiths et al. 1976; Thomson and Stewart 1974). However, the variable deposition in human selenoproteins may be the most important differentiating factor for the species effect (Nève 1991). Food selenium (wheat and meat) appears as a complex medium, since selenium chemical forms are not defined in these supplements, which are characterised only by their total selenium content (Thomson et al. 1985; Levander et al. 1983; Van der Torre et al. 1991). In meat, the form of selenium depends on the form of selenium consumed by the animal (Beilstein and Whanger 1988). Using the example of the Finnish population it was shown that a national selenium fertilisation programme can result in a significant increase of the internal selenium burden in the population (Alfthan et al. 2015).

Table 24.3 Selenium levels in other biological materials of general population

Region	Population	Period[a]	Concentration (mean ± standard deviation (range))	References
Selenium in urine				
Bangladesh	Adults in high-As area (*n* = 128)	2007	15 ± 1.3 µg/g creatinine	Yoshida et al. (2015)
Brazil	Children, 3–6 years, Macapá (*n* = 41)	2014	270 ± 120 µg/L (110–470 µg/L)	Martens et al. (2015)
	Children, 2–6 years, Belém (*n* = 88)	2014	40 ± 10 µg/L (20–100 µg/L)	
Chile	Women in high-As area (*n* = 93)	1998–2000	28.3 ± 13.9 µg/L (5.9–67.5 µg/L)	Christian et al. (2006)
China	Pop. in low-Se area (*n* = 22)	1985	26.1 ± 48.3 µg/day	Yang et al. (1989a)
	Pop. in high-Se area (*n* = 28)	1985	566 ± 238 µg/day	
The Czech Republic	Females in low-Se area (*n* = 60)	1987–1998	11.6 ± 5.2 µg/L	Kvicala et al. (1999)
	Males in low-Se area (*n* = 74)	1987–1998	11.6 ± 4.5 µg/L	
	Girls in low-Se area (*n* = 60)	1987–1998	13.1 ± 5.5 µg/L	
	Boys in low-Se area (*n* = 59)	1987–1998	13.1 ± 5.3 µg/L	
Germany	Adults (*n* = 18)	1981	16.0 ± 4.6 µg/L (9–23 µg/L)	Schierling et al. (1982)
Germany	Adults (*n* = 24)	1988	14.8 ± 6.9 µg/L (3.2–26.3 µg/L)	Oster and Prellwitz (1990)
			16.5 ± 5.4 µg/day (9.5–29.3 µg/day)	
			13.0 ± 3.8 µg/g C (6.3–20.0 µg/g C)	
Germany	Adults (*n* = 47)	2012	10.4 µg/L[b]; 25.9 µg/L[c] (3.5–39.6 µg/L)	Jäger et al. (2013)
			15.7 µg/g crea.[b]; 30.4 µg/g[c] (8.5–39.1 µg/g)	
Germany	Male adults (*n* = 20)	2013	23 µg/g creatinine[b]; 50 µg/g[c] (12–50 µg/g)	Göen et al. (2015)
Germany	Adults (*n* = 20)	2017	18.7 µg/g creatinine[b] (9.20–40.6 µg/g)	Greiner et al. (2018)
India	Adults (*n* = 15)	2000	5.2 ± 1.46 µg/L[d] (2.9–8.3 µg/L)	Raghunath et al. (2002)
Poland	Adolesc. in low-Se area (*n* = 41)	1981–1983	14 ± 6 µg/g creatinine	Wasowicz et al. (2003)
	Adults in low-Se area (*n* = 62)	1981–1983	11 ± 5 µg/g creatinine	

(continued)

Table 24.3 (continued)

Region	Population	Period[a]	Concentration (mean ± standard deviation (range))	References
USA	Adults in high-Se area ($n = 44$)	1985–1986	123 ± 80.5 µg/day (23.7–395 µg/day)	Swanson et al. (1990)
USA	Pop. in S. Dakota, Wyoming ($n = 49$)	1985–1986	87.7 ± 36.3 µg/day (24.5–199 µg/day)	Longnecker et al. (1991)
	Pop. in seleniferous areas ($n = 29$)	1995–1996	188 ± 111 µg/day (66.3–469 µg/day)	
	Pop. in seleniferous areas ($n = 64$)	1996–1997	218 ± 123 µg/day (24.5–554 µg/day)	
USA	Adult population ($n = 261$)	2010	55.5 ± 20.1 µg/g creatinine	Combs et al. (2011)
Selenium in toenails				
Brazil	Children, 3–6 years, Macapá ($n = 41$)	2014	3.43 ± 1.81 µg/g (0.89–8.43 µg/g)	Martens et al. (2015)
	Children, 2–6 years, Belém ($n = 88$)	2014	1.29 ± 0.52 µg/g (0.31–2.16 µg/g)	
China	Pop. in low-Se area ($n = 18$)	1985	0,71 ± 0.14 µg/g	Yang et al. (1989a)
	Pop. in medium-Se area ($n = 66$)	1985	2.72 ± 2.68 µg/g	
	Pop. in high-Se area ($n = 33$)	1985	12.8 ± 6.03 µg/g	
France	Pop. in low-Se area ($n = 36$)	2005–2006	0.53 ± 0.10 µg/g	Barron et al. (2012)
	Pop. in high-Se area ($n = 36$)	2005–2006	0.61 ± 0.12 µg/g	
Hungary	Blood donors ($n = 211$)	1991	0.56 ± 0.18 µg/g	Alfthan et al. (1992)
New Zealand	Pop. in low-Se area ($n = 14$)	1982	0.26 ± 0.09 µg/g	Morris et al. (1983)
Saudi Arabia	Children, 3–16 years ($n = 513$)	2003–2004	0.58 ± 0.20 µg/g	Al-Saleh et al. (2006)
USA	Citizen of South Dakota ($n = 15$)	1982	1.17 ± 0.35 µg/g	Morris et al. (1983)
	Citizen of Georgia ($n = 24$)	1982	0.81 ± 0.14 µg/g	
	Citizen of Boston ($n = 9$]	1982	0.74 ± 0.13 µg/g	
USA	Adults in high-Se area ($n = 44$)	1985–1986	1.20 ± 0.24 µg/g (0.82–2.20 µg/g)	Swanson et al. (1990)
USA	Pop. in high-Se area ($n = 142$)	1985–1987	1.55 ± 0.58 µg/g (0.84–3.82 µg/g)	Longnecker et al. (1991)
USA, northwestern	Adults, partly suppl. ($n = 220$)	2001	1.02 ± 0.21 µg/g	Satia et al. (2006)

(continued)

Table 24.3 (continued)

Region	Population	Period[a]	Concentration (mean ± standard deviation (range))	References
Venezuela	Women in low-Se area (n = 32)	1993	1.64 ± 0.30 µg/g	Brätter et al. (1997)
	Women in medium-Se area (n = 36)	1993	2.61 ± 0.80 µg/g	
	Women in high-Se area (n = 37)	1993	4.26 ± 1.53 µg/g	
Selenium in hairs				
China	Pop. in low-Se area (n = 57)	1985	0.69 ± 0.38 µg/g	Yang et al. (1989a)
	Pop. in medium-Se area (n = 68)	1985	3.76 ± 3.63 µg/g	
	Pop. in high-Se area (n = 65)	1985	14.16 ± 8.38 µg/g	
Brazil	Children, 3–6 years, Macapá (n = 41)	2014	0.89 ± 0.24 µg/g (0.44–1.35 µg/g)	Martens et al. (2015)
	Children, 2–6 years, Belém (n = 88)	2014	0.31 ± 0.10 µg/g (0.12–0.50 µg/g)	
The Czech Republic	Males in low-Se area (n = 31)	1987–1998	0.27 ± 0.04 µg/g	Kvicala et al. (1999)
Germany	Adults (n = 24)	1988	0.31 ± 0.11 µg/g	Oster and Prellwitz (1990)
India	Adults (n = 15)	1995	0.78 ± 0.18 µg/g (0.45–0.99 µg/g)	Srivastava et al. (1997)
Poland, northern	Adults (n = 34)	2000	0.30 µg/g[b]; 0.30 ± 0.11 µg/g	Ha'c et al. (2002)
Turkey, eastern	Lactating women (n = 21)	2007	0.33 ± 0.04 µg/g	Özdemir et al. (2008)
	Neonates (n = 21)	2007	1.12 ± 0.19 µg/g	
Selenium in breast milk				
Poland	Lactating women, mature milk (n = 41)	1998–1999	9.2 ± 3.6 µg/L	Wasowicz et al. (2001)
Poland, national survey	Lactating women (n = 905)	1999	10.2 ± 2.82 µg/L (3.0–23.4 µg/L)	Zachara and Pilecki (2000)
Saudi Arabia	Lactating women (n = 117)	1996	17.6 ± 9.23 µg/L (1.2–83.5 µg/L)	Al-Saleh et al. (1997)
Turkey, eastern	Lactating women (n = 30)	2007	68.6 ± 7.8 ng/g	Özdemir et al. (2008)
Venezuela	Women in low-Se area (n = 52)	1993	42.9 ± 11.3 µg/L (20–72 µg/L)	Brätter et al. (1997)
	Women in medium-Se area (n = 39)	1993	56.6 ± 25 µg/L (36–102 µg/L)	

(continued)

Table 24.3 (continued)

Region	Population	Period[a]	Concentration (mean ± standard deviation (range))	References
	Women in high-Se area ($n = 34$)	1993	112 ± 36.5 µg/L (50–198 µg/L)	
USA	Lactating women, mature milk ($n = 25$)	2003	41.8 ± 6.66 µg/L	Hannan et al. (2005)
Selenium in saliva				
India	Adults ($n = 20$)	2000	2.0 ± 1.32 µg/L[d] (1.3–3.5 µg/L)	Raghunath et al. (2002)

[a]Year before submission of the publication, if assessment period was not stated
[b]Median
[c]95th percentile
[d]Geometric mean ± geometric standard deviation

Moreover, selenium absorption, distribution, metabolism and elimination may depend on basic selenium status. For example, subjects with a low selenium status seem to adjust selenium retention due to modification of urinary excretion (Robinson et al. 1985) and exhibit a modified selenium distribution between organs and tissues which may ensure the maintenance of important selenium-dependent functions. On the other hand, the way the intestinal selenium absorption mechanisms adapt to increased selenium intake in subjects with differing usual selenium intake is not well documented (Nève 1991). Such differences attenuate over the long term (after several weeks, depending on the degree of selenium deficiency), after the internal selenium reservoirs have been saturated.

In several studies, the levels of selenium HBM parameters were proved for gender differences. However, the results were not consistent for any of the parameters (Nève 1991). Undeniably gender differences in haematocrit and creatinine excretion can affect the distribution and standardisation of selenium levels. Nevertheless, the complexity of gender effects may cancel each other, which presents gender as an unimportant factor for internal selenium levels.

In contrast, age should be considered as a relevant determinant of internal selenium levels. A significant difference was demonstrated for selenium levels in children and adults (see Tables 24.2 and 24.3). Comparative data of the same population showed significantly lower Se-P levels in children compared to adults. In contrast, Se-U levels (expressed in µg/L) were higher in children compared to adults (Kvicala et al. 1999). Nevertheless, it has to be pointed out that Se-P levels increase during the early adolescence. In plasma samples of Polish children taken in the period 1980–1982, the mean Se-P levels were 41 µg/L in 2–12-month-aged infants, 55 µg/L in 1–3-year-old children, 62 µg/L in 3–7-year-old children and 77 µg/L in 7–15-year-old children. The effect was confirmed for the first three age groups but vanished for the eldest group in the subsequent survey of 1990–1991 (Wasowicz et al. 2003). Also Iranian children older than 4 years presented higher Se-P levels than young children of the same population (Safaralizadeh et al. 2007). Another study, which investigated the postnatal period in particular, revealed deceasing Se-P levels within the 4 first postnatal months, and a more intensive increase afterwards (Muntau et al. 2002). Age exhibits a weak determinant for the internal Se levels for the adult population too. In a French national survey a significant increase of Se-P was found for females, whereas an age effect was not recognised for males (Arnaud et al. 2006). A small increasing trend of Se-P by age was also indicated in young Australian adults. However, a significant decrease of Se-P was found for individuals older than 80 years (Lymbury et al. 2008). Nevertheless, other studies of Se-P levels in Korean and Italian adults did not show differences between the age groups (Kim et al. 2009; Sesana et al. 1992). The internal Se level of pregnant women decreases during pregnancy, but recovers within several weeks postnatally (Levander et al. 1987; Wasowicz et al. 2001). Further determinants are alcohol consumption, which results in lower Se-P levels (Chen et al. 2006; Gundacker et al. 2006), and active smoking, which exhibits lower internal selenium levels in smokers compared to non-smokers (Swanson et al. 1990; Laclaustra et al. 2009).

Assessment of Non-dietary Exposure/Occupational Exposure

The general determinants of the selenium HBM parameter have to be considered when investigating individuals who might be exposed by special sources (environmental contamination, occupational exposure). Selenium is used in the form of different compounds and purity grades in the glass industry, the colour pigment production, the digital X-ray technique, the pharmaceutical and photographic industry, fertilisers and the electronic industry based on the semiconductive properties of selenium.

Studies on occupational selenium exposure are rare. They were conducted in Germany, Canada, Taiwan, England and India. As described above, the basic level of selenium is influenced by the geographic location of the population. Different parameters were used to evaluate the internal selenium load, whereby urine was the most frequently analysed medium.

20 Workers of a selenium-processing plant in Germany were exposed to selenium concentrations in air from 8 to 950 µg/m³, with a median of 110 µg/m³. In this plant raw selenium was reprocessed to standard selenium and to selenium with a very low amount of impurities. Compared to 20 age-matched controls of the same region, the selenium concentration in plasma and post-shift urine was significantly increased. The exposed workers were examined once more after an exposure-free period of at least 2 weeks. Then their selenium plasma and urine level decreased and reached the level of the controls. The concentration of selenium in urine responded more sensitively to the occupational exposure than the concentration of selenium in plasma (Göen et al. 2015).

In England, 1517 urine samples of 200–300 selenium-exposed workers engaged in rectifier manufacture and 793 control samples were analysed. The workers were exposed to fumes of elemental red selenium and selenium dioxide. Every 3 months they were asked for a urine sample. The highest average selenium concentrations were found in workers involved in the grinding process (336 μg/L), followed by annealing (142 μg/L), special processes (123 μg/L), punching (115 μg/L) and scraping (108 μg/L). Selenium in air was only determined when there were indications of unusually high exposures. Under regular conditions selenium in air was not analysed. Control samples were obtained from pre-employment examinations of persons applying for a job in the factory. In the urine of the controls, an average selenium content of 34 μg/L was detected (Glover 1967).

Steel production workers and quality control workers in Taiwan also showed significantly higher urinary selenium levels than controls (Horng et al. 1999).

Srivastava et al. (1997) found significantly higher levels of selenium in the hair of 19 exposed subjects who were occupied with the manufacture and maintenance of drums used in photocopy machines. 15 subjects working in another part of the same factory and belonging to the same socioeconomic status served as controls. The average concentration of selenium in air was comparable to the one in the German factory described by Göen et al. (2015). However, very high concentrations in air were found during the sieving operation of the raw material (18,040 μg/m³), which was done three times a week for 1.5–2 h by one subject on a rotational basis. Consistent with the results of Glover (1967) in urine, high air concentrations were found in the lathe/grinding process. Complaints of weakness and fatigue were more frequent in the exposed workers than in the controls (Srivastava et al. 1997).

Rajotte et al. (1996) analysed selenium in urine and plasma of 20 selenium-exposed workers of a copper refinery and of 20 controls. Interestingly, plasma selenium concentrations in exposed workers were significantly lower than those of the control group. In urine, there was no significant difference between both groups. The exposed workers reported more often on metallic taste, loss of weight, generalised cutaneous eruptions, hand, wrist and neck redness and skin burns. Two of the workers with cutaneous eruptions proposed other working conditions (dry air, moist hands) as a reason for their condition. One worker attributed the skin burns to nitric and sulfuric acids. There is no more information about the level of exposure and about the control group.

In a Canadian silver refinery, records about urinary analyses for selenium and tellurium concentrations were evaluated. There was no additional air sampling and the selenium exposure was not specified. Controls were not included (Berriault and Lightfood 2011).

Studies about chronic occupational exposures are summarised in Table 24.4. Except in the study of Rajotte et al. (1996), higher selenium concentrations were found in occupationally exposed workers when compared with an appropriate control group. Considering the large range of selenium concentrations in the normal populations of different regions and countries, the differences between the occupationally exposed group and the controls must be put into perspective, especially in plasma.

Table 24.4 Selenium levels in occupationally exposed workers

Region	Exposure	Study population	Selenium concentration (mean ± standard deviation (range))		Material	References
			Exposed workers	Controls		
Germany	Selenium-processing plant	Exposed workers (n = 20)	110 µg/m³ [a] (8–950 µg/m³)		Air	Göen et al. (2015)
			118 µg/L [a] (49–182 µg/L)	76 µg/L [a] (52–102 µg/L)	Plasma	
			107 µg/g creatinine [a] (16–816 µg/g creatinine)	23 µg/g creatinine [a] (12–50 µg/g creatinine)	Urine post-shift	
England	Selenium rectifier manufacture	Exposed workers (1517 samples from 200–300 workers; repeated measurements)	84 µg/L	34 ± 24 µg/L (0–150 µg/L)	Urine	Glover (1967)
Taiwan	Steel production and quality control	Steel production (n = 23), quality control (n = 23), internal controls (n = 23)	Steel production workers: 67.7 ± 27.4 µg/L (24.1–114 µg/L) Quality control workers: 52.6 ± 23.7 µg/L (21.9–107 µg/L)	33.2 ± 12.9 µg/L (13.0–58.9 µg/L)	Urine	Horng et al. (1999)
India	Manufacturing of photocopy machines	Exposed workers (n = 19)	120 µg/m³ (47–202 µg/m³)		Air	Srivastava et al. (1997)
			1.44 ± 0.37 µg/g (1.02–2.37 µg/g)	0.78 ± 0.18 µg/g (0.45–0.99 µg/g)	Hair	
Canada	Copper refinery	Exposed workers (n = 20)	137 ± 17.3 µg/L (114–174 µg/L)	155 ± 18.8 µg/L (120–187 µg/L)	Plasma	Rajotte et al. (1996)
			92.9 ± 42.8 µg/L (34.0–190 µg/L)	74.3 ± 25.3 µg/L (26.7–118 µg/L)	Urine	
Canada	Silver refinery	Exposed workers (n = 77)	49.8 ± 22.0 µg/g creatinine (14–126 µg/g creatinine)		Urine	Berriault and Lightfood (2011)

[a]Median

There are several case reports about occupationally caused selenium intoxica-
tions. One acute fatal selenium poisoning after an eruptive explosion while neutral-
ising selenic acid with caustic soda was reported (Schellmann et al. 1986). The
victim had a selenium concentration in the plasma of 18,400 µg/L and of 2110 µg/L
in urine. In a non-exposed group ($n = 10$) the median in plasma was 75 µg/L (range
32–102) and 24 µg/L (range 20–34) in urine. Another worker, who was employed in
a manufacture of drums used in photocopy machines, suffered from alopecia uni-
versalis. He had a selenium concentration of 500 µg/L in blood and 2.04 µg/g in the
nail. It was concluded that the alopecia may have been affected or caused by the
occupational exposure to selenium (Srivastava et al. 1995). Diskin et al. (1979)
described a patient with a chronic granulomatous hypersensitivity lung disease after
long-term selenium exposure. He had been employed in selenium refining for
50 years and showed reddish orange hair and red fingernails because of this exposure. Abnormal high selenium contents were found in the lung, the peribronchial
nodes, the hair and the nails.

Biological Limit Values

A toxicological evaluation of high selenium concentrations in biological materials
needs limit values, which indicate the threshold between the tolerable and non-
tolerable internal exposure. Up to now, only one biological limit value exists, which
was evaluated by the German Permanent Senate Commission for the Investigation
of Health Hazards in the Work Area (MAK commission) for the assessment of
occupational exposure to selenium and its inorganic compounds. The so-called biological tolerance value (BAT) was set to 150 µg selenium/L plasma, "at which the
health of an employee generally is not adversely affected even when the person is
repeatedly exposed during long periods" (DFG 2014). The BAT was evaluated considering the incidence of type 2 diabetes (T2D) during a long-term selenium supplementation study in the United States (Stranges et al. 2007). In the study a daily
supplementation of 200 µg selenium results in a significantly increased T2D risk in
individuals of highest selenium status, whereas the T2D risk was not significantly
increased in supplemented individuals with low and median basic plasma selenium
levels. These results imply that the acceptable external exposure to selenium may be
associated with the general selenium status of the population.

Conclusion

The internal selenium level differs between the populations in different geographic
locations due to the selenium content in the soil of the region and the resultant selenium burden of the regional food. The difference in the selenium status is reflected
by almost all of the human biomonitoring parameters. Most of the parameters

contain selenium bound in protein structures, which are generated under physiological control. However, the slow kinetics of most of these physiological processes imply a low sensitivity of most of the parameters for short-time variation of the selenium intake. Additionally, some excretion parameters, e.g. selenium in nails and hairs, are not balanced anymore after production, but persist several weeks or months after excretion. On the other hand, the variance in toxicokinetics of different selenium compounds and the small therapeutic margin demand a high specificity for the exposure to different selenium species. Again, parameters which only consist of protein-bound selenium are disadvantaged for specific diagnostics.

For diagnosis of individual short-time exposure to selenium compounds, the determination of selenium in urine presents the highest grade of both sensitivity and specificity. The urinary selenium level responds very quickly on any excess of selenium intake. Moreover, the urinary excretion contains a high share of low-molecular selenium species whose composition relates to the chemical composition of the selenium intake. Thus, a species analysis of the urinary selenium allows for a specific diagnosis of the selenium exposure.

However, several processes of selenium metabolism and toxicity are still not entirely understood, which also affects the validity and evidence of human biomonitoring parameters. In conjunction with a further exploration of these issues the diagnostic value of human biomonitoring parameters of selenium may advance.

References

Achouba A, Dumas P, Ouellet N, Lemire M, Ayotte P. Plasma levels of selenium-containing proteines in Inuit adults from Nunavik. Environ Int. 2016;96:8–15.

Alfthan G, Bogye G, Aro A, Feher J. The human selenium status of Hungary. J Trace Elem Electrolytes Health Dis. 1992;6:233–8.

Alfthan G, Eurola M, Ekholm P, Venäläinen ER, Root T, Korkalainen K, Hartikainen H, Salminen P, Hietaniemi V, Aspila P, Aro A, for the Selenium Working Group. Effects of nationwide addition of selenium to fertilizers on foods, and animal and human health in Finland: from deficiency to optimal selenium status of the population. J Trace Elem Med Biol. 2015;31:142–7.

Al-Saleh I, Al-Doush I, Faris R. Selenium levels in breast milk and cow's milk: a preliminary report from Saudi Arabia. J Environ Pathol Toxicol Oncol. 1997;16:41–6.

Al-Saleh I, Billedo G, El-Doush I, El-Din Mohamed G, Yosef G. Selenium and vitamins status in Saudi children. Clin Chim Acta. 2006;368:99–109.

Arnaud J, Prual A, Preziosi P, Favier A, Hercberg S. Selenium determination in human milk in Niger: influence of maternal status. J Trace Elem Electrolytes Health Dis. 1993;7:199–204.

Arnaud J, Bertrais S, Roussel AM, Arnault N, Ruffieux D, Favier A, Berthelin S, Estaquio S, Galan P, Czernichow S, Hercberg S. Serum selenium determination in French adults: the SU.VI.M.AX study. Br J Nutr. 2006;95:313–20.

Barron E, Migeot V, Séby F, Ingrand I, Potin-Gautier M, Legube B, Rabouan S. Selenium exposure in subjects living in areas with high selenium concentrated drinking water: results of a French integrated exposure assessment survey. Environ Int. 2012;40:155–61.

Bates CJ, Thane CW, Prentice A, Delves HT, Gregory J. Selenium status and associated factors in a British National Diet and Nutrition Survey: young people aged 4-18 y. Eur J Clin Nutr. 2002;56:873–81.

Beilstein MA, Whanger PD. Glutathione peroxidase activity and chemical forms of selenium in tissues of rats given selenite or selenomethionine. J Inorg Biochem. 1988;33(1):31–46.

Bendahl L, Gammelgaard B. Separation and identification of Se-methylselenogalactosamine – a new metabolite in basal human urine - by HPLC-ICP-MS and CE-nano-ESI-(MS). J Anal At Spectrom. 2004;19:950–7.

Berriault CJ, Lightfood NE. Occupational tellurium exposure and garlic odour. Occup Med. 2011;61:132–5.

Brantsæter AL, Haugen M, Thomassen Y, Ellingsen DG, Yderrsbond TA, Hagve TA, Alexander J, Meltzer HM. Exploration of biomarkers for total fish intake in pregnant Norwegian women. Public Health Nutr. 2009;13:54–62.

Brätter P, Negretti de Brätter VE, Recknagel S, Brunetto R. Maternal selenium status influences the concentration and binding pattern of zinc in human milk. J Trace Elem Med Biol. 1997;11:203–9.

Burk RF, Hill KE. Regulation of selenium metabolism and transport. Annu Rev Nutr. 2015;35:109–34.

Burk RF, Hill KE, Motley AK. Plasma selenium in specific and non-specific forms. Biofactors. 2001;14:107–14.

Chen CJ, Lai JS, Wu CC, Lin TS. Serum selenium in adult Taiwanese. Sci Total Environ. 2006;357:448–50.

Christian WJ, Hopenhayn C, Centeno JA, Todorov T. Distribution of urinary selenium and arsenic among pregnant women exposed to arsenic in drinking water. Environ Res. 2006;100:115–22. https://doi.org/10.1016/j.envres.2005.03.009.

Combs GF Jr, Watts JC, Jackson MI, Johnson LK, Zeng H, Scheett AJ, Uthus EO, Schomburg L, Hoeg A, Hoefig CS, Davis CD, Milner JA. Determinants of selenium status in healthy adults. Nutr J. 2011;10:75.

Dawber R. Fingernail growth in normal and psokiatic subjects. Br J Nutr. 1970;82:454–7.

van der Torre HW, Van Dokkum W, Schaafsma G, Wedel M, Ockhuizen T. Effect of various levels of selenium in wheat and meat on blood Se status indices and on Se balance in Dutch men. Br J Nutr. 1991;65(1):69–80.

Devereux G, McNeill G, Newman G, Turner S, Craig L, Marindale S, Helms P, Seaton A. Early childhood wheezing symptoms in relation to plasma selenium in pregnant mothers and neonates. Clin Exp Allergy. 2007;37:1000–8.

DFG - Deutsche Forschungsgemeinschaft. List of MAK and BAT values 2014. Commission on the Investigation of Health Hazards of Substances in the Work Area. Report No. 50. Wiley-VCH, Weinheim. 2014. doi: https://doi.org/10.1002/9783527682010.oth2.

Diskin CJ, Tomasso CL, Alper JC, Glaser MK, Fliegel SE. Long-term selenium exposure. Arch Intern Med. 1979;139:824–6.

Dorea JG. Selenium and breast-feeding. Br J Nutr. 2002;88:443–61.

Dörner K, Schneider K, Sievers E, Schulz-Lell G, Oldings HD, Schaub J. Selenium balance in young infants fed on breast milk and adapted cow's milk formula. J Trace Elem Electrolytes Health Dis. 1990;4:37–40.

Francesconi KA, Pannier F. Selenium metabolites in urine: a critical overview of past work and current status. Clin Chem. 2004;50:2240–53.

Gammelgaard B, Bendahl L. Selenium speciation in human urine samples by LC- and CEICP-MS - separation and identification of selenosugars. J Anal At Spectrom. 2004;19:135–42.

Gammelgaard B, Jøns O. Determination of selenite and selenate in human urine by ion chromatography and inductively coupled plasma mass spectrometry. J Anal At Spectrom. 2000;15:945–9.

Gammelgaard B, Madsen KG, Bjerrum J, Bendahl L, Jøns O, Olsen J, Sidenius U. Separation, purification and identification of the major selenium metabolite from human urine by multidimensional HPLC-ICP-MS and APCI-MS. J Anal At Spectrom. 2003;18:65–70.

Geyer AS, Onumah N, Uyttendaele H, Scher RK. Modulation of linear nail growth to treat diseases of the nail. J Am Acad Dermatol. 2004;50:229–34.

Gil F, Hermández AF. Toxicological importance of human biomonitoring of metallic and metalloid elements in different biological samples. Food Chem Toxicol. 2015;80:287–97.

Glover JR. Selenium in human urine: a tentative maximum allowable concentration for industrial and rural population. Ann Occup Hyg. 1967;10:3–14.

Glover JR. Selenium and its industrial toxicology. IMS Ind Med Surg. 1970;39:50–4.

Göen T, Schaller B, Jäger T, Bräu-Dümler C, Schaller KH, Drexler H. Biological monitoring of exposure and effects in workers employed in a selenium-processing plant. Int Arch Occup Environ Health. 2015;88:623–30.

Golubkina NA, Alfthan GV. The human selnelium status in 27 regions of Russia. J Trace Elem Med Biol. 1999;13:15–20.

Greiner A, Göen T, Hildebrand J, Feltes R, Drexler H. Low resorption of selenium and absence of adverse effects in workers exposed to high air levels of inorganic selenium. Toxicol Lett. 2018; https://doi.org/10.1016/j.toxlet.2018.06.1214.

Griffiths NM, Stewart RDH, Robinson MF. The metabolism of [^{75}Se]selenomethionine in four women. Br J Nutr. 1976;35:373–82.

Gundacker C, Komarnicki G, Zödl B, Forster C, Schuster E, Wittmann K. Whole blood mercury and selenium concentrations in a selected Austrian population: does gender matter? Sci Total Environ. 2006;372:76–86. https://doi.org/10.1016/j.scitotenv.2006.08.006.

Ha'c E, Krechniak J, Szyszko M. Selenium levels in human plasma and hair in Northern Poland. Biol Trace Elem Res. 2002;85:277–85.

Hagmar L, Persson-Moschos M, Åkesson B, Schütz A. Plasma levels of selenium, selenoprotein P, and glutathione peroxidase and their correlations to fish intake and serum levels of thyrotropin and thyroid hormones: a study on Latvian fish consumser. Eur J Clin Nutr. 1998;52:796–800.

Hannan MA, Dogadkin NN, Ashur IA, Markus WM. Copper, selenium and zinc concentrations in human milk during the first three weeks of lactation. Biol Trace Elem Res. 2005;107:11–20.

Haratake M, Fujimoto K, Hirakawa R, Ono M, Nakayama M. Hemoglobin-mediated selenium export from red blood cells. J Biol Inorg Chem. 2008;13:471–9.

He K. Trace elements in nails as biomarkers in clinical research. Eur J Clin Invest. 2011;41:98–102.

Horng CJ, Tsai JL, Lin SR. Determination of urinary arsenic, mercury, and senelium in steel production workers. Biol Trace Elem Res. 1999;70:29–40.

Hughes K, Chua LH, Ong CN. Serum selenium in the general population of Singapore, 1993 to 1995. Ann Acad Med Singapore. 1998;27:520–3.

Jäger T, Drexler H, Göen T. Ion pairing and ion exchange chromatography coupled to ICP-MS to determine selenium species in human urine. J Anal At Spectrom. 2013;28:1402–9. https://doi.org/10.1039/c3ja50083g.

Jäger T, Drexler H, Göen T. Human metabolism and renal excretion of selenium compounds after oral ingestion of sodium selenate dependent on trimethylselenium ion (TMSe) status. Arch Toxicol. 2016a;90:149–58.

Jäger T, Drexler H, Göen T. Human metabolism and renal excretion of selenium compounds after oral ingestion of sodium selenite and selenized yeast dependent on trimethylselenium ion (TMSe) status. Arch Toxicol. 2016b;90:1069–80.

Jitaru P, Pret M, Cozzi C, Turetta C, Cairns W, Seraglia R. Speciatio analysis of selenoproteins in human serum by solid-phase extraction and affinity HPLC hyphenated to ICP-quadrupole MS. J Anal At Spectrom. 2008;23:402–6.

Kempson IM, Lombi E. Hair analysis as a biomarker for toxicolgoy, disease and health status. Chem Soc Rev. 2011;40:3915–40.

Kim YJ, Galindev O, Sei JH, Bae SM, Im H, Wen L, Seo YR, Ahn WS. Serum selenium level in healthy koreans. Biol Trace Elem Res. 2009;131:103–9.

Kuehnelt D, Kienzl N, Traar P, Le NH, Francesconi KA, Ochi T. Selenium metabolites in human urine after ingestion of selenite, L-selenomethionine, or DL-selenomethionine: a quantitative case study by HPLC/ICPMS. Anal Bioanal Chem. 2005;383:235–46.

Kvicala J, Zamrazil V, Jiránek V. Characterization of selenium status in inhabitants in the region Ústi nad Orlici, Czech Republik by INAA of blood serum and hair and fluorimetric analysis of urine. Biol Trace Elem Res. 1999;71-72:31–9.

Labunskyy VM, Hatfield DL, Gladyshev VN. Selenoproteins: molecular pathways and physiological roles. Physiol Rev. 2014;94:739–77.

Laclaustra M, Navas-Acien A, Stranges S, Ordovas JM, Guallar E. Serum selenium concentrations and diabetes in U.S. adults: National Health and Nutrition Examination Survey (NHANES) 2003-2004. Environ Health Perspect. 2009;117:1409–13.

Lemire M, Mergler D, Fillon M, Passos CJS, Guimarães JRD, Davidson R, Lucotte M. Elevated blood selenium levels in the Brazilian Amazon. Sci Total Environ. 2006;366:101–11.

Lemire M, Fillon M, Barbosa F, Guimarães JRD, Mergler D. Elevated levels of selenium in the typical diet of Amazonian reverside population. Sci Total Environ. 2010;408:4076–84.

Letsiou S, Lu Y, Nomikos T, Antonopoulou S, Panagiotakos D, Pitsavos C, et al. High-throughput quantification of selenium in individual serum proteins from a healthy human population using HPLC on-line with isotope dilution inductively coupled plasma-MS. Preteomics. 2010;10:3447–57.

Levander OA, Alfthan G, Arvilommi H, Gref CG, Huttunen JK, Kataja M, Koivistoinen P, Pikkarainen J. Bioavailabiality of selenium to Finnish men as assessed by platelet glutathione peroxidase activity and other blood parameters. Am J Clin Nutr. 1983;37:887–97.

Levander OA, Moser PB, Morris VC. Dietary selenium intake and selenium concentrations of plasma, erythrocytes, and breast milk in pregnant and postpartum lactating and nonlactating women. Am J Clin Nutr. 1987;46(4):694–948.

Longnecker MP, Taylor PR, Levander OA, Howe SM, Veillon C, MacAdam PA, Patterson KY, Holden JM, Stampfer MJ, Morris JS, Willett WC. Selenium in diet, blood, and toenails in relation to human health in a seleniferous area. Am J Clin Nutr. 1991;53:1288–94.

Lymbury R, Tinggi U, Griffiths L, Rosenfeldt F, Perkins AV. Selenium status of the Australian population: effect of age, gender and cardiovascular disease. Biol Trace Elem Res. 2008;126(Suppl. 1):S1–S10.

Mark SD, Qiao YL, Dawsey SM, Wu YP, Katki H, Gunter EW, Fraumeni JF, Blot WJ, Dong ZW, Taylor PR. Prospective study of serum selenium levels and incident esophageal and gastric cancer. J Natl Cancer Inst. 2000;92:1733–63.

Martens IBG, Cardosa B, Hare DJ, Niedzwiecki MM, Lajolo FM, Martens A, Cozzolino SMF. Selenium status in preschool children receiving a Brazil nut-enriched diet. Nutrition. 2015;31:1339–43.

Martin RF, Janghorbani M, Young V. Kinetics of a single administration of [74]Se-Selenite by oral and intravenous routes in adult humans. J Parentaer External Nutr. 1988;12:31–355.

Michalke B, Schramel P. Application of capillary zone electrophoresis-inductively coupled plasma mass spectrometry and capillary isoelectric focusing-inductively coupled plasma mass spectrometry for selenium species. J Chromatogr A. 1998;807:71–80.

Michalke B, Rossbach B, Göen T, Schäferhenrich A, Scherer G. Saliva as a matrix for human biomonitoring in occupational and environmental medicine. Int Arch Occup Environ Health. 2015;88:1–44.

Moreno-Reyes R, Suetens C, Mathieu F, Begaux F, Zhu D, Rivera MT, Boelaert M, Néve J, Perlmutter N, Vanderpas J. Kashin-Beck osteoarthropathy in rural Tibet in relation to selenium and iodine status. N Engl J Med. 1998;339:1112–20.

Morris JS, Stampfer MJ, Willett W. Dietary selenium in humans. Toenails as an indicator. Biol Trace Elem Res. 1983;5:529–37.

Muntau AC, Streiter M, Kappler M, Röschinger W, Schmid I, Rehnert A, Schramel P, Roscher AA. Age-related reference values for serum selenium concentrations in infants and children. Clin Chem. 2002;48:555–60.

Nahapetian AT, Young VR, Janghorbani M. Measurement of trimethylselenonium ion in human urine. Anal Biochem. 1984;140:56–62.

Navarro-Alarcon M, Cabrera-Vique C. Selenium in food and the human body: a review. Sci Total Environ. 2008;400:115–41. https://doi.org/10.1016/j.scitotenv.2008.06.024.

Nève J. Methods in determination of selenium status. J Trace Elem Electrolytes Health Dis. 1991;5:1–7.

Ogra Y, Hatano T, Ohmichi M, Suzuki KT. Oxidative production of monomethylated selenium from the major urinary selenometabolite, selenosugar. J Anal At Spectrom. 2003;18:1252–5.

Olmez I, Gulovali MC, Gordon GE, Henkin RI. Trace elements in human parotid saliva. Biol Trace Elem Res. 1988;17:259–70.

Oster O, Prellwitz W. The renal excretion of selenium. Biol Trace Elem Res. 1990;24:119–46.

Özdemir HS, Karadas F, Pappas AC, Cassey P, Oto G, Tuncer O. The selenium levels in mothers and their neonates using hair, breast milk, meconium, and maternal and umbilical cord blood in Van Basin. Biol Trace Elem Res. 2008;122:206–15.

Parshukova O, Potolitsyna N, Shadrina V, Chernykh A, Bojko E. Features of selenium metabolism in humans living under the conditions of North European Russia. Int Arch Occup Environ Health. 2014;87:607–14.

Raghunath R, Tripathi RM, Mahapatra S, Sadasivan S. Selenium status in biological matrices in adult population of Mumbai, India. Sci Total Environ. 2002;285:21–7.

Rajotte BJ, P'an AY, Malick A, Robin JP. Evaluation of selenium exposure in copper refinery workers. J Toxicol Environ Health. 1996;48(3):239–51.

Reilly C. Selenium in food and health. New York: Springer; 2006.

Reyes LH, Marchante-Gayón JM, Alonso JHJG, Sanz-Medel A. Quantitative speciation of selenium in humn serum by affinity chromatography coupled to post-column isotope dilution analysis ICP-MS. J Anal At Spectrom. 2003;18:1210–6.

Robinson M, Rea HM, Friend GM, Stewart DH, Snow C, Thomson CD. On supplementing the selenium intake of New Zealanders. 2. Prolonged metabolic experiments with daily supplements of selenomethionine, selenite and fish. Br J Nutr. 1978;39:589–600.

Robinson JR, Robinson MF, Levander OA, Thomson CD. Urinary excretion of selenium by New Zealander and North American human subjects on differing intakes. Am J Clin Nutr. 1985;41:1023–31.

Robinson M, Thomson CD, Jenkinson CP, Luzhen G, Whanger PD. Long-term supplementation with selenate and selenomethionine: urinary excretion by New Zealand women. Br J Nutr. 1997;77:551–63.

Safaralizadeh R, Kardar GA, Pourpak Z, Moin M, Zare A, Teimourian S. Serum concentration of selenium in healthy individuals living in Tehran. Nutr J. 2005;4:32.

Safaralizadeh R, Sirjani M, Pourpak Z, Kardar GA, Teimourioan S, Shams S, Namdar Z, Kazemnejad A, Moin M. Serum selenium concentration in healthy children living in Tehran. Biofactors. 2007;31:127–31.

Sánchez C, López-Jurado M, Aranda P, Llopis J. Plasma levels of copper, manganese and selenium in an adult population in southern Spain : influence of age, obesity and lifestyle factors. Sci Total Environ. 2010;408(2010):1014–20.

Satia JA, King IB, Morris JS, Stratton K, White E. Toenail and plasma levels as biomarkers of selenium exposure. Ann Epidemiol. 2006;16:53–8.

Schellmann B, Raithel HJ, Schaller KH. Acute fatal selenium poisoning. Arch Toxicol. 1986;59:61–3.

Schierling P, Oefele C, Schaller KH. Bestimmung von Arsen und Selen in Harnproben mit der Hydrid-AAS-Technik. Ärztl Lab. 1982;28:21–7.

Sesana G, Baj A, Toffoletto F, Sega R, Ghezzi L. Plasma selenium levels of the general populatoin of an area in northern Italy. Sci Total Environ. 1992;120:97–102.

Spina A, Guallar E, Rayman MP, Tigbe W, Kandala NB, Stranges S. Anthropometric indices and selenium status in British adults: the U.K. National Diet and Nutrition Survey. Free Rad Biol Med. 2013;65:1315–21.

Srivastava AK, Gupta BN, Bihari V, Gaur JS. Generalized hair loss and selenium exposure. Vet Human Toxicol. 1995;37:468–9.

Srivastava AK, Gupta BN, Bihari V, Gaur JS, Mathur N. Hair selenium as a monitoring tool for occupational exposure in relation to clinical profile. J Toxicol Environ Health. 1997;51:437–45.

Stranges S, Marshall JR, Natarajan R, Donahue RP, Trevisan M, Combs GF, Cappuccio FP, Ceriello A, Reid ME. Effects of long-term selenium supplementation on the incidence of type 2 diabetes: a randomized trial. Ann Intern Med. 2007;147:217–23.

Swanson CA, Longnecker MP, Veillon C, Howe SM, Levander OA, Taylor PR, McAdam PA, Brown CC, Stampfer MJ, Willett WC. Selenium intake, age, gender, and smoking in relation to indices of selenium status of adults residing in a seleniferous area. Am J Clin Nutr. 1990;52:858–62.

Thomson CD, Stewart RDH. The metabolism of [^{75}Se]selenite in young women. Br J Nutr. 1974;32:47–57.

Thomson CD, Ong LK, Robinson MF. Effects of supplementation with high-selenium wheat bread on selenium, glutathione peroxidase and related enzymes in blood components of New Zealand residents. Am J Clin Nutr. 1985;41:1015–23.

Thomson CD, Robinson MF, Butler JA, Whanger PD. Long-term supplementation with selenite and selenomethionine: selenium and glutathione peroxidase in blood components of New Zealand women. Br J Nutr. 1993;69:577–88.

Van Cauwenbergh R, Robbrecht H, Van Vlaslaer V, Deelstra H. Comparison of the selenium content of healthy adults living in the Antwerp region (Belgium) with recent literature data. J Trace Elem Med Biol. 2004;18:99–112.

Villain M, Cirimele V, Kintz P. Hair analysis in toxicology. Clin Chem Lab Med. 2004;42:1265–72.

Vinceti M, Wei ET, Malagoli C, Bergomi M, Vivoli G. Adverse health effects of selenium in humans. Rev Environ Health. 2001;16:233–51.

Wasowicz W, Gromadzinska J, Szram K, Rydzynski K, Cieslak J, Pietrzak Z. Selenium, zinc and copper concentrations in the blood and milk of lactating women. Biol Trace Elem Res. 2001;79(2001):221–3.

Wasowicz W, Gromadzinska J, Rydzynski K, Tamczak J. Selenium status of low-selenium area residens: polish experrience. Toxicol Lett. 2003;137:95–101.

Wolters M, Hermann S, Golf S, Katz N, Hahn A. Selenium and antioxidant vitamin status of elderly German women. Eur J Clin Nutr. 2006;60:85–91. https://doi.org/10.1038/sj.ejcn.1602271.

Xia Y, Zhao Z, Zhu L, Whanger PD. Metabolism of selenate and selenomethionine by a selenium-deficient population of men in China. J Nutr Biochem. 1992;3:202–10.

Yaemsiri S, Hou N, Slining MM, He K. Growth rate of human fingernails and toenails in healthy American young adults. J Eur Acad Dermatol Venereol. 2010;24:420–3.

Yang G, Zhou R, Yin S, Gu L, Yan B, Liu Y, Liu Y, Li X. Studies of safe maximal daily dietary intake in a seleniferous area in China. J Trace Elem Electrolytes Health Dis. 1989a;3:77–87.

Yang G, Yin S, Zhou R, Gu L, Yan B, Lin Y, Liu Y. Studies of safe maximum daily dietary Se-intake in a seleniferous area in China. Part II: relation between Se-intake and the manifestation of clinical signs and certain biochemical alterations in blood and urine. J Trace Elem Electrolytes Health Dis. 1989b;3:123–31.

Yoshida N, Inaoka T, Sultana N, Ahmad SA, Mabachi A, Shimizu H, Watanabe C. Non-monotonic relationship between arsenic and selenium excretion and its implication on arsenic methylation pattern in a Bangladeshi population. Environ Res. 2015;140:300–7.

Zachara BA, Pilecki A. Selenium concentration in the milk of breast-feeding mothers and its geographic distribution. Environ Health Perspect. 2000;108:1043–6.

Zaichick VA, Tsyb AF, Bagirov S. Neutron activation analysis of saliva application in clinical chemistry, environmental and occupational toxicology. J Radioanal Nucl Chem. 1995;195:123–32.

Chapter 25
Bioanalytical Chemistry of Selenium

Yasumitsu Ogra, Yasumi Anan, and Noriyuki Suzuki

Abstract Selenium (Se) is an interesting element for bioanalytical chemists. Se forms Se-containing compounds having Se-carbon covalent bond(s), i.e., selenometabolites in its metabolic pathway. In this chapter, the analytical techniques for the speciation and identification of unique selenometabolites in animals are highlighted. First, the instruments required for analyses are overviewed. In particular, hyphenated techniques consisting of high-performance liquid chromatography and inductively coupled plasma (tandem) mass spectrometry (ICP-MS) or electrospray ionization (tandem) mass spectrometry are focused on. Second, laser ablation hyphenated with ICP-MS for Se imaging is briefly overviewed. Then, advanced techniques of nuclear magnetic resonance (NMR) spectroscopy for Se analysis are mentioned with an application to a biological sample.

Keywords Speciation · LC-ICP-MS(/MS) · LC-ESI-MS(/MS) · NMR · Selenoprotein P · Glutathione peroxidase · Selenosugar · Selenocyanate · Selenomethionine

Introduction

Selenium (Se) has interesting characteristics in terms of not only biology but also analytical chemistry due to the following reasons: (1) Se exists in an ultra-trace amount as an essential element, suggesting that the detection itself is challenging. (2) In plants, Se is not an essential element, and shares almost metabolic pathways of sulfur (S) that is the same group 16 element as Se and is an essential element of plants. This indicates that Se-substituted metabolites of S-containing metabolites

Y. Ogra (✉) · N. Suzuki
Laboratory of Toxicology and Environmental Health, Graduate School of Pharmaceutical Sciences, Chiba University, Chiba, Japan
e-mail: ogra@chiba-u.jp; ogra@ac.shoyaku.ac.jp

Y. Anan
Laboratory of Health Chemistry, Showa Pharmaceutical Sciences, Tokyo, Japan

© Springer International Publishing AG, part of Springer Nature 2018   495
B. Michalke (ed.), *Selenium*, Molecular and Integrative Toxicology,
https://doi.org/10.1007/978-3-319-95390-8_25

are present in plants. Contrary to plants, Se is an essential element in animals, and is metabolized in its specific pathway, suggesting that unique Se-specific metabolites are found and expected in animals. These indicate that variety kinds of selenometabolites are expected in nature. (3) Se consists of six naturally occurring isotopes, i.e., ^{74}Se, 0.89%; ^{76}Se, 9.36%; ^{77}Se, 7.63%; ^{78}Se, 23.8%; ^{80}Se, 49.6%; and ^{82}Se, 8.73%. The fact facilitates the scanning of Se-containing species by mass spectrometry. (4) ^{77}Se is one of the nuclides detectable by nuclear magnetic resonance (NMR) spectroscopy. On the other hand, analytical instruments for the Se detection have been well developed. For instance, atomic absorption spectrometry (AAS), atomic fluorescence spectrometry (AFS), inductively coupled plasma-atomic emission spectrometry (ICP-AES), and ICP-mass spectrometry (ICP-MS) are used for the detection of Se as an element. Electrospray ionization (ESI) or atmospheric pressure chemical ionization (APCI)-mass spectrometry has also been used. As ESI and APCI are softer ionization sources than ICP, they can provide molecular information of selenometabolites (Ogra 2008). For solid identifications such as determination of absolute configuration of selenometabolite, ^{1}H NMR has been used. As mentioned above, ^{77}Se NMR is also applicable for the characterization of Se in biological samples.

In this chapter, the analytical techniques of Se in biological samples are addressed. First, the speciation and the identification of Se by HPLC coupled with mass spectrometry are overviewed. Namely, the techniques used for the speciation of serum selenoproteins are mentioned. Then, the identification of selenometabolites is also mentioned. Second, the Se imaging by laser ablation (LA)-ICP-MS is overviewed. Finally, ^{77}Se NMR used for selenometabolites is mentioned.

Hyphenated Techniques

HPLC Coupled with Mass Spectrometry

The hyphenated technique is the most frequently used analytical technique for speciation analysis. The term "speciation" of an element (metal or metalloid) is defined as the distribution of an element among defined chemical species in a system, whereas speciation analysis is defined as the analytical activities undertaken to identify and/or measure the quantities of one or more chemical species in a sample (Templeton et al. 2000). The hyphenated technique for metal/metalloid speciation consists of two analytical techniques: the separation technique and the detection technique (Becker and Jakubowski 2009). Chromatography (Szpunar and Łobiński 2002) and capillary electrophoresis (Prange and Pröfrock 2005) are generally used as the separation technique. Among these separation techniques, chromatography, in particular, HPLC, is the most commonly used. Then, ICP-MS is the most frequently used separation technique for Se speciation.

ICP is a hard ionization source for the generation of ions of elemental atoms, and the generated ions are sampled by a mass spectrometer. Single-quadrupole, triple-quadrupole, time-of-flight (TOF), and sector-field (SF) mass spectrometers have been employed with ICP. ICP equipped with a single-quadrupole mass spectrometer, i.e., ICP-MS, is the most widely used among the ICP-mass spectrometers. ICP-MS is a powerful tool for Se detection because its high-energy argon plasma efficiently ionizes Se for the detection by the mass spectrometer. Because of easy hyphenation with HPLC, LC-ICP-MS is the technique of choice for speciation of biological samples.

Speciation of Selenoproteins

Two selenoproteins, extracellular glutathione peroxidase (GPX3), and selenoprotein P (SELENOP) were detected in animal plasma (Borglund et al. 1988; Akesson and Martensson 1988; Persson-Moschos et al. 1995). In addition to GPX3 and SELENOP, Se-containing protein(s) were also detected. A Se-containing protein is a protein that has Se incorporated into its peptide sequence as selenomethionine (SeMet) (Jitaru et al. 2010). The most abundant Se-containing protein in human plasma is albumin (Daniels 1996). However, some studies have indicated that no or little albumin is detected in blood plasma of experimental animals compared to human plasma (Òscar and Łobiński 2007; Kobayashi et al. 2001; Koyama et al. 1996). This can be explained by the fact that human ingests Se mainly as SeMet, whereas the major Se species in experimental animals is inorganic Se, such as selenite and selenate, which are used as feed additive.

Herein, speciation of serum selenoproteins by LC-ICP-MS/MS is shown. The elution profiles of Se in rat serum obtained by ICP-tandem mass spectrometry (ICP-MS/MS) and ICP-single mass spectrometry (ICP-MS) were compared (Fig. 25.1). Two major Se peaks were detected. According to the Western blotting, the faster and the latter are assigned as GPX3 and SELENOP, respectively (Anan et al. 2013). Because body nutritional status of Se reflects the peak heights of these serum selenoproteins (Takahashi et al. 2017), this technique is applicable to evaluate Se deficiency clinically. Although ICP-MS is a powerful tool to detect Se, the interference by polyatomic ions is an ineluctable disadvantage. The three most abundant Se isotopes, ^{80}Se (49.6%), ^{78}Se (23.8%), and ^{76}Se (9.36%), suffer from interference by several polyatomic ions originating from the plasma source argon (Ar), namely, ^{40}Ar^{40}Ar$^+$, ^{40}Ar^{38}Ar$^+$, and ^{38}Ar^{38}Ar$^+$, respectively. In addition, interference by ^{40}Ar^{37}Cl$^+$ on ^{77}Se is not avoidable when chloride exists as the matrix in a sample, such as biological samples. Thus, the less abundant ^{82}Se isotope (8.73%) is the most frequently used among the Se isotopes for Se detection by ICP-MS. To overcome those problems, an ICP-MS equipped with a collision/reaction cell was developed. In the detection of Se, several techniques that use a collision/reaction cell are available (Sloth and Larsen 2000). For instance, hydrogen (H_2), helium (He), and methane (CH_4) gases are used alone or in combination as the collision/reaction gas (Sloth et al. 2003; Darrouzès et al. 2005; Guo et al. 2013). However, those gases often reduce the sensitivity of Se detection. The use of H_2 leads to

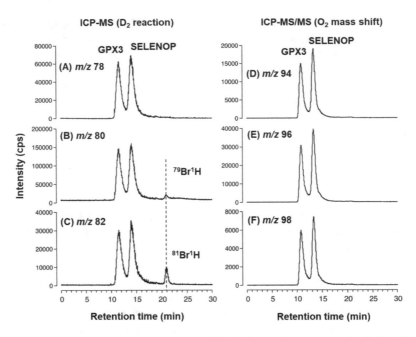

Fig. 25.1 Elution profiles of Se in rat serum. A 200 μL aliquot of a serum sample obtained from a male Wistar rat was injected into a Shodex Asahipak GS-520HQ column (7.5 i.d. × 300 mm, with a guard column, 7.5 i.d. × 75 mm, Showa Denko, Tokyo, Japan), and then eluted with 50 mmol/L Tris–HCl, pH 7.4, at a flow rate of 0.6 mL/min. The eluate was monitored by ICP-MS (**A–C**) or ICP-MS/MS (**D, E**) at M/Z 78 (**A**), 80 (**B**), 82 (**C**), 94 (**D**), 96 (**E**), and 98 (**F**)

another problem in the detection of Se in extracellular fluid, such as plasma/serum and urine: as extracellular fluid contains substantial amounts of bromine (Br) as the matrix, newly generated polyatomic interferences originating from the matrix of Br and the reaction gas of H_2, i.e., $^{79}Br^1H^+$ and $^{81}Br^1H^+$, adversely affect the detection of ^{80}Se and ^{82}Se, respectively. The use of deuterium (D_2) in place of H_2 enabled us to avoid those interferences because the interferences were shifted to m/z 81 ($^{79}Br^2D^+$) and m/z 83 ($^{81}Br^2D^+$) (Ogra et al. 2005). The D_2 reaction mode was practically effective for the detection of Se in extracellular fluid. However, a new problem arose that hindered the accurate measurement of the isotope ratios of Se: D_2 reacted with Se in the reaction cell to generate $^{78}Se^2D^+$ and $^{80}Se^2D^+$ that interfered with ^{80}Se and ^{82}Se, respectively.

As shown in Fig. 25.1B, C, the peak corresponding to BrH was well separated from the peaks of the two selenoproteins. The problem caused by D_2 was the interference by SeD as depicted in Fig. 25.2C, and this interference was not avoidable even though speciation was applied to the Se determination. Indeed, the signal at m/z 80 overlapped with the signal for $^{78}Se^2D^+$, and the signal at m/z 82 was more severely affected than that at m/z 80 because ^{80}Se had a larger abundance than ^{78}Se (Fig. 25.3A). ICP-MS/MS was used under the O_2 mass shift mode for Se speciation (Fig. 25.2D). At the first quadrupole (Q1), the ions detected at m/z 78, 80, and 82 were eliminating Br (m/z 81 and 83). Then, O_2 was introduced into the reaction/col-

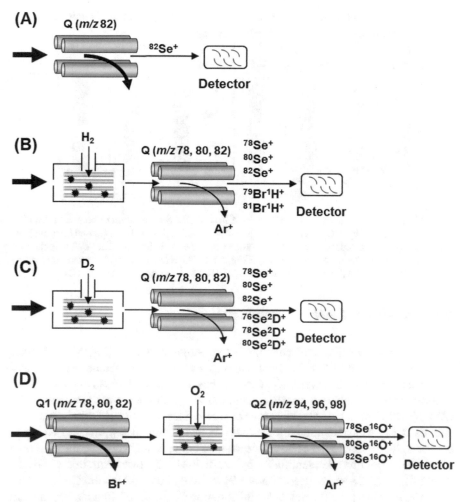

Fig. 25.2 Schematic diagram of the detection of Se in extracellular fluid by ICP-MS under normal (**A**), H₂ (**B**), and D₂ (**C**) modes, and ICP-MS/MS under the O₂ mass shift mode (**D**)

lision cell to collide with dimerized Ar ions, such as $^{38}Ar^{38}Ar^{+}$, $^{38}Ar^{40}Ar^{+}$, and $^{40}Ar^{40}Ar^{+}$, and to shift m/z for the detection of Se at 94, 96, and 98 at the second quadrupole (Q2). No interference originating from BrH was detected on the elution profiles obtained by ICP-MS/MS under the O₂ mass shift mode (Fig. 25.2D–F). In addition, the peak heights of the two serum selenoproteins obtained by ICP-MS/MS were more accurate than those obtained by ICP-MS for the three Se isotopes (Fig. 25.3B). Consequently, ICP-MS/MS is a more powerful tool for the speciation of Se in biological samples than ICP-MS. ICP-SF-MS instruments can be operated in high-resolution mode, where ^{77}Se—but not the other, more abundant selenium isotopes—can be completely resolved from respective interferences (e.g., $[^{40}Ar^{37}Cl]^{+}$, $[^{40}Ar^{36}Ar^{1}H]^{+}$). Though Se speciation at ^{77}Se is usually not interfered with ICP-SF-MS, detection is less sensitive due to the lower isotopic abundance.

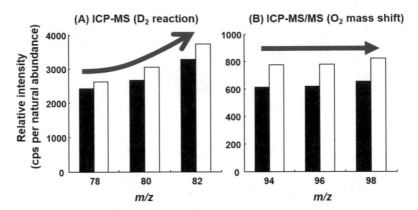

Fig. 25.3 Effect of O mass shift mode by ICP-MS/MS on the Se speciation of rat serum. Relative intensity was defined by counts per second (cps) of the peak heights of GPX3 (closed columns) and SELENOP (open columns) divided by the isotope ratio of each Se isotope. The peak heights were calculated from the elution profiles shown in Fig. 25.1. The relative intensities were obtained by ICP-MS with the D reaction mode (**A**) and ICP-MS/MS with the mass-shift mode (**B**)

Identification of Selenometabolites

In the preceding section, the speciation of selenoproteins by LC-ICP-MS(/MS) is mentioned. LC-ICP-MS is also applicable to analyze selenometabolites with low molecular weight. However, LC-ICP-MS has one crucial disadvantage. Since ICP-MS provides only elemental information of metabolites, the identification by LC-ICP-MS is effective only when the retention times of samples could be matched with those of certified or authentic species (standard compounds). In other words, if the authentic Se compound of an unknown metabolite is not available, the unknown metabolite would not be identifiable by LC-ICP-MS. To overcome this disadvantage, ESI- or APCI-MS is used. Since ESI and APCI are softer ionization sources than ICP, they can provide molecular information (Ogra 2008). In addition, tandem mass spectrometry (MS/MS) and multistage cascade of mass spectrometry (MS^n) enable structure elucidation. Indeed, ESI-MS-MS and ESI-MS^n have been available for the identification of unknown selenometabolites. However, ESI-MS has two weak points compared with ICP-MS. First, the detection limit of ESI-MS for Se-containing compounds is inferior to that of ICP-MS (Anan et al. 2015b). Second, ESI-MS is severely affected by the sample matrix. More elaborate pretreatment is required for the analysis by ESI-MS than that by ICP-MS. Thus, the complementary use of ESI-MS and ICP-MS is the best approach to the identification of unknown selenometabolites. It is difficult for mass spectrometry to distinguish enantiomers and diastereomers. NMR spectroscopy, in contrast, can rigorously define the structure and/or configuration of a chemical species; thus, it is regarded as the most valuable technique for identification, and can be utilized for the precise identification of metabolites. However, NMR spectroscopy requires more stringent purification methods and a higher concentration of sample than ESI-MS. Thus, this technique seems to be not always applicable to the identification of trace selenometabolites in animal and plant samples.

In this section, two identifications of unique selenometabolites in animals are shown.

Selenosugars

Se utilized in a body is mostly excreted in urine. Within the nutritional level and the low toxicity level, the major urinary metabolite is *Se*-methylseleno-*N*-acetylgalactosamine (MeSeGalNAc, selenosugar 1, or SeSugar1) as identified by LC-ICP-MS, ESI-MS-MS, and NMR (Kobayashi et al. 2002). The mass spectra of the fragment ions of SeSugar1 obtained by LC-ESI-MS are indicated in Fig. 25.4. Three precursor ions, m/z 298, 300, and 302, representing Se isotopes, ^{78}Se, ^{80}Se, and ^{82}Se, respectively, were extracted with the first quadrupole MS and then introduced into a collision cell to obtain their fragment ions. Thereafter, the fragment ions were detected with the second quadrupole MS. At low collision energies, all the parent ions produced the same major product ion at m/z 204, suggesting that a Se-containing moiety was cleaved off from each of the parent ions (Fig. 25.5A–C). Because the difference in m/z between the precursor ion and the fragment ion was 96, the common fragment ion was assumed to be a result of the removal of CH_3SeH from the precursor ion, and the presence of a methylselenyl group (CH_3Se-) in SeSugar1 was suggested. A minor product ion appearing at m/z 186 could be easily assigned to the fragment ion that appeared after the loss of H_2O from the major product ion at m/z 204. At high collision energies, common fragment ions

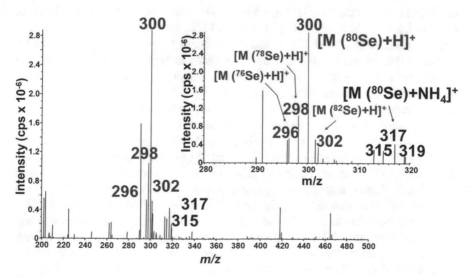

Fig. 25.4 LC-ESI-MS spectrum of the major urinary selenometabolite in positive ion mode. Red indicates the molecular ions containing Se isotopes. The insert is the enlarged around m/z 280–320

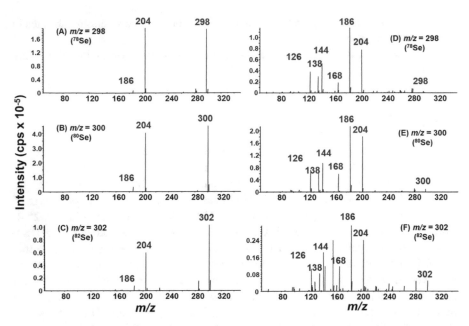

Fig. 25.5 Collision-induced dissociation mass spectra (ESI-MS/MS) of the major urinary seleno-metabolite (SeSugar1) in urine of Se-administered rat. The dissociation of each Se-containing molecular ion, i.e., m/z 298 (^{78}Se, **A** and **D**), 300 (^{80}Se, **B** and **E**), or 302 (^{82}Se **C** and **F**), was induced in the collision cell with 10 (**A–C**) and 20 eV (**D–F**) collision energies and then each fragment ion was detected with the second mass spectrometer. Blue and red indicate the precursor and product ions, respectively

originating in the precursor ions appeared at m/z 186, 144, 138, and 126. Three of the four fragment ions, m/z 186, 144, 126, and 108, were assigned to $[204 – H_2O]^+$, $[204 – CH_3COOH]^+$, $[144 – H_2O]^+$, and $[144 – 2H_2O]^+$, respectively (Fig. 25.5D–F). Although the assignment of m/z 138 was assigned in the literature, it has still been ambiguous (Letsiou et al. 2007). The major urinary selenometabolite could be deconvoluted by ESI-MS/MS, as shown in Fig. 25.6a. However, as mentioned above, the configuration of sugar moiety was unable to be decided. NMR spectroscopy was performed to achieve the complete identification.

The ^{1}H NMR spectrum of the nearly purified urinary metabolite exhibited two characteristic methyl signals ascribable to the CH_3Se group at the C1 position and the CH_3CONH group at the C2 position in the hexosamine unit (as shown in Fig. 25.6B). Furthermore, the coupling constant of protons between C3 and C4 positions indicated that the hexosamine unit is of the galactosamine type. Proton-decoupling experiments as well as analysis of the multiplicity of all the proton signals in addition to ^{1}H–^{13}C correlation studies suggested that the major urinary metabolite is a previously uncharacterized selenosugar, 1β-methylseleno-N-acetyl-d-galactosamine. The proposed structure was confirmed as shown in Fig. 25.6b.

In addition to the major urinary selenosugar, SeSugar1, minor selenosugars, such as *Se*-methylseleno-*N*-acetylglucosamine (MeSeGlcNAc, selenosugar 2, or

(A)

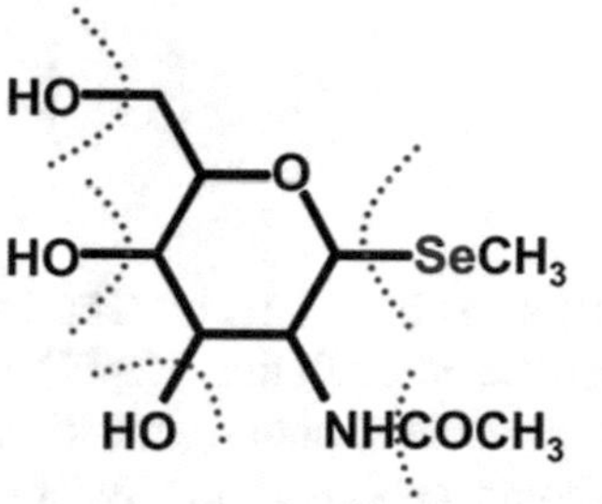

m/z	assignment
300	[M+H]$^+$
204	$300 - CH_3SeH$
186	$204 - H_2O$
168	$204 - 2H_2O$
144	$204 - CH_3COOH$
138	?
126	$204 - CH_3COOH - H_2O$
108	$204 - CH_3COOH - 2H_2O$

(B)

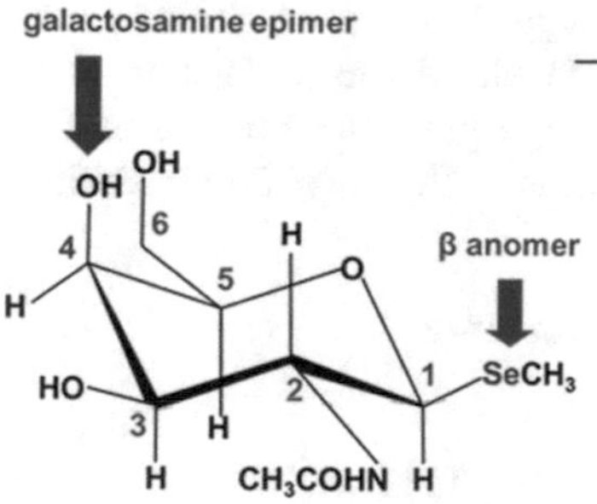

galactosamine epimer

Position	δ (number of protons, multiplicity, coupling constants) Urinary Se metabolite
1	4.61 (1H, d, J = 10.4 Hz)
2	4.13 (1H, t, J = 10.4 Hz)
3	3.54 (1H, dd, J = 10.4, 3.3 Hz)
4	3.89 (1H, d, J = 3.0 Hz)
5	3.49 (1H, dd, J = 6.0, 5.9 Hz)
6	3.76 (1H, dd, J = 11.5, 6.9 Hz) 3.69 (1H, dd, J = 11.5, 5.2 Hz)
1- Me	2.08 (3H, s)
2- Ac	1.96 (3H, s)

Fig. 25.6 Summary of results obtained by mass spectrometry and NMR spectroscopy. Assignment of fragment ions by LC-ESI-MS/MS (**A**). The assignment of fragment ions is summarized in table. ^{1}H NMR spectral data of the major urinary selenometabolite (**B**). Assumed structures based on LC-ESI-MS/MS and NMR are depicted in panels (**A**) and (**B**), respectively

SeSugar2) and *Se*-methylselenogalactosamine (MeSeGalNH$_2$, selenosugar 3, or SeSugar3), were identified in urine by ESI-MS-MS (Gammelgaard et al. 2003; Francesconi and Pannier 2004). *Se*-glutathionylseleno-*N*-acetylgalactosamine (GSSeGalNAc) was also identified in the liver of experimental animals by ESI-MS-MS (Kobayashi et al. 2002). This selenosugar is recognized as the precursor of the major urinary selenosugar, SeSugar1.

The second major urinary metabolite is trimethylselenonium ion (TMSe), which is simply the methylated compound of selenide. Initially, it was thought that TMSe appeared in urine when Se exceeding the nutritional level was ingested (Kraus et al. 1985; Byard 1969; Francesconi and Pannier 2004; Janghorbani et al. 1999). It was reported recently that there is a specific group of people who constantly excrete TMSe, in addition to the major selenosugar, in urine (Kuehnelt et al. 2006, 2015; Jager et al. 2016).

Selenocyanate

The Se metabolism in mammalian cultured cells has been unclear. Thus, we performed the speciation analysis of Se in human hepatoma cell line, HepG2, exposed with sodium selenite. The major peak appearing at the retention time of 35.6 min was assigned to an unknown selenium metabolite present in the supernatant of HepG2 cells exposed to 10 μM sodium selenite (Fig. 25.7A). The retention time of the selenium metabolite did not match the retention times of any of the authentic standards of selenium metabolites reported previously. As the metabolite could be a novel selenium metabolite, we attempted to identify it by molecular mass spectrometry. We analyzed the unknown selenometabolite by ESI quadrupole time-of-flight mass spectrometry (ESI-Q-TOF-MS). Signals composing the isotope pattern of Se were obtained, and the peak at m/z 106 was assigned to a ^{80}Se-containing molecular ion, as observed in the negative ion mode by ESI-MS. As the molecular mass of 106 seemed to be too small for MS-MS analysis as a precursor ion, we used ESI-Q-TOF-MS to determine the elemental composition of the novel Se metabolite based

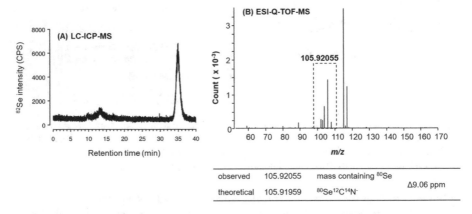

	observed	105.92055	mass containing ^{80}Se	
				Δ9.06 ppm
	theoretical	105.91959	^{80}Se^{12}C^{14}N$^-$	

Fig. 25.7 Elution profiles of selenium by LC-ICP-MS and mass spectrum obtained by ESI-Q-TOF-MS in the supernatant of HepG2 cells. HepG2 cells were exposed to 10 μM sodium selenite for 24 h. The cytosolic fraction for selenium speciation was obtained by ultracentrifugation of the homogenate. A 20 μL aliquot of the supernatant was applied to LC-ICP-MS to analyze the distribution of selenium (**A**). The multimode size-exclusion column (Shodex GS-520HQ) was eluted with 50 mM Tris–HCl, pH 7.4, at a flow rate of 0.6 mL/min. The eluate was introduced directly into the ICP-MS nebulizer to detect selenium at m/z 82. A 5.0 μL aliquot of sample was continuously introduced with 0.3% ammonia into the ion source of ESI-Q-TOF-MS by a syringe pump at a flow rate of 0.1 mL/min. The ions were detected in the negative ion mode (**B**). Signals composing a Se-isotope pattern are highlighted by broken lines. Table shows the difference between observed and theoretical masses

on its exact molecular mass. We speculated that the negative ion at m/z 106 was [^{80}SeCN]$^-$, i.e., selenocyanate. The observed mass containing ^{80}Se in the sample was 105.92055, and the theoretical mass of ^{80}SeCN$^-$ is 105.91959 (Fig. 25.7B). The difference between the observed and theoretical masses was 9.06 ppm. This indicated that the novel selenometabolite found in mammalian cultured cells was selenocyanate. Selenocyanate can be formed in all mammalian cell lines we tested such as human embryonic kidney cells (HEK293), pheochromocytoma cells of the rat adrenal medulla (PC12), mouse hepatoma cells (hepa1-6), rat liver cell (RL34), and fibroblast-like cells from a monkey kidney (COS7). No enzymes were required to form selenocyanate, suggesting that highly reactive endogenous cyanide could be participated in the biosynthesis of selenocyanate. We named highly reactive endogenous cyanide-reactive cyanogen species (RCNS). Because selenocyanate was less toxic than selenite and cyanide, selenocyanate seems to be biosynthesize to detoxify selenite. In addition, selenocyanate was assimilated into selenoproteins and selenometabolites in rats in the same manner as selenite (Anan et al. 2015a). Thus, selenocyanate can be utilized as a nutritional source of Se.

Laser Ablation Coupled with ICP-MS

Laser ablation coupled with ICP-MS, i.e., LA-ICP-MS, is now being used for mapping and imaging of trace elements in biological samples. LA-ICP-MS is also one of the hyphenated techniques, and has some advantages over LC-ICP-MS. Since LC-ICP-MS gives us information about chemical species in a soluble fraction, it is difficult to provide spatial information such as a tissue distribution of elements.

The spatial resolution and elemental sensitivity is almost comparable to X-ray fluorescence (XRF) and secondary ion mass spectrometry (SIMS), respectively. The mapping of selenoproteins on a gel plate of electrophoresis was reported (Sonet et al. 2018). Selenoproteins on 1D or 2D gel plate are specifically detected by the technique (Cruz et al. 2018; Galano et al. 2013). Selenoproteins contain Se as selenocysteine in their primary structure. Therefore, denatured gel is applicable to separate and detect selenoproteins. Because a trace amount of Se exists in animal tissue, it is difficult to visualize the Se distribution on animal tissues by a conventional LA-ICP-MS. The Se imaging on a Se-enriched plant was successfully reported (Maciel et al. 2014).

NMR

Nuclear magnetic resonance (NMR) spectroscopy is used for the investigation of typical elements, such as ^{1}H, ^{13}C, ^{19}F, and ^{31}P, and is, in principle, applicable to almost all of the metallic elements on the periodic table. ^{77}Se is one of the nuclides detectable by NMR spectroscopy because of its relatively high NMR receptivity.

Thus, ^{77}Se NMR spectroscopy has been utilized for the identification of Se compounds in organic chemistry (Lardon 1970). Although ^{77}Se NMR spectroscopy is a reliable tool for the identification of organic and inorganic Se compounds, it has been rarely used in biological samples because of their presence in ultra-trace amounts. However, Se seems to be suitable to evaluate recent NMR techniques for biological research. Recent advances in NMR instrumentation and measurement techniques have enabled us to investigate Se compounds routinely without the need for special knowledge or equipment.

Chemical Shifts of Selenocompounds by Direct Detection

Similarly to ^{1}H and ^{13}C NMR chemical shifts, the ^{77}Se NMR chemical shifts are definitive for compounds containing ^{77}Se (Tan et al. 1988). The chemical shifts of Se compounds having reduced Se (-II) are observed in the relatively high-field region, and those having oxidized Se (from +IV to +VI) are observed in the low-field region. This can be explained by the fact that nuclei in the high-electron-density region are more shielded from the applied field than those in the low-electron-density region. For the Se speciation by NMR spectroscopy, dimethylselenide is used as chemical shift reference ($\delta = 0$) (Luthra et al. 1983). The chemical structures of Se compounds in our library of selenometabolites are shown in Fig. 25.8. The chemical shifts measured by an NMR instrument (ECZ600, JEOL, Tokyo, Japan) are also shown in Fig. 25.8. Important selenometabolites, such as selenoamino acids, a selenosugar, and methylated Se metabolite, were observed in the narrow region from 0 to 300 ppm. The full width at half maximum of each ^{77}Se signal was so narrow that each Se compound could be identified on the basis of its own chemical shift like a fingerprint. Hence, we propose that the region is named "bio-selenium region."

Advanced Techniques for Application of ^{77}Se NMR Spectroscopy in Biological Samples

The indirect measurement by heteronuclear multiple bond correlation (HMBC) spectroscopy with ^{1}H nuclides is the effective technique to enhance ^{77}Se signal intensity (Zhang and Vogel 1994; Schroeder et al. 1995; Block et al. 2004; Kövér et al. 2011). Because the two-dimensional correlation spectrum of ^{77}Se and ^{1}H could be obtained, this method would provide decisive information for chemical structure determination. Furthermore, because this technique is an inverse detection experiment using ^{1}H nuclei, the S/N ratio is markedly increased, namely, the sensitivity obtained at 50 mM would be the same as that obtained at 200 μM. These advanced techniques for ^{77}Se detection by NMR spectroscopy are useful for biological

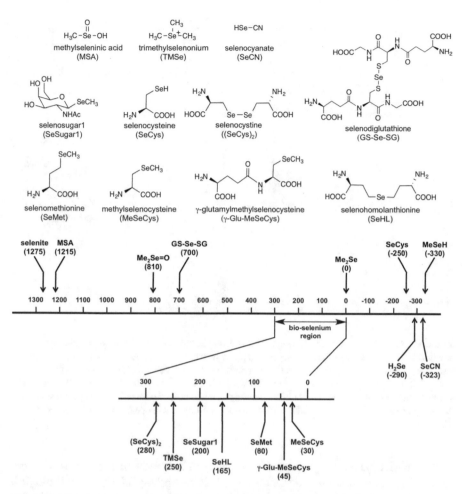

Fig. 25.8 Chemical structures and chemical shifts of Se compounds in our library of selenometabolites measured by NMR (ECZ600, JEOL)

samples. As an example of an application of ^{77}Se NMR spectroscopy for a biological sample, the HMBC spectrum of [77]Se and ^{1}H of Se compound(s) in a dietary Se supplement ("Yeast-Free" Selenium 200 μg, Vitamin World®, New York, USA) is shown in Fig. 25.9.

^{77}Se NMR spectroscopy was used for biological samples in some literatures. Mobli et al. carried out ^{77}Se NMR measurements to determine the pKa values of selenocysteine residues incorporated into a bioactive peptide hormone and a neurotransmitter, and demonstrated that the pKa values of selenocysteine residues in peptide were substantially lower than those of free selenocysteine (Mobli et al. 2011). Schaefer et al. employed the ^{77}Se NMR technique to probe the local electronic environment of reactive selenocysteine residues by preparing [77]Se-enriched proteins (Schaefer et al. 2013).

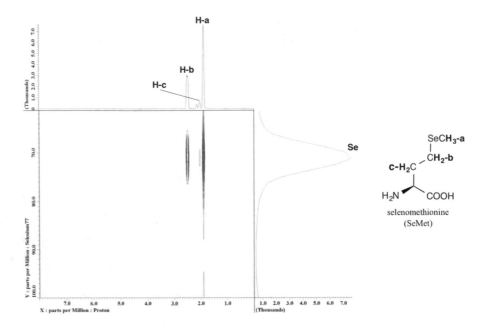

Fig. 25.9 Heteronuclear multiple bond correlation spectrum of Se compound in dietary supplement in D_2O. Five tablets of the dietary Se supplement were ground and extracted with a water and methanol mixture (1,1). The extract was lyophilized, and the lyophilizate was dissolved in D_2O. The HMBC spectrum of the lyophilizate corresponded to that of selenomethionine. The result coincided with the ingredient label showing that selenomethionine is the major Se species in the supplement. (This figure is taken from Suzuki and Ogra, with permission (Suzuki and Ogra 2017))

^{77}Se NMR spectroscopy provides concrete information of the chemical structures of selenometabolites, although the NMR receptivity of ^{77}Se in a biological sample is unsatisfactory compared with the sensitivity in mass spectrometry. The use of enriched stable isotopes is one of the ways to overcome the disadvantages of NMR spectroscopy.

Conclusion

The complementary use of LC-ICP-MS(/MS), LC-ESI-MS(/MS), and NMR would be the best analytical approach for the identification of unknown selenometabolites. In addition, LA-ICP-MS can give us imaging data for Se distribution in a tissue and a separation gel plate of electrophoresis. Further development of the measurement technique and instrumentation is expected to lead to the widespread use of these techniques in selenometabolome.

Acknowledgments This study was supported by JSPS KAKENHI Grant Numbers 24659022, 26293030, 15K14991, and 16H05812, and a grant from the Food Safety Commission, Cabinet Office, Government of Japan (Research Program for Risk Assessment Study on Food Safety, No 1601).

References

Akesson B, Martensson B. Heparin interacts with a selenoprotein in human plasma. J Inorg Biochem. 1988;33(4):257–61.

Anan Y, Hatakeyama Y, Tokumoto M, Ogra Y. Chromatographic behavior of selenoproteins in rat serum detected by inductively coupled plasma mass spectrometry. Anal Sci. 2013;29(8):787–92.

Anan Y, Kimura M, Hayashi M, Koike R, Ogra Y. Detoxification of selenite to form selenocyanate in mammalian cells. Chem Res Toxicol. 2015a;28(9):1803–14. https://doi.org/10.1021/acs.chemrestox.5b00254.

Anan Y, Nakajima G, Ogra Y. Complementary use of LC-ICP-MS and LC-ESI-Q-TOF-MS for selenium speciation. Anal Sci. 2015b;31(6):561–4. https://doi.org/10.2116/analsci.31.561.

Becker JS, Jakubowski N. The synergy of elemental and biomolecular mass spectrometry: new analytical strategies in life sciences. Chem Soc Rev. 2009;38:1969–83.

Block E, Glass RS, Jacobsen NE, Johnson S, Kahakachchi C, Kaminski R, Skowronska A, Boakye HT, Tyson JF, Uden PC. Identification and synthesis of a novel selenium-sulfur amino acid found in selenized yeast: rapid indirect detection NMR methods for characterizing low-level organoselenium compounds in complex matrices. J Agric Food Chem. 2004;52:3761–71.

Borglund M, Akesson A, Akesson B. Distribution of selenium and glutathione peroxidase in plasma compared in healthy subjects and rheumatoid arthritis patients. Scand J Clin Lab Invest. 1988;48(1):27–32. https://doi.org/10.3109/00365518809085390.

Byard JL. Trimethyl selenide. A urinary metabolite of selenite. Arch Biochem Biophys. 1969;130:556–60.

Cruz ECS, Susanne Becker J, Sabine Becker J, Sussulini A. Imaging of selenium by laser ablation inductively coupled plasma mass spectrometry (LA-ICP-MS) in 2-D electrophoresis gels and biological tissues. Methods Mol Biol. 2018;1661:219–27. https://doi.org/10.1007/978-1-4939-7258-6_16.

Daniels LA. Selenium metabolism and bioavailability. Biol Trace Elem Res. 1996;54(3):185–99. https://doi.org/10.1007/bf02784430.

Darrouzès J, Bueno M, Lespès G, Portin-Gautier M. Operational optimisation of ICP - octopole collision/reaction cell - MS for applications to ultratrace selenium total and speciation determination. J Anal At Spectrom. 2005;20:88–94.

Francesconi KA, Pannier F. Selenium metabolites in urine: a critical overview of past work and current status. Clin Chem. 2004;50:2240–53.

Galano E, Mangiapane E, Bianga J, Palmese A, Pessione E, Szpunar J, Lobinski R, Amoresano A. Privileged incorporation of selenium as selenocysteine in Lactobacillus reuteri proteins demonstrated by selenium-specific imaging and proteomics. Mol Cell Proteomics. 2013;12(8):2196–204. https://doi.org/10.1074/mcp.M113.027607.

Gammelgaard B, Grimstrup Madsen K, Bjerrum J, Bendahl L, Jøns O, Olsen J, Sidenius U. Separation, purification and identification of the major selenium metabolite from human urine by multi-dimensional HPLC-ICP-MS and APCI-MS. J Anal At Spectrom. 2003;18:65–70.

Guo W, Hu S, Wang Y, Zhang L, Hu Z, Zhang J. Trace determination of selenium in biological samples by CH4-Ar mixed gas plasma DRC-ICP-MS. Microchem J. 2013;108:106–12.

Jager T, Drexler H, Goen T. Human metabolism and renal excretion of selenium compounds after oral ingestion of sodium selenite and selenized yeast dependent on the trimethylselenium ion (TMSe) status. Arch Toxicol. 2016;90(5):1069–80. https://doi.org/10.1007/s00204-015-1548-z.

Janghorbani M, Xia Y, Ha P, Whanger PD, Butler JA, Olesik JW, Daniels L. Quantitative significance of measuring trimethylselenonium in urine for assessing chronically high intakes of selenium in human subjects. Br J Nutr. 1999;82(4):291–7.

Jitaru P, Goenaga-Infante H, Vaslin-Reimann S, Fisicaro P. A systematic approach to the accurate quantification of selenium in serum selenoalbumin by HPLC-ICP-MS. Anal Chim Acta. 2010;657(2):100–7. https://doi.org/10.1016/j.aca.2009.10.037.

Kobayashi Y, Ogra Y, Ishiwata K, Takayama H, Aimi N, Suzuki KT. Selenosugars are key and urinary metabolites for selenium excretion within the required to low-toxic range. Proc Natl Acad Sci U S A. 2002;99(25):15932–6.

Kobayashi Y, Ogra Y, Suzuki KT. Speciation and metabolism of selenium injected with 82Se-enriched selenite and selenate in rats. J Chromatogr B Biomed Sci Appl. 2001;760(1):73–81.

Kövér KE, Kumar AA, Rusakov YY, Krivdin LB, Illyés T-Z, Szilágyi L. Experimental and computational studies of $^nJ(^{77}Se, {}^1H)$ selenium-proton couplings in selenoglycosides. Magn Reson Chem. 2011;49:190–4.

Koyama H, Kasanuma Y, Kim CY, Ejima A, Watanabe C, Nakatsuka H, Satoh H. Distribution of selenium in human plasma detected by high performance liquid chromatography-plasma ion source mass spectrometry. Tohoku J Exp Med. 1996;178(1):17–25.

Kraus RJ, Foster SJ, Ganther HE. Analysis of trimethylselenonium ion in urine by high-performance liquid chromatography. Anal Biochem. 1985;147(2):432–6.

Kuehnelt D, Engstrom K, Skroder H, Kokarnig S, Schlebusch C, Kippler M, Alhamdow A, Nermell B, Francesconi K, Broberg K, Vahter M. Selenium metabolism to the trimethylselenonium ion (TMSe) varies markedly because of polymorphisms in the indolethylamine N-methyltransferase gene. Am J Clin Nutr. 2015;102(6):1406–15. https://doi.org/10.3945/ajcn.115.114157.

Kuehnelt D, Juresa D, Kienzl N, Francesconi KA. Marked individual variability in the levels of trimethylselenonium ion in human urine determined by HPLC/ICPMS and HPLC/vapor generation/ICPMS. Anal Bioanal Chem. 2006;386:2207–12.

Lardon M. Selenium and proton nuclear magnetic resonance measurements on organic selenium compounds. J Am Chem Soc. 1970;92:5063–6.

Letsiou S, Nischwitz V, Traar P, Francesconi KA, Pergantis SA. Determination of selenosugars in crude human urine using high-performance liquid chromatography/atmospheric pressure chemical ionization tandem mass spectrometry. Rapid Commun Mass Spectrom. 2007;21:343–51.

Luthra NP, Dunlap RB, Odom JD. The use of dimethyl selenide as a chemical shift reference in ^{77}Se NMR spectroscopy. J Magn Reson. 1983;52:318–22.

Maciel BC, Barbosa HS, Pessoa GS, Salazar MM, Pereira GA, Goncalves DC, Ramos CH, Arruda MA. Comparative proteomics and metallomics studies in Arabidopsis thaliana leaf tissues: evaluation of the selenium addition in transgenic and nontransgenic plants using two-dimensional difference gel electrophoresis and laser ablation imaging. Proteomics. 2014;14(7-8):904–12. https://doi.org/10.1002/pmic.201300427.

Mobli M, Morgenstern D, King GF, Alewood PF, Muttenthaler M. Site-specific pKa determination of selenocysteine residues in selenovasopressin by using ^{77}Se NMR spectroscopy. Angew Chem Int Ed. 2011;50:11952–5.

Ogra Y. Integrated strategies for identification of selenometabolites in animal and plant samples. Anal Bioanal Chem. 2008;390:1685–9.

Ogra Y, Ishiwata K, Suzuki KT. Effects of deuterium in octopole reaction and collision cell ICP-MS on detection of selenium in extracellular fluids. Anal Chim Acta. 2005;554:123–9.

Òscar P, Łobiński R. Investigation of the stability of selenoproteins during storage of human serum by size-exclusion LC–ICP-MS. Talanta. 2007;71:1813–6.

Persson-Moschos M, Huang W, Srikumar TS, Akesson B, Lindeberg S. Selenoprotein P in serum as a biochemical marker of selenium status. Analyst. 1995;120(3):833–6.

Prange A, Pröfrock D. Application of CE–ICP–MS and CE–ESI–MS in metalloproteomics: challenges, developments, and limitations. Anal Bioanal Chem. 2005;383:372–89.

Schaefer SA, Dong M, Rubenstein RP, Wilkie WA, Bahnson BJ, Thorpe C, Rozovsky S. [77]Se erichment of poteins expands the biological NMR toolbox. J Mol Biol. 2013;425:222–31.

Schroeder TB, Job C, Brown MF, Glass RS. Indirect detection of selenium-77 in nuclear magnetic resonance spectra of organoselenium compounds. Magn Reson Chem. 1995;33:191–5.

Sloth JJ, Larsen EH. The application of inductively coupled plasma dynamic reaction cell mass spectrometry for measurement of selenium isotopes, isotope ratios and chromatographic detection of selenoamino acids. J Anal At Spectrom. 2000;15:669–72.

Sloth JJ, Larsen EH, Bügel SH, Moesgaard S. Determination of total selenium and [77]Se in isotopically enriched human sample by ICP-dynamic reaction cell-MS. J Anal At Spectrom. 2003;18:317–22.

Sonet J, Mounicou S, Chavatte L. Detection of selenoproteins by laser ablation inductively coupled plasma mass spectrometry (LA-ICP MS) in immobilized pH gradient (IPG) strips. Methods Mol Biol. 2018;1661:205–17. https://doi.org/10.1007/978-1-4939-7258-6_15.

Suzuki N, Ogra Y. ^{77}Se NMR Spectroscopy for speciation analysis of selenium. In: Ogra Y, Hirata T, editors. Metallomics -recent analytical techniques and applications. New York: Springer; 2017. p. 147–56.

Szpunar J, Łobiński R. Multidimensional approaches in biochemical speciation analysis. Anal Bioanal Chem. 2002;373:404–11.

Takahashi K, Suzuki N, Ogra Y. Bioavailability comparison of nine bioselenocompounds in vitro and in vivo. Int J Mol Sci. 2017;18(3):506. https://doi.org/10.3390/ijms18030506.

Tan K-S, Arnold AP, Rabenstein DL. Selenium-77 nuclear magnetic resonance studies of selenols, diselenides, and selenenyl sulfides. Can J Chem. 1988;66:54–60.

Templeton DM, Ariese F, Cornelis R, Danielsson L-G, Muntau H, van Leeuwen HP, Łobiński R. Guidelines for terms related to chemical speciation and fractionation of elements. Definitions, structural aspects, and methodological approaches (IUPAC Recommendations 2000). Pure Appl Chem. 2000;72:1453–70.

Zhang M, Vogel HJ. Two-dimensional NMR studies of selenomethionyl calmodulin. J Mol Biol. 1994;239:545–54.

Index

Printed in the United States
By Bookmasters